Noltenius · Manual of Oncology
Volume 1

Volume 1
Soft Tissues – Retroperitoneum – Nerves – Gastrointestinal
Tract – Liver – Gallbladder – Pancreas – Head and
Neck – Salivary Glands – Thyroid – Mediastinum – Lung –
Brain – Pituitary Gland – Eye

Volume 2
Breast – Bone – Skin – Lymph Nodes and Spleen – Kidney –
Urinary tract – Prostate – Testicle – Ovary – Vulva – Vagina –
Uterus – Adrenal Gland and Paragangliomas

Manual
of Oncology

Volume 1

With 1747 Histological Figures

Harald W. Noltenius

Professor of Pathology and Head,
Department of Pathology
Allgemeines Krankenhaus St. Georg,
University of Hamburg

Former Chairman of the Department of
Pathology, American University of Beirut

Urban & Schwarzenberg
Baltimore – Munich 1981

Urban & Schwarzenberg, Inc.
7 East Redwood Street
Baltimore, Maryland 21202
USA

Urban & Schwarzenberg
Pettenkoferstraße 18
D-8000 München 2
Germany

German Edition: Systematik der Onkologie, Urban & Schwarzenberg, München–Wien–Baltimore 1981.

Address of the author:
Harald W. Noltenius, Professor
Allgemeines Krankenhaus St. Georg
Lohmühlenstraße 5
D-2000 Hamburg 1
West Germany

Library of Congress Cataloging in Publication Data

Noltenius, Harald.
    Manual of oncology.

    Translation of Systematik der Onkologie.
    Includes bibliographical references and index.
    1. Oncology – Classification – Handbooks, manuals, etc.
I. Title. [DNLM: 1. Neoplasms. QZ200 N798s]
RC258.N6413   616.99′2   80-18972
ISBN 0-8067-1331-3

ISBN 0-8067-1311-9 Vol. 1 Baltimore

ISBN 3-541-71311-9 Vol. 1 München

ISBN 0-8067-1331-3 Complete set Baltimore

ISBN 3-541-71331-1 Complete set München

Printed in Germany by Passavia, Passau

To my Daughter Catherine Noltenius

Preface

Optimal treatment for cancer patients has long been a major concern of the physician. It is a concern that requires a multidisciplinary international approach at all levels, from teaching and research to most aspects of diagnosis and treatment.

To this end, MANUAL OF ONCOLOGY presents the tumors listed with their morphological appearance, clinical symptoms, biological behavior, principles of treatment, prognosis, and references to current literature.

In an effort to maximize the book's use in the world scientific community, all tumors are labeled according to international (WHO) nomenclature, including the M and T numbers and TNM and p-TNM (UICC) classifications. This nomenclature was chosen after an intensive study of English language literature, the ICD-O, and terminology proposed by WHO. In the process of standardizing, some tumor designations have been omitted. We hope, however, that the reader will agree with our selection in nomenclature and concentrate on the larger aim of this manual – to transcend the limitations of both language and specialty and to advance international cooperation and progress in the pursuit of optimal cancer treatment.

These lines bring to a close a difficult undertaking that spanned several years. During this period I received invaluable support from the members of the Department of Pathology of the Allgemeines Krankenhaus St. Georg, Hamburg. Most of my collaborators in this endeavor were actively engaged, maintaining a tumor registry, conducting histological tumor seminars, reproducing new slides for photography and electron microscopy, composing the manuscript, checking the German and English versions with each other, determining receptors for hormones and immunological markers on tumor cells, assaying HCG and alpha-fetoprotein, and preparing cell cultures of the tumors. Those who did not participate actively nevertheless played an important part, enthusiastically assuming the increased load of daily work that ensued.

I wish to express my gratitude to all involved and to acknowledge in particular *R. Bergmann, G. Gottschalk, H. Köppen, I. Krehain, S. Krüger, E. Maetschke, H. Mai, M. Matz-Prankel,* and *M. Penssler-Beyer.*

I am indepted to Dr. *J. Petersen-Frey* and Dr. *H. Haenisch* for their help with the index and for reading and correcting the proofs.

My special thanks go to *E. M. Jagfeld,* Essen, West Germany, whose technical and artistic skill is evident in many of the photographs.

Several colleagues have contributed to this book by offering histological slides from their own material.

Prof. Dr. *H. J. Colmant,* Hamburg University, Neuropathology, Chairman, gave advice and material for the tumors of the central nervous system.

Prof. *E. Sprenger,* Kiel, Chairman of the Department of Cytology, helped us with problems of cytology and contributed a number of photographs and legends.

Dr. *G. Schwendemann,* Department of Neuropathology, Hamburg University, performed the electron microscopy included in this book.

It is difficult to express adequately my indebtedness to Dr. *C. Tetzner,* who offered to me her continuous support, her competent help, and loyalty.

Last but not least, on behalf of all co-workers, I would like to acknowledge the fruitful cooperation we enjoyed with our publishers. In particular our thanks to *Michael Urban,* Urban und Schwarzenberg Verlag, Baltimore–München, and Prof. Dr. *H.J. Clemens,* who gave us important advice and encouragement.

We hope that this work will be useful to our colleagues in hospitals oncological centers, to those who in their practice as family doctors detect tumors and care later for the patients, and to students, who might find that this book helps to ease the study of tumors.

Hamburg, Autumn 1980   Harald W. Noltenius

Contents

Acknowledgments

We are grateful to those colleagues who have contributed to this book by giving us histological slides for the following figures:

Prof. Colmant (brain tumors): Figs. 762, 766, 768, 769, 773-776, 778, 780-790, 792, 793, 795, 796, 799, 800, 803-809, 811, 813-815, 817, 820, 822, 824, 825, 827, 833-838, 840-843, 845-851, 835-857, 859-861, 872-874, 880-881 (neuropathology).

Prof. Sprenger (cytology): Figs. 201, 424, 576, 606, 607, 688, 689, 726, 739, 759, 920, 1219, 1314, 1400, 1401, 1527, 1659 and inset Figs. 1671 and 1687.

Dr. Hüsselmann: Figs. 253-255, 315-317, 517, 692, 703, 706-708, 720, 736, 737, 740, 741, 745-748, 1187, 1188, 1480, 1482, 1483, 1626, 1627.

Prof. Könn: Figs. 104-106, 691, 744, 1440, 1502, 1503.

Dr. Donath (odontogenic tumors): Figs. 547, 548, 550-561.

Dr. Saeger (pituitary tumors): Figs. 866-870.

The work on ultrastructure and membrane and intracellular receptors of tumor cells was supported by grants from the Stiftung Volkswagenwerk and the Deutsche Forschungsgemeinschaft.

Prof. Dr. Hans-Joachim Colmant, Professor and Chairman,
Abteilung für Neuropathologie und experimentelle Hirnforschung,
Universitätskrankenhaus Eppendorf, D-2000 Hamburg

Dr. med. Günter Schwendemann, Associate Professor,
Abteilung für Neuropathologie und experimentelle Hirnforschung,
Universitätskrankenhaus Eppendorf, D-2000 Hamburg

Prof. Ernst Sprenger, Professor and Chairman,
Abteilung für Zytopathologie,
Klinikum der Christian-Albrechts-Universität, D-2300 Kiel

Dr. med. Helmuth Hüsselmann,
Head of the Dept. of. Pathology,
Allgemeines Krankenhaus Harburg, D-2000 Hamburg

Prof. Dr. med. Günter Könn, Professor and Chairman,
Pathologisches Universitätsinstitut,
Krankenhaus "Bergmanns Heil", D-4630 Bochum

Priv. Doz. Dr. med. Wolfgang Saeger, Associate Professor,
Head of the Dept. of. Pathology,
Marienkrankenhaus, D-2000 Hamburg

Priv. Doz. Dr. med.Karl Donath, Associate Professor,
Pathologisches Institut,
Universitätskrankenhaus Eppendorf, D-2000 Hamburg

Mrs. Eva-Maria Jagdfeld, Photography.
D-4300 Essen-Holsterhausen.

Introduction

The book is divided into chapters, each concerned with a different organ of the human body (for example, tumors of the lung, tumors of the breast, etc.). Each chapter begins with an enumeration of all tumors arising in the named organ; the listed sequence is kept throughout the chapter. The tumor list is followed by a short introductory text, which discusses the peculiarities of the tumors of that organ. For example, with breast cancer the possibility of determining hormone receptors is mentioned; for bone tumors the importance of cooperation between the members of different disciplines is discussed.

The TNM (p-TNM) classification is included in most instances in the introduction.

Nomenclature

All of the tumor names follow the international classification of tumorous diseases; the most frequent synonyms and the WHO classification are also given. When there was doubt and especially when classification was still under discussion, several classifications were mentioned (for example, in the case of malignant lymphomas or tumors of the testis).

The tumor histology key number (ICD-O), the M number, and the anatomical topographic number (T) [9, 16] were added to the tumor denotation.

The M number defines a tumor independent of language. For instance, M-8140/0 stands for a benign adenoma; in this case /0 defines the tumor as benign, whereas /1 would indicate that the biological nature of the tumor was not clear. /2 means "carcinoma in situ," /3 stands for an infiltrating malignant tumor, and /6 marks a metastasis from a malignant tumor.

Therefore, M-8140/0 – adenoma

        M-8140/2 – adenocarcinoma in situ

        M-8140/3 – infiltrating adenocarcinoma

        M-8140/6 – metastasis from adenocarcinoma.

/9 indicates that a malignant tumor has been found, but that it is is not clear whether this tumor is a primary neoplasm or a metastatic lesion.

The localization of the tumor is indicated by the topographic T number. For example, M-8140/3, T156.1 means adenocarcinoma of the gallbladder.

M and T numbers are found in the margins of the text. The most important T numbers are given at the end of each volume.

---

[9] ICD-O 1978.
[16] UICC 1976.

1

General remarks

This section contains the statistical specifications of a tumor, that is, the incidence, the distribution between the sexes, the peak ages of its occurrence, and particular sites. Peculiarities of the tumors are found under "further information."

Macroscopy

The macroscopic appearance of a tumor is described; in some cases problems of differential diagnosis are mentioned here.

Knowledge of the macroscopic appearance of a tumor is important during excision for frozen sections, for routine histology, and also for the surgeon discovering tumors during operations.

Microscopy

The histological picture of a tumor is discussed with the help of photographic illustration. When histology is being discussed, highly magnified micrographs are included occasionally to show particularities of the tumor cells, especially of the nuclei. This combination of histology and nuclear changes should help to strengthen the link between histology and cytology.

All tumors occurring in specific organs are mentioned in the corresponding chapters; however, to avoid redundancy we have not given the histological description in every chapter. For example, the histological appearance of hemangiomas in the liver is described in the chapter on tumors of the liver, and further details are given in the chapter on soft tissue tumors. When the histology is not mentioned, a page reference is given.

Electron microscopy, histochemistry, immunohistochemistry

Further possible methods of characterizing tumors are not mentioned for each tumor. They are generally mentioned when these methods could be of diagnostic importance. Furthermore, additional particularities of tumors that could lead to a further subdivision of the tumor type and induce further investigation are mentioned: the presence of hormone receptors in tumor cell membranes, the presence of immunological markers in tumor tissue or tumor cells, the amount of lymphocytes in tumor tissue, the level of carcinoembryonic antigen (CEA), the specific appearance of tumor cells in cell cultures, etc.

Cytology

The cytological diagnosis of malignant tumors is of great importance, especially for early detection. Important books covering this topic have been published.

To underline the importance of linking histology and cytology, we have added some cytological illustrations to the histological descriptions.

Differential diagnosis

This section contains facts that could facilitate the separation between different types of tumors or tumor-like lesions. The section contains, therefore, mostly morphological features, especially histological findings. However, differential diagnosis of malignant tumors by electron microscopy and occasionally the importance of clinical indications or other facts have also been included in this section. This includes immunohistochemistry; cytochemistry; the evaluation of tumor products such as alpha-fetoprotein (AFP), CEA, and human chorionic gonadotropin (HCG); direct evidence for hormone production; and the appearance of paraneoplastic syndromes.

Recommendations for how to differentiate the tumors have been summarized at the end of every organ chapter.

Staging

In most instances the staging is mentioned in the introduction to each chapter. This staging is based on the TNM classification and in particular on the P-TNM classification published by the UICC.

Grading

The grade of malignancy of a tumor often can be evaluated by the distinctness of the organoid growth pattern of a tumor, the number of mitotic figures, and the number and degree of nuclear atypias.

The grades are specified by description (well differentiated, moderately differentiated, poorly differentiated, and anaplastic) or by G numbers:

G 1 – well differentiated
G 2 – moderately differentiated
G 3 – poorly differentiated
G 4 – undifferentiated, anaplastic [9, 16].

The therapeutic consequences and the prognosis are determined mostly by the stage of the tumor and less frequently by the grade. However, high grade malignant tumors are more frequently found initially in an unfavorable stage than are tumors of low grade malignancy.

Spread

In this section the basic outlines of the most frequent spread of a specific tumor are discussed. The frequency with which spread is found at the time of diagnosis and the most frequent sites of metastatic lesions from a specific tumor are listed.

---

[9] ICD-O-DA 1978.
[16] UICC 1976.

Clinical findings

Clinical symptoms are described according to their different forms:
a) general symptoms due to the malignant growth,
b) local symptoms due to tumor growth (for example, pain in bone tumor),
c) roentgenological findings and angiographic changes,
d) paraneoplastic appearances,
e) serological observations,
f) the detection of tumor products [7], and
g) peculiarities in family history.

Treatment

Therapeutic decisions should be the result of a team concerned with oncology [3]. This book is intended to facilitate this teamwork.

The section on therapy contains the outlines of major methods of treating malignant tumors by surgery, radiotherapy [15], chemotherapy [1], immunotherapy [14], and hormone therapy. Social problems and other aspects of attending tumor patients such as psychological guidance [5] are not discussed. We also did not discuss possible complications of the tumor therapy: The reader is referred to the pertinent literature and monographs [2, 4, 8, 10, 12] where more detailed information can easily be found.

Intensive research on how to treat malignant tumors must be done. Some new techniques in surgery or irradiation and new efficient chemotherapeutic drugs have been developed [17], but the fundamental therapy of tumors has remained constant over many years. Therefore, we do not feel that the section on therapy is threatened with obsolescence [13]. Today the most vital part of the treatment of tumors is still their early diagnosis. When discussing therapy we kept in mind that not only the length of survival but also the quality of life is important.

While discussing radiotherapy the term gray has been used: 1 Gy = 100 rads [15].

Prognosis

Here again, it has been made clear that a good prognosis is linked to an early diagnosis.

Besides statistical features [6], the importance of determining the spread of the tumor at the time of diagnosis is stressed. To this aim the resection margins should be examined, the lymph nodes should be closely studied, and the depth of tumor infiltration into the tissue should be determined by the pathologist.

[1] Alberto 1978.
[2] Brunner and Nagel 1979.
[3] Brunner et al. 1978.
[4] Dold and Sack 1975.
[5] Fiore 1979.
[6] Gehan 1975.
[7] Goldenberg et al. 1978.
[8] Harrison 1977.
[10] Israël and Chahinian 1975.
[12] Kärcher 1975.
[13] Krokowski 1979.
[14] Oettgen 1977.
[15] Rassow and Harder 1977.
[17] Wrighton 1979.

Further information

This final section contains particularities of a specific tumor or of very rare tumors that are related to the neoplasm under discussion. Also, peculiar or very rare behaviors of the tumor reported in the literature are mentioned. This section gives information to stimulate the reader to further reading.

References

[1] Alberto, P.: Curabilité des tumeurs malignes: Valeur et limites de la chimiothérapie. Schweiz. med. Wschr. *108* (1978) 1930-1934.

[2] Brunner, K. W., und G. A. Nagel (Hrsg.): Internistische Krebstherapie, 2. Aufl. Springer, Berlin–Heidelberg–New York 1979.

[3] Brunner, K., L. Eckmann, H. J. Senn und P. Veraguth: Interdisziplinäre Behandlungsplanung bei Krebskrankheiten. Schweiz. med. Wschr. *108* (1978) 1331-1333.

[4] Dold, U. W., und H. Sack: Praktische Tumortherapie. Die Behandlung maligner Organtumoren und Systemerkrankungen. Thieme, Stuttgart 1975.

[5] Fiore, N.: Fighting cancer – One patient's perspective. New Engl. Journal of Med. *300* (1979) 284-289.

[6] Gehan, E. A.: Statistical methods for survival time studies. Cancer therapy: Prognostic factors and criteria of response, edited by M. J. Staquet, Raven Press, New York 1975.

[7] Goldenberg, D. M., R. M. Sharkey, and F. J. Primus: Immunocytochemical detection of carcinoembryonic antigen in conventional histopathology specimens. Cancer *42* (1978) 1546-1553.

[8] Harrison, T. R.: Principles of internal medicine. Eighth Ed. McGraw-Hill Book Company, New York, Düsseldorf etc. 1977.

[9] ICD-O, International Classification of Diseases for Oncology. First Ed. WHO, Geneva 1976.

Deutsche Ausgabe: Springer, Berlin–Heidelberg–New York 1978.

[10] Israël, L., and P. Chahinian: Mensuration of response. Cancer therapy: Prognostic factors and criteria of response, edited by M. J. Staquet, Raven Press, New York 1975.

[11] Jungi, W. F., R. C. Rohner und B. Widmer: Zusammenarbeit zwischen praktizierendem Arzt, Regionalspital und onkologischem Zentrum. Schweiz. med. Wschr. *108* (1978) 1334-1336.

[12] Kärcher, K. H.: Krebsbehandlung als interdisziplinäre Aufgabe. Springer, Berlin–Heidelberg–New York 1975.

[13] Krokowski, E.: Befindet sich die kurative Krebstherapie in der Sackgasse? Dtsch. med. Wschr. *104* (1979) 326-329.

[14] Oettgen, H. F.: Immunotherapy of cancer. N. Engl. J. Med. *297* (1977) 484-491.

[15] Rassow, J., und D. Harder: Zur Einführung der radiologischen Maßeinheiten Gray und Becquerel. Strahlentherapie *153* (1977) 509-512.

[16] UICC, International Union against cancer. Union internationale contre le Cancer. TNM, Klassifizierung der malignen Tumoren und allgemeine Regeln zur Anwendung des TNM-Systems. 2. Aufl. Springer, Berlin–Heidelberg–New York 1976. – 3. engl. Aufl. Ed. by M. H. Harmer, Geneva 1978.

[17] Wrighton, R. J.: Cancer chemotherapy. Journal of the Royal Society of Medicine *72* (1979) 1-2.

5

1 Soft tissue tumors

Soft tissue tumors show a great variability in their histological appearance, which is responsible for difficulties in the classification of these tumors. The typing of these tumors often requires special staining, such as periodic acid-Schiff (PAS), reticulin stain, or Heidenhain acid-hematoxylin. Sometimes electron microscopy or tumor cell cultures in vitro must be used.

The classification of soft tissue tumors was established by Stout and Lattes [109], who centered many of these tumors around the proliferating histiocytes. Since 1969 there has been an official WHO typing of the soft tissue tumors [42]. Because of the unstable microscopic appearance of soft tissue tumors, it is sometimes difficult to separate the malignant tumors from the nonmalignant neoplasms. For this reason it has been said that soft tissue tumors are probably the "most inadequately treated of all tumors" [1, 109].

Tumors of the peripheral nerves are varieties of soft tissue tumors in which nerve fibers and Schwann's cells form a typical growth pattern. However, it might be difficult to separate the peripheral nerve tumors from the soft tissue tumors, especially when the malignant varieties develop. Chapter 3 discusses the tumors of the peripheral nerves.

Recently, a clinical and pathological staging system has been developed, in which the grading of the tumor has been incorporated [101].

The histological grading is based on the cellularity of the tumor, on the number of mitotic figures, on the production of extracellular substances like mucoid substance or collagen fibers, and on the cellular pleomorphism.

This staging system has been applied to extraskeletal tumors, which originate in the soft tissue:

Alveolar soft part sarcoma, angiosarcoma, extraskeletal chondrosarcoma, extraskeletal osteosarcoma, fibrosarcoma, leiomyosarcoma, liposarcoma, malignant fibrous histiocytoma, malignant mesenchymoma, malignant schwannoma, rhabdomyosarcoma, sarcoma not designated by a special type, synovial sarcoma. The staging is composed of

T   size of the primary tumor
N   regional lymph nodes
M   distant metastases
G   histological grade of malignancy.

T – primary tumor

T 0   = no evidence of primary tumor
T 1   = tumor 5 cm or less in its greatest dimension
T 2   = tumor more than 5 cm in its greatest dimension but without extension to bone, major blood vessels, or major nerves
T 3   = tumor with extension to bone, major blood vessels, or major nerves
T x   = the minimal requirements to assess the primary tumor cannot be met (clinical examination and radiography)

[1] Ackerman and Rosai 1974.
[42] Enzinger 1969.
[101] Russell et al. 1977.
[109] Stout and Lattes 1967.

N – regional lymph nodes

N 0   = no evidence of regional lymph node involvement
N 1   = evidence of involvement of regional lymph nodes
N x   = the minimal requirements to assess the regional lymph nodes cannot be met (clinical examination and radiography)

M – distant metastases

M 0   = no evidence of distant metastases
M 1   = evidence of distant metastases
M x   = the minimal requirements to assess the presence of distant metastases cannot be met (clinical examination and radiography)

pTNM – postsurgical histopathological classification
the pTNM categories correspond to the TNM categories

G – histopathological grading

G 1   = high degree of differentiation
G 2   = medium degree of differentiation
G 3   = low degree of differentiation or undifferentiated
G x   = grade cannot be assessed

Stage grouping

Stage I a	G 1	T 1	N 0	M 0
Stage I b	G 1	T 2	N 0	M 0
Stage II a	G 2	T 1	N 0	M 0
Stage II b	G 2	T 2	N 0	M 0
Stage III a	G 3	T 1	N 0	M 0
Stage III b	G 3	T 2	N 0	M 0
Stage III c	any G	T 1, T 2	N 1	M 0
Stage IV a	any G	T 3	any N	M 0
Stage IV b	any G	any T	any N	M 1

The treatment of malignant soft tissue tumors is based on surgery; irradiation therapy, chemotherapy, and immunotherapy are still being investigated clinically.

The details of treatment depend on the stage and the type of soft tissue tumor.

It has been reported, for instance, that in some tumors the combination of surgery and radiotherapy (about 60 Gy in 6 weeks) is effective [114].

The application of monochemotherapy (adriamycin [52] or combined chemotherapy (for instance, with cyclophosphamide + vincristine + adriamycin + DTIC or high dose methotrexate + citrovorum factor rescue) has been useful, especially in cases of advanced tumors [52, 60, 91-93, 103, 127].

[52] Frei III et al. 1978.
[60] Huber and Grünewald 1978.
[91] Pinedo et al. 1978.
[92] Pinedo and Kenis 1977.
[93] Pinedo and Voûte 1977.
[103] Schmidt et al. 1978.
[114] Suit et al. 1975.
[127] Wilbur 1975.

Tumors of the fibrous tissue

M-7610/0

1. Fibromatosis (WHO)

General Remarks

Site: Fibromatosis can develop at different sites (see following pages).
Fibromatosis rarely develops in the peritoneal cavity, the retroperitoneum, the orbit, the mediastinum, and the viscera organs. In most instances, it originates in the superficial soft tissues, often in the immediate neighborhood of skeletal muscle fibers.

Macroscopy

Fibromatosis is a firm, whitish, ill-defined lesion. The cut surface shows a whorled architecture.
Fibromatosis can be a large or small tumor-like lesion.

Histology

Fibromatosis is composed of large collagen fibers, which are formed by well-differentiated fibroblasts. The cells do not have signs of malignancy. Mitotic figures are rare.
The fibromatosis is poorly separated from the surrounding tissue and gives an aggressive microscopic appearance because of the extension of the collagen fibers into the surrounding fat tissue or muscle fibers (Figs. 1 and 2).

Differential Diagnosis

1. Fibromatosis **with fibrosarcoma (well differentiated):**
   Fibrosarcomas might have few cells with the signs of cellular malignancy (Figs. 24 and 25).
   In fibrosarcomas there are areas of high cellularity, and the number of mitoses is higher than in fibromatosis.
   The appearance of hyperchromatic nuclei is helpful in diagnosis of the fibrosarcoma.
2. The histological picture of fibromatosis does not necessarily predict the biological behavior of the lesion, which might recur.

Treatment

Radical excision of the lesion with a safe margin.

Prognosis

Cure if the excision is sufficient.
Possibility of recurrences in the case of insufficient removal of the lesion.

Further Information

a) Fibromatosis can be induced by irradiation:
   "Irradiation fibromatosis" (WHO).
   This lesion shows collagen fibers and cells with the signs of nuclei atypias due to the previous irradiation.
   Occasionally, differential diagnosis from a malignant mesenchymal tumor may therefore be necessary.

M-7617/0

b) Fibromatosis can develop after scar formation:
   "Cicatricial fibromatosis" (WHO).
   This lesion contains large collagen fibers and few cells (Fig. 3).

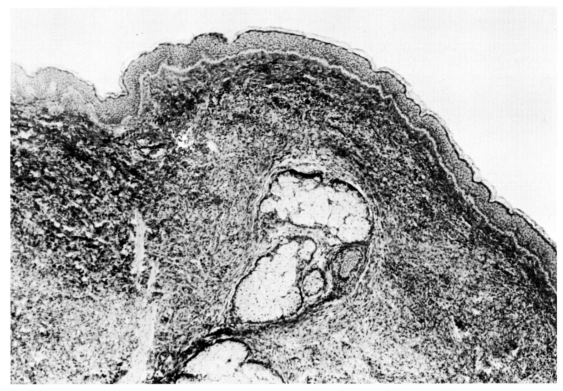

Fig. 1. Subepithelial fibromatosis: Ill-defined network of collagen fibers (33-year-old female, × 40).

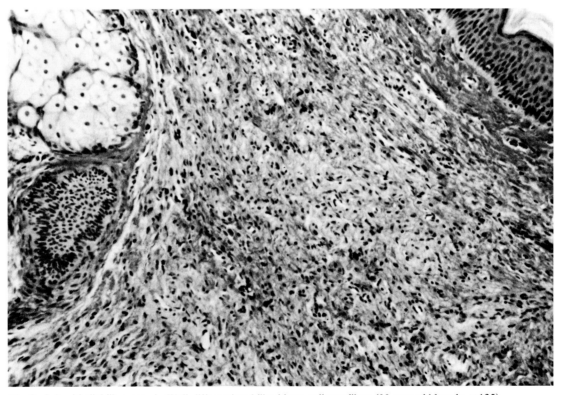

Fig. 2. Subepithelial fibromatosis: Well-differentiated fibroblasts, collagen fibers (33-year-old female, × 125).

M-4972/0
T 173.0

c) Keloid (WHO)

This lesion is composed of large collagen fibers that are glassy (Fig. 4).
This lesion tends to recur.

d) Fibromatosis of the omentum and mesentery is observed in association with multiple osteomas and polyposis coli in **Gardner's syndrome.**

M-7610/0
T 171.2

e) Palmar fibromatosis (WHO)
(Dupuytren's contracture)

T 171.3

f) Plantar fibromatosis (WHO)

General Remarks

Incidence: These are relatively rare lesions. Palmar fibromatosis is more frequently observed than plantar fibromatosis.
Age: Palmar and plantar fibromatosis are mainly observed in adults after the 5th decade.
Sex: Both sexes are equally affected in plantar fibromatosis. Palmar fibromatosis more often affects males.
Site: This fibromatosis can be a solitary lesion. However, multiple fibromatoses involving both sides especially palmar and simultaneously the palmar and plantar areas are observed frequently.

Histology

This form of fibromatosis is composed of collagen fibers and numerous cells (Fig. 5).
The nuclei of the cells are spindle-shaped and regular (Fig. 6).

Electron Microscopy

Cytoplasmic fibrils similar to those in smooth muscle cells and deformed nuclei.
This picture corresponds to contractile cells [53].

Differential Diagnosis

1. Palmar (plantar) fibromatosis **with fibrosarcoma** (Figs. 21 to 25).
2. Palmar (plantar) fibromatosis **with Kaposi's sarcoma** (Figs. 84 to 88).
3. Palmar (plantar) fibromatosis **with melanoma** (Fig. 1198).
4. Palmar (plantar) fibromatosis **with synovial sarcoma** (Figs. 129 to 132):
   Because of the foci of high cellularity, the differential diagnosis from malignant tumors must be solved.
   In palmar (plantar) fibromatosis there are no signs of malignancy.
   Sarcomas are rare in the palmar and plantar sites [4].

Clinical Findings

Contraction of fingers or toes in adults.

Treatment

Resection of the lesion.

Prognosis

Recurrence in the case of incomplete excision.

Further Information

M-7610/0
T-187.4

1. There is a report of **multiple congenital mesenchymal hamartomas** that involved the head, neck, trunk, and all four extremities, leading to multiple contractions [11].
2. Palmar and plantar fibromatosis can be combined with fibromatosis of the penis **(Peyronie's disease).**

---

[4] Allen et al. 1955.
[11] Benjamin et al. 1977.
[53] Gabbiani and Majno 1972.

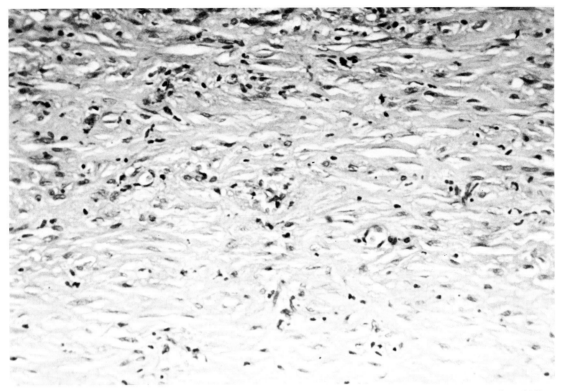

Fig. 3. Cicatricial fibromatosis: Large collagen fibers, few fibroblasts, remnants of capillaries (76-year-old male, × 200).

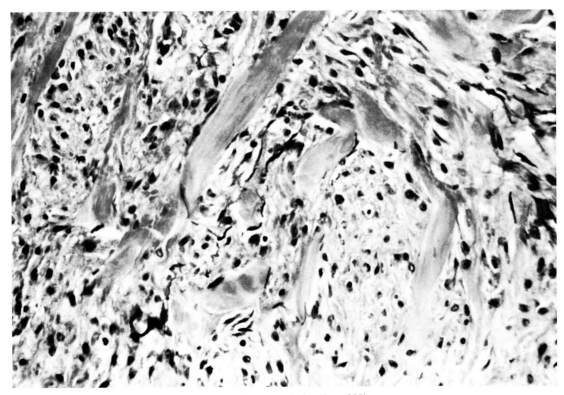

Fig. 4. Keloid: Homogenized large collagen fibers (33-year-old female, × 200).

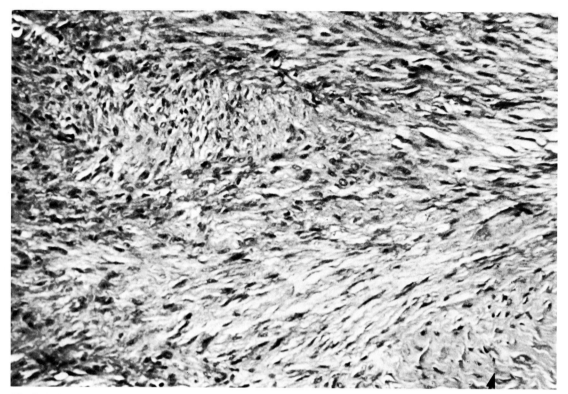

Fig. 5. Palmar fibromatosis: Bundles of fibroblasts with collagen fibers in the palmar fascia (arrow) (× 125).

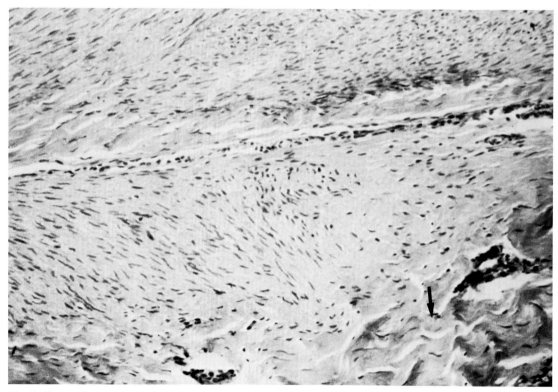

Fig. 6. Plantar fibromatosis: Numerous small fibroblasts and collagen fibers in the plantar fascia (arrow) (10-year-old male, × 125).

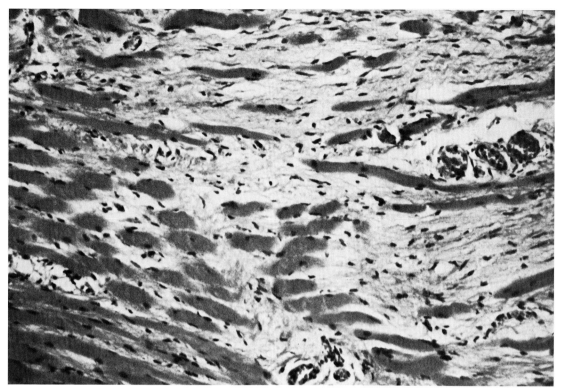

Fig. 7. Fibromatosis colli: Loose collagen fibers with fibroblasts growing into the skeletal muscle bundles (dark) (× 125).

Fibromatosis

M-7610/0
T 187.4

g) Penile fibromatosis
   (Peyronie's disease – WHO)

General Remarks

Incidence: This is a rare lesion.
Age: The main age group is between 40 and 65 years of age.
Site: Dorsal surface of the penis.

Macroscopy

Hard, circumscribed lesion.

Histology

Fibromatosis originating in the fascial structures of the sheath, extending between the tunica albuginea and corpus cavernosum. The corpus cavernosum is separated by the fibromatosis from the tunica albuginea.

Clinical Findings

Painful penile curvature at the site of the lesion and penile erection.

Treatment

Small doses of irradiation.
Steroids.
Excision [128].

M-7610/0
T 171.0

h) Fibromatosis colli (WHO)
   (congenital torticollis)

General Remarks

Incidence: This is a rare lesion.
Age: The lesion is observed at birth or develops a few weeks after birth.
Site: This fibromatosis develops in the sternomastoid muscle.
Further notes: The lesion is often combined with congenital anomalies of a different nature.
Fibromatosis colli is often preceded by a difficult delivery.

Histology

The skeletal muscle fibers of the sternomastoid muscle (in the lower one-third) are separated from each other by the fibromatosis, which is of a medium cellularity (Fig. 7).

Treatment

Surgical resection of the involved muscle is in most instances required.
Rarely, spontaneous regression has been observed.

M-7615/0

i) Juvenile aponeurotic fibroma
   (calcifying fibroma – WHO)

General Remarks

Incidence: This is a rare disease.
Age: Mainly children, followed by adolescents and young adults, are affected.
Site: The usual site of this is the volar side of the hands, followed by the plantar sides of the feet.

---

[128] Wild et al. 1979.

18

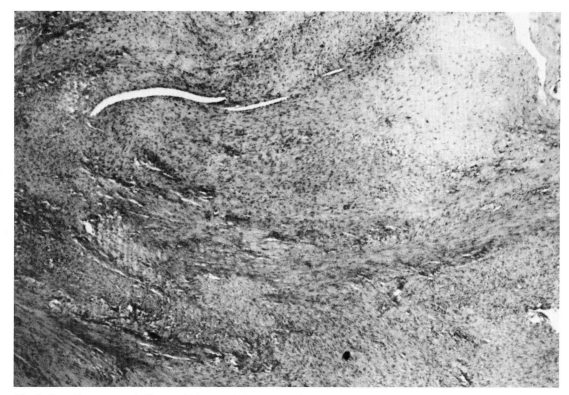

Fig. 8. Juvenile aponeurotic fibroma (16-year-old female, × 40).

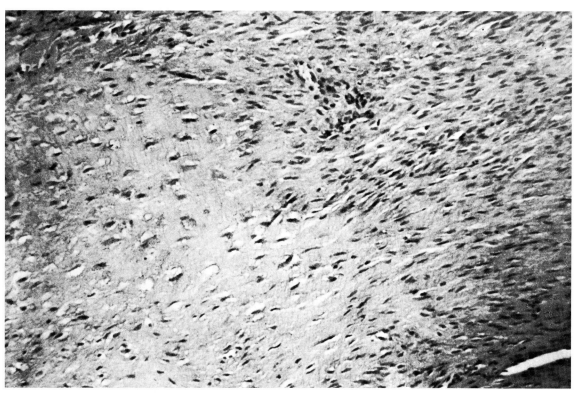

Fig. 9. Juvenile aponeurotic fibroma: Chondroid metaplasia (16-year-old female, × 125).

Histology	The fibromatosis develops in the aponeurotic tissue (the subcutaneous fat and the muscles). The lesion can contain chondroid metaplastic tissue and calcifications (Figs. 8 and 9).
Treatment	Surgery to completely remove the lesion.
Prognosis	Excellent, if the entire lesion has been removed. Recurrences are observed after incomplete surgical excision.

M-7610/0
T 171.2

k) Infantile digital fibromatosis

General Remarks

Incidence: This is a very rare lesion.
Age: The fibromatosis becomes apparent during early childhood or is found at birth.
Site: End phalanges of the fingers and toes, exterior surface.
Further notes: This lesion might be of viral origin.

Histology This is a fibromatosis with cells containing eosinophilic inclusions in their cytoplasm.

Treatment The lesions are removed.

Prognosis Infantile digital fibromatosis has a high recurrence rate [99].

M-7610/0

l) Congenital generalized fibromatosis (WHO)

This lesion consists of multiple mesenchymal nodules, which are composed mainly of collagen fibers and fibroblasts. These nodules are observed at birth or develop during the 1st year of life.
Besides the superficial part of the body the visceral organs might be involved.
The tumor can be fatal.
There is a hereditary component in this disease [9, 33].
In congenital fibromatosis of the skeleton, the tumor cells resemble primitive fibroblasts [66].

m) Fibromatosis hyalinica multiplex juvenilis

This is a variety of congenital generalized fibromatosis.
These are lesions that develop after birth.
After surgical excision they recur.
These lesions are very rare and are usually observed in the trunk, the head, and the neck in the subcutaneous region.
These tumor-like lesions grow rapidly [135].

[9] Bartlett et al. 1961.
[33] Drescher et al. 1967.
[66] Kindblom and Angervall 1978.
[99] Reye 1965.
[135] Woyke et al. 1970.

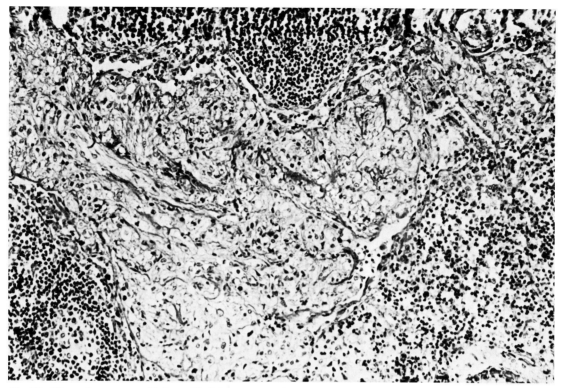

Fig. 10. Fibrous hamartoma of infancy: Nodule composed of loose fibrous tissue (2-month-old boy, several nodules in the deep dermal tissue, shoulder, × 125).

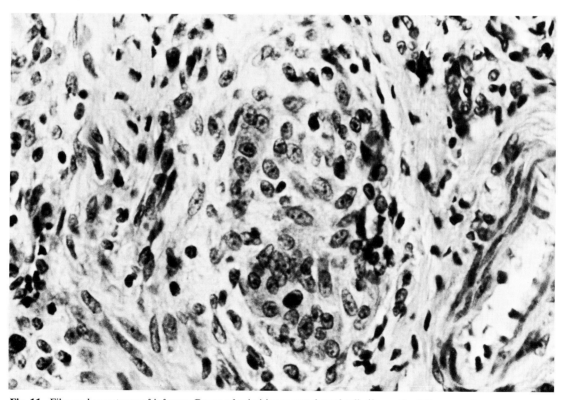

Fig. 11. Fibrous hamartoma of infancy: Group of primitive mesenchymal cells (2-month-old boy, spontaneous regression of the nodule in the following 7 months, no recurrences, × 310).

Fibromatosis

M-9351/0

n) Fibrous hamartoma of infancy (WHO)

General Remarks

Incidence: This is a very rare lesion.
Age: The lesion develops during the first 2 years of life.
Sex: Males are more frequently affected than females.
Site: Fibrous hamartomas are solitary tumors in the axilla, shoulder, or arm.

Macroscopy

The lesion is poorly circumscribed and has a whitish cut surface surrounding yellowish, fatty areas.

Histology

The tumor is composed of mature adipose tissue, well-differentiated fibrous tissue, and cellular areas, resembling primitive mesenchyma [39, 41, 98] (Figs. 10 and 11).

M-7613/0

o) Nodular fasciitis
    (pseudosarcomatous fibromatosis – WHO)

General Remarks

Incidence: This is a relatively rare lesion.
Age: All ages can be affected.
The lesion is usually observed in young adults, with the peak occurrence during the 4th decade.
Sex: Both sexes are affected equally.
Site: Nodular fasciitis develops mostly in the neck region, trunk, and upper extremities.

Macroscopy

The lesion is a hard nodule associated with the fascia.
The lesion has ill-defined borders toward the surrounding soft tissue.

Histology

The lesion contains numerous fibroblasts (Fig. 12). There are many mitoses. The fibroblasts grow in an edematous or mucoid stroma. There are numerous blood vessels and inflammatory cells [83] (Fig. 13).
The fibroblasts may have bizarre nuclei (Fig. 14).
The lesion infiltrates the surrounding fat tissue and the muscle (Figs. 14 and 15).

Electron Microscopy

In nodular fasciitis the proliferating cells contain myofilaments in addition to basement membrane-like material (myofibroblasts) [130].

Differential Diagnosis

Nodular fasciitis (pseudosarcomatous fasciitis) **with fibrosarcoma** (Fig. 23):
This differential diagnosis is very important because the high cellularity, the high number of mitotic figures (rapid growth clinically), and the occasional occurrence of bizarre nuclei (Figs. 16 and 17), in addition to the signs of infiltration into the surrounding tissue, are suggestive of a malignant tumor.

---

[39] Enzinger 1965.
[41] Enzinger 1968.
[83] Meister et al. 1978.
[98] Reye 1956.
[130] Wirman 1976.

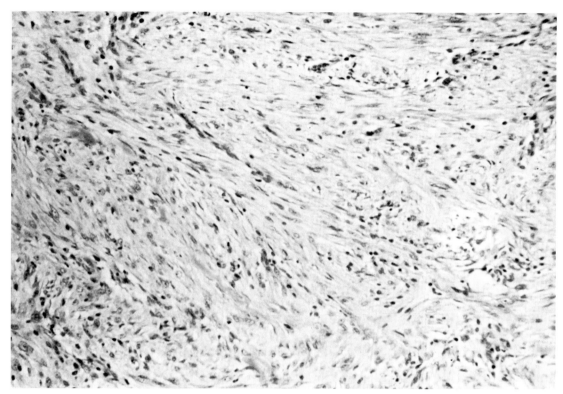

Fig. 12. Nodular fasciitis: Upper part of the lesion with interlacing collagen bundles and fibroblasts. Discrete inflammatory cell infiltration (28-year-old female, × 125).

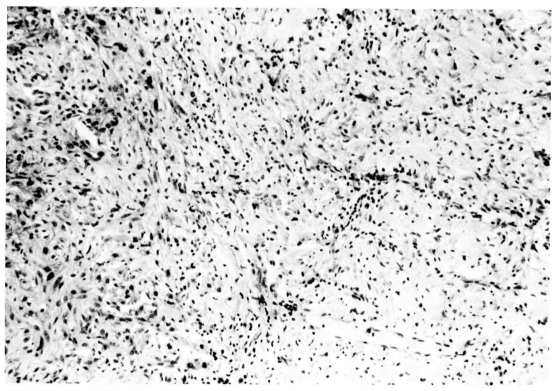

Fig. 13. Nodular fasciitis: Numerous capillaries and inflammatory cells (deep area toward the fat tissue) (69-year-old female, × 125).

23

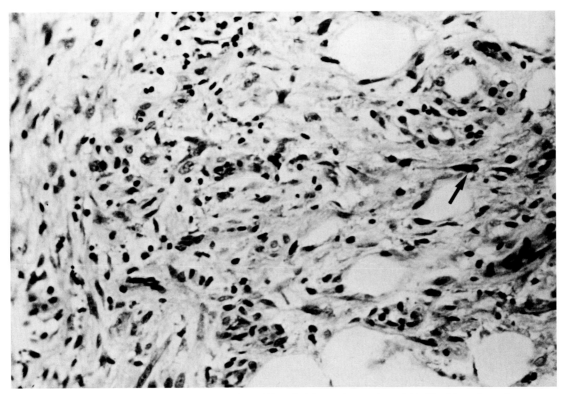

Fig. 14. Nodular faciitis: Pseudoinfiltration of the tissue. Note dark hyperchromatic nuclei in fibroblasts (arrow) (28-year-old female, × 200).

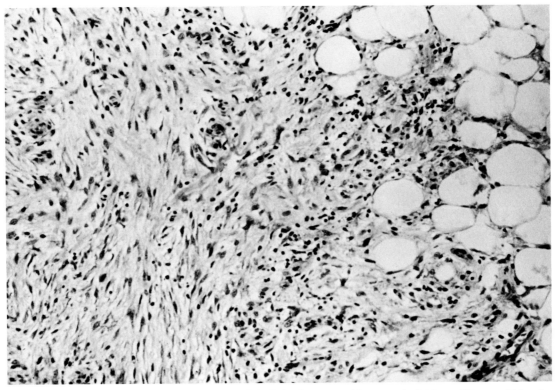

Fig. 15. Nodular fasciitis: The inflammatory nature of the lesion becomes evident near the fat tissue (28-year-old female, × 125).

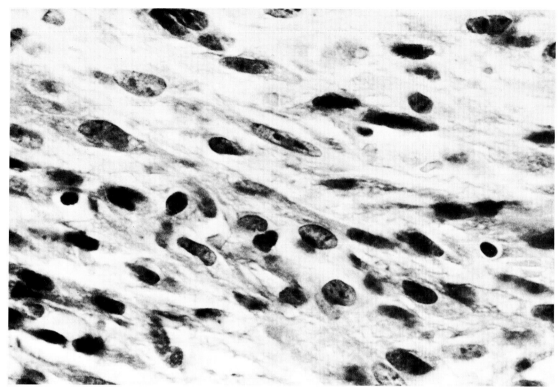

Fig. 16. Pseudosarcomatous fasciitis: Oval, large nuclei with some irregularity (28-year-old female, × 600).

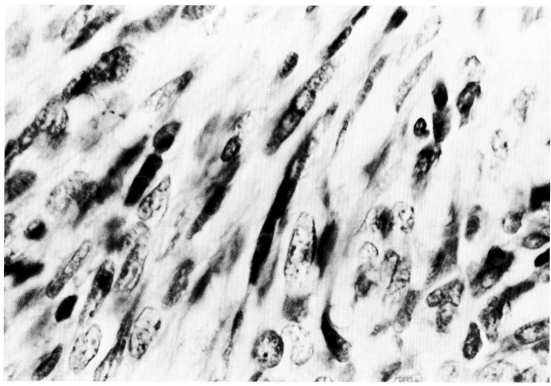

Fig. 17. Pleomorphic malignant nuclei in fibrosarcoma (× 600).

Nodular fasciitis

Differential Diagnosis

Differentiating features of nodular fasciitis are:
– No hyperchromatic (malignant) nuclei.
– Inflammatory cells and capillary growth (especially toward the margin of the lesion).

Clinical Findings

Nodular fasciitis presents as a rapidly growing nodule, which is painful. The lesion grows in the subcutaneous tissue.

Treatment

Removal of the lesion.

Prognosis

This is a benign lesion with an excellent prognosis.

Further Information

The proliferating cells in nodular fasciitis are most probably myofibroblasts [130].

---

[130] Wirman 1976.

M-9160/0
T 147.9

2. Nasopharyngeal fibroma
(juvenile angiofibroma – WHO)

General Remarks
Incidence: This is a rare tumor.
Age: The majority of the patients are in the 2nd or 3rd decades.
Sex: The tumor affects males.
Site: The tumor develops in the nasal space or from the wall of the nasopharyngeal cavity.

Macroscopy
The tumor is soft and easily bleeds when touched.

Histology
The tumor is composed of numerous ectatic blood vessels, which are surrounded by a loose connective tissue (Fig. 474).

Treatment
Surgical removal.

Prognosis
The tumor shows a tendency to recur.
Spontaneous regression may be observed.

M-8820/0

3. Elastofibroma (WHO)

General Remarks
Incidence: This is a very rare lesion.
Age: Elderly patients are affected most often.
Site: In almost all instances the tumor develops at the lower border of the scapula and the ribs.

Macroscopy
The tumor can be rather large.

Histology
The tumor is composed of collagen fibers and elastic fibers.
These elastic fibers are broken into small fragments, which are eosinophilic.

Treatment
Excision of the tumor.

Prognosis
Excellent. No recurrences.

Further Information
Most probably this is not a tumor, but a reaction of elastic fiber tissue to trauma.

M-8822/1

4. Abdominal fibromatosis (WHO)
(desmoid tumor, abdominal desmoid, musculoaponeurotic fibromatosis)

**General
Remarks**

Incidence: This is a relatively rare lesion.
Age: The tumor grows mainly in young women during (or after) pregnancy.
Men and children can also be affected **("juvenile fibromatosis").**
Site: Abdominal fibromatosis originates from the musculoaponeurotic region of the rectus muscle and the adjacent muscles.

M-8821/1

5. Extraabdominal desmoid
(fibromatosis or aggressive fibromatosis) (WHO)

This tumor affects young adults and children.
Extraabdominal musculoaponeurotic fibromatosis is mainly observed in the shoulder girdle, the thigh and buttock, and the head and neck area [24, 44].

Macroscopy

This is a firm lesion that is poorly differentiated from the surrounding soft tissue. The tumor can be of different sizes.

Histology

Musculoaponeurotic fibromatosis is composed of collagen fibers, which are large and dominate the picture (Fig. 18). The fibroblasts are spindle-shaped and small (Fig. 19). Atypical cells are missing, and mitotic divisions are observed rarely.
The tumor extends into the surrounding fat tissue and into the muscle fibers.

**Differential
Diagnosis**

1. Musculoaponeurotic fibromatosis **with fibrosarcoma (well-differentiated)** (Fig. 23):
   In fibrosarcomas there are atypical cells and a higher cellularity than in fibromatosis.
2. Musculoaponeurotic fibromatosis **with dermatofibrosarcoma protuberans** (Figs. 41 to 43):
   The dermatofibrosarcoma shows a very cellular tissue with atypical cells growing in a cartwheel pattern.

**Clinical
Findings**

Firm tumor in the abdominal or extraabdominal site in young adults (or in children).

Treatment

Radical removal of the tumor with a large, safe margin.
Surgical excision is also used in cases of recurrence [24, 61].
No radiation therapy.

Prognosis

This fibromatosis recurs frequently. There are no metastases. Recurrences are observed more frequently in extraabdominal fibromatosis than in abdominal fibromatosis [61].
Recurrences can be controlled by surgical excision in most instances.

[24] Conley et al. 1966.
[44] Enzinger and Shiraki 1967.
[61] Hunt et al. 1960.

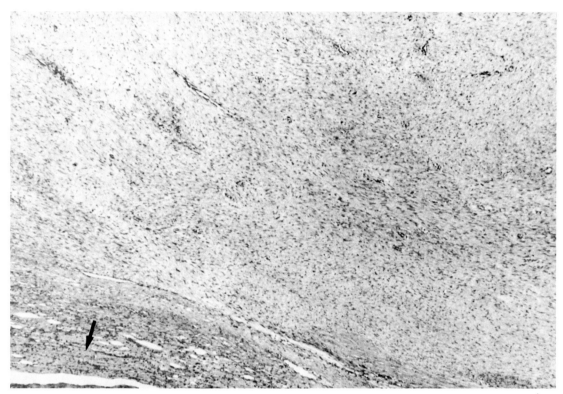

Fig. 18. Abdominal fibromatosis (desmoid): Numerous fibroblasts and collagen fibers, developing in skeletal muscle (arrow) (76-year-old male, × 40).

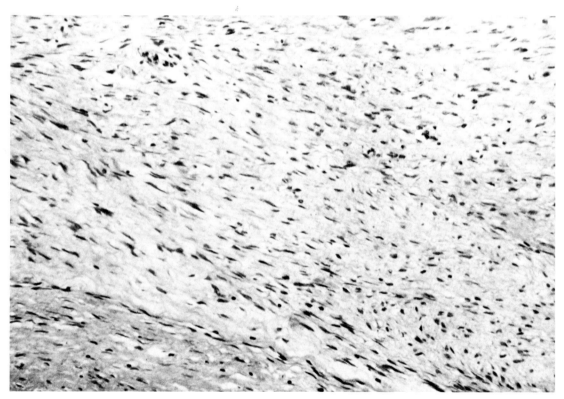

Fig. 19. Abdominal fibromatosis (desmoid): Numerous small fibroblasts without nuclear atypias and collagen bundles (76-year-old male, × 125).

M-8810/0

6. Fibroma (WHO)

M-8810/0   These are benign, common tumors of the skin surface or of the mucous membranes.

M-8851/0   The tumor can contain numerous or few collagen fibers (fibroma durum and fibroma molle **(fibrolipoma)** – WHO) (Fig. 20).
Fibromas are covered by the corresponding cells (epidermis or mucosa).
The tumor can be removed surgically [49].

---

[49] Feldman and Meyer 1976.

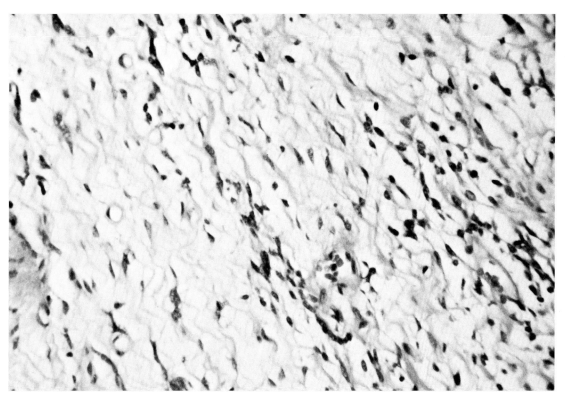

Fig. 20. Fibroma: Interlacing bundles of collagen fibers, regular fibroblasts (× 200).

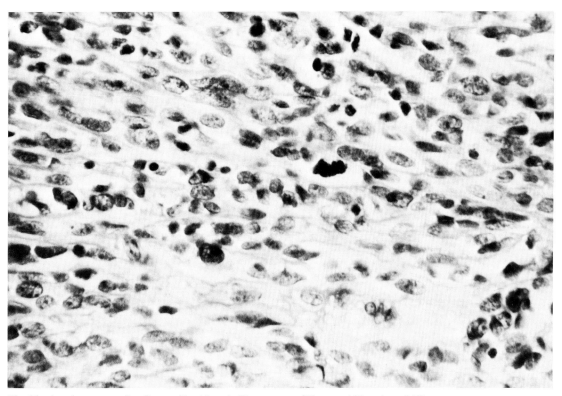

Fig. 21. Another aspect of malignant fibroblasts in fibrosarcoma (72-year-old female, × 310).

M-8810/3

7. Fibrosarcoma (WHO)

**General
Remarks**

Incidence: About 40% of malignant soft tissue tumors are fibrosarcomas.
Age: Patients of any age can be affected including infants and children [106]; however, the majority of the tumors grow in adults.
Sex: Males are affected more frequently than females.
Site: The majority of fibrosarcomas grow in the superficial and deep soft tissues of the head, neck, extremities, and torso.
However, other areas of the body may be affected: central nervous system, breast, liver, lung, thyroid, prostate, kidney, urinary bladder, vulva, vagina, omentum, tendon, mesentery, periosteum, bone, mediastinum, retroperitoneum [109].

Macroscopy

Fibrosarcomas are grayish-whitish soft tumors. The cut surface shows necroses and bleeding. The tumor infiltrates into the surrounding soft tissue parts.

Histology

The tumor is composed of malignant fibroblasts. They can show a smaller or higher number of regular or atypical mitotic figures (Figs. 21 and 22).
The tumor cells have hyperchromatic nuclei of different sizes and shapes (Figs. 23 and 24).
The tumor cells invade the surrounding tissue.
Fibrosarcomas contain numerous reticulin fibers. These fibers often surround single tumor cells (Fig. 25).

**Electron
Microscopy**

Endoplasmic reticulum, sometimes dilated, and microfilaments (Figs. 26 to 28).

**Differential
Diagnosis**

1. Fibrosarcoma, well differentiated, **with fibromatosis** (especially in young patients and children) (Figs. 1 to 7):
   In fibrosarcomas, hyperchromatic nuclei are observed. There are more mitotic figures than in fibromatosis.
2. Fibrosarcoma, poorly differentiated **with other undifferentiated sarcomas:**
   – pleomorphic fibrous histiocytoma (Figs. 45 to 48),
   – synovial sarcoma (Figs. 129 to 132),
   – malignant schwannoma (Figs. 169 to 175),
   – soft tissue sarcoma (Figs. 124 to 128),
   – rhabdomyosarcoma (Figs. 111 to 122),
   – malignant melanoma (Fig. 1216).
   An important help in determining the origin of the sarcoma is evidence that the individual tumor cells are surrounded by reticulin fibers (fibrosarcoma).
   Malignant giant cells are not frequently observed in fibrosarcoma.

---

[106] Soule and Pritchard 1977.
[109] Stout and Lattes 1967.

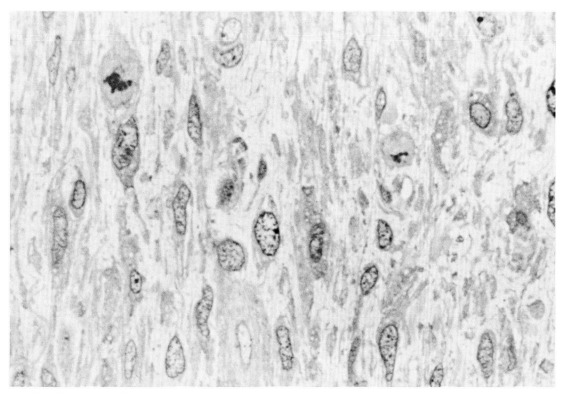

Fig. 22. Fibroblasts in fibrosarcoma: Coarse chromatin, marked nuclear pleomorphism, atypical mitoses, cytoplasmic processes (79-year-old male, × 800).

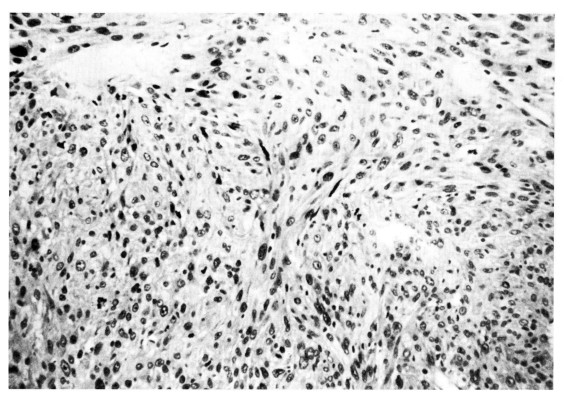

Fig. 23. Fibrosarcoma: Interlacing bundles of malignant fibroblasts (40-year-old female, × 125).

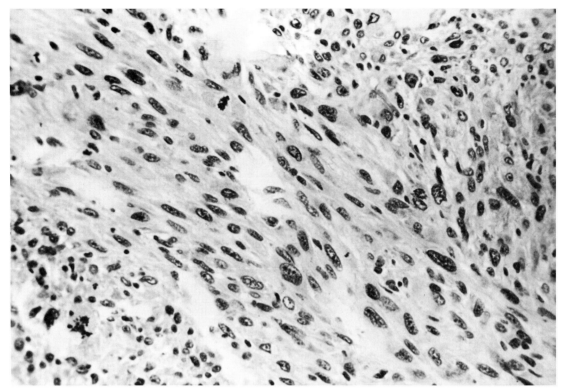

Fig. 24. Fibrosarcoma: Atypical fibroblasts and atypical mitotic figures (40-year-old female, × 200).

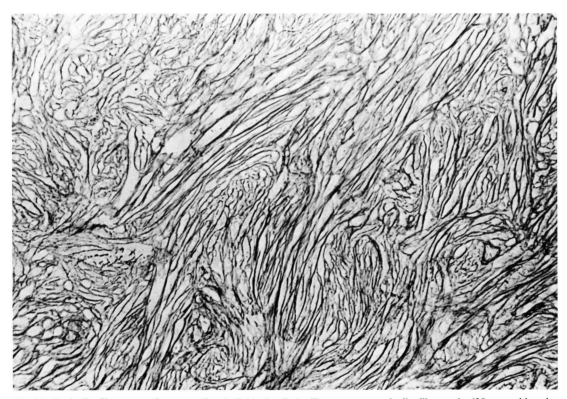

Fig. 25. Reticulin fiber network surrounding individual cells in fibrosarcoma; reticulin fiber stain (29-year-old male, × 125).

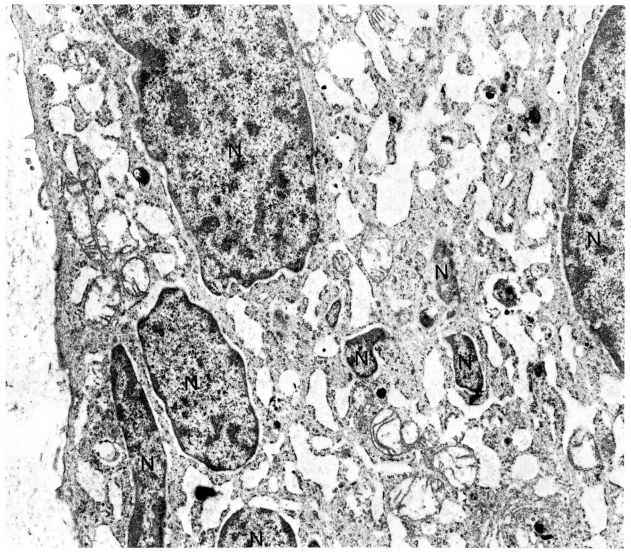

Fig. 26. Fibrosarcoma: Multinucleated giant cell with several profiles of the nuclei (N). The cytoplasm contains numerous dilated cisterns of rough endoplasmic reticulum. Few swollen mitochondria (× 14,400) (see also Figs. 27 and 28).

Fibrosarcoma

Staging   See Introduction, page 11.

Grading   See Introduction, page 11.
High numbers of mitotic divisions in a sarcoma correlate with an increased incidence of metastases [122].

Spread   Fibrosarcomas disseminate mainly by a hematogenous route.

Clinical
Findings   Rapidly growing soft tumor with symptoms according to the site of its origin.

Treatment   Radical **surgery.**
Frequently fibrosarcomas are of low radiosensitivity. Fast neutron therapy might be effective [51 a].
Chemotherapy can be tried with DTIC, vincristine, cyclophosphamide, and adriamycin or with DTIC and adriamycin [72, 90, 92].

Prognosis   The prognosis is determined by the stage of the tumor. The 5-year survival rate for Stage I is approximately 70%; for Stage IV it is less than 10%.
Fibrosarcomas in children have a considerably better prognosis than those in adults because of the low rate of recurrence and metastasis.
Fibrosarcomas in children: 39% recur,
9% metastasize,
13% cause death.
Fibrosarcomas in adults: 75% recur,
25% metastasize,
50% cause death.
Although fibrosarcomas in children and infants have a better prognosis than do tumors in adults, a prolonged follow-up after treatment is needed [19].

[19] Chung and Enzinger 1976.
[51a] Franke 1979.
[72] Krementz et al. 1977.
[90] Perevodchikova et al. 1977.
[92] Pinedo and Kenis 1977.
[122] Van Der Werf-Messing and van Unnik 1965.

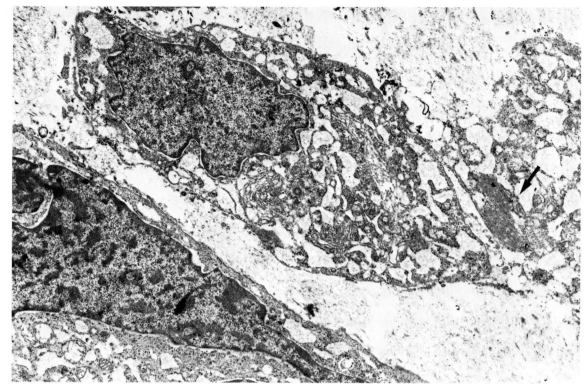

Fig. 27.

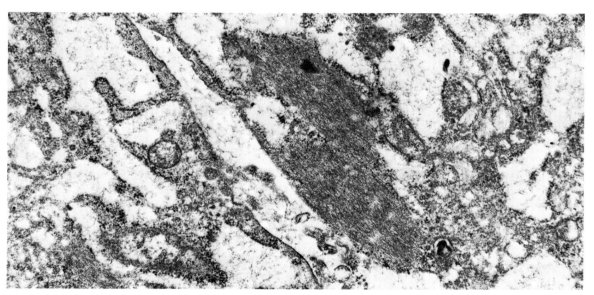

Fig. 28.

Figs. 27 and 28. Fibrosarcoma: Tumor cells with dilated cisterns of rough endoplasmic reticulum and intracytoplasmatic bundles of microfilaments (arrow and Fig. 28) (Fig. 27, × 6600; Fig. 28, × 25,500).

Histiocytic tumors [109]

8. Benign histiocytoma

M-8832/0
T 173.9

General
Remarks

Incidence: This is a frequently observed tumor in the skin.
Age: The tumor affects all ages.
Sex: There is no sex difference.

Macroscopy

The skin lesion may be soft or firm, has a whitish cut surface, and is round or oval.
The tumor is well delineated from the surrounding tissue.

Histology

The tumor is composed of collagen bundles ("cartwheel") and histiocytes (Fig. 29). The histiocytes have regular nuclei, which are clear (Figs. 30 and 31). The cytoplasm is abundant and may be foamy and contain iron pigment. Between the histiocytes, fibroblasts can be found [126].

The collagen structures occasionally can dominate the picture and imitate fibromatosis (Fig. 32):

M-8830/0

Fibrous histiocytoma
(dermatofibroma) (fibroxanthoma – WHO)

Occasionally the histiocytoma contains numerous cells that have a foamy cytoplasm. Between these foamy cells numerous histiocytes with siderin and giant cells are observed.

This lesion can be called:

M-8831/0

Xanthomatosis
(xanthoma – WHO).

Occasionally in the eyelids these histiocytomas are composed entirely of foamy histiocytes:

Xanthelasma
(xanthoma diabeticorum) (xanthoma – WHO) (Figs. 33 and 34).

---

[109] Stout and Lattes 1967.
[126] Weiss et al. 1978.

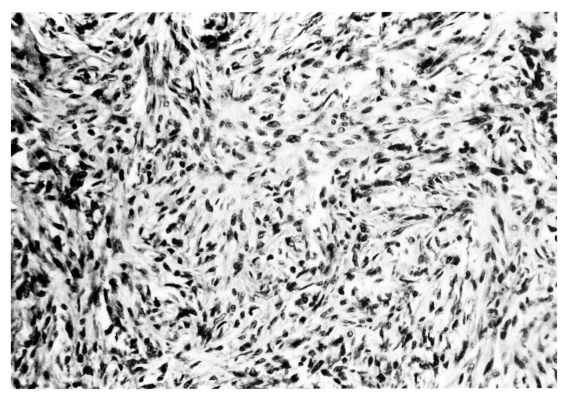

Fig. 29. Benign histiocytoma: Fibroblasts, histiocytes, collagen fibers form interlacing bundles (52-year-old female, × 200).

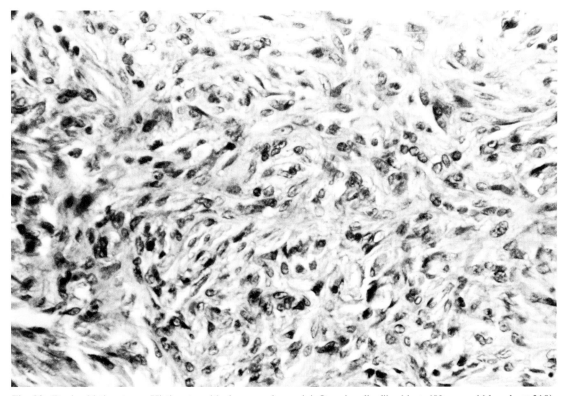

Fig. 30. Benign histiocytoma: Histiocytes with clear, regular nuclei. Occasionally, fibroblasts (52-year-old female, × 310).

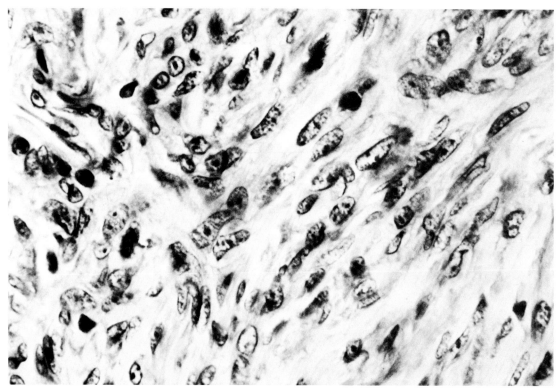

Fig. 31. Benign histiocytoma (52-year-old female, × 600).

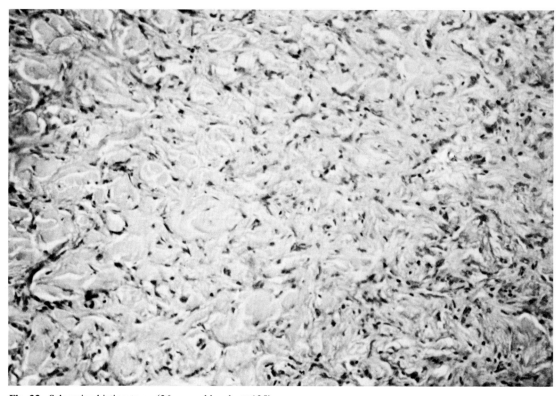

Fig. 32. Sclerosing histiocytoma (36-year-old male, × 125).

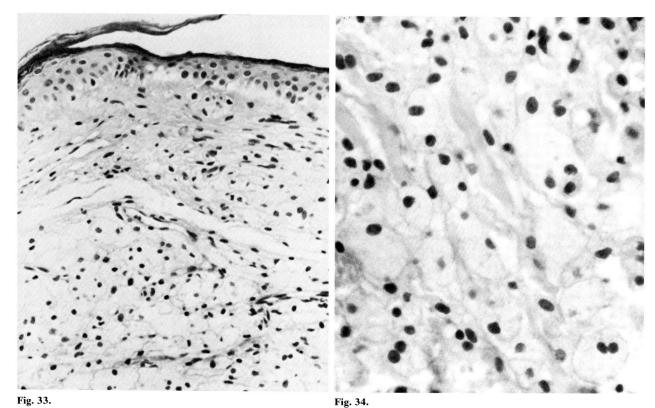

Fig. 33.   Fig. 34.

Figs. 33 and 34. Xanthelasma: Group of foamy cells underneath the covering epidermis (48-year-old female, eyelid, Fig. 33, × 200; Fig. 34, × 310).

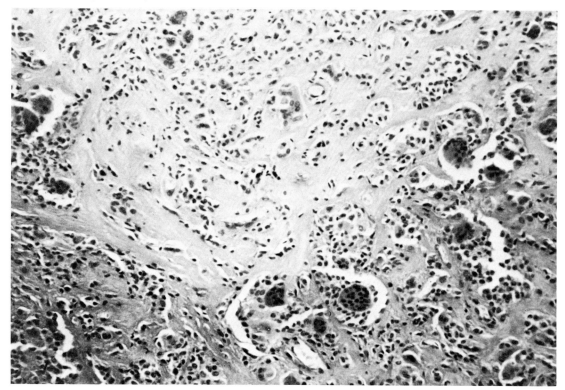

Fig. 35. Benign histiocytic giant cell tumor (tendon sheath) (35-year-old female, × 125).

M-8830/0

9. Benign histiocytic giant cell tumor (of tendon sheaths)
(nodular tenosynovitis – WHO)

General Remarks

Incidence: This is a rather common soft tissue tumor.

Age: Young or middle-aged patients are usually affected.

Sex: Females are affected more frequently than males.

T 171.2
T 171.3

Site: The majority of these tumors develop between the ankle and the toe tips or between the wrist and the finger tips.

Histology

The tumor is very cellular and contains numerous benign histiocytic giant cells (Figs. 35 and 36).

In a number of histiocytes, siderin is deposited. There are nests of foamy histiocytes (Figs. 37 and 38).

Differential Diagnosis

Due to the cellularity of this tumor it must occasionally be differentiated from **sarcoma.** The histiocytes always have regular nuclei. There is no sign of infiltration.

Treatment

Removal of the tumor.

Prognosis

Excellent.

After incomplete removal, giant cell tumors recur.

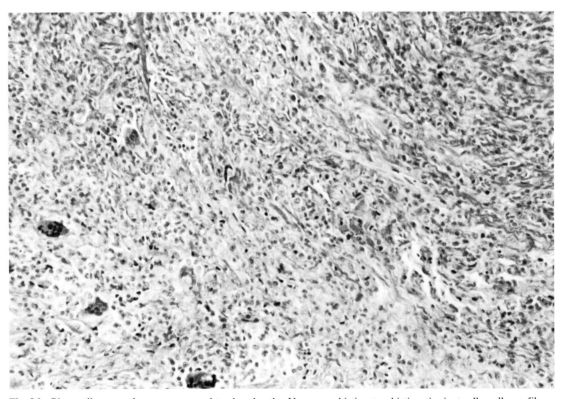

Fig. 36. Giant cell tumor of aponeuroses and tendon sheaths: Numerous histiocytes, histiocytic giant cells, collagen fibers (29-year-old male, × 125).

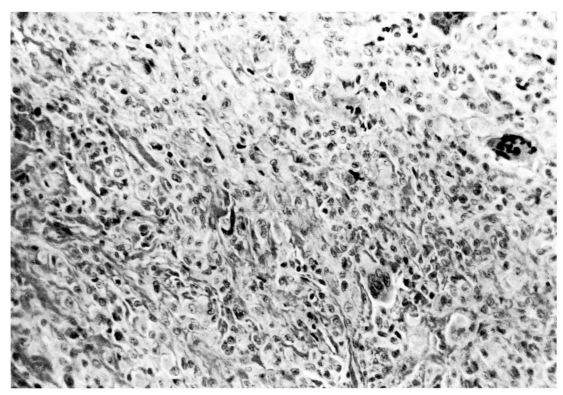

Fig. 37. Giant cell tumor of aponeuroses and tendon sheaths: Numerous histiocytes with regular nuclei, occasionally foamy cytoplasm, some histiocytic giant cells, collagen fibers (29-year-old male, × 200).

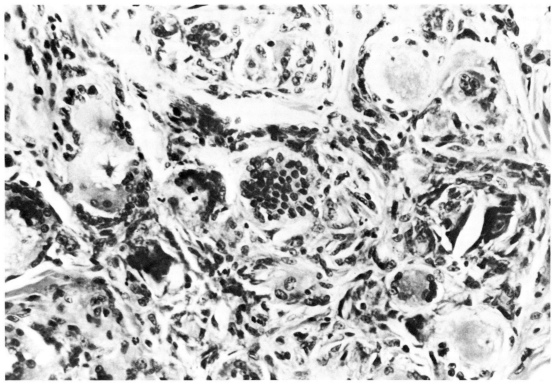

Fig. 38. Giant cells in giant cell granuloma with foreign bodies (44-year-old female, × 200).

M-4783/0

10. Villonodular pigmented synovitis
(nodular tenosynovitis – WHO)

**General
Remarks**

Incidence: Villonodular synovitis is a relatively rare tumor (see Bone tumors, page 1112).
Age: In most instances the tumor affects young adults.
Site: Usually villonodular synovitis is a lesion at the knee joint.
This lesion can, however, also be observed in the ankle, the shoulder, and the hip.
Villonodular synovitis affects almost always only one articulation.
Further notes:
a) Villonodular synovitis develops in the synovia or bursa.
b) Villonodular synovitis can be considered a variety of giant cell histiocytoma.

Macroscopy

The lesion is soft and brownish.

Histology

Villonodular synovitis is composed of histiocytes that contain abundant amounts of siderin pigment (Fig. 39).
The tumor contains many benign histiocytic giant cells (Fig. 40). Nests of lymphocytes are observed.

**Differential
Diagnosis**

Villonodular synovitis **with sarcoma:**
Due to the high cellularity and the numerous giant cells, the microscopic appearance of a malignant tumor can be mimicked:
– fibrosarcoma (Figs. 21 to 25),
– synovial sarcoma (Figs. 129 to 132),
– osteogenic sarcoma (Figs 993 to 996),
– malignant giant cell tumor (Figs. 1048 to 1050).
In villonodular synovitis there are no signs of malignant nuclei in the giant cells or in the stroma cells.
In doubtful cases clinical findings and radiographs are helpful.

Treatment

Villonodular synovitis is removed completely by operation. Recurrences are observed in cases of incomplete excision.
Villonodular synovitis can also be treated by irradiation.

Prognosis

This is a benign lesion.

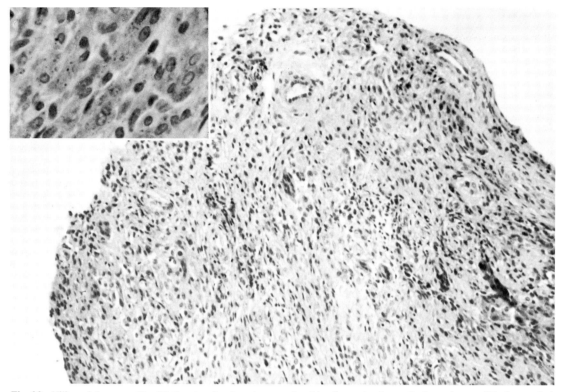

Fig. 39. Villonodular synovitis: Histiocytes, few lymphocytes, few blood vessels, giant cells. Iron pigment (black granules) in histiocytes (× 125; inset × 200, iron stain).

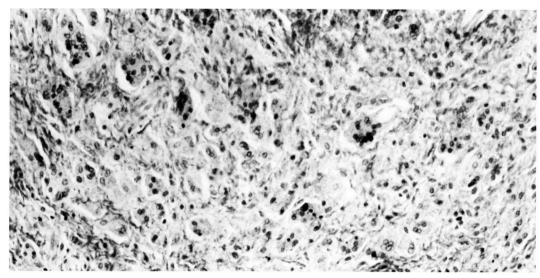

Fig. 40. Numerous histiocytic giant cells (benign) in villonodular synovitis (× 200).

M-8832/0
T 173.9

11. Fibrous histiocytoma, vascular variety

(sclerosing hemangioma-Wolbach) (sclerosing hemangioma; dermatofibroma – WHO)

This histiocytoma contains numerous blood vessels between the collagen fibers and the histiocytes.
Occasionally this picture might simulate a hemangioma with regressive changes.
This is a benign lesion, which can be excised surgically.

M-8832/1, 3
T 173.9

12. Dermatofibrosarcoma protuberans (WHO)
(dermatofibroma protuberans)

General Remarks

Incidence: This is a rare histiocytic tumor.
Age: Patients of all ages can be affected.
Sex: Females are affected slightly more often than males.
Site: The tumor can develop in the skin or in deeper tissues.
In most instances dermatofibrosarcoma protuberans develops on the anterior surface of the body away from the midline.
The tumor can be solitary or multiple nodular lesions.

Macroscopy

The tumor is hard and poorly differentiated from the surrounding tissue.

Histology

The tumor is very cellular. The tumor cells are fibroblasts derived from histiocytes [109] (Fig. 41).
The tumor cells are surrounded by reticulin fibers (Fig. 42). The tumor cells are arranged in a so-called cartwheel (whorled, storiform) pattern [117] (Fig. 43).

Electron Microscopy

The nuclei of the tumor cells are multisegmented [7].

Differential Diagnosis

Dermatofibrosarcoma protuberans **with fibrosarcoma** (Figs. 21 to 25):
In dermatofibrosarcoma protuberans there are no nuclei atypias (Fig. 44).
The characteristic cartwheel architecture of the tumor identifies the dermatofibrosarcoma protuberans.

Clinical Findings

Dermatofibrosarcoma protuberans is large with infiltration of the surrounding tissue.
The tumor grows slowly over many years.

Treatment

Complete excision of the tumor.
Great probability of recurrence in cases of incomplete excision.

Prognosis M-8832/3

This is almost always a benign lesion; however, rarely malignant development with metastases has been observed [14, 42].

Further Information

1. It is debated whether the Schwann's cell could be involved in the origin of dermatofibrosarcoma protuberans [58].

M-8832/0, 1

2. Dermatofibroma (see Histiocytoma, page 38).

[7] Auböck 1975.
[14] Brenner et al. 1975.
[42] Enzinger 1969.
[58] Harkin and Reed 1969.
[109] Stout and Lattes 1967.
[117] Taylor and Helwig 1962.

Dermatofibrosarcoma protuberans

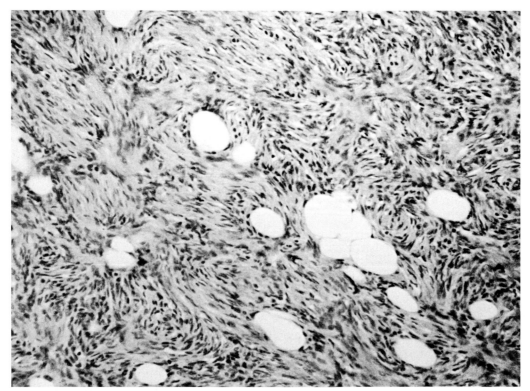

Fig. 41. Dermatofibrosarcoma protuberans: Numerous histiocytes (fibroblasts) infiltrating the fat tissue (66-year-old male, alive after 20 years of follow-up, × 125).

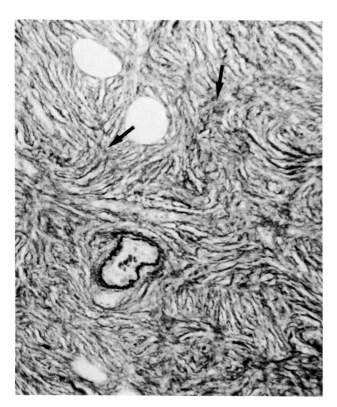

Fig. 42. Dermatofibrosarcoma protuberans: Reticulin fibers demonstrating the storiform growth pattern (center, arrows) (66-year-old male, reticulin fiber stain, × 125).

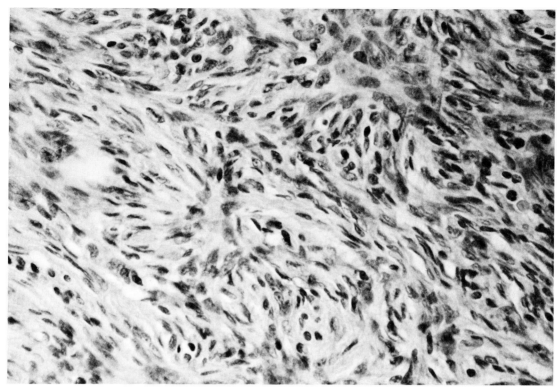

Fig. 43. Dermatofibrosarcoma protuberans: Regular nuclei of histiocytes and fibroblasts, storiform pattern of cells and fibers (66-year-old male, × 200).

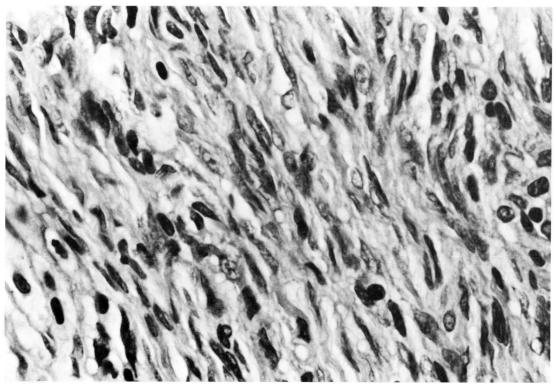

Fig. 44. Dermatofibrosarcoma protuberans: Regular nuclei (66-year-old male, × 600).

M-8830/3

13. Malignant fibrous histiocytoma
(malignant fibroxanthoma – WHO, pleomorphic fibrous xanthoma)

**General
Remarks**

Incidence: This is a rare, malignant, soft tissue tumor.
Age: This tumor develops mostly in adults.
Sex: Both sexes are affected equally.
Site: Malignant fibrous histiocytoma can develop in any part of the body: skin, mediastinum, bone, retroperitoneum, breast.

Histology

The tumor is composed of malignant cells with hyperchromatic nuclei, numerous mitotic figures, pleomorphic cells and giant cells (Figs. 45 and 46). The tumor resembles reticulum cell sarcoma [109] (Fig. 47). In the very cellular tumor tissue, the cells are arranged in a storiform cartwheel pattern (Fig. 48). Between the histiocytic cells there are fibroblasts [80]. On reticulin stain the lack of reticulin fibers is observed [75].

**Electron
Microscopy**

The cytoplasm in malignant fibrous histiocytoma contains few organelles; occasionally there are dilated cisternae of rough endoplasmatic reticulum. The cytoplasm might contain actin-like filaments with dense bodies. The nuclei are slightly lobulated. Frequently there are prominent nucleoli. The chromatin can be clumped.
In some cells a Golgi apparatus or numerous mitochondria can be found. Lysosomes are present, and Langerhans' granules are seemingly exceedingly rare or do not exist. Desmosomes are scant [2, 116].

**Differential
Diagnosis**

1. Malignant fibrous histiocytoma **with reticulosarcoma** (Figs. 1042 to 1044).
2. Malignant fibrous histiocytoma **with plemorphic rhabdomyosarcoma** (Figs. 111 to 114).
3. Malignant fibrous histiocytoma **with liposarcoma** (Figs. 61 to 69).
4. Malignant fibrous histiocytoma **with fibrosarcoma** (Figs. 21 to 25).
   Helpful for the diagnosis of malignant fibrous histiocytoma is the storiform growth pattern of the tumor and the lack of reticulin fibers. (Reticular cell sarcoma and fibrosarcoma have tumor cells that are individually surrounded by reticulin fibers).
   Pleomorphic rhabdomyosarcoma is indicated by the striated cytoplasm.
   In liposarcoma one might finally encounter remnants of the malignant fat cells (in cases of very undifferentiated liposarcoma).

Spread

Lymphatic spread into regional lymph nodes. Hematogenous spread, especially to the lung [105].

Staging

See Introduction, page 11.

Grading

See Introduction, page 11.

---

[2] Alguacil-Garcia et al. 1977.
[75] Kyriakos and Kempson 1976.
[80] Limacher et al. 1978.
[105] Soule and Enriquez 1972.
[109] Stout and Lattes 1967.
[116] Taxy and Battifora 1977.

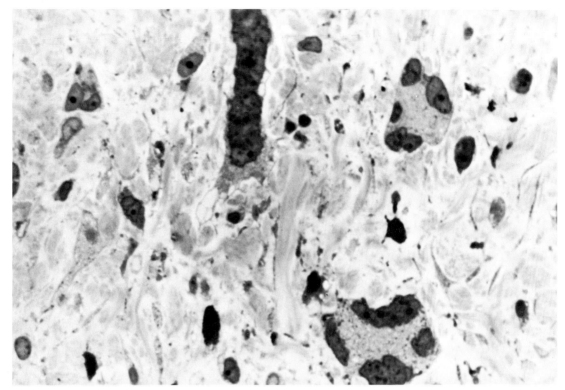

Fig. 45. Malignant histiocytoma (74-year-old male, × 600).

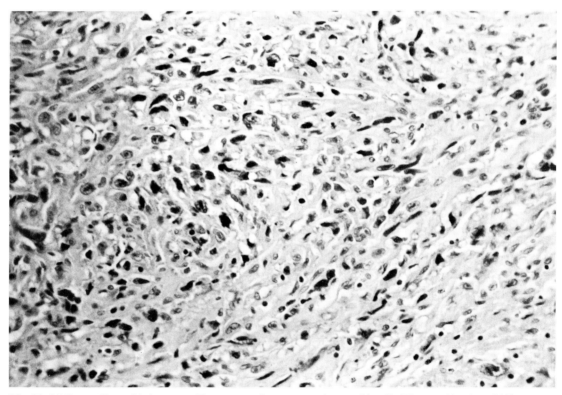

Fig. 46. Malignant fibrous histiocytoma: Numerous malignant, very pleomorphic cells (29-year-old male, × 200).

51

Malignant histiocytoma

Treatment   Radical **surgery.**
Radiation therapy.
It has been reported that **chemotherapy** with cyclophosphamide combined with vincristine, adriamycin, and DTIC gives a response in 33% of the cases [77, 78].

Prognosis   The individual prognosis depends on the stage of the tumor at the time of diagnosis.
The 5-year survival rate for Stage I tumors is about 80%. For Stage IV tumors it is less than 10%.

[77] Langsam et al. 1978.
[78] Leite et al. 1977.

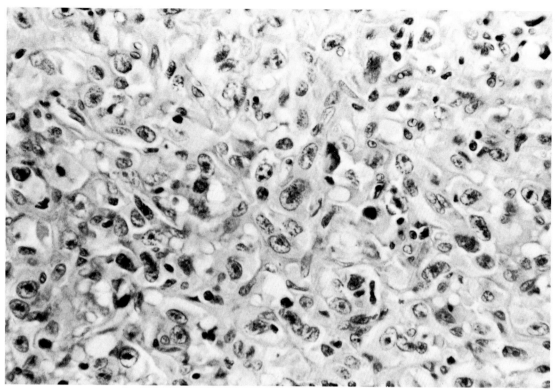

Fig. 47. Malignant fibrous histiocytoma: Malignant histiocytes with large nuclei (differential diagnosis with reticulosarcoma), only few reticulin fibers in malignant fibrous histiocytoma (29-year-old male, × 310).

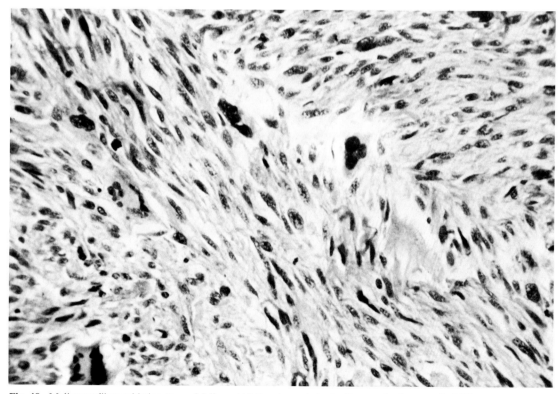

Fig. 48. Malignant fibrous histiocytoma: Malignant histiocytes and giant cells, cartwheel pattern (× 200).

M-8840/0, 1, 3

14. Myxoma (WHO)

(myxosarcoma)

General Remarks	**Incidence:** This is a very rare tumor. **Age:** Almost all myxomas occur in adults. **Sex:** Males and females are affected equally. **Site:** Myxomas develop in the superficial soft tissue areas: Fingertips, around the thighs, and in the pelvic girdle. About 20% of myxomas grow in the skeletal muscle [48].
Macroscopy	Small or large tumors without a capsule. The tumor seems to be well delineated from the surrounding tissue. The cut surfaces contain cysts in a mucoid substance. Myxomas are solitary tumors.
Histology	The tumor is composed of a loose tissue that contains few stellate cells. The cells have long fibrillary processes. The ground substance shows a mucin-carmine-positive staining. The tumor contains few blood vessels. There are almost no mitoses (Figs. 49 and 50).
Differential Diagnosis	1. Myxoma **with malignant soft tissue tumors undergoing myxomatous changes** [67], for instance neurofibromas (Figs. 176 to 179), rhabdomyosarcoma (Figs. 111 to 122), and liposarcomas (Fig. 63). 2. Myxoma **with localized myxomatous changes in the soft tissue with cyst formation. Ganglion** (WHO): Cysts in ganglion are not lined by cells. There is no communication between the cyst of a ganglion and the joint. Ganglions develop in the soft tissue of a joint capsule or a tendin sheath (Figs. 51 and 52). 3. Myxoma **with localized myxoedema** (WHO): Localized myxoedema might be associated with thyroid dysfunction.
Clinical Findings	Slow-growing tumor.
Treatment	Complete surgical excision.
Prognosis	In cases of incomplete excision, recurrences have been observed. There are no metastases. The prognosis is excellent [38].
Further Information	1. Myxomas can also be observed at other sites: for instance, the jaws, the heart, the parotid gland, the orbit muscle, the ileum, and the aorta. 2. There are some reports of myxomas associated with fibrous dysplasia of the bone [62, 131].

[38] Enzinger 1965.
[48] Feldman 1979.
[62] Ireland et al. 1973.
[67] Kindblom et al. 1979.
[131] Wirth et al. 1971.

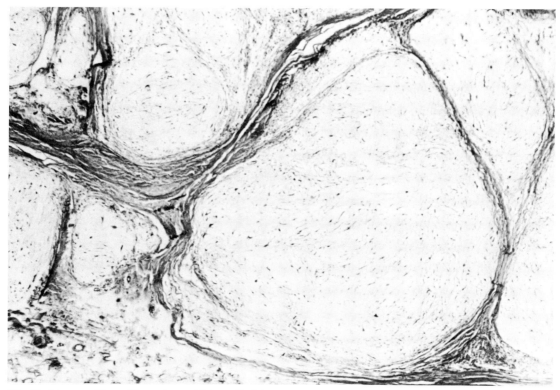

Fig. 49. Myxoma: Nests of loose tissue with few cells (55-year-old male, × 30).

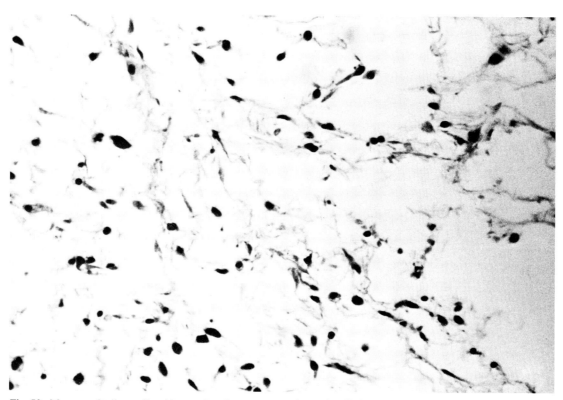

Fig. 50. Myxoma: Stellate cells with cytoplasmic processes and occasionally hyperchromatic nuclei (72-year-old female, × 200).

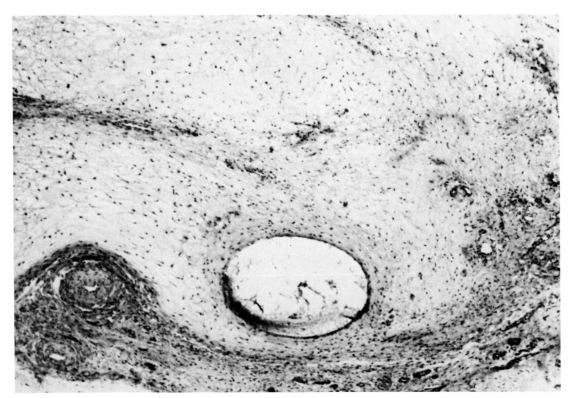

Fig. 51. Ganglion: Beginning cyst formation in myxomatous tissue (× 50).

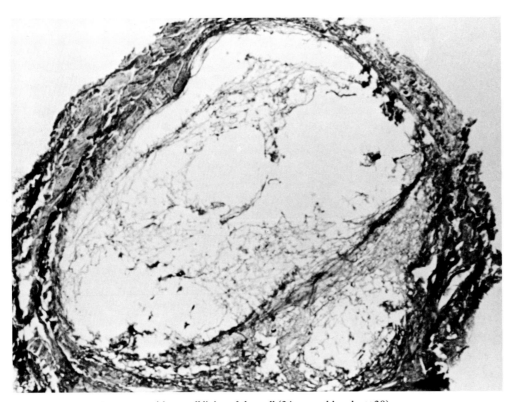

Fig. 52. Ganglion: Large cyst without cell lining of the wall (34-year-old male, × 30).

Tumors of the fat tissue

M-8850/0

15. Lipoma (WHO)

General Remarks

Incidence: This is a frequently observed, benign, soft tissue tumor.
Age: Lipomas can be observed in patients at any age; the peak age seems to be during the 5th and 6th decades.
Sex: There is no sex difference.
Site: Any site can be affected.
The majority of lipomas grow in the superficial soft tissues and the skin.

Macroscopy

The tumor can be small or very large. The cut surface is yellow with some grayish parts. The tumor is encapsulated.

Histology

Lipomas are composed of mature fat tissue (Figs. 53 and 54).

Treatment

If necessary, surgical excision.

Prognosis

Excellent. There is no malignant transformation of lipomas.

Further Information

According to the site, the age of the patient, and the clinical symptoms, some varieties of benign tumors of the fat tissue have been established:

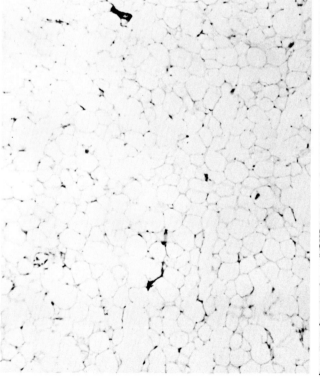

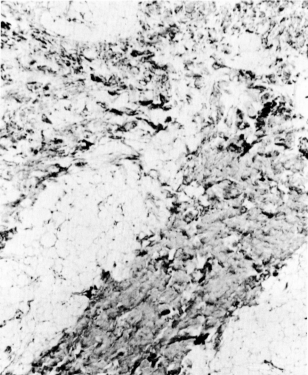

Fig. 53. Lipoma: Mature fat tissue (×30).

Fig. 54. Lipoma with collagen bundles (fibrolipoma) (×30).

57

16. Lipoma dolorosa

This tumor is painful. Histologically there is no connection with the nerves. The tumor contains mature fat tissue.

17. Intramuscular lipoma
(infiltrating lipoma – WHO)

In these cases the fat tissue of mature cells infiltrates the striated muscles (Fig. 55). Differential diagnosis from well-differentiated liposarcoma might be required: The benign lesion does not contain signs of nuclei atypias [47].

M-8870/0

18. Myelolipoma (WHO)

The lesion is rare and is composed of fat tissue and hematopoietic tissue.
This tumor can be observed in the adrenal gland (choristoma), the pelvis, or the retroperitoneum (Figs. 1726 and 1727).

19. Multiple symmetric lipomas

These tumors are regular lipomas composed of mature fat tissue. The tumors grow in a symmetrical arrangement.

---

[47] Evans et al. 1979.

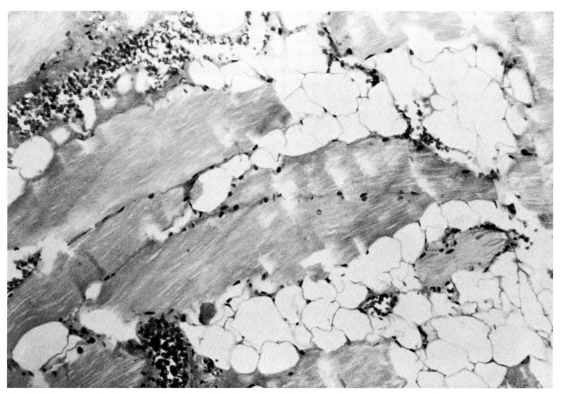

Fig. 55. Intramuscular lipoma: Infiltration of fat tissue into skeletal muscle. No nuclear atypias (72-year-old male, × 125).

20. Lipomas in deeper sites

Occasionally lipomas can develop in deeper sites. They can be considered varieties of benign mesenchymomas [109].

M-8880/0

21. Hibernoma (WHO)

General Remarks

Incidence: Hibernomas are rare benign tumors.
Site: The tumor develops in the axilla, abdominal wall, popliteal space, back, neck, mediastinum, and thigh.

Macroscopy

Hibernomas have a brown cut surface and are soft.

Histology

The tumor is composed of uniform cells that have a vacuolated cytoplasm (Fig. 56). This cytoplasm contains lipid.
The tumor cells have a lobular growth pattern.

Electron Microscopy

The tumor cells are similar to fat cells observed in the glands of hibernating animals [16].

**M-8860/0
(T 189.0)**

22. Angiomyolipoma (WHO)

This is a tumor of the kidney, in which mature fat cells grow in combination with angiomas (Fig. 57) (see Tumors of the kidney, Figs. 1329 and 1330).

---

[16] Brines and Johnson 1949.
[109] Stout and Lattes 1967.

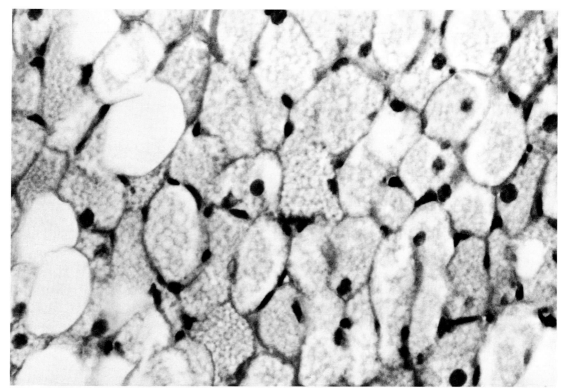

Fig. 56. Hibernoma: Vacuolated cytoplasm of tumor cells (15-year-old male, × 400).

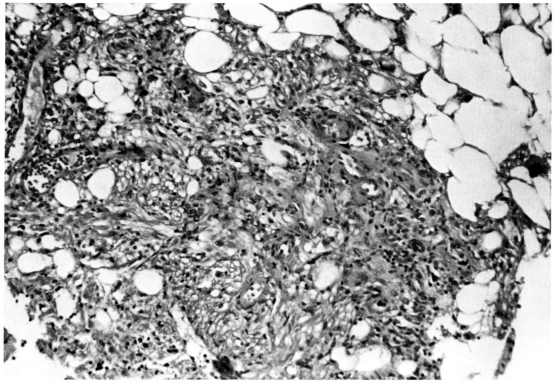

Fig. 57. Angiomyolipoma of kidney (× 125).

M-8861/0, 1

23. Angiolipoma

This tumor is composed of mature fat tissue with numerous blood vessels (Fig. 58).

These nodular tumors are painful and multiple.

The majority of the tumors occur in adolescents.

M-8881/0

24. Lipoblastomatosis (WHO)
(fetal lipoma; embryonal lipoma; lipoblastoma)

**General
Remarks**

Lipoblastomatosis is observed mainly in infants and children. It is exceedingly rare in adults [109, 123].

Macroscopy

The tumor is soft, yellowish-grayish, and lobulated. The tumor is often well separated from the surrounding tissue; often, however, there seems to be infiltration into the normal tissue.

Histology

The tumor is composed of small, embryonal fat cells, which have a large regular nucleus at the periphery of the cell. There are no signs of malignant atypical nuclei.

The embryonal fat cells (lipoblasts) grow in a myxomatous tissue. They are lobulated by delicate collagen fibers (Fig. 59) [123].

**Differential
Diagnosis**

Lipoblastomatosis **with liposarcoma** (Figs. 61 to 69):

In lipoblastomatosis there are no malignant cells.

Lipoblastomas occur in very young patients.

**Further
Information**

Lipomas in children are rare.

If they occur, they are observed mainly in the central nervous system, the retroperitoneum, and the mediastinum.

---

[109] Stout and Lattes 1967.
[123] Vellios et al. 1958.

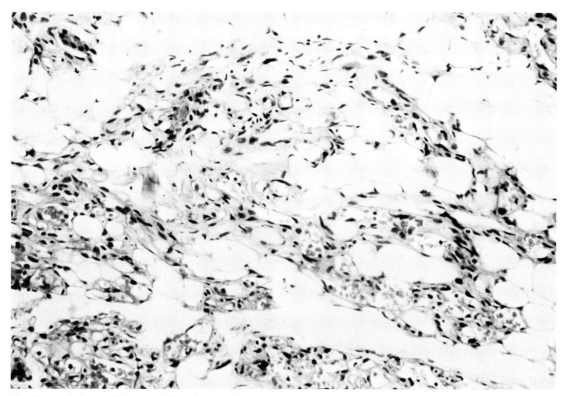

Fig. 58. Angiolipoma (35-year-old female, × 125).

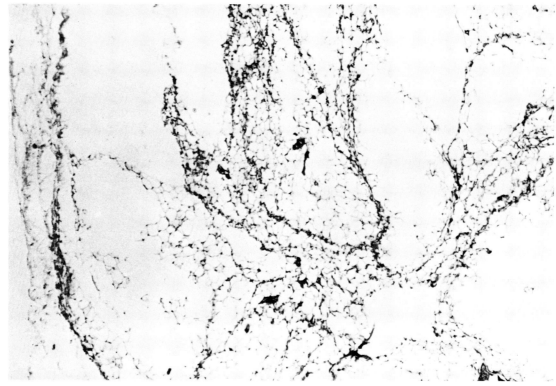

Fig. 59. Lipoblastomatosis (8-year-old female, × 30).

M-7410/3

25. Diffuse lipomatosis (WHO)

**General
Remarks**

This is a very rare lesion, which is mainly observed in children and shows great rarity in adults.

Site: Diffuse lipomatosis can involve parts of the trunk or large areas of an extremity.

Histology

The tumor contains mature fat tissue. The cells are without signs of malignancy.

M-8850/3

26. Liposarcoma (WHO)

**General
Remarks**

Incidence: Liposarcoma is the most frequently observed malignant soft tissue tumor in adults.

Age: Peak age is during the 6th decade.

Liposarcomas occur mostly in adults; they are only very rarely observed in children [36].

Site: Liposarcomas can develop at any site. The tumor is often observed in the retroperitoneum, thigh, popliteal fossa, shoulder, and mesenteric region [97].

Macroscopy

Liposarcomas can exhibit different aspects on gross inspection due to different degrees of differentiation.

The cut surface can be yellowish or almost whitish. The tumor might be firm or myxoid.

The tumor has no capsule and often seems to be well separated from the surrounding tissue.

The tumor can have a slimy surface, or the surface is lobulated resembling cerebral convolutions.

Liposarcomas can be very large.

Histology

Liposarcomas are composed of malignant lipoblasts. The nuclei are hyperchromatic, and mitotic figures are observed. The cytoplasm can contain fat. In these instances the nucleus is in a peripheral position in the cell and is compressed to a crescent-like shape.

Liposarcomas have distinct grades of differentiation. In poorly differentiated liposarcomas it might be difficult to detect fat vacuoles in the cytoplasm. In these instances the number of mitotic figures and nuclei atypias is high.

Occasionally the liposarcoma contains numerous blood vessels and areas with abundant collagen fibers (differential diagnosis with fibrosarcoma).

Myxoid change in liposarcomas is observed frequently.

[36] Enterline et al. 1960.
[97] Reszel et al. 1966.

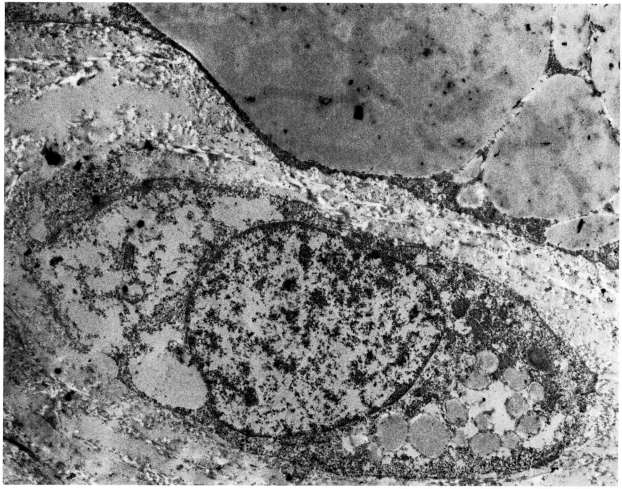

Fig. 60. Liposarcoma: Several lipid droplets in a malignant cell (lower part, right corner). Large lipid inclusions in another tumor cell (upper right corner) with remnants of cytoplasmic structures between the inclusions and a small rim of cytoplasm at the periphery of the inclusions (×7500).

Liposarcoma

Electron Microscopy

The cells of a pleomorphic liposarcoma may contain large amounts of non-membrane-bound lipid droplets of different sizes and shapes in the cytoplasm.

The nuclei might contain fatty droplets (Fig. 60).

Centrioles and autophagocytic inclusions are in close proximity to the nuclei [27, 48].

Differential Diagnosis

1. Liposarcoma, well differentiated, **with lipoma** (Figs. 53 to 59):
   Liposarcomas contain hyperchromatic nuclei and mitotic figures.
2. Liposarcoma **with other sarcomas:**
   Rhabdomyosarcoma, fibrosarcoma, malignant fibrous histiocytoma.
3. Liposarcoma **with myxoma** (Figs. 49 and 50) (especially in cases in which myxomatous areas dominate the picture of the liposarcoma):
   Liposarcomas contain numerous blood vessels; myxomas contain few blood vessels.

Staging

See Introduction, page 11.

Grading

The grading of liposarcomas is important because there is a correlation between the degree of differentiation and the survival rates [46].

Liposarcomas can be graded as

M-8851/3

– **well-differentiated liposarcoma** with large fat droplets in the cytoplasm and hyperchromatic nuclei at the periphery of the cell (Figs. 61 and 62).

M-8852/3

– **myxoid liposarcoma:**
This is the most frequently observed variety of liposarcomas: Malignant cells grow in a myxoid ground substance with positive PAS staining (Fig. 63).

M-8853/3

– **round cell liposarcoma:**
This is a rather poorly differentiated liposarcoma, which contains fat droplets. The nuclei are round and of different sizes (Fig. 64).

M-8854/3

– **pleomorphic liposarcoma:**
In these instances the tumor cells may or may not contain vacuoles in their cytoplasm. The tumor cells are of different sizes. The nuclei are often large, with strong hyperchromasia and numerous atypical mitotic figures (Figs. 65 to 69) [42, 46].

M-8855/3

– **liposarcoma, mixed type:**
Combination of the above-mentioned subtypes.

Spread

Liposarcoma, well differentiated: Metastases are rare (less than 5%).

Poorly differentiated liposarcoma: Metastases are frequent; into the lung, liver, and skeleton.

---

[27] Desai et al. 1978.
[42] Enzinger 1969.
[46] Enzinger and Winslow 1962.
[48] Feldman 1979.

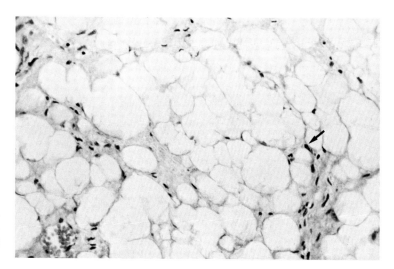

Fig. 61. Liposarcoma, well differentiated: Occasionally hyperchromatic malignant nuclei (arrow) (72-year-old male, × 200).

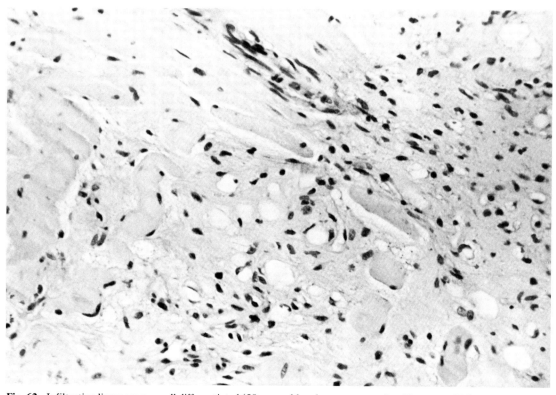

Fig. 62. Infiltrating liposarcoma, well differentiated (58-year-old male, recurrence after 15 years, × 200).

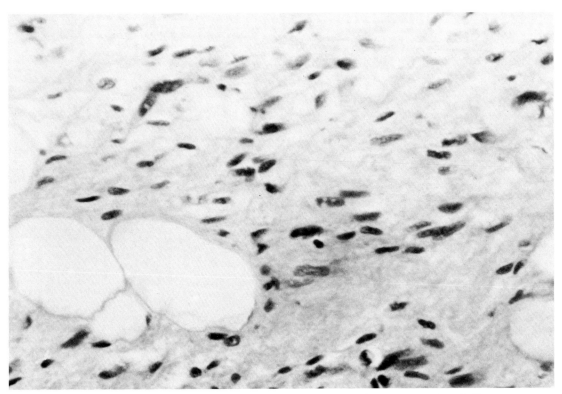

Fig. 63. Myxoid liposarcoma: Tumor cells growing in myxoid ground substance (72-year-old male, × 310).

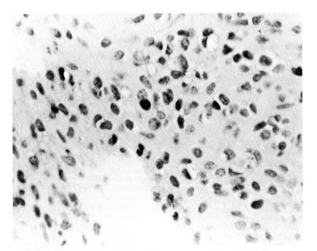

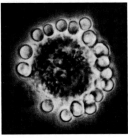

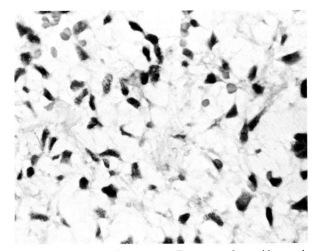

Fig. 64. Round cell liposarcoma: Remnants of fat vacuoles, malignant, round nuclei. Inset: EA-rosette forming cell in a liposarcoma (Fc receptors) (58-year-old male, × 400; inset, × 625).

Fig. 65. Pleomorphic liposarcoma: Remnants of myxoid ground substance (× 400).

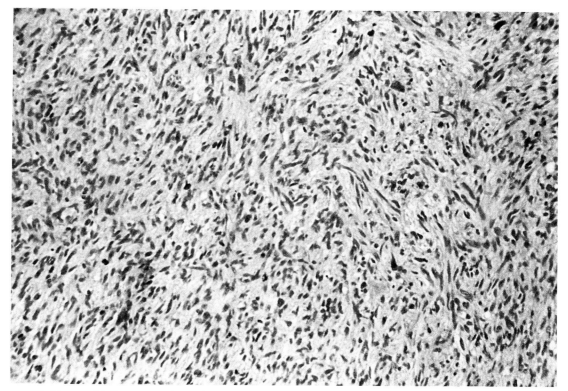

Fig. 66. Pleomorphic liposarcoma: Resemblance with fibrosarcoma (× 125).

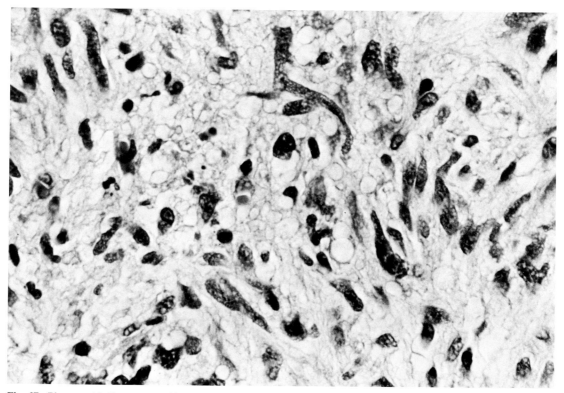

Fig. 67. Pleomorphic liposarcoma: Numerous vacuoles in tumor cells, marked pleomorphism of nuclei (× 400).

Liposarcoma

Treatment

Surgery:
The tumor should be resected with a large safe margin.
To decrease the rate of recurrences, postoperative **irradiation** has been recommended, up to 70 Gy [113].

Prognosis

Myxoid liposarcomas and well-differentiated liposarcomas show a strong tendency to recur, especially if the tumor is not resected entirely. Metastases are rare.

Poorly differentiated liposarcomas (pleomorphic and round cell liposarcoma) metastasize frequently (metastases in about 40% of the cases) [109].

The 5-year survival rate for well-differentiated liposarcoma is about 70%. The 5-year survival rate for poorly differentiated liposarcoma is about 18% [46].

In the individual case the stage of the tumor at the time of diagnosis is important for the 5-year survival rate (staging, see Introduction, page 11).

Stage I,   5-year survival rate about 80%

Stage III, 5-year survival rate about 35%

Stage IV, 5-year survival rate less than 10%.

[46] Enzinger and Winslow 1962.
[109] Stout and Lattes 1967.
[113] Suit et al. 1973.

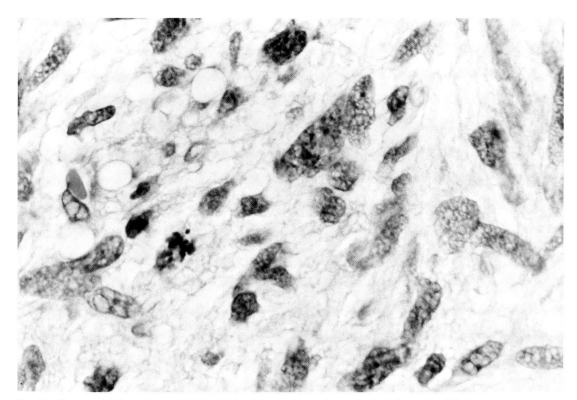

Fig. 68. Pleomorphic liposarcoma: Extreme nuclear pleomorphism, atypical mitotic figures (× 800).

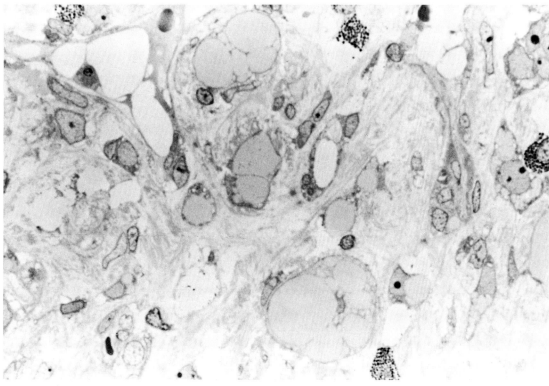

Fig. 69. Liposarcoma, with fat droplets in tumor cells (38-year-old male, × 600).

Tumors and tumor-like lesions of the blood vessels (WHO)

M-9131/0

27. Hemangioma
(capillary hemangioma, juvenile hemangioma – WHO)

General Remarks

Incidence: This is a rather frequently observed, benign, soft tissue tumor.

Age: The majority of hemangiomas appear in early years of life; they often are present at birth or develop in the months after birth.

Site: The majority of hemangiomas grow in the skin; 50% are located in the neck area and the head.

Histology

The tumor contains numerous capillaries that are packed closely together. The lining endothelial cells are regular (Figs. 70 and 71).

M-9130/0

28. Benign hemangioendothelioma (WHO)

This tumor is in most instances structured as a capillary hemangioma; however, other vascular formations may be observed.

The tumor is very cellular and the large endothelial cells show numerous mitotic figures.

The lining of the vascular spaces can show multilayered cells. However, there are no signs of malignancy.

This **strawberry-type of capillary hemangioma** grows rapidly after birth.

This benign hemangioendothelioma regresses spontaneously after a few months or several years.

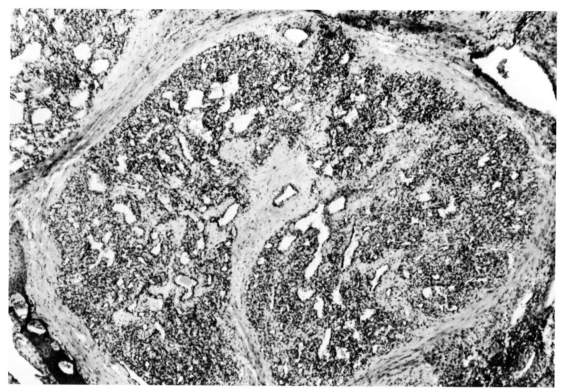

Fig. 70. Partly lobulated hemangioma of mainly capillary type (50-year-old male, × 40).

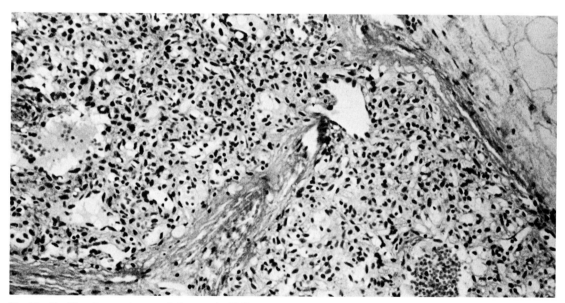

Fig. 71. Capillary hemangioma; cellular type (× 125).

M-9121/0

29. Cavernous hemangioma (WHO)

This tumor is composed of dilated capillaries that are lined by regular endothelial cells (Fig. 72).

The tumor can appear in parenchymal tissue like the liver, brain, kidney, and lung; usually it is observed in the skin.

M-7554/0

Cavernous hemangioma of the portwine type (nevus flammeus)

This cavernous hemangioma is observed at birth and develops mainly in the skin of the face, thorax, neck, and extremities.

This hemangioma does not show spontaneous regression, but grows with the patient and becomes very large.

For these reasons, this hemangioma is often difficult to treat. Cavernous hemangiomas of the portwine type are radioresistant.

M-9122/0

30. Venous hemangioma (WHO)

Hemangiomas composed of venous vessels are rare.

Histologically, they show blood vessels of different sizes, lined by regular cells. The wall of these blood vessels contains fibrous tissue and smooth muscle fibers (Fig. 73).

M-9123/0

31. Racemose (cirsoid) hemangioma (WHO)

This tumor occurs rarely. Histologically, it is composed of veins and arteries.

The wall of the blood vessels is thick and tortuous.

This tumor often shows foci of thromboses and calcifications (Figs. 74 to 76).

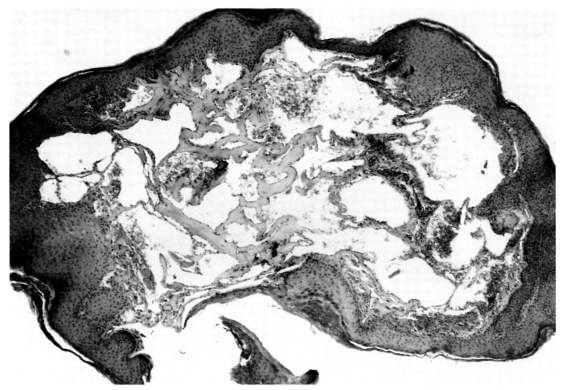

Fig. 72. Cavernous hemangioma (39-year-old female, × 50).

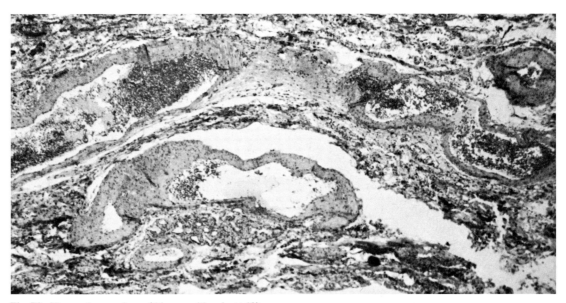

Fig. 73. Venous hemangioma (66-year-old male, × 40).

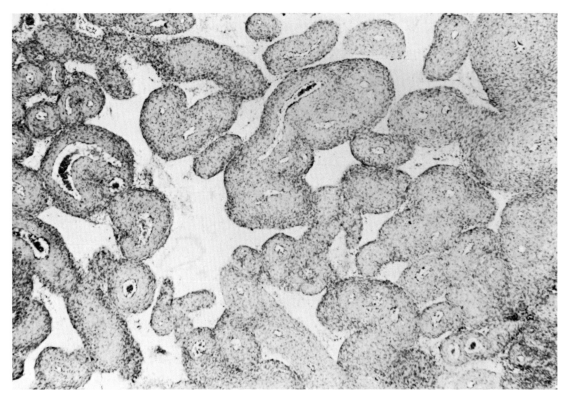

Fig. 74. Angiomatous hamartoma (× 40).

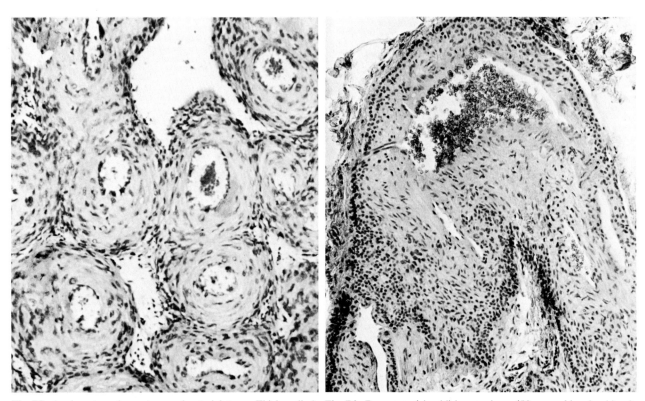

Fig. 75. Angiomatous hamartoma of arterial type: Thick-walled blood vessels, regular endothelial layer (× 125).

Fig. 76. Racemose (cirsoid) hemangioma (59-year-old male, skin of right forearm, × 125).

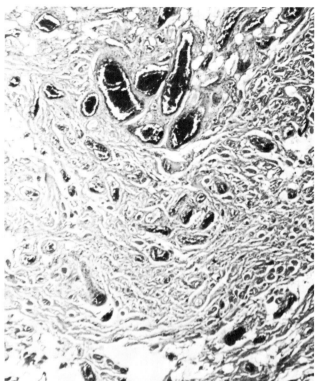

Fig. 77. Intramuscular hemangioma (×40).

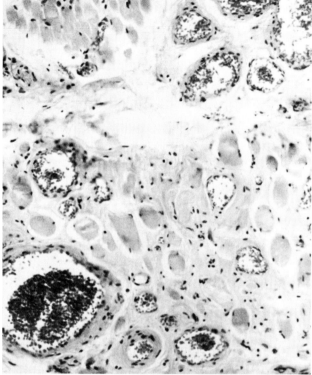

Fig. 78. Intramuscular hemangioma: Thin- and thick-walled blood vessels (35-year-old male, ×125).

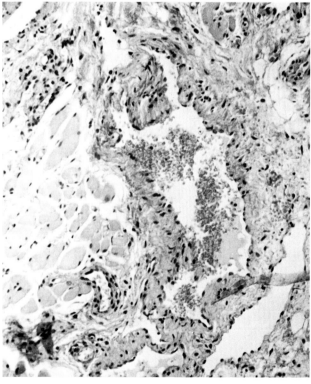

Fig. 79. Intramuscular hemangioma: Angiectatic blood vessels, some of venous type (36-year-old female, ×125).

M-9132/0

32. Intramuscular hemangioma (WHO)
(diffuse angiomatosis)

This tumor is composed of areas containing hemangiomas of the capillary, cavernous, or arteriovenous type.

The blood vessels grow in the skeletal muscle, eventually mimicking a malignant, infiltrating growth (Figs. 77 to 79).

Differential diagnosis from **angiosarcomas** becomes necessary if the lesion is very cellular and has hyperchromatic nuclei, numerous mitotic figures, papillary growth into the lumen of the blood vessels, and occasionally even infiltration of the perineural spaces (Figs. 82 and 83).

However, intramuscular hemangioma is almost always a benign lesion, which metastasizes only in exceedingly rare cases [3].

M-7631/4

33. Systemic hemangiomatosis (WHO)

Occasionally the parenchymal tissue can be involved by hemangiomatous disease, which might originate at several foci or involve the tissue diffusely.

This disease is observed mainly in the brain:

Sturge-Weber's disease
von Hippel-Lindau's disease,
Mafucci syndrome,
Bourneville syndrome (see Tumors of the brain).

A widespread systemic hemangiomatosis is

Rendu-Osler-Weber's disease, in which multiple hemangiomas cause severe bleeding (intestinal bleeding, hemoptysis) (telangiectasia hereditaria).

---

[3] Allen and Enzinger 1972.

M-4444/0

34. Hemangioma of the granulation tissue type
(granuloma pyogenicum) (WHO)

Granuloma pyogenicum is an inflammatory reaction most probably due to a discrete traumatic lesion of the tissue.

The "tumor" is ulcerated and histologically shows capillaries embedded in edematous tissue and surrounded by inflammatory cells (Figs. 80 and 81). Granuloma pyogenicum is a lesion of adult patients with an initially rapid growth.

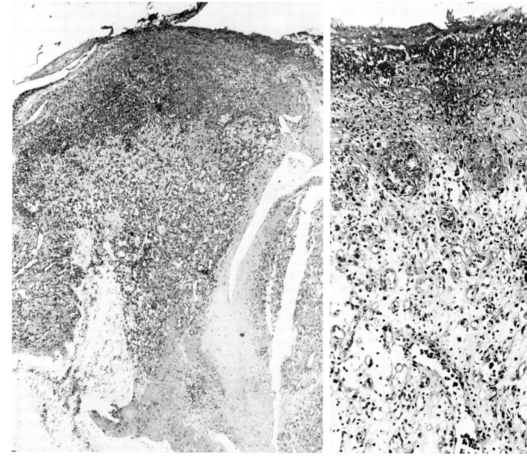

Fig. 80. Hemangioma of granulation tissue type (granuloma pyogenicum) (32-year-old female, × 50).

Fig. 81. Hemangioma of granulation tissue type (granuloma pyogenicum) (32-year-old female, × 125).

79

M-9120/3
M 9130/3

35. Malignant hemangioendothelioma
(angiosarcoma) (WHO)
(hemangioendothelial sarcoma)

**General
Remarks**

Incidence: Angiosarcomas are very rare malignant tumors of the soft tissue.
Age: The tumor can occur at any age.
Sex: Males and females are affected equally.
Site: Angiosarcomas can grow in the breast, liver, spleen [8], lung, thyroid, and skeletal muscle.

Macroscopy

In most instances this is a reddish tumor, which shows on gross inspection the probability of containing numerous blood vessels. However, occasionally the tumor might be whitish-grayish, and there is macroscopically no evidence for a tumor composed of blood vessels.

Histology

The tumor is composed of malignant endothelial cells. These cells show numerous mitotic figures and hyperchromasia of the pleomorphic nuclei (Fig. 82).
The tumor cells grow inside anastomosing capillaries in a multilayered arrangement (Fig. 83). Occasionally the lumen of the blood vessels can be almost occluded. Giant cells can be observed.

**Differential
Diagnosis**

1. Angiosarcoma **with benign hemangioendothelioma in infants** (or children)
   Angiosarcoma **with benign hemangiomas** (Figs. 70 and 71).
   Angiosarcoma **with hemangiopericytoma** (Figs. 89 to 91):
   Staining of the reticulin fibers reveals the position of the malignant cells: inside the reticulin fibers near the lumen of the capillaries (Fig. 83).
   The tumor cells contain malignant nuclei, which are not present in benign hemangiomas.
2. Angiosarcoma **with malignant tumors containing numerous blood vessels:**
   Occasionally malignant tumors are very vascular (for instance, renal cell carcinomas, osteogenic sarcomas, choriocarcinomas). Again the use of reticulin fiber staining will give the correct diagnosis of angiosarcoma.
3. Angiosarcoma **with intramuscular angiomatosis** (Figs. 77 to 79):
   In intramuscular angiomatosis there are no signs of malignancy. In some instances diagnosis based on the histological picture alone might be very difficult.
   It is, however, known that intramuscular angiomatosis is almost never malignant.
4. Angiosarcoma **with intravascular angiomatosis in thrombus organization:**
   Occasionally the organization of thrombotic material in blood vessels might mimic a malignant growth because of numerous mitotic figures and a very cellular tissue.
   This intravascular angiomatosis is limited to the vascular lumen [102].

---

[8] Autry and Weitzner 1975.
[102] Salyer and Salyer 1975.

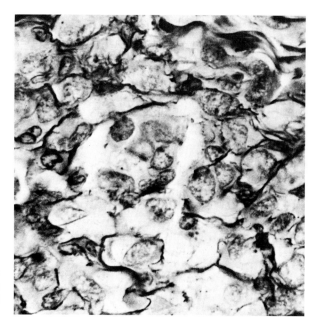

Fig. 82. Malignant hemangioendothelioma (angiosarcoma): Malignant tumor cells of endothelial type inside blood vessels (reticulin stain, 55-year-old female, ×500).

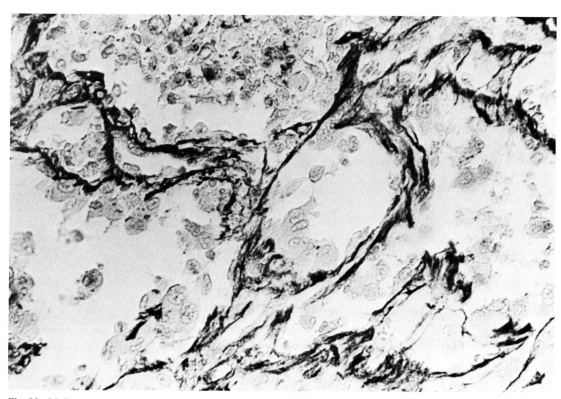

Fig. 83. Malignant hemangioendothelioma (angiosarcoma): Malignant cells growing into the lumen of blood vessels (reticulin stain, ×200).

**Differential
Diagnosis**

5. Angiosarcoma **with capillary angiomatosis** (capillary hemangioma):
In these hemangiomas, thrombi are frequently observed. The mesenchyma infiltrating these thrombi might mimic a malignant tumor [81, 102].

6. Angiosarcoma **with Masson's "vegetant intravascular hemangioendothelioma":**
This hemangioendothelioma of Masson is composed of endothelial cells that grow into the lumen of the blood vessels in a papillary pattern.
These papillary formations are supported by fibrous tissue. There are no signs of malignant cells [74].

Staging

See Introduction, page 11.

Spread

Lymphatic and hematogenous spread.

**Clinical
Findings**

Swelling of the affected area.

Treatment

Radical **surgery.**
Chemotherapy seems to have almost no effect [30].

Prognosis

Frequent recurrences. Poor prognosis.
The death rate for adults with angiosarcoma is about 50%; for children it is about 25%.
Angiosarcomas of the breast are almost always fatal. The 5-year survival rate for Stages I to IV tumors is approximately 10 to 20%.

**Further
Information**

1. There is one report of a circumscribed angiosarcoma originating from the endothelial cells in the arteria femoralis [79].
2. Recently one angiosarcoma was observed in the radial nerve [15].
3. Hemangioendotheliosarcoma in the liver can be induced by polyvinylchloride (PVC) [81].
4. There is one case with intravascular papillary endothelial hyperplasia, mimicking an angiosarcoma or granulation tissue [73].

[15] Bricklin and Rushton 1977.
[30] Dolf and Sack 1976.
[73] Kreutner et al. 1978.
[74] Kuo et al. 1976.
[79] Leu and Sulser 1976.
[81] Makk et al. 1976.
[102] Salyer and Salyer 1975.

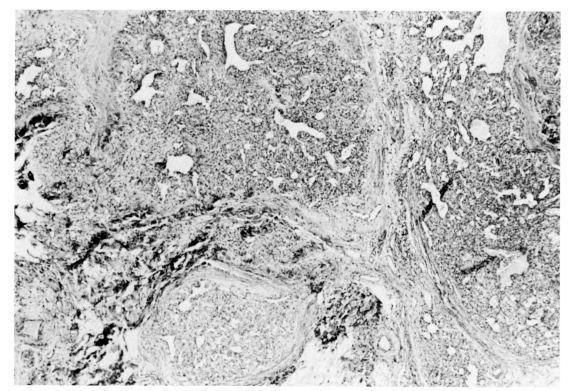

Fig. 84. Kaposi's sarcoma: Lobulated growth pattern (53-year-old male, × 30).

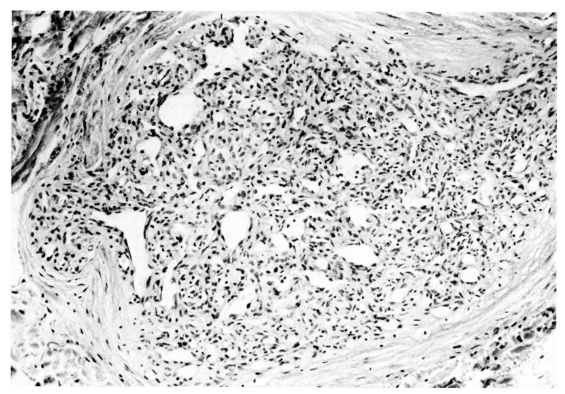

Fig. 85. Kaposi's sarcoma: Capillaries and mesenchymal cells (53-year-old male, × 125).

M-9140/3

36. Kaposi's sarcoma (WHO)

**General
Remarks**

Incidence: Kaposi's sarcoma is a rare tumor.

Age: The peak age is during the 5th through 8th decades.

The tumor occurs rarely in children (less than 4% of the cases).

Sex: 70 to 90% of Kaposi's sarcomas occur in males.

Site: Kaposi's sarcoma can be observed anywhere in the body. The most common sites are the skin of lower extremities; the head, neck, and scalp; the viscera (brain, lung, liver); bone; the rectum; and the lymph nodes.

Further notes:

a) Kaposi's sarcoma is observed frequently in blacks in certain areas in Africa.

b) It is still debated whether Kaposi's sarcoma is a true neoplasm.

c) Kaposi's sarcoma is occasionally associated with malignant lymphoma.

Macroscopy

Skin nodules in Kaposi's sarcoma are bluish-red.

Histology

The tumor is composed of two components: capillaries and spindle-shaped mesenchymal cells (Figs. 84 to 86).

Occasionally the picture is dominated by the blood vessels, which can proliferate with signs of malignant behavior (Fig. 87) [13].

Occasionally the tumor is dominated by the mesenchymal cells, which can produce reticulin fibers, giving to the lesion the aspect of a fibrosarcoma (Fig. 88).

Between these mesenchymal cells histiocytes with hemosiderin pigment are found.

Occasionally the endothelial cells are large, and they can narrow the lumen of the capillaries.

**Differential
Diagnosis**

1. Kaposi's sarcoma **with fibrosarcoma** (Figs. 21 to 25).
2. Kaposi's sarcoma **with angiosarcoma** (Figs. 82 and 83) (according to the dominant two tissue components in Kaposi's sarcoma).
3. Kaposi's sarcoma **with glomus tumor** (Fig. 94 and 95):

   Important for the diagnosis is evidence for both components: capillaries with hyperplastic endothelial cells and mesenchymal cells in the intercapillary spaces.

Spread

The tumor can involve all viscera and the lymph nodes.

Treatment

Surgery:

Surgical excision.

Radiation therapy:

Low dose irradiation of the skin lesion (25 Gy in 3 weeks) [17, 59, 65].

Chemotherapy:

Kaposi's sarcoma reacts with high sensitivity to chemotherapeutic drugs, as do other soft tissue sarcomas.

Actinomycin D and cyclophosphamide have been used [124].

---

[13] Braun-Falco et al. 1976.
[17] Brunner and Nagel 1979.
[59] Holecek and Harwood 1978.
[65] Kim et al. 1977.
[124] Vogel et al. 1971.

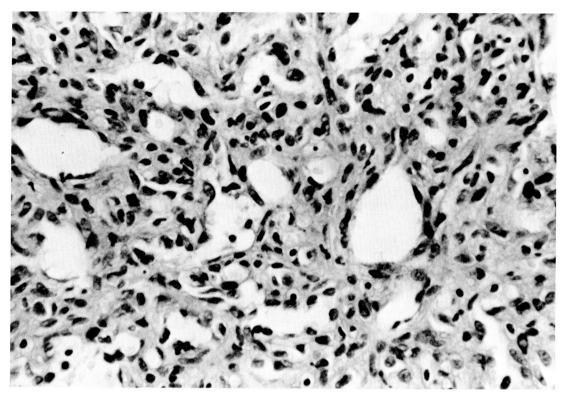

Fig. 86. Kaposi's sarcoma: Malignant mesenchymal cells and large epithelial cells (53-year-old male, × 310).

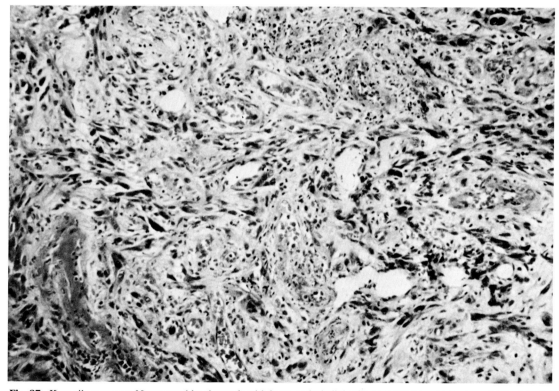

Fig. 87. Kaposi's sarcoma: Numerous blood vessels with large endothelial cells, separated by mesenchymal (fibroblastic) cells (× 125).

Kaposi's sarcoma

Prognosis

Kaposi's sarcoma is a slowly progressing tumorous disease, which finally becomes fatal because of metastasis.

In children no fatal Kaposi's sarcoma has been reported [35].

Further Information

1. It has been reported that Kaposi's sarcoma is associated frequently with prior immunosuppressive therapy [69].
2. The cell of origin in Kaposi's sarcoma might be an undifferentiated adventitial cell [56].

[35] Dutz and Stout 1960.
[56] Gokel et al. 1976.
[69] Klepp et al. 1978.

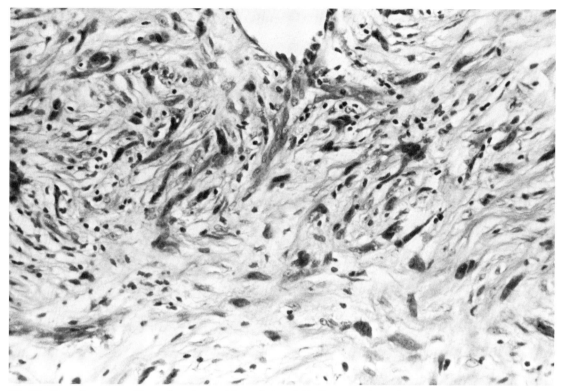

Fig. 88. Kaposi's sarcoma: Mesenchymal part with atypical nuclei in fibroblasts (× 200).

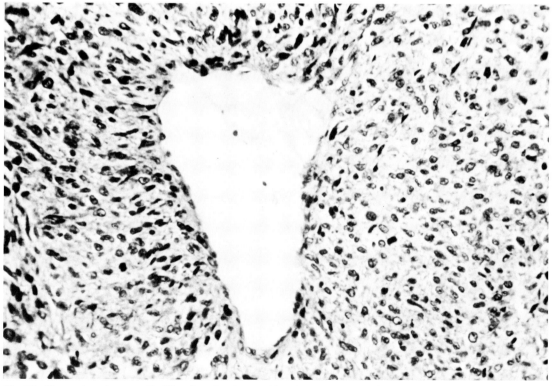

Fig. 89. Hemangiopericytoma: Proliferation of pericytes with rather regular nuclei (62-year-old female, × 200).

M-9150/0,1

37. Benign hemangiopericytoma (WHO)

General Remarks

Incidence: Hemangiopericytomas are rare soft tissue tumors.
Age: All ages can be affected; 10% of the patients are younger than 15 years old.
Sex: Males and females are affected equally.
Site: Hemangiopericytomas can grow at any site. In most instances this tumor grows subcutaneously or intramuscularly. The tumor can develop in the nose, the uterus, the lung, the retroperitoneal space, the orbit, the bone, the liver, the brain, the kidney, and the gastrointestinal tract.
It is debated whether certain meningiomas could be hemangiopericytomas (Fig. 828) (see Tumors of the brain, page 810).

Macroscopy

This is a rather soft, encapsulated tumor, which is well demarcated from the surrounding tissue.

Histology

The tumor is composed of proliferating benign pericytes. The cells are spindle-shaped with an oval nucleus (Fig. 89). Reticulin stain shows that these cells grow at the periphery of the blood vessels and that each tumor cell is surrounded by reticulin fibers (Fig. 90). There are numerous blood vessels in this tumor, which are lined by regular endothelial cells.

Electron Microscopy

The pericytes in hemangiopericytoma (tumor cells) contain rough endoplasmatic reticulum, mitochondria, free polyribosomes, and fine fibrils. The intercellular space is filled with material resembling the basal lamina [100].

Differential Diagnosis

1. Hemangiopericytoma, benign, **with malignant hemangiopericytoma** (Figs. 1716 to 1718):
   The biological behavior of hemangiopericytomas is difficult to predict because there are no clear morphological signs of malignancy.
2. Hemangiopericytoma **with angioma and angiosarcoma** (Figs. 82 and 83):
   In cases of hemangiopericytoma the reticulin stain will show proliferating adventitial cells and normal endothelial cells (Fig. 91).

Clinical Findings

Swelling of the affected area without pain.
The tumor can be visualized by angiographic studies [5].

Treatment

Aggressive **surgery** with complete surgical removal of the tumor.
Radiation therapy:
Although hemangiopericytomas are considered to have a low sensitivity to irradiation, it has been recommended to try postoperative high dose radiation therapy especially for malignant hemangiopericytoma [29, 76, 85].
Chemotherapy [133]: Adriamycin alone or in a combination drug regimen.

---

[5] Angervall et al. 1978.
[29] Döring and Graudins 1975.
[76] Lal et al. 1976.
[85] Mira et al. 1977.
[100] Reyes et al. 1977.
[133] Wong and Yagoda 1978.

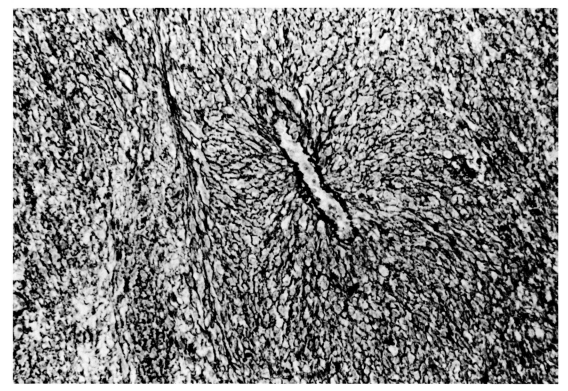

Fig. 90. Hemangiopericytoma: Pericytes are surrounded by reticulin fibers (62-year-old female, × 125).

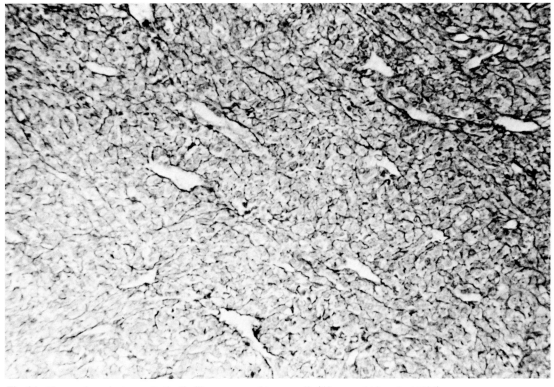

Fig. 91. Hemangiopericytoma: Reticulin fibers surround tumor cells (69-year-old female, × 125).

Hemangiopericytoma

Prognosis

Hemangiopericytomas are usually benign tumors; however, in 10 to 20% of the cases the tumor metastasizes:

M-9150/3

Malignant hemangiopericytoma (WHO):

Histologically the malignant hemangiopericytoma might show occasionally some signs of cellular malignancy and a high number of mitotic figures (Figs. 92 and 93); however, there is usually almost no histological proof that the hemangiopericytoma might be malignant.

It is therefore important to consider a hemangiopericytoma as possibly malignant even without any histological signs of a malignant biological behavior.

90

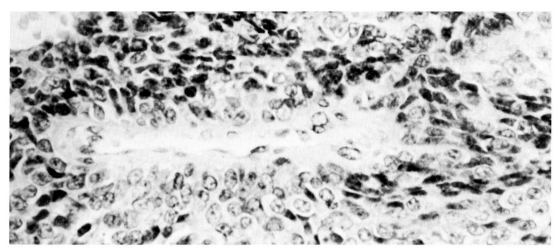

Fig. 92. Hemangiopericytoma: Pericytes with atypical nuclei (malignant?) (× 310).

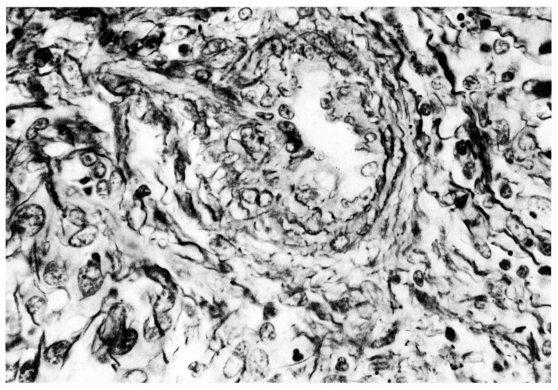

Fig. 93. Hemangiopericytoma: Pericytes with large atypical nuclei, surrounded by reticulin fibers (malignant?) (55-year-old female, × 500).

M-8711/0

38. Glomus tumor (WHO)
(glomangioma, Popoff tumor)

General Remarks

Incidence: These are uncommon, benign soft tissue tumors.

Age: The majority of patients are in the 3rd through 5th decades. Children however, can be affected, often by multiple glomus tumors [70].

Sex: Glomus tumor of the finger is considerably more frequently observed in females than in males [68].

For glomus tumors at other sites there is a male predominance.

Site: The majority of glomus tumors occur in the fingers (subungual) and hand; they can also be observed in the deeper soft tissue areas and very rarely in the stomach, heart, lymph nodes, vagina, mediastinum, uterus, bone, and periosteum.

Further notes:
– Glomus tumors are a variety of hemangiopericytoma.
– Occasionally glomus tumors have a familial occurrence.

Macroscopy

The tumor is small and firm.

Histology

The tumor is composed of blood vessels and chords of regular cells, which grow between the blood vessels (Fig. 94). The blood vessels have a thick wall, with regular endothelial cells (Fig. 95). The lumen of these blood vessels might be narrowed. The pericytes surrounding the blood vessels have formed chords. Between the cells different amounts of connective tissue can be found. Furthermore, there are some smooth muscle cells [107].

Differential Diagnosis

1. Glomus tumor **with hemangiopericytoma** (Figs. 89 and 90).
2. Glomus tumor **with Kaposi's sarcoma** (Figs. 84 to 88).
3. Glomus tumor **with angiosarcoma** (Figs. 82 and 83):
   In glomus tumor there are no signs of malignancy.
   The clinical findings and the localization are helpful.

Clinical Findings

This is a small tumor often associated with paroxysmal pain.

Treatment

Removal of the tumor.

Prognosis

Excellent, very rare recurrences.

[68] King 1954.
[70] Kohout and Stout 1961.
[107] Stout 1935.

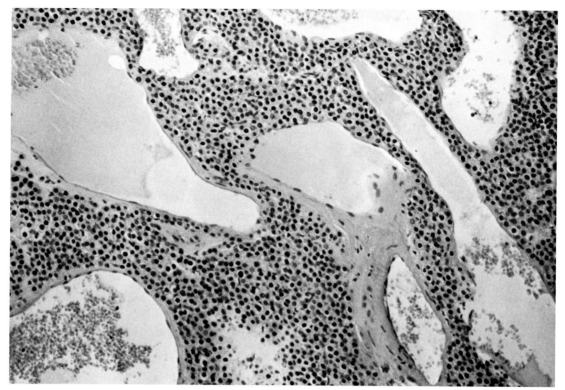

Fig. 94. Glomus tumor: Another aspect of proliferating intervascular pericytes (71-year-old male, × 125).

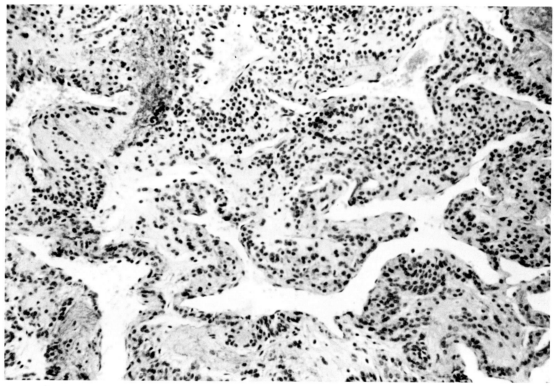

Fig. 95. Glomus tumor: Thick-walled blood vessels, separated by strands of pericytes (71-year-old male, × 125).

M-9170/0

39. Lymphangioma
(capillary, cavernous, cystic) (WHO)

General Remarks

Incidence: Lymphangiomas are rare.

Age: The tumor can be detected at any age.

Because lymphangiomas seem to be malformations, certain of these lesions are observed in infants and children.

Sex: Males and females are affected equally.

M-9171/0

Site: Capillary lymphangiomas develop mostly in the subdermal tissue, the mouth, the mediastinum, and the tongue. These lesions are rare.

M-9172/0
M-9173/0

Cavernous and cystic lymphangiomas: Neck, omentum, mesentery, and retroperitoneum; very rarely in the liver, kidney, and adrenal gland.

Macroscopy

According to the size, lymphangiomas present as soft cystic lesions.

Histology

The tumor is composed of lymph vessels, which might contain some lymphocytes. The lining cells are flat and regular.

The lymph vessels are embedded in a loose connective tissue (Figs. 96 to 98).

Differential Diagnosis

Lymphangioma **with hemangioma:**

In cases of capillary lymphangioma the differential diagnosis with capillary hemangioma might be difficult.

Clinical Findings

Swelling of the affected region.

Treatment

Surgical excision. Some lymphangiomas regress spontaneously.

Prognosis

Excellent. No recurrences.

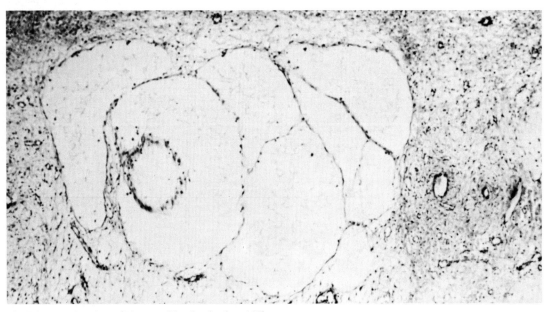

Fig. 96. Lymphangioma (70-year-old male, cheek, × 125).

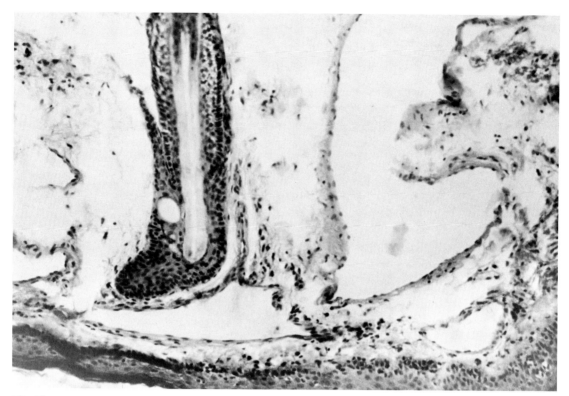

Fig. 97. Lymphangioma (×60).

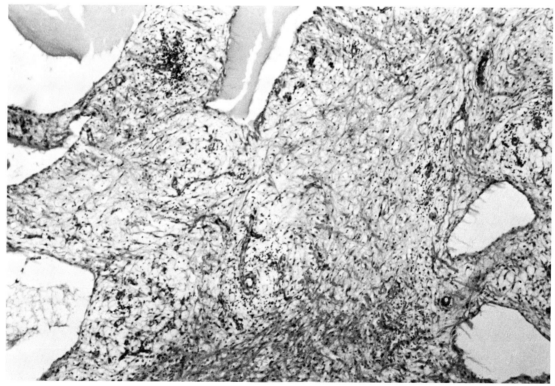

Fig. 98. Lymphangioma with loose connective tissue (×80).

M-9174/0

40. Lymphangiomyoma (WHO)
(lymphangiopericytoma)

**General
Remarks**

Incidence: Lymphangiopericytoma is a rare lesion.
Age: The tumor can occur at any age.
Sex: Lymphangiopericytomas are almost always observed in females.
Site: The tumor occurs in the mediastinum and occasionally also in the lymph nodes.

Histology

The tumor corresponds to the hemangiopericytoma, with proliferating pericytes and smooth muscle cells, surrounding the dilated lymph vessels.

**Clinical
Findings**

The lymphangiopericytoma is closely associated with the lymphatic tracts (development of chylothorax).

Treatment

Surgical removal, eventually irradiation.

**Further
Information**

Lymphangiopericytomas might be associated with tuberous sclerosis. The prognosis is determined accordingly [86].

M-9170/3

41. Lymphangiosarcoma (WHO)

**General
Remarks**

Incidence: The tumor seems to develop only secondary to chronic lymph stasis.
Therefore the tumor seems to develop exclusively after radical mastectomy (months or years later) (see Tumors of the breast).

Macroscopy

The lesion extends into the subcutaneous tissue of the region with chronic lymph stasis. There are grayish-reddish nodules.

Histology

The tumor is composed of malignant endothelial cells, which give a great similarity to the picture observed in angiosarcoma. The tumor does not contain blood in the lumen of the malignant lymph vessels.

Staging

See Introduction, page 11.

Grading

See Introduction, page 11.

Treatment

Radical **surgery.**

Prognosis

The prognosis of lymphangiosarcoma is very poor [134].

---

[86] Monteforte Jr. and Kohnen 1974.
[134] Woodward et al. 1972.

Tumors of the muscles

M-8890/0

42. Leiomyoma (WHO)

General Remarks

Incidence: Leiomyomas are common, soft tissue tumors.
Site: Leiomyomas have a preference for certain sites:

T 179.9

a) Leiomyoma of the uterus (Figs. 99 and 100) (see page 1766)
b) Leiomyomas of the gastrointestinal tract (Fig 249) (see page 238)

M-8891/0,1

43. Epithelioid leiomyoma
(bizarre leiomyoma; leiomyoblastoma) (WHO)

Leiomyomas of the gastrointestinal tract can be composed of cells that have a clear cytoplasm, distinct cell borders, and large, slightly pleomorphic nuclei in the center of the cells (Fig. 101).

Leiomyomas and bizarre epithelioid leiomyomas can also be observed in the omentum, the mesentery, the retroperitoneum, and the deeper and superficial parts of the soft tissue.

These superficial leiomyomas are composed of smooth muscle bundles, which form interlacing structures.

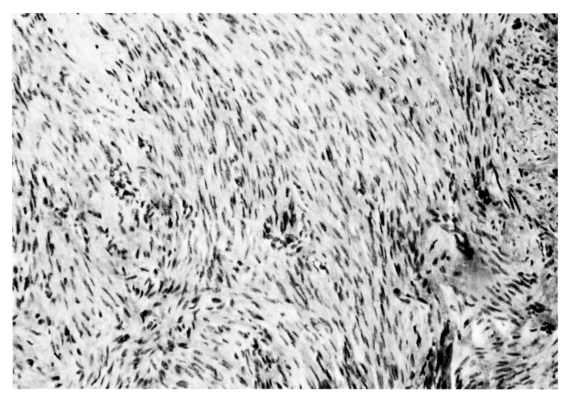

Fig. 99. Leiomyoma (46-year-old female, uterus, × 125).

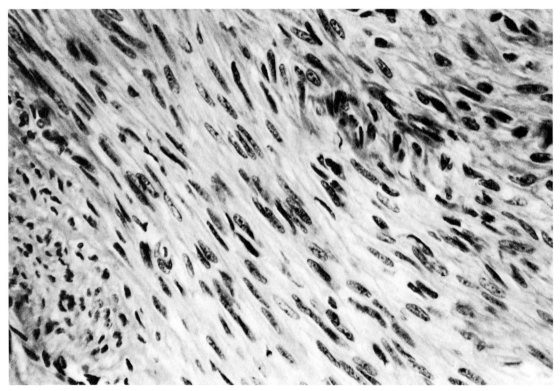

Fig. 100. Leiomyoma: Nuclei with slight to moderate signs of atypia, no mitotic figures (46-year-old female, uterus, × 310).

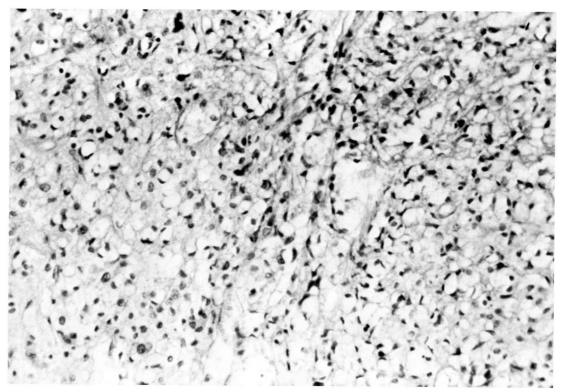

Fig. 101. Epithelioid leiomyoma (66-year-old female, stomach, × 200).

M-8894/0

44. Vascular leiomyoma
(angiomyoma) (WHO)

Vascular leiomyomas are painful tumors. They grow in the wrist or ankle region (superficial leiomyomas).

This tumor affects females almost exclusively.

On histological analysis the smooth muscle bundles surround numerous blood vessels, which have a thick wall (Figs. 102 and 103).

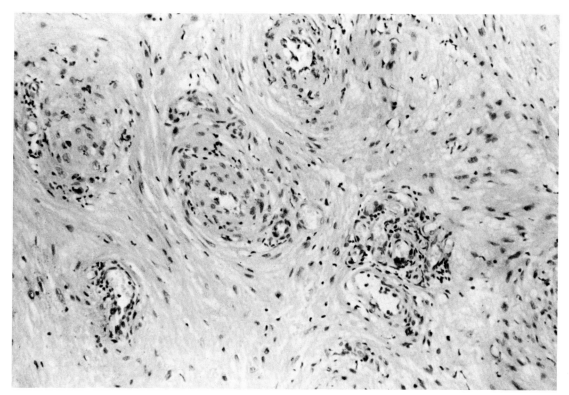

Fig. 102. Vascular leiomyoma (51-year-old female, × 125).

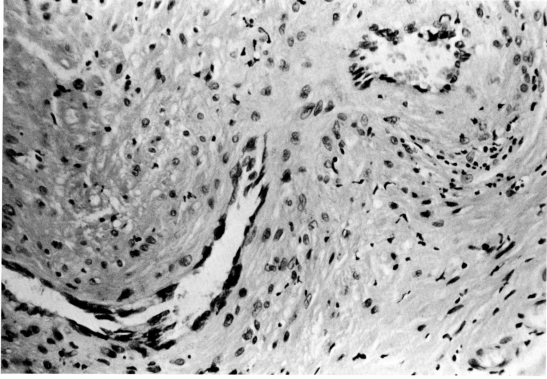

Fig. 103. Vascular leiomyoma (51-year-old female, × 200).

M-8890/3

45. Leiomyosarcoma (WHO)

**General
Remarks**

Incidence: This is a rare soft tissue tumor.
Age: Leiomyosarcomas can be observed at any age, including infancy and childhood.
Sex: Females seem to be affected slightly more often than males.
Site: Leiomyosarcomas can grow at any site:
Uterus, mesentery, retroperitoneum, mediastinum, diaphragma or in a subcutaneous or intramuscular location and in the visceral organs. This tumor can also originate in the wall of large veins (Figs. 104 to 106) [109].
In **infants** this tumor is observed in the urinary bladder and prostate and occasionally in the bone.

Macroscopy

Leiomyosarcomas are very similar to leiomyomas, with a grayish-yellowish cut surface showing interlacing structures. The tumor is well circumscribed and therefore resembles the benign leiomyoma.

Histology

The tumor contains atypical cells that form interlacing bundles. The nuclei are blunt-ended and occasionally can form palisading structures (similar to those observed in neurofibroma).
The tumor cells might have nuclei that are hyperchromatic and pleomorphic.
Important is the appearance of atypical and numerous mitotic divisions (Fig. 107).

**Electron
Microscopy**

Microtubules and microfilaments (Fig. 108).

**Differential
Diagnosis**

1. Leiomyosarcoma **with benign leiomyoma:**
   The differential diagnosis is based on the appearance of mitoses. The number of mitotic figures is more important than the nuclear signs of malignancy, which can be absent in cases of leiomyosarcoma [108] (Figs. 1711 to 1714).
   Besides the degree of mitotic activity the appearance of necroses in the tumor indicates an aggressive behavior [95].
2. Leiomyosarcoma **with malignant schwannoma** (Fig. 169 to 175).

Staging

See Introduction, page 11.

Grading

The number of mitotic figures (together with necroses) indicates the aggressiveness of the tumor (for further information on grading, see page 11).

Spread

1. Hematogenous dissemination into the lung and other organs.
2. Lymphatic spread into the regional lymph nodes.

---

[95] Ranchod and Kempson 1977.
[108] Stout and Hill 1958.
[109] Stout and Lattes 1967.

102

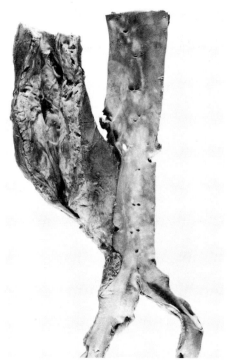

Fig. 104. Leiomyosarcoma of the inferior vena cava (45-year-old male).

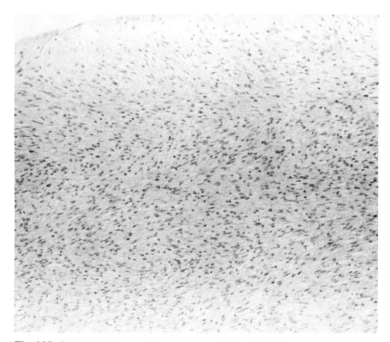

Fig. 105. Leiomyosarcoma of the vena cava inferior (× 125).

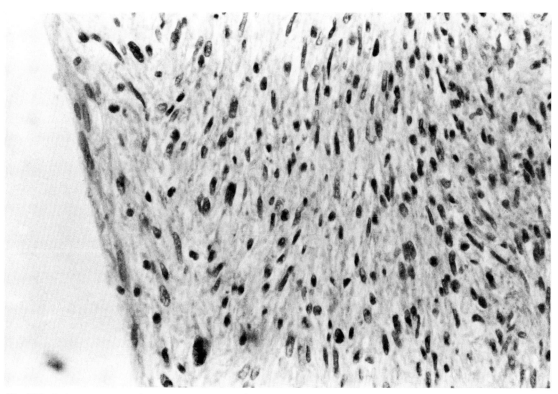

Fig. 106. Leiomyosarcoma of the vena cava inferior (× 310).

Leiomyosarcoma

Treatment

Surgery:

The tumor should be removed entirely.

Unfortunately leiomyosarcomas show a gross aspect of a benign tumor. Incomplete surgical excision might lead to recurrences.

Chemotherapy:

Combined chemotherapy with adriamycin and DTIC can be attempted [92, 111].

Prognosis

Leiomyosarcomas in adults:

The 5-year survival rate for Stage I tumors is 11%;

Stage II, 7%;

Stage III, approximately 3%;

Stage IV, 1%.

The mortality rate for leiomyosarcomas in superficial soft tissue is about 40%.

Leiomyosarcoma of the uterus (see page 1768).

Leiomyosarcomas in children and infants:

These are exceedingly rare. When located in the prostate and urinary bladder, there is a very poor prognosis.

Leiomyosarcomas in superficial parts have an excellent prognosis.

Further Information M-8891/3

1. **Epithelioid leiomyosarcoma** corresponds histologically to the benign epithelioid leiomyoma.

   Epithelioid leiomyosarcoma is the most common type of gastric sarcoma [6] (Figs. 253 and 254).

2. There is a report of an association between multiple pulmonary chondrohamartomas and epithelioid leiomyosarcoma [119].

[6]   Appelman and Helwig 1976.
[92] Pinedo and Kenis 1977.
[111] Subramanian and Wiltshaw 1978.
[119] Tisell et al. 1978.

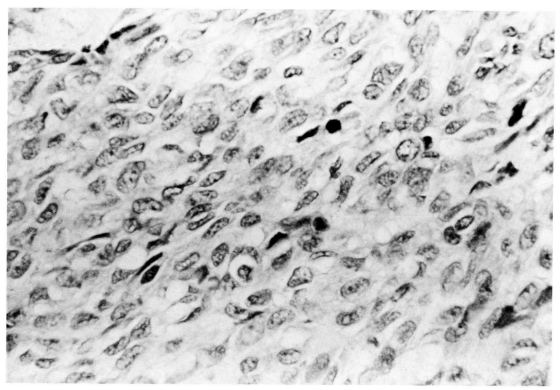

Fig. 107. Leiomyosarcoma: Atypical cells, several mitotic figures (×310).

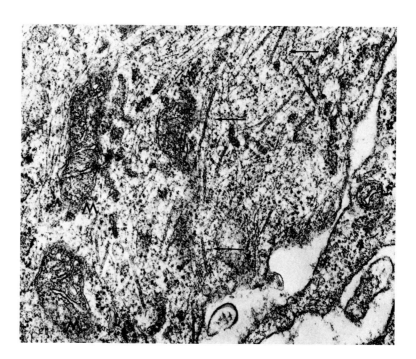

Fig. 108. Leiomyosarcoma: Microtubules (arrow) parallel to microfilaments (×45,000) (Nevaleinen and Linna, Virchows Arch. A Path. Anat. and Histol. *379* (1978) 25-33).

M-8900/0

46. Rhabdomyoma (WHO)

General Remarks

M-8904/0

M-8903/0

Incidence: This is an exceedingly rare, benign soft tissue tumor.

Age: The tumor can be observed in adults:

Adult rhabdomyoma (glycogenic rhabdomyoma, glycogen tumor).

The tumor can occur in young children:

Fetal rhabdomyoma [26, 125].

Site: Rhabdomyomas have been observed in the oral cavity and the surrounding tissues (larynx, uvula, nasal cavity, neck muscles, tongue) and in the vulva.

Rhabdomyomas can also occur in the heart (see page 652).

Histology

The tumor is composed of mature striated muscle fibers.

Cross-striation might be detected occasionally.

In fetal rhabdomyomas the fibers are smaller than those in adult rhabdomyomas, which have a clear (glycogen) cytoplasm.

The nuclei are regular. There is no mitotic activity (Figs. 109 and 110).

Treatment

Removal of the tumor.

Prognosis

Excellent. This is a benign lesion.

[26] Dehner and Enzinger 1972.
[125] Walter and Guerbaoui 1976.

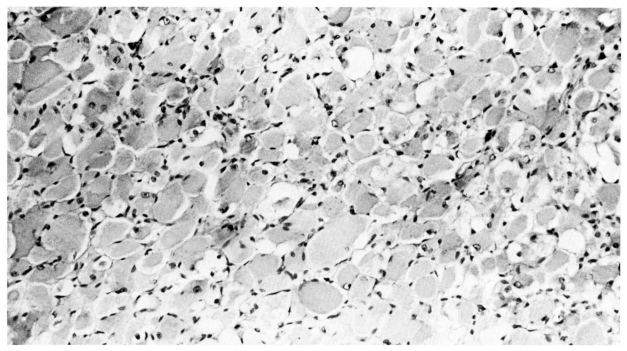

Fig. 109. Rhabdomyoma, adult type: Mature muscle fibers, some with clear cytoplasm. Regular nuclei (50-year-old male, × 125).

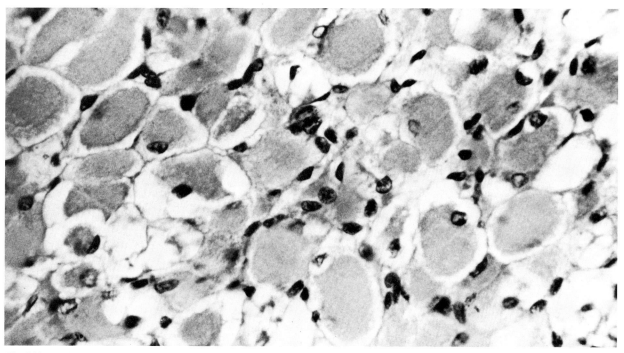

Fig. 110. Rhabdomyoma, adult type: Regular nuclei, partly vacuolated cytoplasm (clear) (50-year-old male, × 310).

M-8900/3

47.-49. Rhabdomyosarcoma (WHO)

General Remarks

Incidence: This is an uncommon, malignant soft tissue tumor. Rhabdomyosarcomas are the most frequent sarcomas in childhood.

Age: According to the growth pattern and the cellular aspects of the tumor cells, rhabdomyosarcomas can be subdivided [57]:

M-8901/3

Pleomorphic rhabdomyosarcoma occurs mainly in **adults.**
The peak age is during the 5th decade.

Embryonal and alveolar rhabdomyosarcomas occur mostly in **infants and children** (see pages 110 and 114).

Site: Pleomorphic rhabdomyosarcoma: The tumor originates in the skeletal muscle usually in the upper extremities, lower extremities, and torso [109].

Embryonal rhabdomyosarcoma: Neck and head region, vagina, urinary bladder, perirectal region (see page 114).

Macroscopy

Soft, large lobulated tumor mass with necroses and a grayish-reddish cut surface.

M-8901/3

47. Pleomorphic rhabdomyosarcoma (WHO)

Histology

The malignant rhabdomyoblasts in this variety of rhabdomyosarcoma are large cells with giant nuclei (Figs. 111 and 112). The cytoplasm of these large cells contains numerous irregularly shaped vacuoles in the periphery, giving a "spider web" appearance to the cells (Fig. 113).

In some tumor cells the nuclei are arranged in a tandem form.

There are numerous mitotic figures and severe nuclei atypias.

The diagnosis of rhabdomyosarcoma is decided by the evidence of cross-striation in the cytoplasm of the tumor cells (or the evidence for longitudinal myofibrils) (Figs. 114 and 115).

Electron Microscopy

In ultrastructural studies the evidence for cross-striation is important for diagnosis [87] (Fig. 116).

Differential Diagnosis

Rhabdomyosarcoma **with other sarcomas:**
– Liposarcoma (Figs. 64 to 69),
– malignant histiocytoma (Figs. 45 to 48),
– malignant lymphoma (see page 1268).
The evidence for rhabdomyosarcoma is based on cross-striation of the tumor cells.

Spread

1. Early hematogenous metastases into the lung, liver, bone, and other organs.
2. Lymph node metastases.

---

[57] Gonzalez-Crussi and Black-Schaffer 1979.
[87] Morales et al. 1972.
[109] Stout and Lattes 1967.

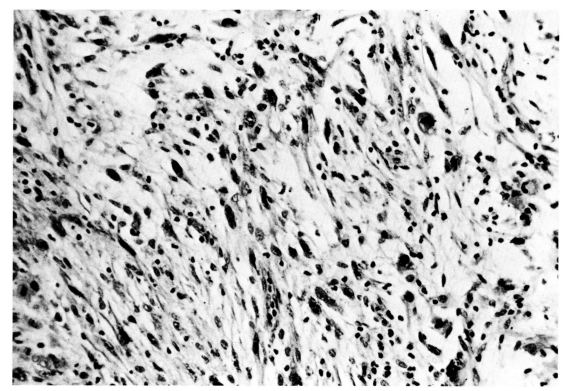

Fig. 111. Pleomorphic rhabdomyosarcoma (77-year-old male, × 125).

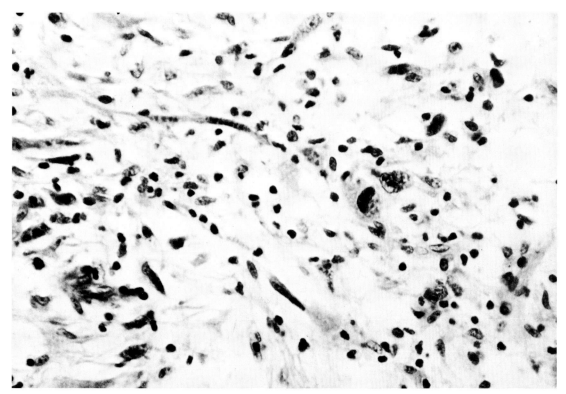

Fig. 112. Pleomorphic rhabdomyosarcoma (77-year-old male, × 200).

Rhabdomyosarcoma

Staging	See Introduction, page 11.
Grading	See Introduction, page 11.
Clinical Findings	According to the site of the tumor growth there are signs of a rapidly growing, malignant tumor.
Treatment	**Surgery:** Radical surgery, depending on the site of the tumor.
Prognosis	The overall 5-year survival rate is about 30%. The 5-year survival rate for Stage IV tumors is less than 1% [112]. According to the histological type, the overall survival rate is about 23 to 29 months [115].

M-8920/3

48. Alveolar rhabdomyosarcoma (WHO)

General Remarks	**Age:** This tumor is observed in children and young adults. The main age group is 10 to 25 years. **Site:** The tumor grows mainly in the extremities (forearm and arm) and in the perirectal and perineal area [45].
Macroscopy	The tumor is soft and has a grayish-whitish, sometimes moiste cut surface with cysts and areas of necroses. Occasionally some tumors seem to be well circumscribed (which is not the case histologically).
Histology	The tumor is composed of small cells that are oval or round. The cells have an acidophilic cytoplasm, in which it is difficult to detect cross-striation (Fig. 117). Occasionally multinucleated tumor giant cells are present. Characteristic of this tumor is the pseudoglandular or alveolar growth pattern (Fig. 118). These alveolar structures can be filled with tumor cells. They are often lined by multilayered cells (Fig. 119). The nucleus is often opposite the site of attachment of the tumor cell to the wall of the alveolar structure.
Electron Microscopy	The majority of the tumor cells in alveolar rhabdomyosarcoma are small and polygonal, containing polyribosomes, variable amounts of glycogen, and small desmosome-like structures [21].

[21] Churg and Ringus 1978.
[45] Enzinger and Shiraki 1969.
[112] Suit and Russell 1977.
[115] Sulser 1978.

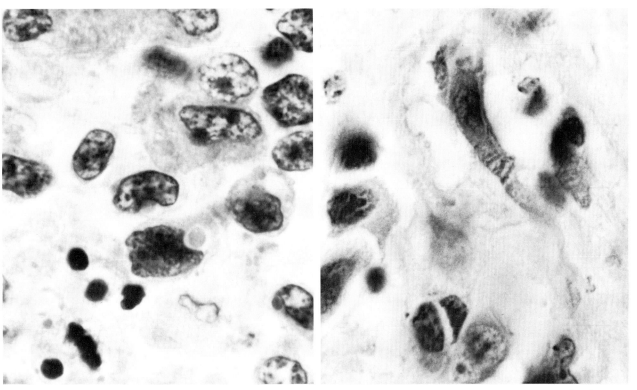

Fig. 113. Pleomorphic rhabdomyosarcoma: Pleomorphic nuclei, vacuolated cytoplasm, mitoses (64-year-old male, × 1250).

Fig. 114. Pleomorphic rhabdomyosarcoma: Cross-striated tumor cells (44-year-old male, × 1250).

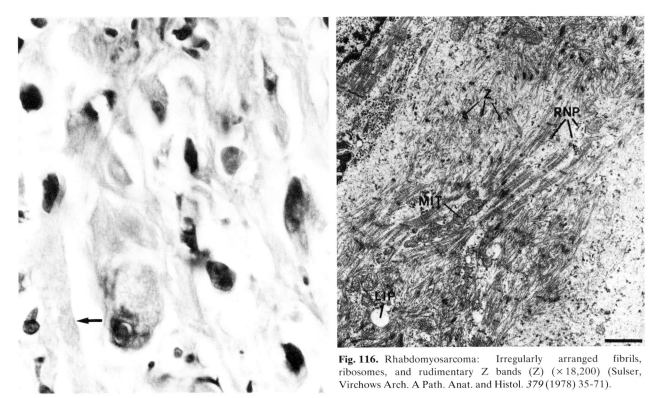

Fig. 115. Pleomorphic rhabdomyosarcoma: Atypical nuclei, vacuolated cytoplasm (spider web), longitudinal fibrils (arrow) (74-year-old male, × 1250).

Fig. 116. Rhabdomyosarcoma: Irregularly arranged fibrils, ribosomes, and rudimentary Z bands (Z) (× 18,200) (Sulser, Virchows Arch. A Path. Anat. and Histol. *379* (1978) 35-71).

Rhabdomyosarcoma

Differential Diagnosis

Alveolar rhabdomyosarcoma **with other malignant tumors:**
– Malignant lymphoma (see page 1268),
– neuroblastoma (due to occasional pseudorosette formations in alveolar rhabdomyosarcoma) (Figs. 1730 and 1731),
– synovial sarcoma (Figs. 129 to 132),
– malignant mesothelioma (Figs. 444 to 446).
The alveolar growth pattern is the most helpful finding for the diagnosis of this tumor.

Staging

See Introduction, page 11.

Grading

See Introduction, page 11.

Spread

Early hematogenous and lymphatic dissemination.

Clinical Findings

According to the site, there are signs of a rapidly growing malignant tumor in children and young adults.

Treatment

A combined modality treatment with surgery, high dose radiation therapy, and chemotherapy has been recommended [34].
Surgery:
The most radical aggressive surgery should be attempted.
Chemotherapy:
Aggressive chemotherapy with a combination, for instance, of vincristine, cyclophosphamide, DTIC, and adriamycin can be tried.
A maintenance adjuvant chemotherapy for subclinical micrometastases may be used [50, 54].
Radiation therapy:
Radiation therapy up to 60 Gy.

Prognosis

The 5-year survival rate for Stage I to IV tumors is less than 1%. Death occurs mainly from metastases into the lung.

---

[34] Dritschilo et al. 1978.
[50] Fernandez et al. 1975.
[54] Ghavimi et al. 1975.

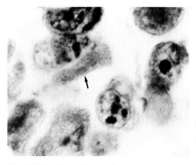

Fig. 117. Alveolar rhabdomyosarcoma: Pleomorphic nuclei, longitudinal fibrils (arrow) and cross-striation (64-year-old male, × 2000).

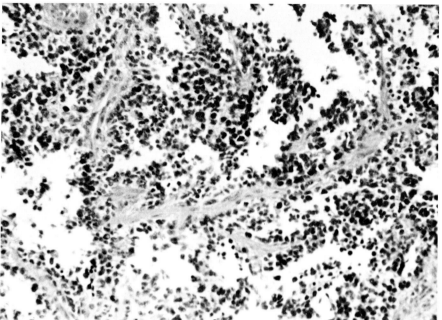

Fig. 118. Alveolar rhabdomyosarcoma (× 125).

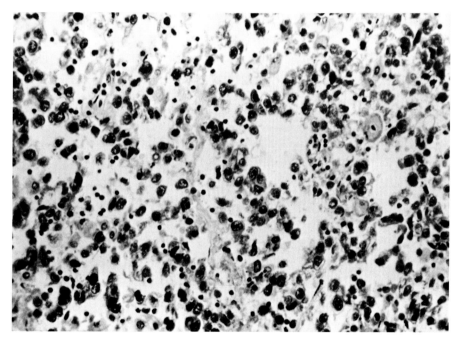

Fig. 119. Alveolar rhabdomyosarcoma (64-year-old male, × 200).

113

M-8910/3

49. Embryonal rhabdomyosarcoma (WHO)
(sarcoma botryoides)

**General
Remarks**

Age: Embryonal rhabdomyosarcomas occur in infants and children. The majority of the patients are 5 years old or younger.

Site: The tumor can originate in the urethra, vagina, urinary bladder, nasopharynx, or bile ducts; it originates rarely in the extremities.

Macroscopy

The tumor grows close to the surface of the organs (subcutaneous tissue and submucosa). The tumor grows exophytically and forms polypoid masses, which give the tumor a grapelike form (botryoid).

The tumor has a whitish-grayish cut surface and is soft and friable.

Histology

The microscopic picture is at low magnification similar to that of edematous tissue with inflammation (Fig. 120).

With higher magnification, malignant rhabdomyoblasts are found, which are spindle-shaped and small (Figs. 121 and 122).

These malignant cells grow preferentially close to the surface underneath the epithelial layer.

The tumor cells might exhibit cross-striation in their longitudinal cytoplasm.

**Differential
Diagnosis**

1. Embryonal rhabdomyosarcoma **with inflammatory polyp** (Fig. 489).
2. Embryonal rhabdomyosarcoma **with myxoma** (Figs. 49 and 50).
3. Embryonal rhabdomyosarcoma **with myxoid liposarcoma** (Fig. 63).
4. Embryonal rhabdomyosarcoma **with malignant lymphoma** (see page 114).
5. Embryonal rhabdomyosarcoma **with amelanotic melanoma** (Figs. 1261 and 1293).
6. Embryonal rhabdomyosarcoma **with undifferentiated carcinoma:**
   The correct diagnosis of embryonal rhabdomyosarcoma is based on the evidence for cross-striation in the tumor cells combined with the youth of the patients.

Spread

Early hematogenous metastases into the bone, bone marrow, lung, and other organs.

Staging

See Introduction, page 11.

Grading

See Introduction, page 11.

Treatment

Aggressive **surgery, chemotherapy,** and **radiation therapy** in a combined modality treatment.

Combination chemotherapy before irradiation might be useful [118].

Chemotherapy:

Several effective drugs and drug combinations are known and occasionally result in a normal life span.

Vincristine + cyclophosphamide + dactinomycin in combination with surgery and irradiation has resulted in 1 to 2 years of disease-free time in about 76% of the cases [28].

---

[28] De Vita Jr. 1977.
[118] Tefft et al. 1977.

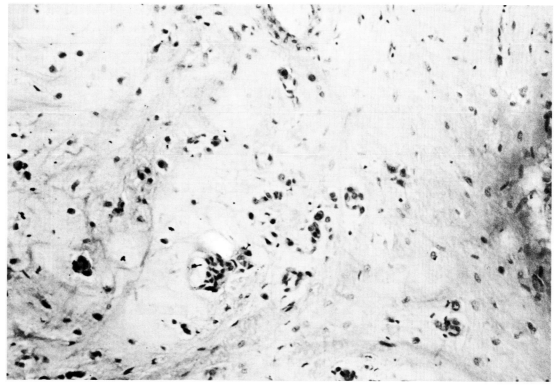

Fig. 120. Embryonal rhabdomyosarcoma (sarcoma botryoides): Foci of tumor cells in a loose tissue of low cellularity (× 125).

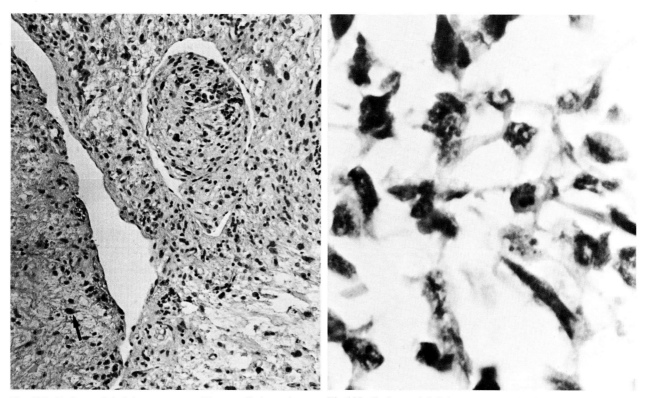

Fig. 121. Embryonal rhabdomyosarcoma: Tumor cells (arrow) (36-year-old female, × 125).

Fig. 122. Embryonal rhabdomyosarcoma: Rather small, often spindle-shaped tumor cells (× 800).

Treatment	Occasionally a favorable response of the tumor has been reported when adriamycin + DTIC has been used [82]. Postoperative and postirradiation chemotherapy has been recommended [63]. In cases of inoperable rhabdomyosarcoma, radiation therapy (up to 60 Gy in 6 weeks) combined with chemotherapy can be attempted.
Prognosis	The 5-year survival rate is about 8% [37].

M-9580/0

50. Granular cell tumor (WHO)
(myoblastoma, Abrikossoff's tumor)

General Remarks	**Incidence:** This is a relatively rare, but not uncommon, benign tumor. **Age:** Granular cell tumor can occur at any age. The majority of patients are in the 4th or 5th decade. **Sex:** Females are affected slightly more often than males. **Site:** The most frequent site is the tongue (about 30%). The tumor may occur elsewhere (lip, mouth, orbit, external auditory canal, skin, subcutaneous tissue, vulva, pituitary stalk, muscles of the extremities, urinary bladder, bile ducts, rectum, appendix) [110].
Macroscopy	Myoblastomas are relatively small, firm tumors with a whitish-yellowish cut surface.
Histology	The tumor is composed of large cells that sometimes have distinct cell borders. The cytoplasm contains coarse granules, which show a PAS-positive staining. The nuclei are small, regular, and dense (Fig. 123).
Electron Microscopy	The granules exhibit the features of lysosomes. Besides 1,2-glycols they contain cerebrosides.
Differential Diagnosis	1. Granular cell tumor **with carcinoma** (especially when located in the breast). 2. Myoblastomas **with squamous cell carcinoma:** Myoblastoma induces a hyperplasia in the covering epidermis, mimicking occasionally infiltrating carcinomas, especially at the site of the tongue (Fig. 465). 3. Myoblastoma **with metastases of a renal cell carcinoma** (Fig. 1304): This differential diagnosis is sometimes required because of the large and clear cytoplasm of the myoblastoma cells.
Treatment	Surgical removal of the tumor.
Prognosis	The great majority of granular cell tumors (myoblastomas) are benign.

---

[37] Enzinger 1963.
[63] Jungi 1978.
[82] Maurus and Otten 1978.
[110] Strong et al. 1970.

116

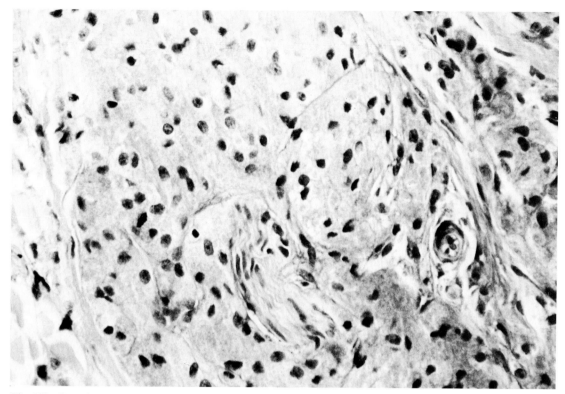

Fig. 123. Granular cell tumor: Regular nuclei, granular cytoplasm (PAS positive) (32-year-old male, × 310).

M-9580/3

Rarely a metastasizing **malignant granular cell tumor** (WHO) is observed.
The tumor is very cellular, and the cells contain the same granules observed in benign myoblastoma.
Malignancy is revealed by hematogenous and lymphatic metastases.

Further Information

There is still controversy over the origin of this tumor: Schwann's cells, smooth muscle cells, ameloblasts [1, 58].

[1] Ackerman and Rosai 1974.
[58] Harkin and Reed 1969.

M-9581/3

51. Alveolar soft part sarcoma (WHO)

General Remarks

Incidence: This is a rare, malignant, soft tissue tumor.
Age: The tumor can be observed at any age: adults, young adults, and children.
Sex: Females are affected more frequently than males.
Site: The majority (about 50%) grow in the extremities, followed by the retroperitoneum, the mesentery, and the omentum.
The tumor has also been discovered in the mediastinum [64] and the oral cavity and at other sites [109].

Macroscopy

The tumor is large and has a yellowish and grayish cut surface. In the firm tumor, areas of hemorrhage and yellowish necroses develop.

Histology

The tumor is composed of large clear cells (Fig. 124). The nuclei are relatively regular, round, and slightly oval with a centrally located nucleolus.
The cytoplasm contains granules (similar to those observed in myoblastoma) (Fig. 125). These granules show a PAS-positive staining and are diastase-resistant.
There are few mitotic figures.
The growth pattern of these tumor cells mimics an endocrine or pseudoglandular architecture (Fig. 126).
Invasion of tumor cells, particularly into the veins, is observed frequently (Fig. 127).

Electron Microscopy

The cytoplasm contains crystals (which can be seen also with PAS stain in light microscopy).

Differential Diagnosis

1. Alveolar soft part sarcoma **with renal cell carcinoma** (Fig. 1304).
2. Alveolar soft part sarcoma **with clear cell carcinoma** (Fig. 1672).
3. Alveolar soft part sarcoma **with paraganglioma** (Fig. 1741).
4. Alveolar soft part sarcoma **with pheochromocytoma** (Fig. 1736).
5. Alveolar soft part sarcoma **with malignant melanoma** (Fig. 1216).
6. Alveolar soft part sarcoma **with malignant sweat gland tumors:**
   A histological aspect with endocrine-like clear cells argues for the diagnosis of carcinoma (Fig. 128).
   Helpful for the diagnosis of an alveolar soft part sarcoma is the presence of PAS-positive, diastase-resistant granules in the cytoplasm; evidence for PAS-positive crystals; and the peculiar growth pattern of the tumor cells.

Spread

1. Hematogenous spread.
2. Early lymphatic spread.

Clinical Findings

This is a tumor that grows slowly and does not cause pain. Because of this growth pattern patients often have metastases at the time of diagnosis.

---

[64] Khan and Nixon 1978.
[109] Stout and Lattes 1967.

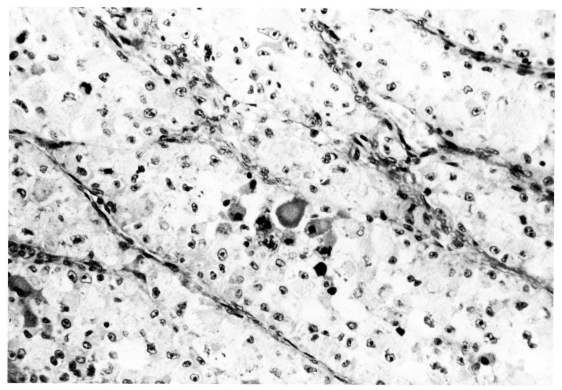

Fig. 124. Alveolar soft part sarcoma (malignant granular cell tumor) (32-year-old male, × 310).

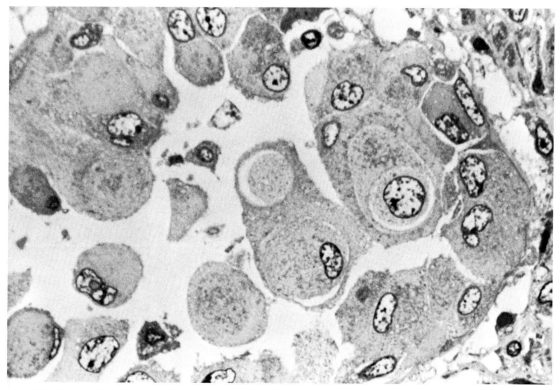

Fig. 125. Tumor cells in alveolar soft part sarcoma: Granulated cytoplasm, pleomorphism of the nuclei, alveolar structure (32-year-old male, × 800).

119

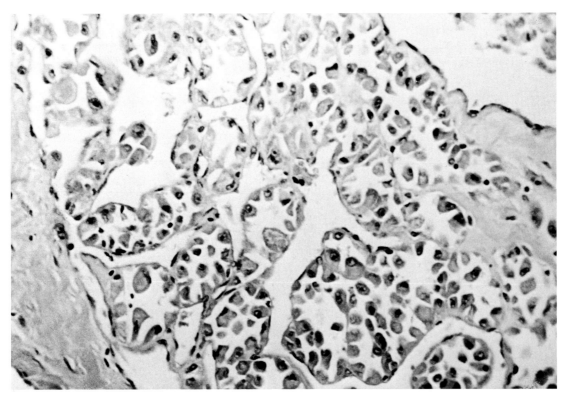

Fig. 126. Alveolar soft part sarcoma: Typical appearance (×200).

Treatment	**Surgery.** **Chemotherapy** [132] (see page 11).
Prognosis	Despite the slow growth of the tumor, alveolar soft part sarcomas are very malignant neoplasms.
Further Information	The originating cell of this tumor has not yet been definitively determined [109]. Probably this soft part sarcoma is a variety of rhabdomyosarcoma [1, 51].

[1] Ackerman and Rosai 1974.
[51] Fisher and Reidbord 1971.
[109] Stout and Lattes 1967.
[132] Wobbes 1978.

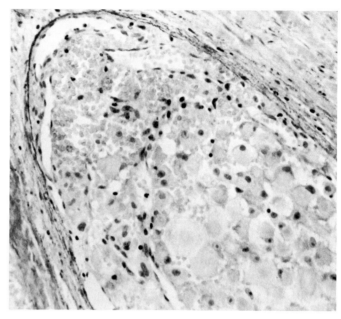

Fig. 127. Blood vessel invasion in alveolar soft part sarcoma: Similarity with cells in pheochromocytoma or renal cell carcinoma (32-year-old male, × 200).

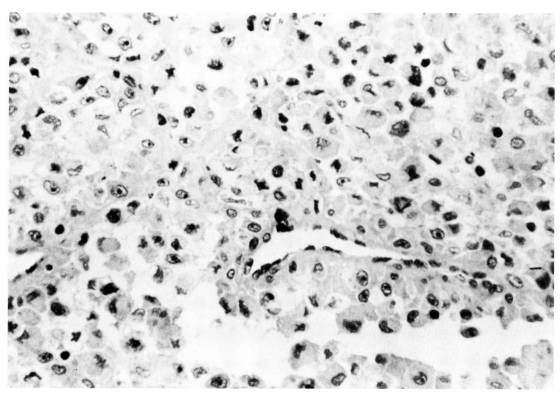

Fig. 128. Alveolar soft part sarcoma: Similarity with epithelial cells (32-year-old male, × 310).

M-9040/3

52. Synovial sarcoma (WHO)
(malignant synovioma)

**General
Remarks**

Incidence: This is a relatively rare tumor.

Age: The tumor most often affects young adults (3rd and 4th decades).
However, younger patients can be affected.

Sex: Males seem to be affected more frequently than females.

Site: The great majority of synovial sarcomas (about 80%) arise in the vicinity of the ankle joints and the knee.

The tumor can also be observed in the elbow, the hip region, the shoulder, and the soft tissue of the head and neck [1, 88].

Macroscopy

The tumor seems to be circumscribed; the cut surface is grayish-reddish and shows calcifications.

The tumor is associated with the joints, bursae, and tendon sheaths. The synovial membrane is almost never occupied by the tumor.

Histology

The tumor is composed of cells that form solid clusters or small tubular structures and clefts (Figs. 129 and 130).

The tumor cells in the solid parts are spindle cells; they are surrounded by reticulin fibers. These tumor cells are similar to those observed in fibrosarcomas (Figs. 131 and 132).

The slits, clefts, and tubular formations are lined by cells that have a more epithelial appearance. These cells contain in their cytoplasm PAS-positive material. This material can also be found in the lumen of the spaces, which are lined by the tumor cells.

**Differential
Diagnosis**

1. Synovial sarcoma **with fibrosarcoma** (Figs. 21 to 25):
   Due to the fibrosarcoma-like picture of the solid parts of the tumor, this differential diagnosis must be determined. The appearance of typical small spaces lined by epithelial-like cells decides for synovial sarcoma.

M-9040/0

2. Synovial sarcoma **with benign synovioma** (WHO):
   This is a tumor-like lesion that is extremely rare.
   Benign synoviomas are found in the capsule of the knee joint.
   Histologically there are slits and clefts; however, in the cells there are no signs of malignancy.
   Therefore the architecture of the benign synovioma is similar to that observed in synovial sarcoma [109].

3. Synovial sarcoma **with villonodular synovitis** (Figs. 39 and 40).

4. Synovial sarcoma **with fibromatosis** (especially plantar fibromatosis) (Fig. 5).

Staging

See Introduction, page 11.

Grading

See Introduction, page 11.

---

[1] Ackerman and Rosai 1974.
[88] Nunez-Alonso et al. 1979.
[109] Stout and Lattes 1967.

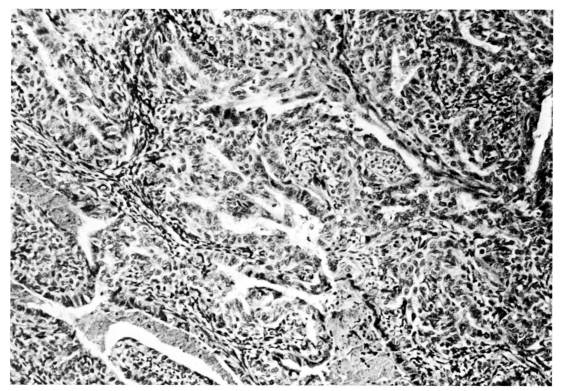

Fig. 129. Synovial sarcoma: The tumor is dominated by a glandular-like arrangement of tumor cells (42-year-old male, ×125).

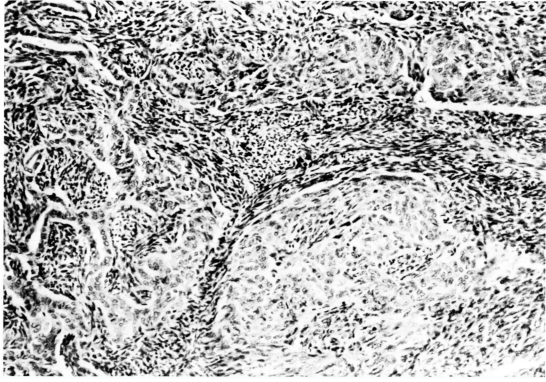

Fig. 130. Synovial sarcoma: Biphasic tumor with tubular and solid growth of tumor cells (fibrosarcoma-like) (42-year-old male, ×125).

Synovial sarcoma

Spread

1. Hematogenous spread into the lung and other organs.
2. Lymphatic spread into the regional lymph nodes.

Clinical Findings

Painful swelling, often related to previous trauma.
There are frequent recurrences after the initial treatment.

Roentgenogram

Occasionally calcification is observed on the roentgenogram.

Treatment

Radical **surgery** [104].
Radiation therapy:
Synovial sarcomas are rather radiosensitive.
Chemotherapy:
A combination with DTIC and adriamycin can be tried [72, 91].

Prognosis

Synovial sarcomas initially grow slowly; however, they are very malignant.
The duration from the onset of symptoms to death is 5 to 7 years [109].
About 50% of synovial sarcomas develop metastases.
The 5-year survival rate for Stages I to IV tumors is approximately 10 to 20%. There are some reports of a 50% 5-year survival rate [121].

[72] Krementz et al. 1977.
[91] Pinedo et al. 1978.
[104] Shiu et al. 1979.
[109] Stout and Lattes 1967.
[121] Van Andel 1972.

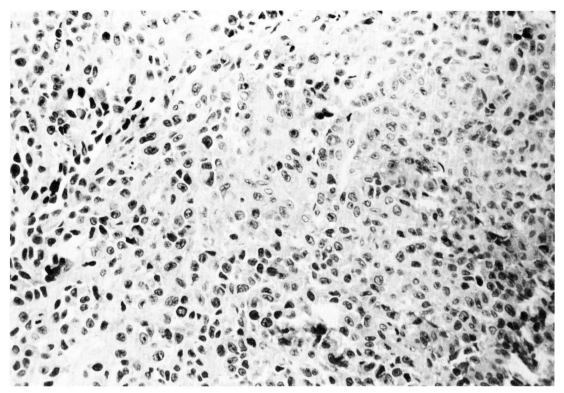

Fig. 131. Synovial sarcoma: Remnants of tubular structures, large solid tumor cell nests (fibrosarcoma-like) (42-year-old male, × 200).

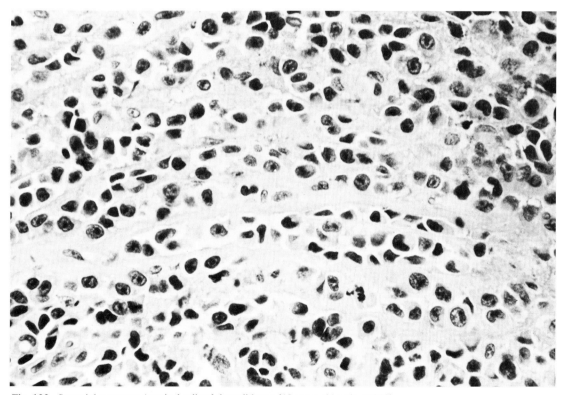

Fig. 132. Synovial sarcoma: Atypical cells of the solid part (42-year-old male, × 310).

M-9044/3
T 171.9

53. Clear cell sarcoma of tendons and aponeuroses (WHO) [40]

General Remarks

Incidence: This is a rare, malignant tumor.
Age: The tumor usually affects young adults.
Site: The tumor develops in the knees and feet, with the majority observed in the feet.
The tumor grows in the immediate neighborhood of aponeuroses and tendons.

Macroscopy

The tumor is well circumscribed and firm and has a grayish cut surface.

Histology

The tumor is composed of cuboidal cells that have a large clear cytoplasm. The tumor cells show signs of atypias and are occasionally multinucleated. The nuclei are clear and have a centrally located, large nucleolus (Fig. 133).
The tumor cells grow in small groups and fascicles, which are surrounded by reticulin fibers.
In the cytoplasm iron pigment can be observed (Fig. 134).

Differential Diagnosis

1. Clear cell sarcoma **with synovial sarcoma** (Figs. 129 to 132).
2. Clear cell sarcoma **with alveolar soft part sarcoma** (Figs. 124 to 127).

Spread

The tumor metastasizes by the hematogenous and lymphatic routes.

Clinical Findings

The tumor shows a slow-growing swelling at the site of growth.

Treatment

Radical **surgery.**

Prognosis

The tumor recurs frequently.
Distant metastases might occur.

Further Information

Most probably the majority of these clear cell sarcomas are "melanomas of the soft part" [10]. A minority of these tumors should be considered malignant tumors of the synovial type [120]. The clear cells of clear cell sarcoma can contain melanosomes [120] (melanotic type).

[10] Bearman et al. 1975.
[40] Enzinger 1965.
[120] Tsuneyoshi et al. 1978.

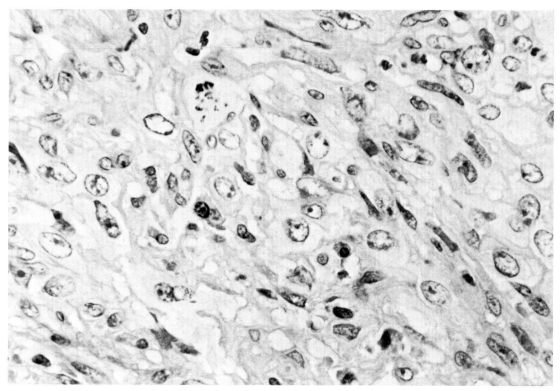

Fig. 133. Clear cell sarcoma of tendons and aponeuroses: Atypical clear nuclei, some of them with prominent nucleolus (34-year-old female, × 400).

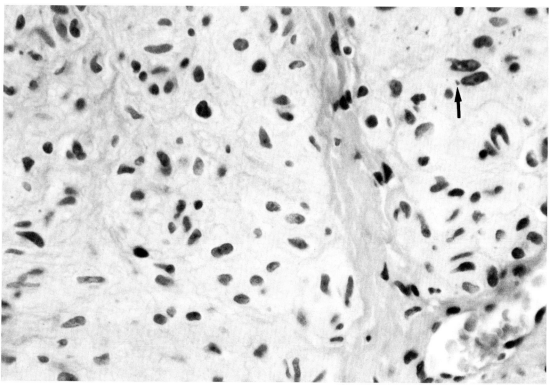

Fig. 134. Nests of cells in clear cell sarcoma: Iron pigment (arrow) (34-year-old female, × 400).

127

M-8804/3

54. Epithelioid cell sarcoma [43]

General Remarks

Incidence: This is a very rare tumor.
Age: The majority of patients are in the 3rd through 6th decades.
Site: The tumor probably originates from the tendon sheaths.

Macroscopy

The tumor has a glassy, whitish cut surface.

Histology

The tumor cells resemble epithelioid cells. The tumor cells have a clear cytoplasm. The cytoplasm is acidophilic.
The tumor cells exhibit signs of malignancy with hyperchromasia of the nuclei and mitotic figures. The tumor cells form small nodules. This growth pattern together with the epithelioidlike structure of the tumor cells can lead to the differential diagnosis of a granulomatous inflammation (Fig. 135).

Spread

The tumor disseminates by the lymphatic and hematogenous routes.

Treatment

Amputation or early wide excision [94].

Prognosis

The average survival time is 8 years.
Local recurrences occur in 85% of the cases.
Distant metastases are observed in 30% of the cases.

Further Information

There is suggestive evidence that the epithelioid sarcoma is derived from synovioblastic mesenchyma [89].

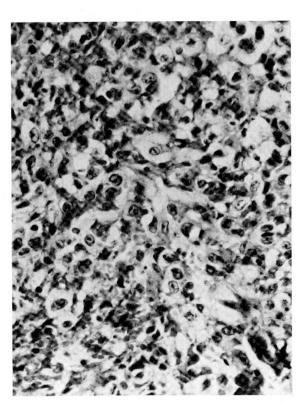

Fig. 135. Epithelioid cell sarcoma: Round and spindle-shaped tumor cells (×120) (Patchefsky et al., Cancer *39* [1977] 143-152).

[43] Enzinger 1970.
[89] Patchefsky et al. 1977.
[94] Prat et al. 1978.

M-8990/0, 1

55. Benign mesenchymoma (WHO)

General Remarks

Benign mesenchymomas develop mainly in the kidney, the perirenal tissue, and the muscles.

The lesion is rare.

Histology

Benign mesenchymomas are composed of different elements of mesenchymal tissue. A constant finding in this lesion is numerous blood vessels with thick walls (Fig. 136). These blood vessels are associated with elements of lipoma, myoma, cartilage, striated muscle, and lymphoid tissue and foci of extramedullary hematopoiesis (Fig. 137).

Treatment

Surgery:

Removal of the tumor.

Prognosis

In cases of incomplete excision recurrences are occasionally observed.

In the recurrence, sometimes only one part of the different components of the mesenchymoma carries on growth.

Further Information

Benign mesenchymoma of the kidney and the perirenal tissue can be associated with tuberous sclerosis.

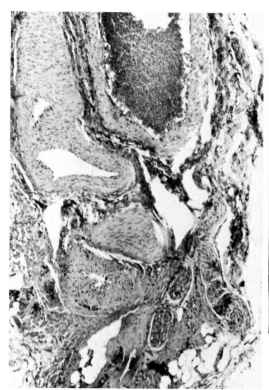

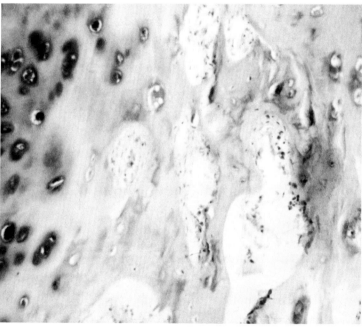

Fig. 137. Benign mesenchymoma: Connective tissue, hematopoietic tissue, bone (41-year-old male, abdominal wall, × 125).

Fig. 136. Benign mesenchymoma: Fat tissue, connective tissue, numerous blood vessels, and nerve fibers (20-year-old male, inguinal region, × 40).

129

M-8990/3

56. Malignant mesenchymoma (WHO)

General Remarks

Incidence: Malignant mesenchymomas are very rare.
Age: The tumor is observed in children and adults.
Sex: In adults, males and females are affected equally.
In children, males are affected more often than females (2:1).
Site: Malignant mesenchymomas develop usually in the extremities; however, this tumor can be observed in the retroperitoneum, mediastinum, torso, head, and neck.

Macroscopy

The tumor is circumscribed without a capsule.

Histology

M-8860/3

The tumor is composed of different types of sarcomas, such as liposarcoma, rhabdomyosarcoma, osteogenic sarcoma, and chondrosarcoma, in various combinations, for instance, angiomyoliposarcoma.

Treatment

Radical excision.

Prognosis

In children the death rate is 40%; in adults it is 60% [109].

M-9080/0, 1, 3

57. Soft tissue teratoma
(dermoid cyst – WHO)
(adult teratoma)

General Remarks

Incidence: Soft tissue teratomas are very rare.
Age: The tumor can be observed at birth or develop in early childhood or in young adults.
Sex: Females are affected more frequently than males.
Site: Soft tissue teratomas can be observed in the sacrococcygeal area, the retroperitoneum, the mediastinum, the neck, the base of the skull, and the pineal region [12, 129].
Further notes: Soft tissue teratomas probably develop from extragonadal germ cells (WHO) [42].

Macroscopy

Soft tissue teratomas are encapsulated lesions of various sizes; occasionally they are very large.
The cut surface shows a lobulated architecture and numerous cysts that contain a clear or yellowish fluid, sebaceous material, and always hairs.

[12] Berry et al. 1969.
[42] Enzinger 1969.
[109] Stout and Lattes 1967.
[129] Willis 1968.

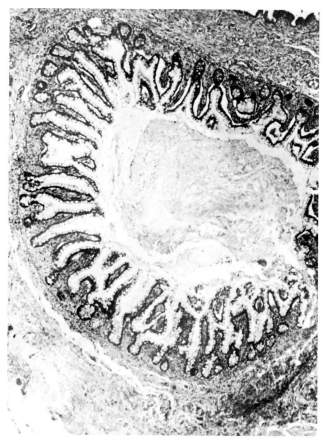

Fig. 138. Teratoma: Areas resembling primitive gut (17-day-old female, sacrococcygeal region, × 40).

Fig. 139. Remnants of gonadal tissue in inguinal region (7-year-old male, × 50).

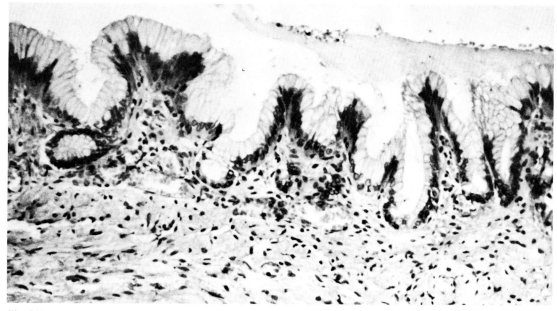

Fig. 140. Teratoma: Wall of a well-differentiated cyst, lined by columnar epithelium (17-day-old female, × 125).

131

Soft tissue teratoma

Histology

The cysts are lined by stratified squamous epithelium; in the wall there are sebaceous glands. In the lumen there are hairs.

The wall and the solid part of the tumor contain cartilage, neural tissue, intestinal or pancreatic areas, or cysts that are lined by respiratory epithelium (Figs. 138 to 142).

The tumor is disseminated by foci of calcification in numerous cases.

Differential Diagnosis

In cases of benign teratoma, areas for possible malignant growth should be ruled out.

Clinical Findings

The symptoms depend on the size and site of the teratoma. Mediastinal teratomas, for instance, can cause coughing; sacrococcygeal or retroperitoneal teratomas can cause malfunctions of the urinary bladder or bowel.

Treatment

Resection of the teratoma.

Prognosis

Most teratomas (about 75%) are benign.
- Sacrococcygeal teratomas at birth: benign [23, 25, 31].
- Sacrococcygeal teratomas discovered after the age of 2 years: often malignant.
- Teratomas in the anterior mediastinum: almost always malignant.

M-9080/3

Malignant teratomas (WHO) present as embryonal carcinoma, teratocarcinoma, choriocarcinoma, or yolk sac tumor [18].

Malignant teratomas have a very poor prognosis [18].

[18] Chretien et al. 1970.
[23] Conklin and Abell 1967.
[25] Dehner 1973.
[31] Donnellan and Swenson 1968.

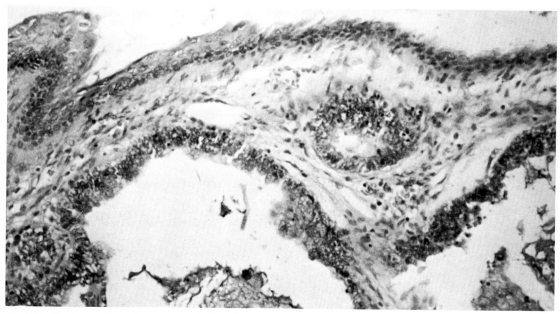

Fig. 141. Teratoma: Several cysts, one of them lined by squamous cells (2-month-old female, sacrococcygeal region, ×200).

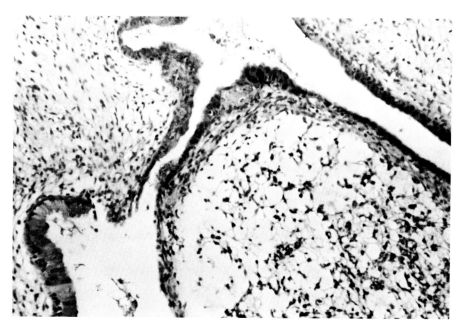

Fig. 142. Teratoma: Primitive mesenchyma; cyst lined by different epithelial cells (2-month-old female, ×200).

133

M-9363/0

58. Pigmented neuroectodermal tumor of infancy

(melanotic progonoma; retinal anlage tumor) (WHO)

General Remarks

Incidence: The melanotic progonoma is a rare, benign lesion.

Site: The main sites are the maxilla, the skull, and the mediastinum [22, 71]. Occasionally the tumor has been observed in the thigh, forearm, epididymis [1], and retroperitoneum.

Macroscopy

The tumors are usually rather small and have a brown-black cut surface. The cut surface contains numerous cysts.

Histology

The tumor is composed of cuboidal cells that contain abundant melanin in their cytoplasm. These structures form glandular-like spaces or tubular formations. The tumor cells are embedded in a connective tissue with numerous collagen fibers (Figs. 143 to 145).

Clinical Findings

According to the site and size of the tumor.

Treatment

Surgical removal.

Prognosis

This is a benign tumor.

Further Information

1. Histologically there is a certain similarity between melanotic neuroectodermal tumors and the fetal pineal gland [32].
2. It seems possible that the origin of the melanotic progonoma is the neural crest.

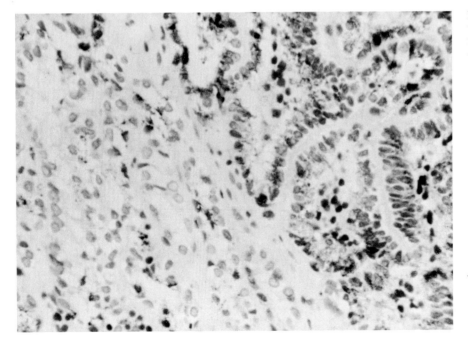

Fig. 143. Pigmented neuroectodermal tumor (retinal anlage tumor): Melanin-containing cells growing in clusters or alveolar structures (22-year-old male, retroperitoneum, ×310).

[1] Ackerman and Rosai 1974.
[22] Clarke and Parsons 1951.
[32] Dooling et al. 1977.
[71] Koudstaal et al. 1968.

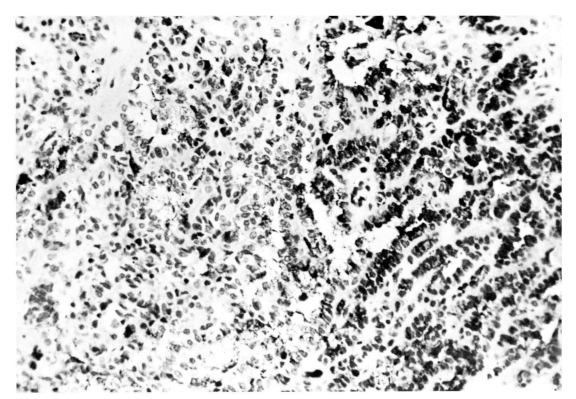

Fig. 144. Another aspect of the pigmented neuroectodermal tumor: Alveolar structures and solid nests of melanin-containing cells (22-year-old male, × 200).

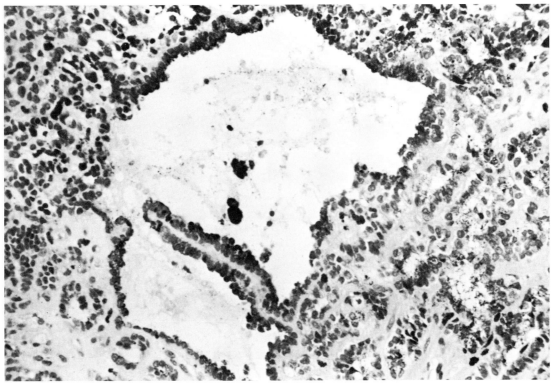

Fig. 145. Larger cystic structures lined by melanin-containing cells in neuroectodermal tumor (22-year-old male, × 200).

135

M-9240/3

59. Chondrosarcoma of soft parts (WHO)

(mesenchymal chondrosarcoma)

Chondrosarcomas in an extraskeletal position are very rare.
The tumor is composed of elements of a chondrosarcoma, similar to those observed in the bone (Figs. 1027 to 1032).
Extraskeletal chondrosarcomas are less malignant than those of the bone.

M-9180/3
T-171.9

60. Osteogenic sarcoma of soft parts (WHO)

**General
Remarks**

Incidence: Extraskeletal osteogenic sarcomas are very rare.
Age: The tumor occurs in adults and children. This osteogenic sarcoma occurs usually at a later age (peak age, 58 years).
Sex: Both sexes are affected equally.
Site: Osteogenic sarcomas are usually found in the extremities and occasionally also in the viscera.

**Differential
Diagnosis**

1. Osteogenic sarcoma **with metaplastic bone in synovial sarcoma or fibrosarcoma.**
2. Osteogenic sarcoma **with myositis ossificans** (Figs. 146, 147, 1005, and 1006).

Prognosis

Extraskeletal osteogenic sarcomas have a very poor prognosis.
The 5-year survival rate is about 25%; the overall median survival time is 20 months [96].
Osteogenic sarcomas can be part of a malignant mesenchymoma.

M-9180/3
T-171.9

61. Osteoma of soft parts (WHO)

This is a very rare tumor.

---

[96] Rao et al. 1978.

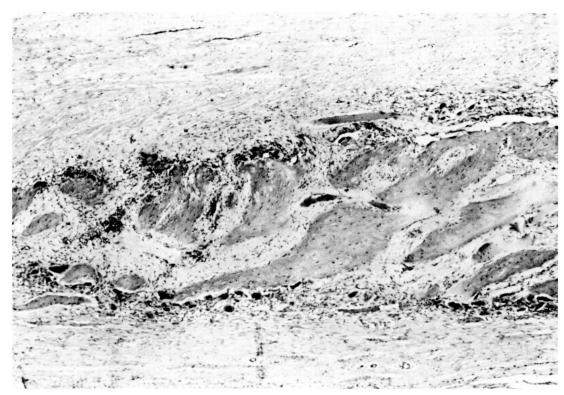

Fig. 146. Myositis ossificans: Osseous metaplasia in skeletal muscle (59-year-old male, × 50).

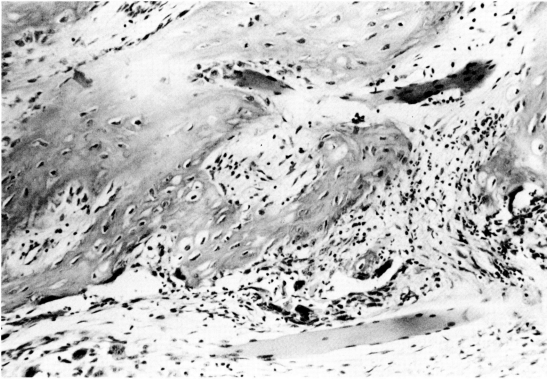

Fig. 147. Myositis ossificans: Metaplastic bone trabeculae with regular osteoblasts in skeletal muscle (59-year-old male, × 125).

M-9220/0
T-171.9

62. Chondroma of soft parts (WHO)

This is a very rare tumor.
Chondromas of soft tissue are benign lesions, which can be excised and are cured.
Chondromas are observed in patients in the 3rd and 4th decades of life. Chondromas grow mainly in the feet and hands [20].

M-7341/0

63. Myositis ossificans (WHO)

This is an osseous metaplasia at the site of skeletal muscle, most probably caused by previous trauma (Figs. 146 and 147) (for histology and differential diagnosis see Bone tumors, page 1100).

M-9054/0

64. Adenomatoid tumor (WHO)

Adenomatoid tumors can occur in the soft tissue.
They are varieties of benign mesotheliomas (see Tumors of the testis) (Figs. 1494 to 1496).

M-9050/0, 1, 3

65. Mesothelioma (WHO)

Mesothelial cells covering the peritoneum and the pleura can be the origin of benign and malignant tumors (see Tumors of the pleura and the peritoneum) (Figs. 442 to 448, 747, and 756).

---

[20] Chung and Enzinger 1978.

M-9260/3
T-171.9

66. Extraskeletal Ewing's sarcoma

Very rarely Ewing's sarcoma originates and grows in the soft tissue [55, 84].

M-9251/3

67. Malignant giant cell tumor of soft parts (WHO)

Occasionally malignant soft tissue tumors contain numerous giant cells, similar to those observed in malignant giant cell tumor of bone.

M-8800/3

68. Unclassified sarcoma (WHO)

M-8803/3

Sarcomas that cannot be classified according to the above-mentioned types are called unclassified sarcomas (WHO) (small round cell sarcoma).

---

[55] Gillespie et al. 1979.
[84] Meister and Gokel 1978.

Recommendations for differential diagnosis in soft tissue tumors

fibromatosis	with	– fibrosarcoma
palmar-plantar fibromatosis	with	– fibrosarcoma – synovial sarcoma – Kaposi's sarcoma – malignant melanoma
idiopathic retroperitoneal fibromatosis (fibrosis) (see page 148)	with	– epithelial or mesenchymal malignant tumors
nodular fasciitis	with	– desmoid – dermatofibrosarcoma protuberans – fibrosarcoma
desmoid	with	– fibrosarcoma – nodular fasciitis
fibrosarcoma	with	– fibromatosis – nodular fasciitis – desmoid – dermatofibrosarcoma protuberans – malignant fibrous histiocytoma – schwannoma – liposarcoma – synovial sarcoma
malignant fibrous histiocytoma	with	– benign histiocytoma – reticulum cell sarcoma – fibrosarcoma – dermatofibrosarcoma protuberans – fibromatosis
villonodular synovitis	with	– synovial sarcoma – malignant giant cell tumor of the bone – osteogenic sarcoma – fibrosarcoma
liposarcoma	with	– lipoblastoma – benign lipoma – fibrosarcoma – myxoma – rhabdomyosarcoma – other poorly differentiated sarcomas

myxoma	with	– localized myxedema – ganglion – chondrosarcoma – rhabdomyosarcoma – other sarcomas – neurofibromas
hemangiopericytoma, benign	with	– malignant hemangiopericytoma – other vascular tumors – angiomas – angiosarcomas – glomus tumor – Kaposi's sarcoma
angiosarcoma	with	– diffuse intramuscular angiomatosis – benign hemangioendothelioma in infants and children – malignant tumors with numerous blood vessels (renal cell carcinoma, osteosarcoma) – benign hemangiomas
Kaposi's sarcoma	with	– benign inflammation – plantar fibromatosis – glomus tumor – hemangiopericytoma – hemangioma – angiosarcoma
leiomyoma	with	– leiomyosarcoma
leiomyosarcoma	with	– benign leiomyoma – fibrosarcoma – liposarcoma (in cases of un-differentiated tumors) – malignant schwannoma
embryonal rhabdomyosarcoma (botryoid sarcoma)	with	– inflammatory polyps – malignant lymphoma – undifferentiated carcinoma – amelanotic melanoma
alveolar rhabdomyosarcoma	with	– malignant lymphoma – alveolar soft part sarcoma – neuroblastoma – undifferentiated sarcoma – synovial sarcoma

pleomorphic rhabdomyosarcoma	with	– other malignant sarcomas with giant cells, including liposarcoma – malignant histiocytoma – pheochromocytoma
granular cell tumor (myoblastoma)	with	– malignant granular cell tumor – metastatic renal cell carcinoma – squamous cell carcinoma
alveolar soft part sarcoma	with	– renal cell carcinoma (metastatic) – clear cell carcinoma – malignant melanoma – pheochromocytoma – paraganglioma – sweat gland carcinoma
synovial sarcoma	with	– fibrosarcoma – benign synovioma – villonodular synovitis – fibromatosis – alveolar rhabdomyosarcoma
epithelioid cell sarcoma	with	– reticulum cell sarcoma – histiocytoma – synovial sarcoma – chronic inflammation

References

[1] Ackerman, L. V., and J. Rosai: Surgical Pathology. Fifth ed. C. V. Mosby Company 1974.

[2] Alguacil-Garcia, A., K. K. Unni, and J. R. Goellner: Malignant giant cell tumor of soft parts. An ultrastructural study of four cases. Cancer 40 (1977) 244-253.

[3] Allen, P. W., and F. M. Enzinger: Hemangioma of skeletal muscle; an analysis of 89 cases. Cancer 29 (1972) 8-22.

[4] Allen, R. A., L. B. Woolner, and R. K. Ghormley: Soft-tissue tumors of the sole; with special reference to plantar fibromatosis. J. Bone Joint Surg. (Am) 37 (1955) 14-26.

[5] Angervall, L., L. G. Kindblom, J. Möller Nielsen, B. Stener, and P. Svendsen: Hemangiopericytoma. A clinicopathologic, angiographic, and microangiographic study. Cancer 42 (1978) 2412-2427.

[6] Appelman, H. D., and E. B. Helwig: Gastric epithelioid leiomyoma and leiomyosarcoma (leiomyoblastoma). Cancer 38 (1976) 708-728.

[7] Auböck, L.: Zur Ultrastruktur fibröser und histiocytärer Hauttumoren (Dermatofibrom, Dermatofibrosarcoma protuberans, Fibroxanthom und Histiocytom). Virchows Arch. A Path. Anat. and Histol. 368 (1975) 253-274.

[8] Autry, J. R., and S. Weitzner: Hemangiosarcoma of spleen with spontaneous rupture. Cancer 35 (1975) 534-539.

[9] Bartlett, R. C., R. D. Otis, and A. O. Laakso: Multiple congenital neoplasms of soft tissues. Report of 4 cases in 1 family. Cancer 14 (1961) 913-920.

[10] Bearman, R. M., J. Noe, and R. L. Kempson: Clear cell sarcoma with melanin pigment. Cancer 36 (1975) 977-984.

[11] Benjamin, S. P. R. D. Mercer, and W. A. Hawk: Myofibroblastic contraction in spontaneous regression of multiple congenital mesenchymal hamartomas. Cancer 40 (1977) 2343-2352.

[12] Berry, C. L., J. Keeling, and C. Hilton: Teratoma in infancy and childhood: A review of 91 cases. J. Pathol. 98 (1969) 241-252.

[13] Braun-Falco, O., C. Schmoeckel und G. Hübner: Zur Histogenese des Sarcoma idiopathicum multiplex haemorrhagicum (M. Kaposi). Eine histochemische und elektronenmikroskopische Studie. Virchows Arch. A Path. Anat. and Histol. 369 (1976) 215-227.

[14] Brenner, W., K. Schaefler, H. Chhabra, and A. Postel: Dermatofibrosarcoma protuberans metastatic to a regional lymph node. Report of a case and review. Cancer 36 (1975) 1897-1902.

[15] Bricklin, A. S., and H. W. Rushton: Angiosarcoma of venous origin arising in radial nerve. Cancer 39 (1977) 1556-1558.

[16] Brines, O. A., and M. H. Johnson: Hibernoma, a special fatty tumor; report of a case. Am. J. Pathol. 25 (1949) 467-479.

[17] Brunner, K. W., und G. A. Nagel: Internistische Krebstherapie. 2. Aufl. Springer, Berlin–Heidelberg–New York 1979.

[18] Chretien, P. B., J. D. Milam, F. W. Foote, and T. R. Miller: Embryonal adenocarcinoma (a type of malignant teratoma) of the sacrococcygeal region; clinical and pathologic aspects of 21 cases. Cancer 26 (1970) 522-535.

[19] Chung, E. B., and F. M. Enzinger: Infantile fibrosarcoma. Cancer 38 (1976) 729-739.

[20] Chung, E. B., and F. M. Enzinger: Chondroma of soft parts. Cancer 41 (1978) 1414-1424.

[21] Churg, A., and J. Ringus: Ultrastructural observations on the histogenesis of alveolar rhabdomyosarcoma. Cancer 41 (1978) 1355 to 1361.

[22] Clarke, B. E., and H. Parsons: An embryological tumor of retinal anlage involving the skull. Cancer 4 (1951) 78-85.

[23] Conklin, J., and M. R. Abell: Germ cell neoplasms of sacrococcygeal region. Cancer 20 (1967) 2105-2117.

[24] Conley, J., W. V. Healey, and A. P. Stout: Fibromatosis of the head and neck. Am. J. Surg. 112 (1966) 609-614.

[25] Dehner, L. P.: Intrarenal teratoma occurring in infancy; report of a case with discussion of extragonadal germ cell tumors in infancy. J. Pediatr. Surg. 8 (1973) 369-378.

[26] Dehner, L. P., and F. M. Enzinger: Fetal rhabdomyoma; an analysis of nine cases. Cancer 30 (1972) 160-166.

[27] Desai, U., C. V. Ramos, and H. B. Taylor: Ultrastructural observations in pleomorphic liposarcoma. Cancer 42 (1978) 1284-1290.

[28] DeVita, V. T. Jr.: In Harrison's „Principles of internal medicine". Eighth Edition. McGraw-Hill Book Company, New York, Düsseldorf etc. 1977.

[29] Döring, L., und J. Graudins: Primäres Hämangioperizytom der Lunge. Thoraxchirurgie 23 (1975) 560-566.

[30] Dold, U. W., und H. Sack: Praktische Tumortherapie. Die Behandlung maligner Organtumoren und Systemerkrankungen. Thieme, Stuttgart 1976.

[31] Donnellan, W. A., and O. Swenson: Benign and malignant sacrococcygeal teratomas. Surgery 64 (1968) 834-846.

[32] Dooling, E. C., J. G. Chi, and F. H. Gilles: Melanotic neuroectodermal tumor of infancy. Its histological similarities to fetal pineal gland. Cancer 39 (1977) 1535-1541.

[33] Drescher, E., S. Woyke, C. Markiewicz, and S. Tegi: Juvenile fibromatosis in siblings (fibromatosis hyalinica multiplex juvenilis). J. Pediatr. Surg. 2 (1967) 427-430.

[34] Dritschilo, A., R. Weichselbaum, J. R. Cassady, N. Jaffe, D. Pead, D. Green, and R. M. Filler: The role of radiation therapy in the treatment of soft tissue sarcomas of childhood. Cancer 42 (1978) 1192-1203.

[35] Dutz, W., and A. P. Stout: Kaposi's sarcoma in infants and children. Cancer *13* (1960) 684-694.

[36] Enterline, H. T., J. D. Culberson, D. B. Rochlin, and L. W. Brady: Liposarcoma – a clinical and pathological study of 53 cases. Cancer *13* (1960) 932-950.

[37] Enzinger, F. M.: Recent trends in soft tissue pathology. In „Tumors of bone and soft tissue". M. D. Anderson Hospital, Houston 1963.

[38] Enzinger, F. M.: Intramuscular myxoma. A review and follow-up study of 34 cases. Am. J. Clin. Pathol. *43* (1965) 104-113.

[39] Enzinger, F. M.: Fibrous hamartoma of infancy. Cancer *18* (1965) 241-248.

[40] Enzinger, F. M.: Clear cell sarcoma of tendons and aponeuroses. An analysis of 21 cases. Cancer *18* (1965) 1163-1174.

[41] Enzinger, F. M.: Fibrous tumors of infancy. In: Tumors of bone and soft tissue. M. D. Anderson Hospital, Houston 1968.

[42] Enzinger, F. M.: Histological typing of soft tissue tumours. WHO, Geneva 1969.

[43] Enzinger, F. M.: Epithelioid sarcoma; a sarcoma simulating a granuloma or a carcinoma. Cancer *26* (1970) 1029-1041.

[44] Enzinger, F. M., and M. Shiraki: Musculo-aponeurotic fibromatosis of the shoulder girdle (extra-abdominal desmoid); analysis of 30 cases followed up for ten or more years. Cancer *20* (1967) 1131-1140.

[45] Enzinger, F. M., and M. Shiraki: Alveolar rhabdomyosarcoma; an analysis of 110 cases. Cancer *24* (1969) 18-31.

[46] Enzinger, F. M., and D. J. Winslow: Liposarcoma; a study of 103 cases. Virchows Arch. *335* (1962) 367-388.

[47] Evans, H. L., E. H. Soule, and R. K. Winkelmann: Atypical lipoma, atypical intramuscular lipoma, and well differentiated retroperitoneal liposarcoma. A reappraisal of 30 cases formerly classified as well differentiated liposarcoma. Cancer *43* (1979) 574-584.

[48] Feldman, P. S.: A comparative study including ultrastructure of intramuscular myxoma and myxoid liposarcoma. Cancer *43* (1979) 512-525.

[49] Feldman, P. S., and M. W. Meyer: Fibroelastic hamartoma (fibroma) of the heart. Cancer *38* (1976) 314-323.

[50] Fernandez C. H., W. W. Sutow, O. R. Merino, and S. L. George: Childhood rhabdomyosarcoma – analysis of coordinated therapy and results. American Journal of Roentgenol. *123* (1975) 588-597.

[51] Fisher, E. R., and H. Reidbord: Electron microscopic evidence suggesting the myogenic derivation of the so-called alveolar soft part sarcoma. Cancer *27* (1971) 150-159.

[51a] Franke, H. D.: Results of clinical applications of fast neutrons at Hamburg-Eppendorf. Eur. J. Cancer (Suppl.) (1979) 51-59.

[52] Frei, E. III, R. Blum, and N. Jaffe: Sarcoma: Natural history and treatment. In: Immunotherapy of cancer: Present status of trials in man; edited by W. D. Terry and D. Windhorst. Raven Press, New York 1978.

[53] Gabbiani, G., and G. Majno: Dupuytren's contracture; fibroblast contraction? An ultrastructural study. Am. J. Pathol. *66* (1972) 131-146.

[54] Ghavimi, F., P. R. Exelby, G. J. D'Angio, W. Cham, P. H. Lieberman, C. Tan, V. Miké, and M. L. Murphy: Multidisciplinary treatment of embryonal rhabdomyosarcoma in children. Cancer *35* (1975) 677-686.

[55] Gillespie, J. J., L. M. Roth, E. R. Wills, L. H. Einhorn, and J. Willman: Extraskeletal Ewing's sarcoma. Histologic and ultrastructural observations in three cases. Am. J. Surg. Path. *3* (1979) 99-108.

[56] Gokel, J. M., R. Kürzel, and G. Hübner: Fine structure and origin of Kaposi's sarcoma. Path. Europ. (Brüssel) *11* (1976) 45-47.

[57] Gonzalez-Crussi, F., and S. Black-Schaffer: Rhabdomyosarcoma of infancy and childhood. Problems of morphologic classification. Am. J. Surg. Path. *3* (1979) 157-171.

[58] Harkin, J. C., and R. J. Reed: Tumors of the peripheral nervous system. Atlas of tumor pathology. A. F. I. P., Washington, D. C. 1969.

[59] Holecek, M. J., and A. R. Harwood: Radiotherapy of Kaposi's sarcoma. Cancer *41* (1978) 1733-1738.

[60] Huber, H., und K. Grünewald: Dacarbazin (DTIC) in der Therapie maligner Erkrankungen. – Eine Übersicht. Wiener klin. Wschr. *90* (1978) 861-864.

[61] Hunt, R. T., H. C. Morgan, and L. V. Ackerman: Principles in the management of extraabdominal desmoids. Cancer *13* (1960) 825-836.

[62] Ireland, D. C. R., E. H. Soule, and J. C. Ivins: Myxoma of soft tissue. A report of 58 patients, 3 with multiple tumors and fibrous dysplasia of bone. Mayo Clinic Proc. *48* (1973) 401 to 410.

[63] Jungi, W. F.: Knochen- und Weichteilsarkome. Schweiz. med. Wschr. *108* (1978) 1350-1355.

[64] Khan, O., and H. H. Nixon: Alveolar soft part sarcoma mimicking a lingual thyroid. A review of the literature and a case report. Z. Kinderchir. *23* (1978) 313-318.

[65] Kim, J. H., E. W. Hahn, N. Tokita, and L. Z. Nisce: Local tumor hyperthermia in combination with radiation therapy. – 1. Malignant cutaneous lesions. Cancer *40* (1977) 161 to 169.

[66] Kindblom, L.-G., and L. Angervall: Congenital solitary fibromatosis of the skeleton. Case report of a variant of congenital generalized fibromatosis. Cancer *41* (1978) 636-640.

[67] Kindblom, L.-G., C. Merck, and L. Angervall: The ultrastructure of myxofibrosarcoma. A study of 11 cases. Virchows Arch. A Path. Anat. and Histol. *381* (1979) 121-139.

[68] King, E. S. J.: Glomus tumour. Australian and New Zealand J. Surg. *23* (1954) 280-295.

[69] Klepp, O., O. Dahl, and J. T. Stenwig: Association of Kaposi's sarcoma and prior immunosuppressive therapy. A 5-year material of Ka-

posi's sarcoma in Norway. Cancer *42* (1978) 2626-2630.

[70] Kohout, E., and A.P. Stout: The glomus tumor in children. Cancer *14* (1961) 555-567.

[71] Koudstaal, J., J. Oldhoff, A.K. Panders, and M.J. Hardonk: Melanotic neuroectodermal tumor of infancy. Cancer *22* (1968) 151 to 161.

[72] Krementz, E.T., R.D. Carter, C.M. Sutherland, and I. Hutton: Chemotherapy of sarcomas of the limbs by regional perfusion. Trans. South. Surg. Assoc. *88* (1977) 63-72.

[73] Kreutner, A., R.M. Smith, and F.A. Trefny: Intravascular papillary endothelial hyperplasia. Light and electron microscopic observations of a case. Cancer *42* (1978) 2304-2310.

[74] Kuo, T.-T., C.P. Sayers, and J. Rosai: Masson's „vegetant intravascular hemangio-endothelioma": A lesion often mistaken for angiosarcoma. Study of seventeen cases located in the skin and soft tissues. Cancer *38* (1976) 1227-1236.

[75] Kyriakos, M., and R.L. Kempson: Inflammatory fibrous histiocytoma. An aggressive and lethal lesion. Cancer *37* (1976) 1584-1606.

[76] Lal, H., B. Sanyal, G.T. Pant, B.L. Rastogi, N.N. Khanna, and K.N. Undupa: Hemangiopericytoma: Report of three cases regarding role of radiation therapy. Am. J. Roentgenol. Radium Ther. Nucl. Med. *126* (1976) 885-891.

[77] Langsam, L.B., G. Fine, and J.L. Ponka: Malignant histiocytomas. Arch. Surg. *113* (1978) 473-476.

[78] Leite, C., J.W. Goodwin, J.G. Sinkovics, L.H. Baker, and R. Benjamen: Chemotherapy of malignant fibrous histiocytoma. A southwest oncology group report. Cancer *40* (1977) 2010-2014.

[79] Leu, H.J., und H. Sulser: Maligner endothelialer Tumor der A. femoralis mit distaler Embolisation. Virchows Arch. A Path. Anat. and Histol. *371* (1976) 153-159.

[80] Limacher, J., C. Delage, and R. Lagacé: Malignant fibrous histiocytoma. Clinicopathologic and ultrastructural study of 12 cases. Amer. J. Surg. Path. *2* (1978) 265-275.

[81] Makk, L., F. Delmore, J.L. Creech Jr., L.L. Ogden, E.H. Fadell, C.L. Songster, J. Clanton, M.M. Johnson, and W.M. Christopherson: Clinical and morphologic features of hepatic angiosarcoma in vinyl chloride workers. Cancer *37* (1976) 149-163.

[82] Maurus, R., and J. Otten: Solid tumors in children. In: Randomized trials in cancer: A critical review by sites, edited by Maurice J. Staquet, Raven Press, New York 1978.

[83] Meister, P., F.-W. Bückmann, and E. Konrad: Nodular fasciitis (analysis of 100 cases and review of the literature). Path. Res. Pract. *162* (1978) 133-165.

[84] Meister, P., and J.M. Gokel: Extraskeletal Ewing's sarcoma. Virchows Arch. A Path. Anat. and Histol. *378* (1978) 173-179.

[85] Mira, J.G., F.C. Chu, and J.G. Fortner: The role of radiotherapy in the management of malignant hemangiopericytoma. Report of eleven new cases and review of the literature. Cancer *39* (1977) 1254-1259.

[86] Monteforte, W.J., Jr., and P.W. Kohnen: Angiomyolipomas in a case of lymphangiomyomatous syndrome: Relationships to tuberous sclerosis. Cancer *34* (1974) 317-321.

[87] Morales, A.R., G. Fine, and R.C. Horn, Jr.: Rhabdomyosarcoma; an ultrastructural appraisal. Pathol. Ann. *7* (1972) 81-106.

[88] Nunez-Alonso, C., E.N. Gashti, and M.L. Christ: Maxillofacial synovial sarcoma. Light- and electron-microscopic study of two cases. Am. J. Surg. Path. *3* (1979) 23-30.

[89] Patchefsky, A.S., R. Soriano, and M. Kostianovsky: Epithelioid sarcoma. Ultrastructural similarity to nodular synovitis. Cancer *39* (1977) 143-152.

[90] Perevodchikova, N.I., M.R. Lichinitser, and V.A. Gorbunova: Phase I clinical study of carminomycin: Its activity against soft tissue sarcomas. Cancer Treat. Rep. *6* (1977) 1705-1707.

[91] Pinedo, H.M., B.A. Chabner, M.G. Nieuwenhuis, and S.A. Rosenberg: Soft tissue sarcoma in adults. In: Randomized trials in cancer: A critical review by sites, edited by Maurice J. Staquet, Raven Press, New York 1978.

[92] Pinedo, H.M., and Y. Kenis: Chemotherapy of advanced soft-tissue sarcomas in adults. Cancer Treatment Reviews *4* (1977) 67-86.

[93] Pinedo, H.M., and P.A. Voûte: Combination chemotherapy in soft tissue sarcomas. In: Recent advances in cancer treatment, edited by H.J. Tagnon and M.J. Staquet. Raven Press, New York 1977.

[94] Prat, J., J.M. Woodruff, and R.C. Marcove: Epithelioid sarcoma. An analysis of 22 cases indicating the prognostic significance of vascular invasion and regional lymph node metastasis. Cancer *41* (1978) 1472-1487.

[95] Ranchod, M., and R.L. Kempson: Smooth muscle tumors of the gastrointestinal tract and retroperitoneum. A pathologic analysis of 100 cases. Cancer *39* (1977) 255-262.

[96] Rao, U., A. Cheng, and M.S. Didolkar: Extraosseous osteogenic sarcoma. Clinicopathological study of eight cases and review of literature. Cancer *41* (1978) 1488-1496.

[97] Reszel, P.A., E.H. Soule, and M.B. Coventry: Liposarcoma of extremities and limb girdles: A study of 222 cases. J. Bone Joint Surg. (Am) *48* (1966) 229-244.

[98] Reye, R.D.K.: A consideration of certain subdermal „fibromatous tumours" of infancy. J. Pathol. Bact. *72* (1956) 149-154.

[99] Reye, R.D.K.: Recurring digital fibrous tumors of childhood. Arch. Pathol. *80* (1965) 228-231.

[100] Reyes, J.W., H. Shinozuka, P. Garry, and P.B. Putong: A light and electron microscopic study of a hemangiopericytoma of the prostate with local extension. Cancer *40* (1977) 1122-1126.

[101] Russell, W.O., J. Cohen, F. Enzinger, S.I. Hajdu, H. Heise, R.G. Martin, W. Meissner, W.T. Miller, R.L. Schmitz, and H.D. Suit:

A clinical and pathological staging system for soft tissue sarcomas. Cancer *40* (1977) 1562 to 1570.

[102] Salyer, W. R., and D. C. Salyer: Intravascular angiomatosis: Development and distinction from angiosarcoma. Cancer *36* (1975) 995-1001.

[103] Schmidt, M., C.-P. Sodomann, C. Gropp und K. Havemann: Behandlung metastasierender Weichteilsarkome mit einer einheitlichen Polychemotherapie aus Cyclophosphamid, Vincristin, Adriamycin und DTIC (CyVADIC). Dtsch. med. Wschr. *103* (1978) 1206-1210.

[104] Shiu, M. H., P. M. McCormack, S. I. Hajdu, and J. G. Fortner: Surgical treatment of tendosynovial sarcoma. Cancer *43* (1979) 889-897.

[105] Soule, E. H., and P. Enriquez: Atypical fibrous histiocytoma, malignant fibrous histiocytoma and epithelioid sarcoma; a comparative study of 65 tumors. Cancer *30* (1972) 128-143.

[106] Soule, E. H., and D. J. Pritchard: Fibrosarcoma in infants and children. Cancer *40* (1977) 1711-1721.

[107] Stout, A. P.: Tumors of the neuromyo-arterial glomus. Am. J. Cancer *24* (1935) 255-272.

[108] Stout, A. P., and W. T. Hill: Leiomyosarcoma of the superficial soft tissues. Cancer *11* (1958) 844-854.

[109] Stout, A. P., and R. Lattes: Soft tissue tumors. „Atlas of tumor pathology." A. F. I. P., Washington, D. C. 1967.

[110] Strong, E. W., R. W. McDivitt, and R. D. Brasfield: Granular cell myoblastoma. Cancer *25* (1970) 415-422.

[111] Subramanian, S., and E. Wiltshaw: Chemotherapy of sarcoma. A comparison of three regimens. Lancet *1* (1978) 683-686.

[112] Suit, H. D., and W. O. Russell: Soft part tumors. Cancer *39* (1977) 830-836.

[113] Suit, H. D., R. G. Martin, and W. W. Sutow: Primary malignant tumors of the bone. In: Clinical pediatric oncology. Mosby, St. Louis 1973.

[114] Suit, H. D., W. O. Russell, and R. G. Martin: Sarcoma of soft tissue: Clinical and histopathologic parameters and response to treatment. Cancer *35* (1975) 1478-1483.

[115] Sulser, H.: Das Rhabdomyosarkom. Alters- und Geschlechtsverteilung, Lokalisation, pathologische Anatomie und Prognose. Virchows Arch. A Path. Anat. and Histol. *379* (1978) 35-71.

[116] Taxy, J. B., and H. Battifora: Malignant fibrous histiocytoma. An electron microscopic study. Cancer *40* (1977) 254-267.

[117] Taylor, H. B., and E. B. Helwig: Dermatofibrosarcoma protuberans; a study of 115 cases. Cancer *15* (1962) 717-725.

[118] Tefft, M., C. H. Fernandez, and T. E. Moon: Rhabdomyosarcoma: Response with chemotherapy prior to radiation in patients with gross residual disease. Cancer *39* (1977) 665-670.

[119] Tisell L.-E., L. Angervall, I. Dahl, C. Merck, and B. F. Zachrisson: Recurrent and metastasizing gastric leiomyoblastoma (epithelioid leiomyosarcoma) associated with multiple pulmonary chondro-hamartomas. Long survival of a patient treated with repeated operations. Cancer *41* (1978) 259-265.

[120] Tsuneyoshi, M., M. Enjoji, and T. Kubo: Clear cell sarcoma of tendons and aponeuroses. A comparative study of 13 cases with a provisional subgrouping into the melanotic and synovial types. Cancer *42* (1978) 243-252.

[121] Van Andel, J. G.: Synovial sarcoma; a review and analysis of treated cases. Radiol. Clin. Biol. *41* (1972) 145-159.

[122] Van Der Werf-Messing, B., and J. A. M. van Unnik: Fibrosarcoma of the soft tissues, a clinicopathologic study. Cancer *18* (1965) 1113-1123.

[123] Vellios, F., M. J. Baez, and H. B. Shumacker: Lipoblastomatosis: A tumor of fetal fat different from hibernoma. Report of a case, with observations on the embryogenesis of human adipose tissue. Am. J. Pathol. *34* (1958) 1149-1155.

[124] Vogel, C. L., C. J. Templeton, A. C. Templeton, J. F. Taylor, and S. K. Kyalwazi: Treatment of Kaposi's sarcoma with actinomycin-D and cyclophosphamide: Results of a randomized clinical trial. Int. J. Cancer *8* (1971) 136-143.

[125] Walter, P., and M. Guerbaoui: Rhabdomyome foetal. Etude histologique et ultrastructurale d'une nouvelle observation. Virchows Arch. A Path. Anat. and Histol. *371* (1976) 59-67.

[126] Weiss, S. W., F. M. Enzinger, and F. B. Johnson: Silica reaction simulating fibrous histiocytoma. Cancer *42* (1978) 2738-2743.

[127] Wilbur, J. R.: Sarcomas. In: Clinical cancer chemotherapy, edited by E. M. Greenspan. Raven Press, New York 1975.

[128] Wild, R. M., C. J. Devine, and C. E. Horton: Dermal graft repair of Peyronie's disease: Survey of 50 patients. J. Urol. *121* (1979) 47-50.

[129] Willis, R. A.: Pathology of tumors. Ed. 4. – Butterworth & Co., Ltd. London 1968.

[130] Wirman, J. A.: Nodular fasciitis, a lesion of myofibroblasts. An ultrastructural study. Cancer *38* (1976) 2378-2389.

[131] Wirth, W. A., D. Leavitt, and F. M. Enzinger: Multiple intramuscular myxomas; another extraskeletal manifestation of fibrous dysplasia. Cancer *27* (1971) 1167-1173.

[132] Wobbes, T.: Alveolar soft part sarcoma. J. Surg. Oncol. *10* (1978) 201-204.

[133] Wong, P. P., and A. Yagoda: Chemotherapy of malignant hemangiopericytoma. Cancer *41* (1978) 1256-1260.

[134] Woodward, A. H., J. C. Ivins, and E. H. Soule: Lymphangiosarcoma arising in chronic lymphedematous extremity. Cancer *30* (1972) 562-572.

[135] Woyke, S., W. Domagala, and W. Olszewski: Ultrastructure of a fibromatosis hyalinica multiplex juvenilis. Cancer *26* (1970) 1157 to 1168.

2 Tumors of the retroperitoneum

M-4900/0
T 158.9

1. Idiopathic retroperitoneal fibrosis
(Ormond's disease, periureteric fibrosis)

**General
Remarks**

Incidence: Idiopathic retroperitoneal fibrosis is a rare tumor-like lesion.
Site: The lesion develops in the midline of the retroperitoneum.

Macroscopy

Hard, whitish mass in the retroperitoneum.

Histology

The lesion contains collagen fibers with fibroblasts (Figs. 148 and 149). They show numerous mitotic figures. The nuclei are regular. Between the collagen fibers and the surrounding blood vessels there are eosinophils, plasma cells, and lymphocytes (Figs. 150 and 151). There are germinal centers.

**Differential
Diagnosis**

Idiopathic retroperitoneal fibrosis **with metastatic carcinoma inducing strong sclerosis** (adenocarcinoma, signet ring cell carcinoma, occasionally malignant lymphoma).

Idiopathic retroperitoneal fibrosis with

M-7610/0
T 158.9

2. Fibromatosis
The fibromatosis contains fibroblasts without inflammatory cells.

Idiopathic retroperitoneal fibrosis with

M-8810/3
T 158.9

3. Fibrosarcoma (Figs. 21 to 25)
Fibrosarcomas contain nuclei with signs of malignancy. However, fibrosarcomas are exceedingly rare in the retroperitoneum.

Idiopathic retroperitoneal fibrosis with

M-8830/0
T 158.9

4. Fibrous histiocytoma (Fig. 29)
(retroperitoneal xanthogranuloma – WHO):

The fibrous histiocytoma (xanthogranuloma) contains fibroblasts, collagen fibers, inflammatory cells, and histiocytes with a foamy cytoplasm.
Fibrous histiocytoma of the retroperitoneum occurs more frequently than idiopathic retroperitoneal fibrosis. Occasionally the fibrous histiocytoma may contain malignant cells:

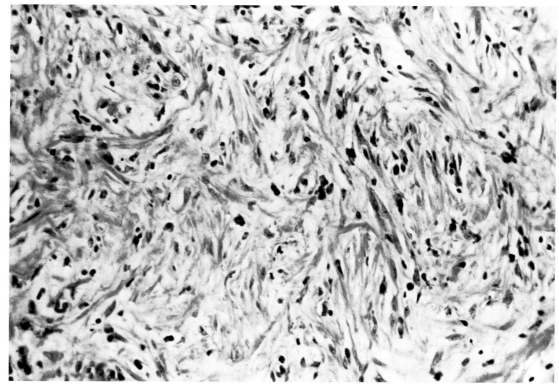

Fig. 148. Idiopathic retroperitoneal fibrosis: Regular fibroblasts, numerous collagen fibers in loose arrangement, some inflammatory cells (37-year-old male, × 200).

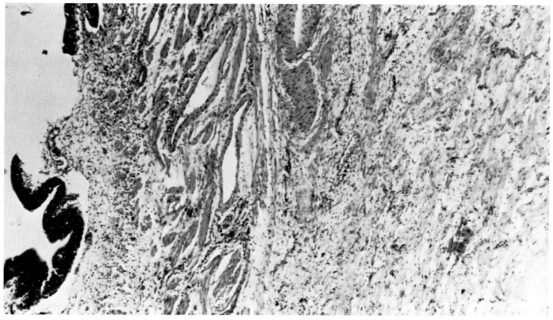

Fig. 149. Idiopathic retroperitoneal fibrosis in the wall of the ureter (37-year-old male, × 40).

149

M-8830/3
T 158.9

5. Malignant fibrous histiocytoma
(malignant fibroxanthosarcoma) (Figs. 45 to 48)

**Clinical
Findings**

Idiopathic retroperitoneal fibrosis induces progressive renal failure due to the final obliteration of the ureter.

Roentgenogram

Medial displacement of the ureters.

Treatment

Surgical intervention.

Prognosis

In the individual case the prognosis depends on the extension of the fibrosis.

**Further
Information**

1. The retroperitoneal fibrosis can be associated with similar lesions at other sites: sclerosing cholangitis, fibrosis in the mediastinum, fibrosis in the orbit, Riedl's thyroiditis [4].
2. There is one case reported in which the fibrosis extended into the brain [9].
3. Very rarely retroperitoneal fibrohistiocytic tumors have been observed in children [5].

M-8850/3
T 158.9

6. Liposarcoma

Liposarcomas in the retroperitoneum can be extremely large. Liposarcoma is the most frequently observed malignant soft tissue tumor of the retroperitoneal space [1, 8].

[1] Binder et al. 1978.
[4] Comings et al. 1967.
[5] Cozzutto et al. 1978.
[8] Evans et al. 1979.
[9] Mende et al. 1974.

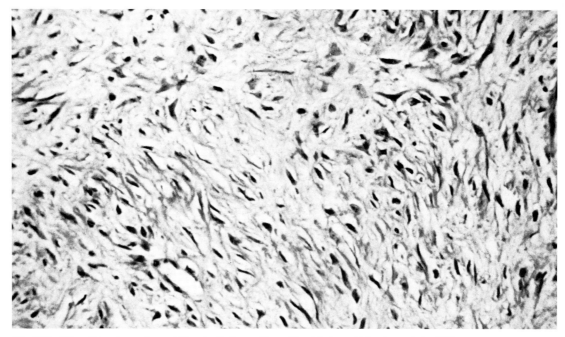

Fig. 150. Idiopathic retroperitoneal fibrosis: Collagen fibers, fibroblasts, and blood vessels (×200).

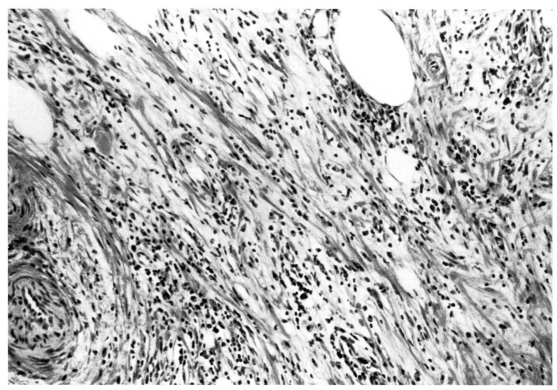

Fig. 151. Idiopathic retroperitoneal fibrosis: Inflammatory cells, collagen fibers, fibroblasts, and blood vessels (37-year-old male, ×125).

M-8890/3
T 158.9

7. Leiomyosarcoma

This is a very malignant tumor with a 2-year survival rate of about 16% [10]. Leiomyosarcomas are the second most frequent malignant soft tissue tumor in the retroperitoneum.

M-8810/3
T 158.9

8. Fibrosarcoma

Occasionally fibrosarcomas, which are exceedingly rare in the retroperitoneum, and leiomyosarcomas can produce insulin-like substances causing hypoglycemia (see Paraneoplastic syndromes, page 424).

M-8900/3
T 158.9

9. Rhabdomyosarcoma

Rhabdomyosarcomas in the retroperitoneal space have an extremely poor prognosis. In most instances the embryonal type of rhabdomyosarcoma occurs in this location.

M-8840/1
T 158.9

10. Myxoma

Myxomas in the retroperitoneum are very rare.

M-8850/0
T 158.9

11. Lipoma

Lipomas are rare in the retroperitoneum.

---

[10] Ranchod and Kempson 1977.

M-8890/0
T 158.9

12. Leiomyoma

Leiomyomas are exceedingly rare in the retroperitoneum.

M-9170/0
T 158.9

13. Lymphangioma

Lymphangiomas in the retroperitoneal space can form small or large cysts. The lymphangiomas are benign tumors.

M-9120/0, 3
T 158.9

14. Angioma and angiosarcoma

These vascular tumors occur very rarely in the retroperitoneum.

M-9540/0
M-9560/0, 3
T 158.9

15. Tumors of peripheral nerves
(neurofibroma, neurilemmoma, malignant neurilemmoma)

These malignant tumors are exceedingly rare in this location.

M-9490/0, 1
M-9500/3
M-8680/1
T-158.9

16. Ganglioneuroma, ganglioneuroblastoma, neuroblastoma, paraganglioma

About 10% of these tumors grow in the retroperitoneal space (see Tumors of the adrenal gland, page 1792).

17. Tumor of the "renal anlage"

Very rarely tumors are observed originating from the renal anlage.
Other tumors can arise from heterotopic adrenal cortical cells.

M-9080/1
T 158.9

18. Benign teratoma

General Remarks

Incidence: Benign teratomas in this location are rare.
Sex: Cystic teratomas are observed mainly in females.
Site: The teratomas are located between the rectum and the sacrum.

Macroscopy

The tumor can be very large and has multiple cysts with hairs and calcifications.

Histology

Teratomas are composed of mature epithelial and mesenchymal cells in an organoid growth pattern (see Figs. 152 to 162).

Treatment

The tumor can be removed surgically, which means cure for the patient [7].

Further Information

1. See Soft tissue tumors, page 130.
2. There is a report of a retroperitoneal teratoma containing elements of a renal cell carcinoma and a Wilms' tumor [2].

M-9080/3
T 158.9

3. **Malignant teratomas** are very rare in the retroperitoneal space: seminomas, embryonal carcinomas, yolk sac tumors [6, 11], choriocarcinoma (Fig. 163).

[2] Carney 1975.
[6] Das et al. 1975.
[7] Engel et al. 1978.
[11] Veraguth et al. 1970.

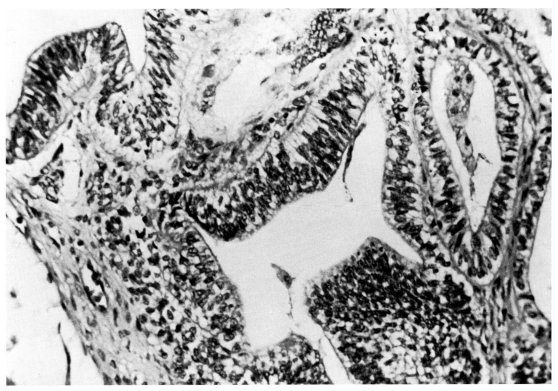

Fig. 152. Benign teratoma: Cysts lined by different layers of different epithelial cells (2-month-old female, × 310).

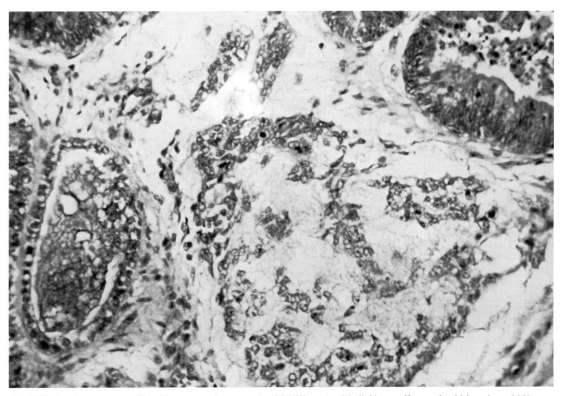

Fig. 153. Benign teratoma: Primitive mesenchyma, cysts with different epithelial layers (2-month-old female, × 200).

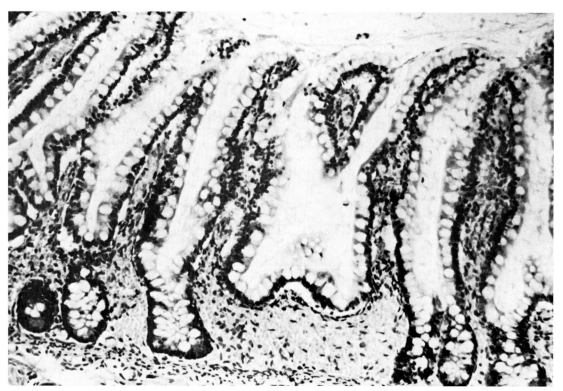

Fig. 154. Benign teratoma: Wall of cyst with colonic-like cell lining (17-day-old female, × 310).

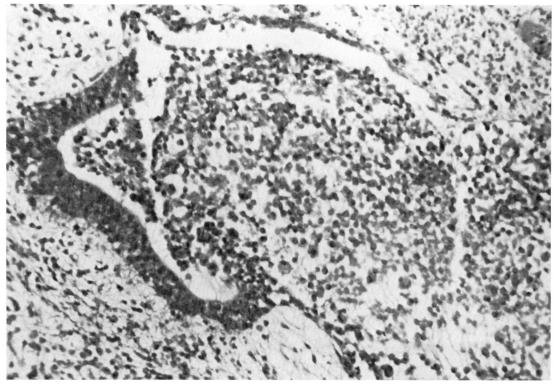

Fig. 155. Benign teratoma: Neuroectodermal tissue component; sacrococcygeal region (2-month-old female, × 200).

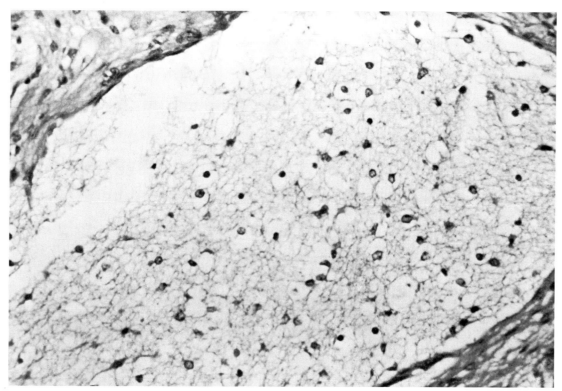

Fig. 156. Benign teratoma: Neural tissue (2-month-old female, × 200).

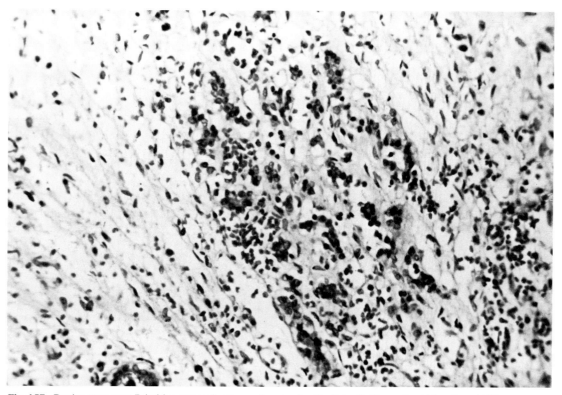

Fig. 157. Benign teratoma: Primitive mesenchyma, small nests of epithelial cells (2-month-old female, × 125).

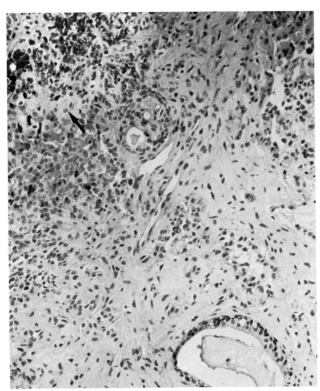

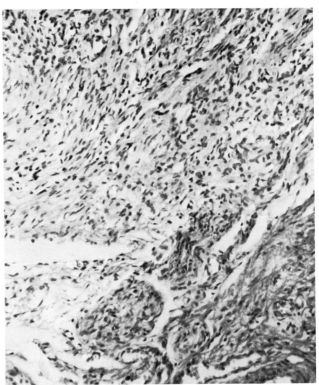

Fig. 158. Benign teratoma: Several cysts, neuroectodermal tissue (arrow) (22-year-old male, × 125).

Fig. 159. Benign teratoma: Connective tissue and small areas of primitive mesenchyma, nerve fibers (17-day-old female, × 125).

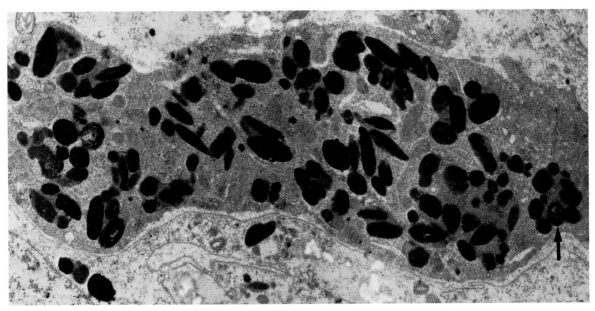

Fig. 160.

Figs. 160 and 161. Retroperitoneal neuroectodermal tumor (retinal anlage): Tumor cells with numerous melanosomes, mostly containing pigment (Fig. 160, × 13,000; Fig. 161, × 75,800).

158

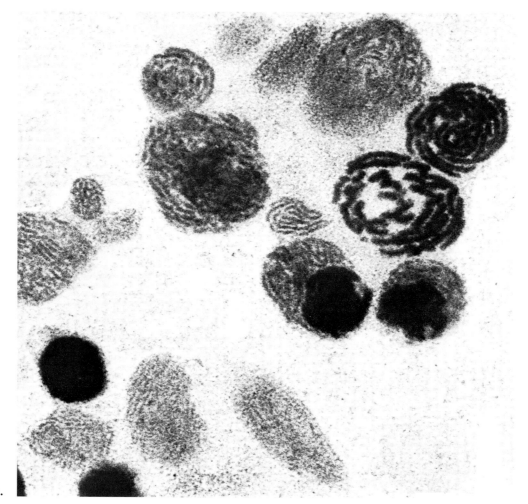

Fig. 161.

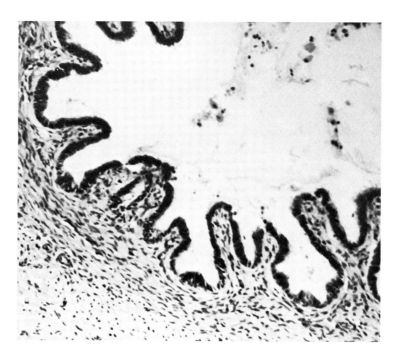

Fig. 162. Benign teratoma: Cyst lined by respiratory epithelium (17-day-old female, × 125).

159

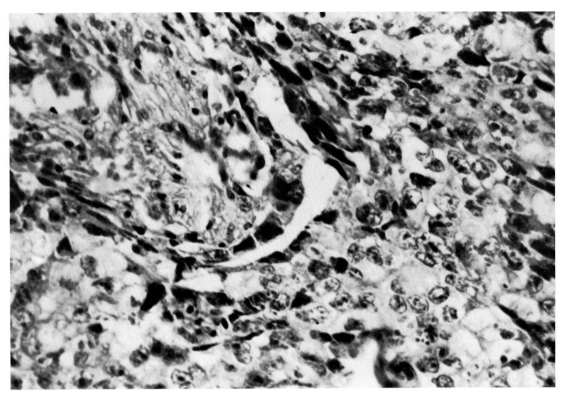

Fig. 163. Choriocarcinoma of the retroperitoneum (19-year-old male, × 310).

M-9370/3, 1
T 158.9

19. Chordoma

Very rarely chordomas can grow in the retroperitoneal space (see Tumors of the bone) (Figs. 1062 to 1066).

M-4318/0
T 158.9

20. Malakoplakia [3]
(Figs. 1396 to 1398)

M-8000/3
T 158.9

21. Unclassifiable tumors
(Fig. 164 a, b)

---

[3] Colby 1978.

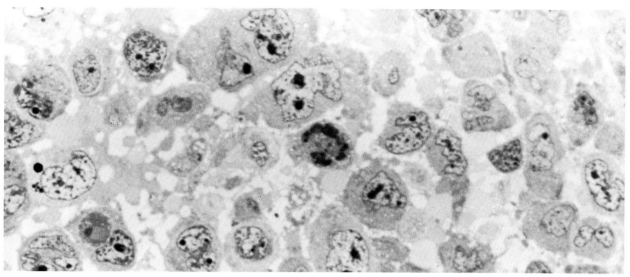

Fig. 164 a.

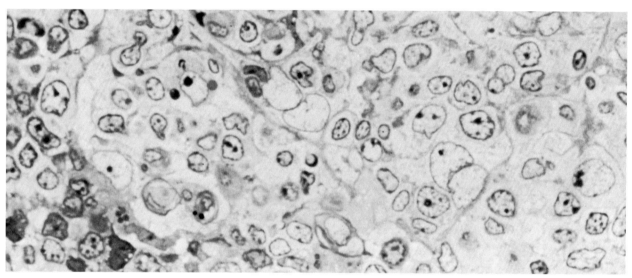

Fig. 164 b.

Fig. 164 a, b. Two types of unclassifiable retroperitoneal malignant soft tissue tumors (30- and 31-year-old males, × 400).

References

[1] Binder, S., B. Katz, and B. Sheridan: Retroperitoneal liposarcoma. Ann. Surg. *187* (1978) 257-261.

[2] Carney, J.A.: Wilms' tumor and renal cell carcinoma in retroperitoneal teratoma. Cancer *35* (1975) 1179-1183.

[3] Colby, T.V.: Malakoplakia. Two unusual cases which presented diagnostic problems. Am. J. Surg. Path. *2* (1978) 377-382.

[4] Comings, D.E., K.B. Skubi, J. van Eyes, and A.G. Motulsky: Familial multifocal fibro-sclerosis; findings suggesting that retroperitoneal fibrosis, mediastinal fibrosis, sclerosing cholangitis, Riedl's thyroiditis and pseudo-tumor of the orbit may be different manifestations of a single disease. Ann. Int. Med. *66* (1967) 884-892.

[5] Cozzutto, C., B. de Bernardi, M. Guarino, A. Comelli, and F. Soave: Retroperitoneal fibrohistiocytic tumors in children. Report of five cases. Cancer *42* (1978) 1350-1363.

[6] Das, S., J.R. Bochetto, and L.I. Alpert: Primary retroperitoneal seminoma. Report of a case and review of the literature. Cancer *36* (1975) 595-598.

[7] Engel, R.M., R.C. Elkins, and B.D. Fletcher: Retroperitoneal teratoma; review of the literature and presentation of an unusual case. Cancer *22* (1968) 1068-1073.

[8] Evans, H.L., E.H. Soule, and R.K. Winkelmann: Atypical lipoma, atypical intramuscular lipoma, and well differentiated retroperitoneal liposarcoma. A reappraisal of 30 cases formerly classified as well differentiated liposarcoma. Cancer *43* (1979) 574-584.

[9] Mende, S., M. Völpel, and I. Rotthauwe: Idiopathic retroperitoneal fibrosis (Ormond's disease) with unusual extension involving the brain. Beitr. Path. *153* (1974) 80-90.

[10] Ranchod, M., and R.L. Kempson: Smooth muscle tumors of the gastrointestinal tract and retroperitoneum. A pathologic analysis of 100 cases. Cancer *39* (1977) 255-262.

[11] Veraguth, P., G.-F. Maillard, and W. MacGee: Retroperitoneal seminomas without evidence of primary growth. Oncology *24* (1970) 193-209.

3 Tumors of peripheral nerves

M-9560/0

1. Neurinoma
(schwannoma, neurilemoma) (WHO)

General Remarks

Incidence: Neurinomas are relatively common tumors, originating from Schwann's cells.

Age: The tumors are observed mainly in adults.

Sex: Males and females are affected equally; however, intracranial schwannomas are seen more often in females.

Site: Neurinomas can develop intracranially (mainly in the cerebellopontine angle) and at other sites such as the neck, mediastinum, flexor surfaces of the extremities, retroperitoneum, posterior spinal roots, and stomach.

Further notes: Neurinomas can be solitary tumors or may be associated with neurofibromatosis.

Macroscopy

Schwannomas are firm tumors. The tumor is well separated from the surrounding tissue and is encapsulated.

The tumor can be small or large; schwannomas are sometimes spheroidal and sometimes lobulated. The cut surface is gray. Occasionally there are thick-walled blood vessels. There are areas of cyst formation or of bleeding.

Occasionally the nerve can be seen at the periphery of the neurinoma.

Histology

The tumor is composed of spindle-shaped cells, which are thin and have tapering ends (Fig. 165). The cytoplasm is pale. There are numerous reticulin fibers surrounding each cell.

The growth pattern of these cells can be subdivided into two types:

a) Antony type A

This growth pattern is characterized by a rather high cellularity; the tumor cells grow in a palisading pattern (Verocay bodies) (Fig. 165).

b) Antony type B

This type of growth pattern is characterized by an edematous, mucinous substance with few cells. Regressive changes with cyst formation can be observed (Fig. 166).

Both types can grow in one tumor, and they are well demarcated from each other (Fig. 167).

Occasionally neurinomas contain numerous blood vessels (Fig. 168).

Electron Microscopy

The tumor cells contain electron-dense basement membrane material, which can cover the surface of the cells [2, 5]. The Antony B-cell contains many mitochondria and lysosomes.

---

[2] Cervós-Navarro et al. 1968.
[5] Mennemeyer et al. 1979.

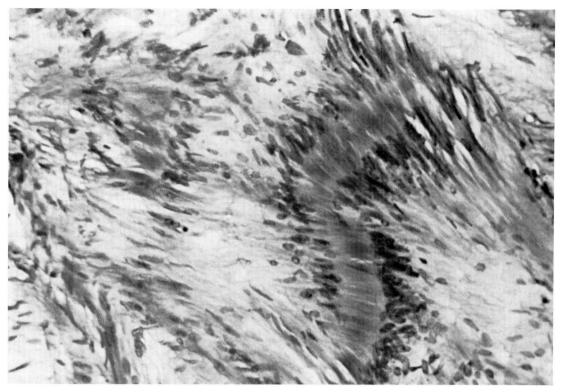

Fig. 165. Neurinoma: Verocay body in Antony type A (× 200).

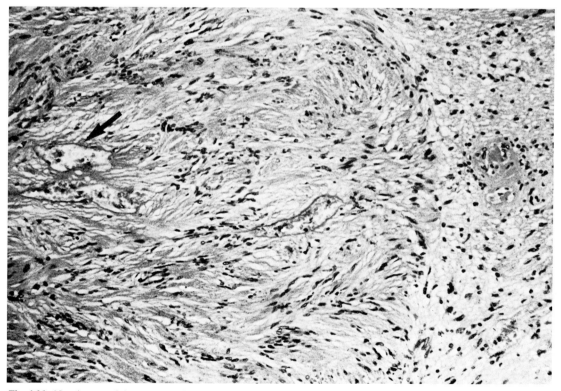

Fig. 166. Neurinoma of Antony type B growth: Beginning cyst formation (arrow) (29-year-old male, von Recklinghausen's disease, × 125).

Neurinoma

Differential Diagnosis

1. Neurinoma **with hemangioma:**
   Occasionally neurinomas contain multiple blood vessels, mimicking a hemangioma.
2. Neurinoma **with leiomyoma:**
   The cells of a leiomyoma have a more abundant cytoplasm. However, the palisading of nuclei is observed at least as frequently as in neurinomas.

Clinical Findings

The symptoms are determined by the size and site of the tumor. Small neurinomas are asymptomatic.
Larger neurinomas can cause pain.
Schwannomas are movable.

Treatment

Surgical removal.

Prognosis

If the neurinoma can be removed surgically the patient is cured; recurrences are rare.
When the neurinoma is removed the nerve of origin should be preserved (if possible).
In the individual case the prognosis is also determined by the site of the tumor (for instance, intracranial neurinomas).
Neurinomas can be part of von Recklinghausen's disease:
In these instances the neurinoma is associated with pigmented skin lesions (café au lait spots) or neurofibromas.

Further Information

Very rarely a primary cardiac neurilemoma can occur [3].

---

[3] Factor et al. 1976.

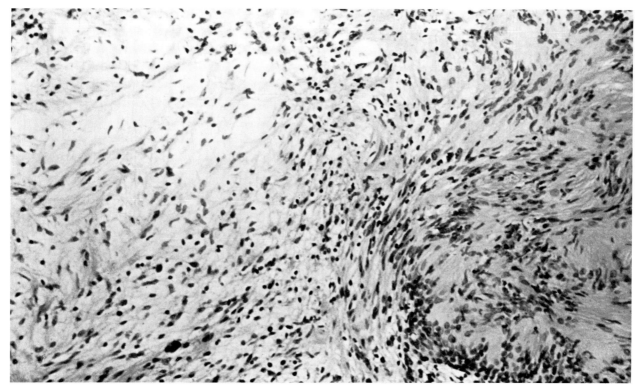

Fig. 167. Neurinoma composed of Antony type A and B pattern (49-year-old female, × 125).

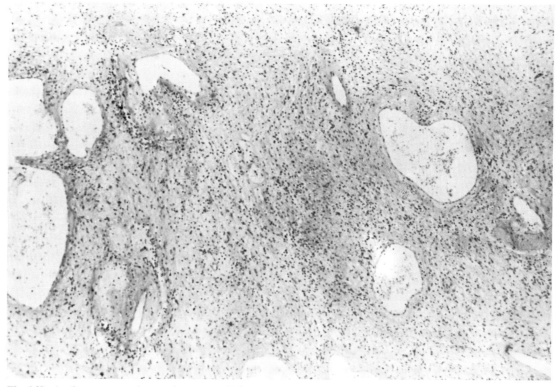

Fig. 168. Angiomatous neurinoma, Antony type B (58-year-old female, × 50).

M-9560/3

2. Malignant schwannoma (WHO)

(malignant neurinoma, malignant neurilemoma, neurofibrosarcoma, neurogenic sarcoma)

**General
Remarks**

Incidence: Malignant schwannomas are rare.
Age: Most of these tumors occur in adults.
Site: The tumor is observed usually in the neck, the buttock, and the forearm.
Further notes: Von Recklinghausen's disease can be complicated by malignant schwannomas [9].

Macroscopy

Malignant neurinomas are large tumors, which may be firm or soft. The cut surface is grayish-whitish with a fleshy appearance.

Histology

The tumor is composed of malignant cells with nuclear atypias. The cells are spindle-shaped. They are surrounded by reticulin fibers. The cells and fibers form interlacing bundles (Figs. 169 to 173).
Giant cells can be observed. The tumor is very similar to fibrosarcoma (Figs. 174 and 175).

**Differential
Diagnosis**

Malignant schwannoma **with other sarcomas:**
The distinction between fibrosarcoma and malignant schwannoma is particularly difficult (Figs. 21 to 25).
The diagnosis of malignant schwannoma should only be accepted when the site of origin (possibly in association with a benign schwannoma) can be demonstrated. The diagnosis of malignant schwannoma can also be accepted in cases of von Recklinghausen's disease [1, 4, 9].

Spread

Early hematogenous metastases.

**Clinical
Findings**

Signs of a rapidly growing malignant tumor with local symptoms according to the size and the site of the tumor.

Treatment

Radical **surgery.**

Prognosis

Malignant schwannomas are very malignant tumors.
Recurrences and distant metastases are observed frequently. The 5-year survival rate for Stages I to IV tumors (see page 11) is approximately 10 to 20%.

**Further
Information**

Rare malignant tumors that are postulated to arise from Schwann's cells:

malignant epithelioid schwannoma [4],

malignant melanocytic schwannoma [4],

**M-8810/3
T 171.9**

nerve sheath fibrosarcoma,

**M-8990/3
T 171.9**

malignant mesenchymoma of nerve sheath origin.

---

[1] Ackerman and Rosai 1974.
[4] Harkin and Reed 1969.
[9] Russell and Rubinstein 1977.

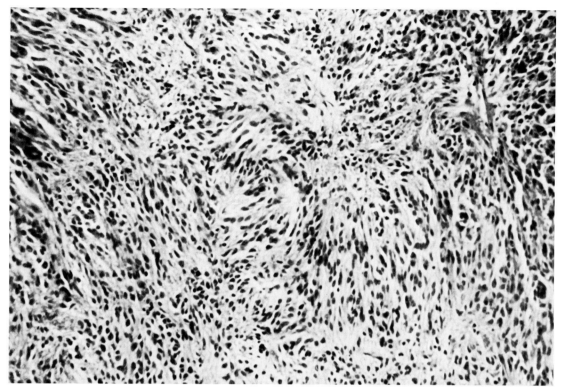

Fig. 169. Malignant schwannoma: Pleomorphic cells with organoid growth pattern (× 125).

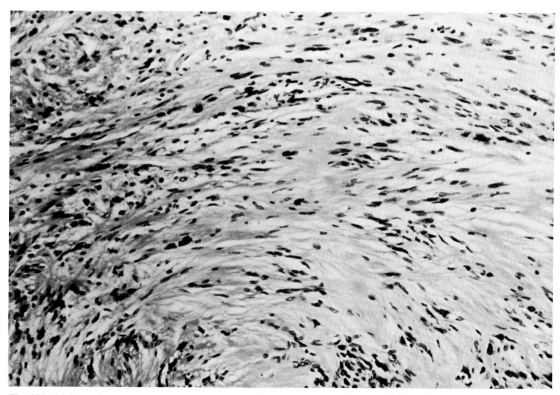

Fig. 170. Malignant schwannoma: Remnants of organoid growth pattern, pleomorphic hyperchromatic nuclei (× 125).

169

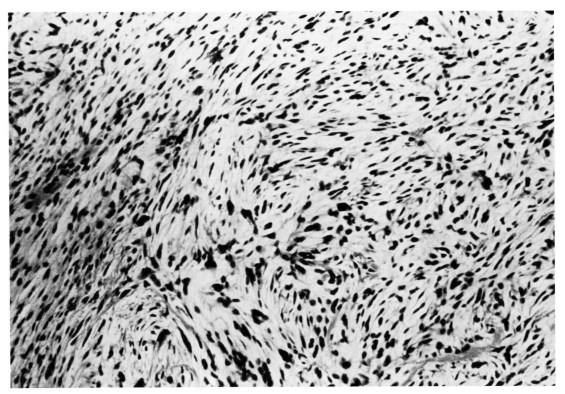

Fig 171. Malignant schwannoma: Hyperchromatic malignant tumor cells growing in an organoid (remnants of Antony A type) growth pattern (68-year-old male, × 125).

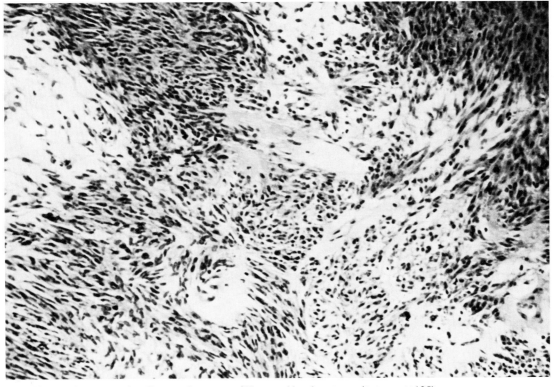

Fig. 172. Another aspect of malignant schwannoma (83-year-old male, retroperitoneum, × 125).

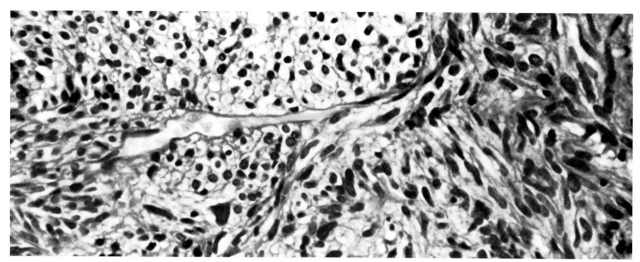

Fig. 173. Malignant schwannoma: Another aspect of organoid growth pattern of malignant cells (83-year-old male, retroperitoneum, × 310).

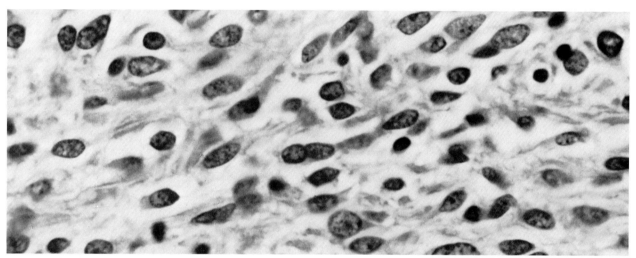

Fig. 174. Malignant schwannoma: Atypical cells similar to those observed in fibrosarcoma (× 600).

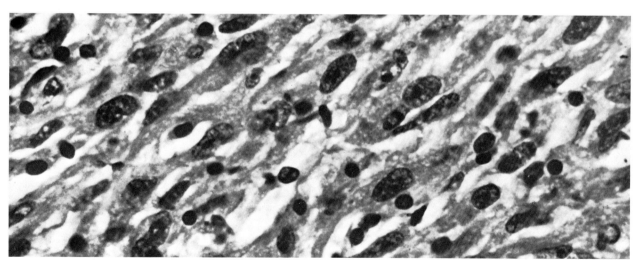

Fig. 175. Pleomorphic malignant tumor cells of a malignant schwannoma (× 600).

M-9540/0

3. Neurofibroma (WHO)

Macroscopy

Neurofibromas are soft tumors that are not encapsulated. The cut surface is grayish.

The neurofibromas in a superficial position are rather small, whereas those in the deeper areas can become large.

Often the nerve of origin enters the tumor.

Histology

The tumor is composed of collagen fibers and Schwann's cells. The collagen fibers form an irregular growth pattern (Figs. 176 and 177). They are embedded in a matrix that stains positive with PAS. The tumor contains numerous reticulin fibers.

The Schwann's cells are numerous. They contain spindle-shaped nuclei, which have tapering ends.

The neurofibroma might contain numerous areas of myxoid degeneration (differential diagnosis with myxoma) (Fig. 178).

Besides the structures of neurofibroma, occasionally fields of a neurinoma can be found with zones of the Antony A type (Fig. 179).

Differential Diagnosis

1. Neurofibroma **with neurinoma:**
    a) Neurofibromas very rarely contain Verocay bodies.
    b) Neurofibromas are not encapsulated (neurinomas are encapsulated).
    c) The ground substance in neurofibromas stains positive with PAS.
2. Neurofibroma **with myxoma.**

Clinical Findings

Local symptoms are determined by the size and site of the tumor.

In most instances neurofibromas occur as part of von Recklinghausen's disease.

A neurofibroma that is not linked with von Recklinghausen's disease is designated "solitary neurofibroma."

Treatment

Surgical excision.

Prognosis

Excellent.

Further Information

It is probable that the neurofibromas originate from Schwann's cells [6-8].

[6] Pineda 1966.
[7] Poirier et Escourolle 1967.
[8] Poirier et al. 1968.

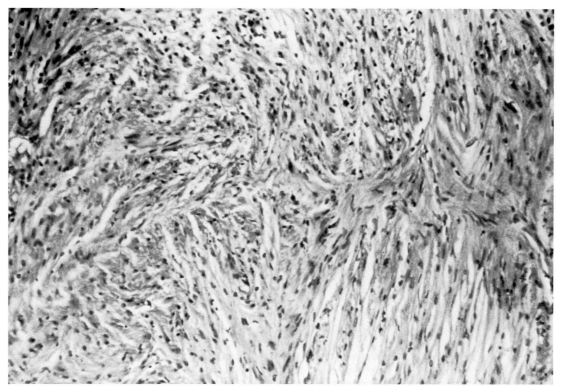

Fig. 176. Neurofibroma in plexiform arrangement with collagen bundles (36-year-old male, von Recklinghausen's disease, × 125).

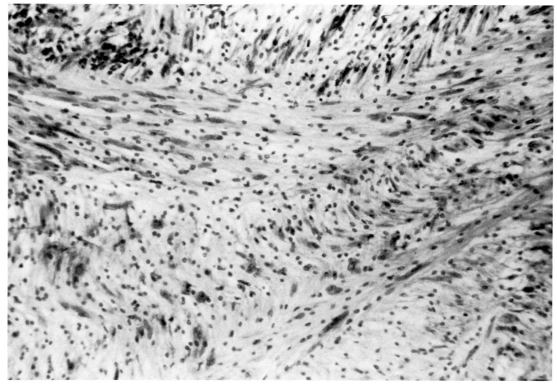

Fig. 177. Cellular neurofibroma in von Recklinghausen's disease (36-year-old male, × 125).

M-9550/1

4. Neurofibromatosis
(von Recklinghausen's disease) (WHO)

Von Recklinghausen's neurofibromatosis is an inherited dominant disease.

The neurofibromatosis can be observed as a forme fruste, which might be so mild that it remains unrecognized clinically.

On the other hand, the presence of several neurofibromas are not necessarily an indication of this hereditary disease.

Numerous tumors other than neurofibromas are observed in von Recklinghausen's disease:

schwannomas, malignant schwannomas, lipomas, meningiomas, pheochromocytomas, ganglioneuromas, medullary carcinomas of the thyroid [1], Wilm's tumors [10], non-ossifying fibromas [4], gliomas, and plexiform neurofibromas.

M-9363/0

5. Melanotic neuroectodermal tumor
(neurocutaneous melanosis syndrome) (WHO)

This benign lesion is observed mainly in children and infants. The disease is congenital but not inherited.

The lesion consists of a combination of giant pigmented nevi of the skin and melanosis of the leptomeninges.

Part of this disease can be the development of malignant melanomas in the brain.

Other cutaneous tumors are blue nevus, cellular blue nevus, and neurofibromas [4].

This tumor might be of a neural crest origin, inasmuch as it can be composed of neuroid structures, cartilage, and melanotic cells [11].

The melanotic neuroectodermal tumor might also be related to von Recklinghausen's disease. (See also Brain tumors and Soft tissue tumors.)

[1] Ackerman and Rosai 1974.
[4] Harkin and Reed 1969.
[10] Stay and Vawter 1977.
[11] Wahlström and Saxén 1976.

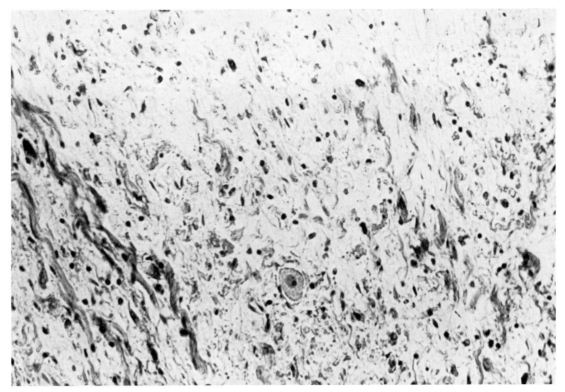

Fig. 178. Neurofibroma: Loose collagen fibers, Schwann's cells, one ganglion cell (× 125).

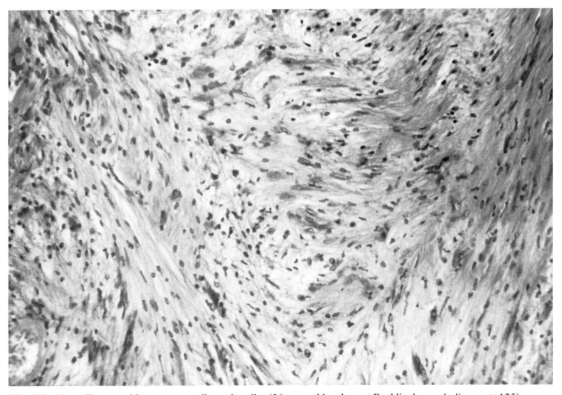

Fig. 179. Neurofibroma with numerous collagen bundles (36-year-old male, von Recklinghausen's disease, × 125).

M-4977/0
(M-9571/0)

6. Traumatic neuroma (WHO)
(amputation neuroma)

Macroscopy

Traumatic neuromas are hard lesions, resembling scar tissue. Often they are encapsulated.

The tumor is of a traumatic origin. The neuroma tissue therefore grows at the site of the traumatic lesion (or amputated nerve).

Histology

Neuromas are composed of tissue that starts growing after a traumatic lesion: collagen fibers, Schwann's cells, and nerve fibers (Fig. 180).

The nerve fibers grow in irregular formations and are embedded in the scar tissue (Fig. 181).

Clinical Findings

Often painful, tumor-like lesion.

Treatment

Surgery.

Further Information

Morton's neuroma:

This neuroma also shows collagen fibers, which are often arranged in an onion bulb growth pattern. The collagen fibers surround the perineural area.

Between the collagen fibers there are arterioles with a thick wall. In the lumen of these blood vessels there are occasionally thrombi.

Morton's neuroma is usually observed in women at the site of the interdigital plantar nerve.

Morton's neuroma is most probably also due to repeated trauma.

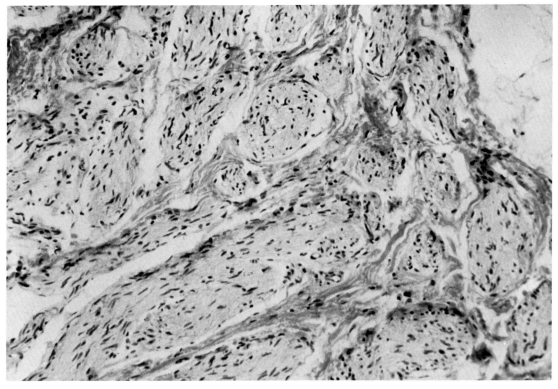

Fig. 180. Neuroma (50-year-old male, × 125).

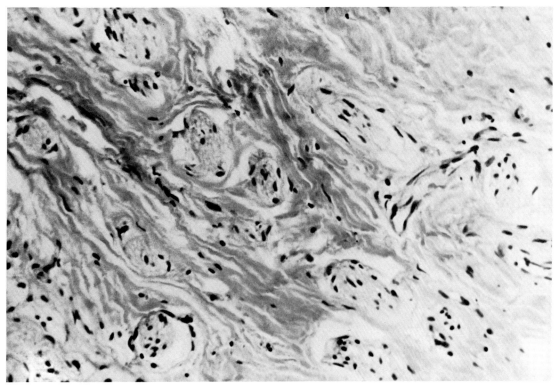

Fig. 181. Neuroma: Fascicles of nerve fibers surrounded by collagen fibers (50-year-old male, × 200).

References

[1] Ackerman, L. V., and J. Rosai: Surgical Pathology. Fifth Edition. C. V. Mosby Company 1974.

[2] Cervós-Navarro, J., F. Matakas und M. C. Lazabo: Das Bauprinzip der Neurinome. Ein Beitrag zur Histogenese der Nerventumoren. Virchows Arch. A Path. Anat. and Histol. *345* (1968) 276-291.

[3] Factor, S., G. Turi, and L. Biempica: Primary cardiac neurilemmoma. Cancer *37* (1976) 883-890.

[4] Harkin, J. C., and R. J. Reed: Tumors of the peripheral nervous system. Atlas of tumor pathology. A. F. I. P., Washington, D. C. 1969.

[5] Mennemeyer, R. P., S. P. Hammar, J. S. Tytus, K. O. Hallman, J. E. Raisis, and D. Bockus: Melanotic schwannoma. Clinical and ultrastructural studies of three cases with evidence of intracellular melanin synthesis. Am. J. Surg. Path. *3* (1979) 3-10.

[6] Pineda, A.: Electron microscopy of the lemmocyte in peripheral nerve tumors (neurolemmomas). J. Neurosurg. *25* (1966) 35-44.

[7] Poirier, J., et R. Escourolle: Ultrastructure des neurinomes de l'acoustique. Z. Mikrosk. Anat. Frschg. *76* (1967) 509-523.

[8] Poirier, J., R. Escourolle, et P. Castaigne: Les neurofibromes de la maladie de Recklinghausen. Étude ultrastructurale et place nosologique par rapport aux neurinomes. Acta Neuropath. (Berl.) *10* (1968) 279-294.

[9] Russell, D. S., and L. J. Rubinstein: Pathology of tumours of the nervous system. Fourth edition. Edward Arnold, London 1977.

[10] Stay, E. J., and G. Vawter: The relationship between nephroblastoma and neurofibromatosis (von Recklinghausen's disease). Cancer *39* (1977) 2550-2555.

[11] Wahlström, T., and L. Saxén: Malignant skin tumors of neural crest origin. Cancer *38* (1976) 2022-2026.

4 Tumors of the esophagus

1. Cancer of the gastrointestinal tract causes more deaths than cancer of any other organ system.
2. The majority of malignant tumors of the esophagus are squamous cell carcinomas.
3. Some lesions of the esophagus might enhance the occurrence of malignant tumor: Plummer-Vinson syndrome, long-standing strictures, and achalasia.
4. There is a very strong geographical difference in the incidence of esophageal cancer: In Europe and the United States about 5% of malignant tumors are carcinomas of the esophagus; in countries of the Arabian Gulf and the Caspian Sea (Iran), this cancer is very frequent.
5. Carcinoma in situ in the squamous cell layer of the esophagus is very rare.
6. Adenocarcinoma of the esophagus is a very rare tumor.
7. Cancer of the esophagus has a poor prognosis.
8. Benign tumors of the esophagus are very rare, and most of them are clinically silent. Among those tumors that cause clinical signs, probably less than 1% are benign [17, 19].

---

[17] Ming 1973.
[19] Moersch and Harrington 1944.

T – primary tumor
Cervical and intrathoracic esophagus

Tis   = preinvasive carcinoma (carcinoma in situ)
T 0   = no evidence of primary tumor
T 1   = tumor that involves 5 cm or less of the esophageal length, that produces no obstruction, that does not involve the entire circumference of the esophagus, and that shows no evidence of extraesophageal spread
T 2   = tumor that involves more than 5 cm of the esophageal length and that shows no evidence of extraesophageal spread or tumor of any size that produces obstruction and/or involves the entire circumference of the esophagus and that shows no evidence of extraesophageal spread
T 3   = tumor with evidence of extraesophageal spread
T x   = the minimal requirements to assess the primary tumor cannot be met (clinical examination, radiography and endoscopy, including bronchoscopy)

N – regional lymph nodes – cervical esophagus
(cervical nodes, including the supraclavicular nodes)

N 0   = no evidence of regional lymph node involvement
N 1   = evidence of involvement of the movable unilateral regional lymph nodes
N 2   = evidence of involvement of the movable bilateral regional lymph nodes
N 3   = evidence of involvement of the fixed regional lymph nodes
N x   = the minimal requirements to assess the regional lymph nodes cannot be met (clinical examination, radiography and endoscopy)

N – regional lymph nodes – intrathoracic esophagus
(mediastinal nodes)

N 0   = no evidence of involvement of the regional lymph nodes in surgical exploration or mediastinoscopy
N 1   = evidence of involvement of the regional lymph nodes on surgical exploration or mediastinoscopy
N x   = it is not possible to assess the regional lymph nodes (i.e., exploratory operation is not done)

M – distant metastases

M 0   = no evidence of distant metastases
M 1   = evidence of distant metastases
M x   = the minimal requirements to assess the presence of distant metastases cannot be met (clinical examination and radiography)

pTNM – postsurgical histopathological classification
pT – primary tumor

pTis   = preinvasive carcinoma (carcinoma in situ)
pT 0   = no evidence of tumor found on histological examination of the specimen
pT 1   = tumor with invasion of the mucosa or submucosa but not the muscle coat
pT 2   = tumor with invasion of the muscle coat
pT 3   = tumor with invasion beyond the muscle coat or with gross invasion of the contiguous structures
           pT 3 a = tumor with invasion beyond the muscle coat
           pT 3 b = tumor with gross invasion of the contiguous structures
pT x   = the extent of invasion cannot be assessed

pN – regional lymph nodes

the pN categories correspond to the N categories

pM – distant metastases

the pM categories correspond to the M categories

Stage grouping

Stage I

cervical and intrathoracic:	T 1	N 0	M 0

Stage II

cervical:	T 1	N 1, N 2	M 0
	T 2	N 0, N 1, N 2	M 0
intrathoracic:	T 2	N 0	M 0

Stage III

cervical:	T 3	any N	M 0
	any T	N 3	M 0
intrathoracic:	any T	N 1	M 0

Stage IV

cervical and intrathoracic:	any T	any N	M 1

M-8070/3
T 150.9

1. Squamous cell carcinoma (WHO)

General
Remarks

Incidence: About 5% of malignant tumors are squamous cell carcinomas of the esophagus.

Of malignant tumors in the esophagus, 90% are squamous cell carcinomas.

Age: The peak age is the 5th and 6th decades.

Sex: Males are affected about 4 times more frequently than females.

T 150.4
T 150.5
T 150.3

Site: The main localizations are the middle third of the esophagus (50%), the lower third (30%), and the upper third (20%).

Macroscopy

Usually the tumor is well demarcated from the surrounding tissue. In most instances the entire circumference of the esophagus is involved. The tumor narrows the lumen of the esophagus.

Cut surface: whitish with infiltration into the wall and the adjacent tissue.

M-8051/3
T 150.9

In most instances the tumor is **ulcerated;**
rarely **verrucous carcinoma** (WHO) is observed [21].

Histology
M-8071/3

The majority of these tumors grow as **well-differentiated (keratinizing) squamous cell carcinoma** (WHO) (Figs. 182 to 184).

Other forms are **moderately differentiated** with discrete keratinization and a marked atypia of the tumor cells (WHO) (Figs. 185 and 186).

M-8020/3

The **poorly differentiated carcinoma** (WHO) lacks foci of keratinization (Fig. 187).

The tumor cells infiltrate the wall and penetrate into the lymphatics.

For the surgeon it is important to know that nests of tumor cells are often observed 4 to 5 cm distal or proximal from the tumor (large resection margin is required).

M-8042/3
T 150.9

Occasionally carcinoma of the esophagus can grow as **oat cell carcinoma** [24].

Differential
Diagnosis

1. Infiltrating carcinoma **with carcinoma in situ or squamous cell hyperplasia in cases of chronic inflammation** (Figs. 183 and 184).
2. Squamous cell carcinoma **with metastatic involvement** of the esophagus from the lymphatics or lymph nodes (primary tumor is often carcinoma of the bronchus).
3. Undifferentiated carcinoma of the esophagus **with undifferentiated adenocarcinoma of the cardia,** infiltrating the esophagus.

Spread

1. At the time of diagnosis more than 50% of the cases have metastases.
2. The majority of metastases are located in regional lymph nodes (paratracheal, parabronchial, posterior mediastinum, paraesophageal, upper deep cervical region, and celiac groups).
3. Hematogenous metastases in the liver and lung and occasionally in the adrenals and other organs [12].

---

[12] Irie et al. 1978.
[21] Oota 1977.
[24] Rosen et al. 1975.

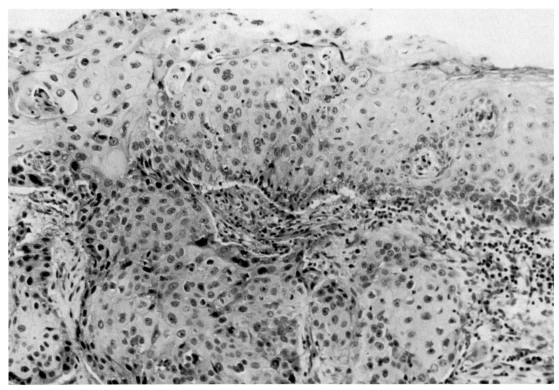

Fig. 182. Keratinized squamous cell carcinoma, well-differentiated, of the esophagus (81-year-old male, × 125).

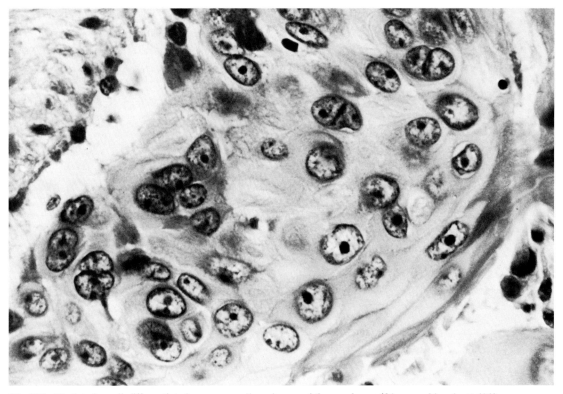

Fig. 183. Nuclei of a well-differentiated squamous cell carcinoma of the esophagus (81-year-old male, × 600).

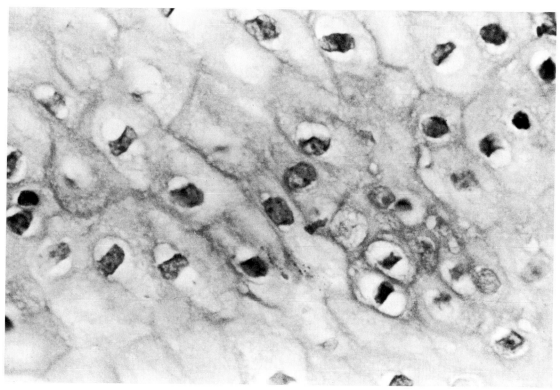

Fig. 184. Squamous cell hyperplasia of the esophagus (57-year-old female, × 600).

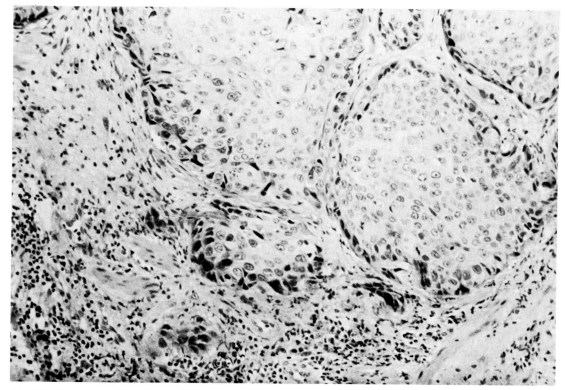

Fig. 185. Squamous cell carcinoma of the esophagus: Discrete keratinization and marked atypia of tumor cells (moderately differentiated) (81-year-old male, × 125).

185

Squamous cell carcinoma

Spread

4. Tumors of the lower third of the esophagus often extend into the submucosal region of the stomach.
5. By lymphatic spread the tumor cells are often found more than 5 cm distant from the tumor: Frozen sections of the operative margins are therefore required!

Clinical Finding

Difficulties in swallowing and dysphagia.
About 70% of the cases have an elevated CEA level [2].

Treatment

Surgery:
Resection of the tumor of the esophagus is mainly indicated for those in the lower third.
Radiation therapy:
This is mostly indicated for tumors in the middle and upper third of the esophagus. The application of up to 60 Gy in 6 weeks has been recommended [23, 29].
Occasionally preoperative irradiation might produce better operative results [15].
Postoperative irradiation is indicated only if the tumor cannot be entirely resected.
In case of nonoperability of the tumor radiation therapy of up to 75 Gy has been applied [28].
Chemotherapy
is only occasionally effective. The role of chemotherapy alone and combined with radiotherapy is still unknown [8].

Prognosis

1. The prognosis is poor. There is no cure potential by surgical or radiation therapy. The 5-year survival rate is about 3 to 10%. A 5-year cure rate of 15% has been obtained very rarely with small tumors of the lower third of the esophagus.
   It has been reported that radiation therapy alone can occasionally give a 20% 5-year survival rate [14, 22].
2. The poor prognosis of this tumor is due to
   a) late symptoms and early tumor spread,
   b) poor response to radiation, and
   c) technical difficulties for the surgeon.
3. The verrucous type of carcinoma might have a better prognosis because of
   a) late lymph node involvement,
   b) limited local invasion [17, 18], and
   c) well-differentiated tumor cells.

Further Information M-8070/2 M-8033/3

1. **Carcinoma in situ** (squamous cell carcinoma in situ – WHO) is a very rare lesion. This lesion, if present, can be observed at multiple sites (Fig. 188).
2. **Pseudosarcoma** (tumor of polyploid appearance – WHO)
   These tumors are squamous cell carcinomas composed of spindle cells, with only rare foci of keratinization. This tumor shows an exophytic growth into the lumen of the esophagus.
3. The incidence of cancer of the esophagus has marked geographic differences [13, 25].

---

[2] Alexander et al. 1978.
[8] Davis Jr. et al. 1978.
[13] Mahboubi 1977.
[14] Marcial et al. 1966.
[15] Marks Jr. et al. 1976.
[17] Ming 1973.
[18] Minielly et al. 1967.
[22] Pearson 1971.
[23] Pearson 1977.
[25] Sadeghi et al. 1977.
[28] Voss and Seeliger 1979.
[29] Wieland and Hymmen 1977.

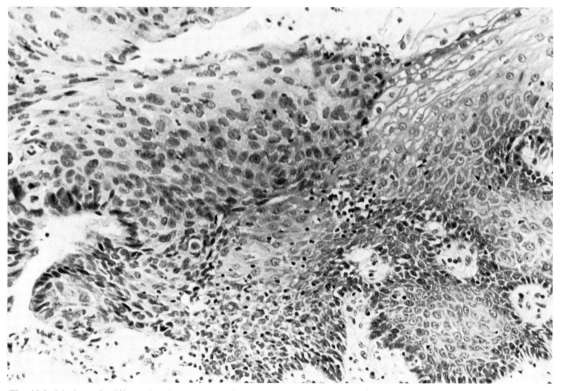

Fig. 186. Moderately differentiated squamous cell carcinoma of the esophagus (55-year-old male, × 160).

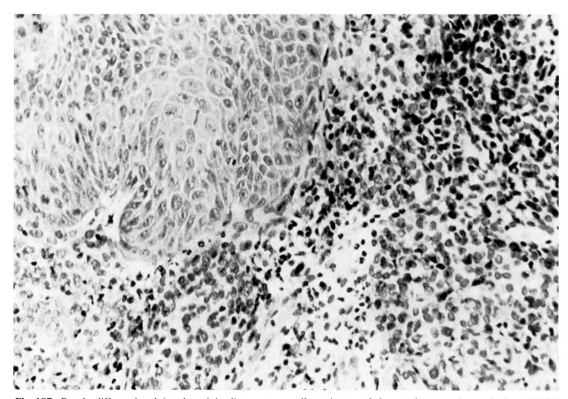

Fig. 187. Poorly differentiated (nonkeratinized) squamous cell carcinoma of the esophagus underneath the epithelial layer (75-year-old male, × 200).

187

M-8140/3
T 150.5

2. Adenocarcinoma of the esophagus (WHO)

General
Remarks

Incidence: This is a very rare tumor.
Site: The tumor usually arises at the esophagogastric junction. Other locations are exceedingly rare [17].
The adenocarcinoma can, however, occur from the esophageal columnar epithelium [4].

Macroscopy

The adenocarcinoma presents as a smooth, ulcerated tumor, infiltrating the wall and narrowing the lumen.

Histology

Adenocarcinoma with different degrees of differentiation:
Well-differentiated or poorly differentiated (WHO).

M-8570/3
M-8200/3
M-8260/3

Occasionally the tumor grows as an **adenoacanthoma** (WHO) [17], or as an
adenoid cystic carcinoma (WHO) [20]
(Fig. 189).
In other instances the tumor grows as a **papillary adenocarcinoma** (WHO).

Differential
Diagnosis

1. In cases of adenocarcinoma the possibility of an **aberrant gastric mucosa** should be ruled out.
2. Primary adenocarcinoma of the esophagus should be separated from **carcinoma of the cardia** (Figs. 190 and 191):
   The adenocarcinoma of the esophagus is surrounded on both sides by squamous epithelial cells.

Staging

See page 182.

Clinical
Findings

Dysphagia.

Spread

Early lymph node metastases.

Treatment

Resection of the tumor (frozen section control of the border!)

Prognosis

The 5-year survival rate is less than 5%.

Further
Information
M-8020/3

Undifferentiated carcinoma (WHO)
The undifferentiated tumor cells do not reveal any organoid pattern.

[4] Berenson et al. 1978.
[17] Ming 1973.
[20] Morson and Dawson 1974.

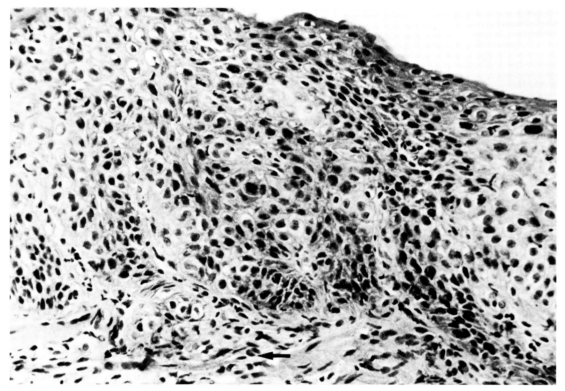

Fig. 188. Carcinoma in situ of the esophagus with beginning infiltration (arrow) (68-year-old male, × 200).

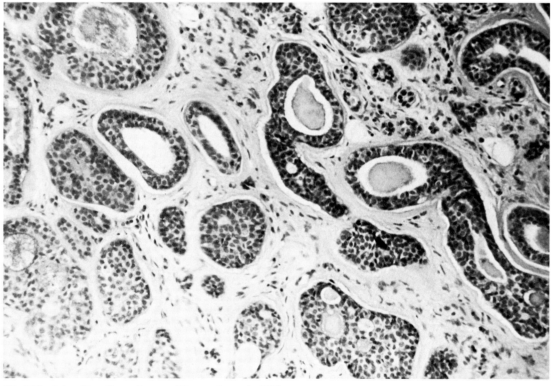

Fig. 189. Adenoid cystic carcinoma of the esophagus (× 200).

M-8890/0
T 150.9

3. Leiomyoma (WHO)

General Remarks

Incidence: This is the most frequent benign tumor of the esophagus.
Age: The peak age is the 3rd to 5th decades.
Sex: Men are affected twice as often as women.
Site: The main site of the tumor is the lower esophagus (about 50%).

Macroscopy

Leiomyomas might be solitary or multiple.
The tumors are firm, growing into the lumen of the esophagus.
Occasionally they surround the circumference, and occasionally they are pedunculated.

Histology

The tumor is composed of smooth muscle fibers with interlacing structures. The nuclei are regular, and mitoses are very rare.

Differential Diagnosis

Benign leiomyoma **with leiomyosarcoma:**
Numerous mitotic figures and signs of infiltration in cases of leiomyosarcoma (Figs. 249 to 254).

Clinical Findings

About 50% of the tumors are asymptomatic.
The remaining cases show dysphagia and substernal pain.

Treatment

Surgery:
Transthoracic enucleation seems to be the treatment of choice. The results of surgery are excellent [26].

[26] Seremetis et al. 1976.

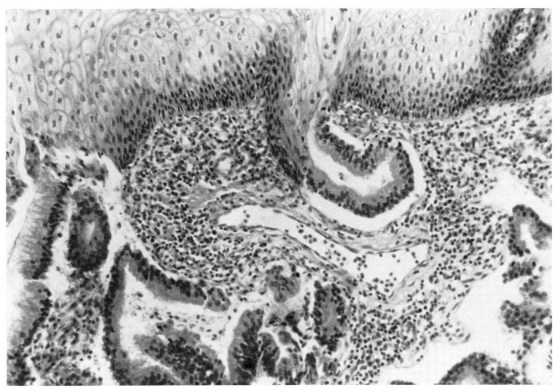

Fig. 190. Adenocarcinoma of the stomach growing underneath the epithelial layer of the esophagus (54-year-old female, ×125).

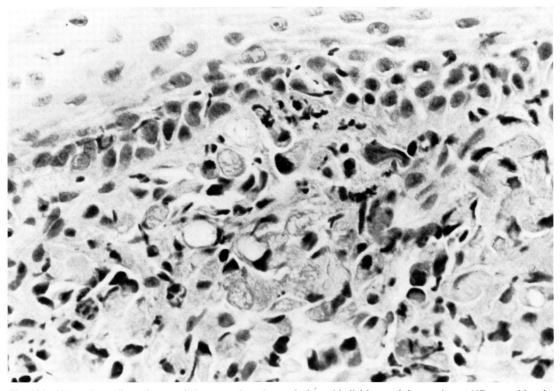

Fig. 191. Signet ring cell carcinoma of the stomach underneath the epithelial layer of the esophagus (67-year-old male, ×400).

191

M-8890/3
T 150.9

4. Leiomyosarcoma (WHO)

General Remarks

Incidence: Leiomyosarcoma is the most frequent malignant mesenchymal tumor in the esophagus.

The overall incidence of malignant mesenchymal tumors of the esophagus is very low.

Age: The peak age is the 6th decade.

Sex: Men are more frequently affected than women.

Site: No site of preferred growth.

Macroscopy

Similar to leiomyoma with extreme narrowing of the lumen.

The mucosa might be ulcerated.

Histology

Growth of atypical smooth muscle fibers. Multiple mitotic figures and signs of infiltration into the wall of the esophagus (Figs. 253 and 254).

Differential Diagnosis

Leiomyosarcoma **with leiomyoma:**

Gross appearance: Ulceration of the mucosa indicates sarcoma.

Histology: A high number of mitoses and infiltration indicates leiomyosarcoma.

Clinical Findings

Substernal pain and dysphagia.

Spread

Lymph node metastases occur late.

Treatment

Surgery:
Surgical resection.
Radiation therapy:
The tumor is radiosensitive (fast neutron therapy)

Prognosis

Relatively good.

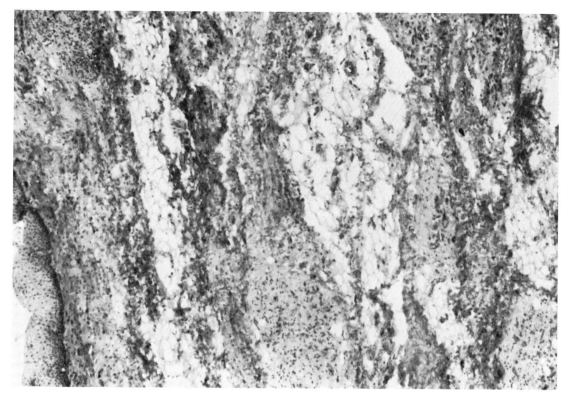

Fig. 192. Fibrovascular polyp of the esophagus (64-year-old male, upper third of the esophagus, × 50).

M-7681/0
T 150.9

5. Fibrovascular polyp
(fibrous polyp – WHO)

General Remarks

Incidence: The second most common benign tumor; however, it is very rare.
Sex: Men are affected more often than women.
Site: In most instances this tumor grows in the upper third of the esophagus.

Macroscopy

The lumen of the esophagus is partially or completely obstructed by a pedunculated tumor, which often shows ulcerations and bleeding.
The tumor can reach the larynx and cause obstruction.
Size of the tumor: Diameter, up to 5 cm; length, 1 to 20 cm!

Histology

The tumor grows underneath the squamous epithelium, which is narrowed, but normally structured. The tumor is composed of collagen fibers with numerous blood vessels (Fig. 192).

Clinical Findings

Dysphagia and occasionally attacks of asphyxia.

Treatment

Removal of the tumor.

Prognosis

Excellent.

M-8052/0
T 150.9

6. Squamous cell papilloma (WHO)

This rare tumor grows in most instances as a sessile lesion (Fig. 1111).

M-8140/0
T 150.9

7. Adenoma

This is an exceedingly rare tumor without functional importance.

M-8430/3
T 150.9

8. Mucoepidermoid carcinoma (WHO)

This type of carcinoma occurs very rarely in the esophagus (Fig. 193).

M-8980/3
T 150.9

9. Carcinosarcoma (WHO)

This tumor is composed of malignant cells of an epithelial and mesenchymal origin (Figs. 1361 to 1364).
Incidence: Very rare; 41 cases have been reported [17].
Age and sex: This tumor has been predominantly observed in men over 50 years old.
Site: The main site is the lower portion of the esophagus.

▷

Fig. 193. Mucoepidermoid carcinoma of the esophagus (91-year-old female, × 125).

Fig. 194a, b. Apudoma of the esophagus: Tumor cells arranged in cords and cell nests (a × 760, b × 700) (Tateichi et al., Virchows Arch. Path. Anat. and Histol. *371* [1976] 283-294).

[17] Ming 1973.

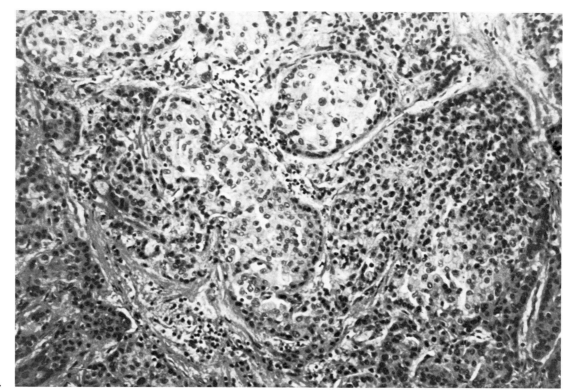

Fig. 193.

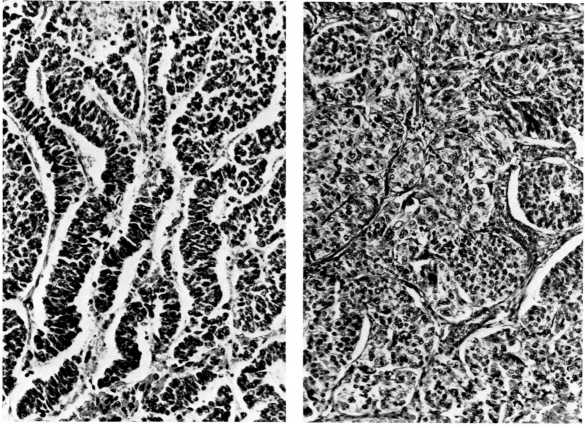

Fig. 194 a.   Fig. 194 b.

10. Multiple carcinomas of the esophagus

The simultaneous appearance of different carcinomas (combination of adenocarcinoma and squamous cell carcinoma and Paget's disease and squamous cell carcinoma) has been reported very rarely [17].

M-8240/1, 3
T 150.9

11. Carcinoid

This tumor occurs very rarely in the esophagus [5] (Fig. 194, a and b).

M-8042/3
T 150.9

12. Oat cell carcinoma [7] (WHO)

This tumor is rare and has a male preponderance.
The site is mainly the lower and midesophagus.
The tumor arises from cells of the APUD series [27].
The tumor cells often have a high content of ACTH [11].

M-8720/3
T 150.9

13. Malignant melanoma (WHO)

In the esophagus this tumor is very rare; about 30 cases have been reported [3] (page 1222).

---

[3] Basque et al. 1970.
[5] Brodman and Pai 1968.
[7] Cook et al. 1976.
[11] Imai et al. 1978.
[17] Ming 1973.
[27] Tateishi et al. 1976.

T 150.9 # Non-epithelial tumors (WHO)

M-9540/0 ## 14. Neurofibroma

This soft tissue tumor is often part of von Recklinghausen's disease (Figs. 176 to 179).

M-9580/0 ## 15. Granular cell tumor [10] (Fig. 123).

This is a very rare tumor in the esophagus.

M-9120/0 ## 16. Hemangioma (Figs. 70 to 79)

M-9170/0 ## 17. Lymphangioma (Figs. 96 to 98)

M-8810/0 ## 18. Fibroma (Fig. 26)

---

[10] Gloor and Clémençon 1975.

M-8850/0

19. Lipoma (Fig. 53)

Fibromas and lipomas of the esophagus are often pedunculated tumors and narrow the lumen.

M-8851/0

20. Fibrolipoma (Fig. 54)

This is a very rare tumor in the esophagus [16].

M-9140/3

21. Kaposi's sarcoma (Figs. 84 to 88)

This tumor might involve the esophagus when systemic spread has occurred.

M-9800/6

22. Leukemic infiltration

Leukemic infiltration can also involve the esophagus.

M-9590/6

23. Malignant lymphoma

The esophagus might be infiltrated by malignant lymphoma.

---

[16] Merck and Weerda 1977.

M-9730/3

24. Extramedullary plasmacytoma

This is exceedingly rare; only one case has been reported [1].

M-8800/3

25. Sarcoma

Sarcomas of the esophagus are exceedingly rare [6].

M-8900/3

Rhabdomyosarcomas have been reported [9].

M-8000/3

26. Unclassified tumors (WHO)

These are tumors that do not reveal by light microscopy their origin from epithelial or mesenchymal cells. They therefore cannot be classified into one of the above-mentioned tumor groups.

When studied by electron microscopy a number of these tumors become classifiable.

27. Tumor-like lesions of the esophagus (WHO)

M-2600/0

a) Aberrant gastric mucosa (gastric heterotopia – WHO)

Islets of aberrant gastric mucosa can appear at the level of the squamous cell epithelium (Fig. 195).

This heterotopia should not be mistaken for adenocarcinoma!

[1] Ahmed et al. 1976.
[6] Chiara and Wanke 1971.
[9] DeMuth Jr. 1956.

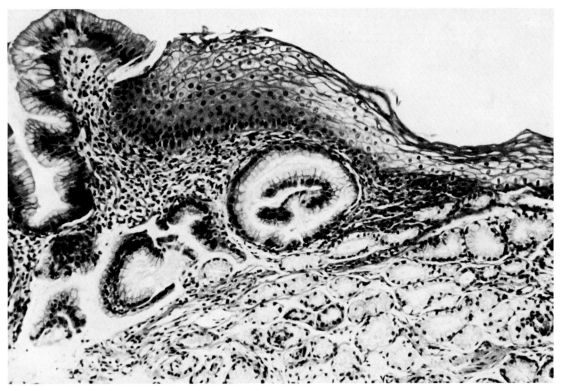

Fig. 195. Keratosis with islets of gastric mucosa in the esophagus (35-year-old male, × 125).

b) Chronic inflammation combined with intestinal metaplasia of squamous cells of the esophagus and benign hyperplasia

This lesion should not be mistaken for carcinoma in situ or infiltrating tumor.
There is no keratinization of the squamous cell epithelium in the esophagus (Figs. 196 and 197).

c) Cysts

– **Inclusion cyst:**
    This cyst is lined by different types of epithelial cells.
M-3340/0   – **Retention cyst:**
    This is lined by flat epithelium or by hyperplastic squamous cells.
– **Cysts of developmental origin:**
    They are lined by different kinds of epithelial cells (bronchial ciliated epithelium or intestinal epithelium).
    In most instances these are located outside of the wall.

200

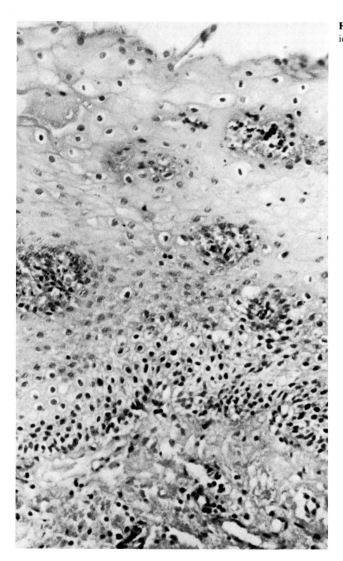

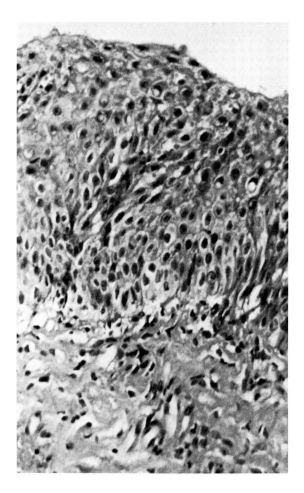

Fig. 197. Hyperplasia of the esophageal squamous cell layer with some dysplastic cells (67-year-old male, × 200).

Recommendations for differential diagnosis in tumors of the esophagus

infiltrating squamous cell carcinoma	with	– chronic inflammation combined with benign squamous cell hyperplasia – carcinoma in situ – infiltration of a squamous cell carcinoma into the esophagus
adenocarcinoma of the esophagus	with	– adenocarcinoma of the stomach infiltrating the esophagus – intestinal metaplasia of the cells of the esophagus in cases of chronic inflammation – aberrant gastric mucosa
benign leiomyoma	with	– leiomyosarcoma
chronic inflammation of the esophagus	with	– malignant lymphoma – leukemic infiltration – plasmacytoma – hemangioma – Kaposi's sarcoma – fibroma

References

[1] Ahmed, N., S. Ramos, J. Sika, H.H. LeVeen, and V.A. Piccon: Primary extramedullary esophageal plasmocytoma. First case report. Cancer *38* (1976) 943-947.

[2] Alexander, J.C., P.B. Chretien, A.L. Dellon, and J. Snyder: CEA levels in patients with carcinoma of the esophagus. Cancer *42* (1978) 1492-1497.

[3] Basque, G.J., J.E. Boline, and J.B. Holyoke: Malignant melanoma of the esophagus: First reported case in a child. Am. J. Clin. Pathol. *53* (1970) 609-611.

[4] Berenson, M.M., R.H. Riddell, D.B. Skinner, and J.W. Freston: Malignant transformation of esophageal columnar epithelium. Cancer *41* (1978) 554-561.

[5] Brodman, H.R., and B.N. Pai: Malignant carcinoid of the stomach and distal esophagus. Review of the literature and a case report. Am. J. Dig. Dis. *13* (1968) 677-681.

[6] Chiari, H., und M. Wanke: Oesophagus. In: Spezielle pathologische Anatomie. Band II, Teil 1. Hrsg.: W. Doerr, G. Seifert, E. Uehlinger, Springer, Berlin–Heidelberg–New York 1971.

[7] Cook, M.G., V. Eusebi, and C.M. Betts: Oatcell carcinoma of the oesophagus: A recently recognized entity. J. Clin. Pathol. *29* (1976) 1068-1073.

[8] Davis, H.L., Jr., D.D. von Hoff, M. Rozencweig, H. Handelsman, W.T. Soper, and F.M. Muggia: Gastrointestinal cancer: Esophagus, stomach, small bowel, colorectum, pancreas, liver, gallbladder, and extrahepatic ducts. In: Randomized trials in cancer: A critical review by sites, edited by M. J. Staquet, Raven Press, New York 1978.

[9] DeMuth, W.E., Jr.: Rhabdomyosarcoma of the esophagus. J. Thoracic Surg. *32* (1956) 115-118.

[10] Gloor, F., and G. Clémençon: Granular cell tumors ("myoblastomas") of the esophagus. Endoscopy *7* (1975) 239-242.

[11] Imai, T., Y. Sannohe, and H. Okano: Oat cell carcinoma (apudoma) of the esophagus. A case report. Cancer *41* (1978) 358-364.

[12] Irie, K., E. Austin, and L. Morgenstern: Solitary meningocerebral metastasis from squamous cell carcinoma of the esophagus. A case report. Cancer *42* (1978) 2461-2465.

[13] Mahboubi, E.: The epidemiology of oral cavity, pharyngeal and esophageal cancer outside of North America and Western Europe. Cancer *40* (1977) 1879-1886.

[14] Marcial, V.A., J.M. Tomé, J. Ubiñas, A. Bosch, and J.V. Correa: The role of radiation therapy in esophageal cancer. Radiology *87* (1966) 231-239.

[15] Marks, R.D., Jr., H.J. Scruggs, and K.M. Wallace: Preoperative radiation therapy for carcinoma of the esophagus. Cancer *38* (1976) 84-89.

[16] Merck, W., und H. Weerda: Über ein Fibrolipom des Ösophagus. HNO *25* (1977) 204-205.

[17] Ming, S.C.: Tumors of the esophagus and stomach. Atlas of tumor pathology. A.F.I.P., Washington, D.C. 1973.

[18] Minielly, J.A., E.G. Harrison, Jr., R.S. Fontana, and W.S. Payne: Verrucous squamous cell carcinoma of the esophagus. Cancer *20* (1967) 2078-2087.

[19] Moersch, H.J., and S.W. Harrington: Benign tumors of the esophagus. Ann. Otol. *53* (1944) 800-817.

[20] Morson, B.C., and I.M.P. Dawson: Gastrointestinal pathology. Blackwell Scientific Publication. Oxford–London–Edinburgh–Melbourne 1974.

[21] Oota, K.: Histological typing of gastric and oesophageal tumours. WHO, Geneva 1977.

[22] Pearson, J.G.: The value of radiotherapy in the management of squamous oesophageal cancer. Br. J. Surg. *58* (1971) 794-798.

[23] Pearson, J.G.: The present status and future potential of radiotherapy in the management of esophageal cancer. Cancer *39* (1977) 882-890.

[24] Rosen, Y., S. Moon, and B. Kim: Small cell epidermoid carcinoma of the esophagus. An oatcell-like carcinoma. Cancer *36* (1975) 1042-1049.

[25] Sadeghi, A., S. Behmard, H. Shafiepoor, and E. Zeighmani: Cancer of the esophagus in southern Iran. Cancer *40* (1977) 841-845.

[26] Seremetis, M.G., W.S. Lyons, V.C. DeGuzman, and J.W. Peabody, Jr.: Leiomyomata of the esophagus. An analysis of 838 cases. Cancer *38* (1976) 2166-2177.

[27] Tateishi, R., K. Taniguchi, T. Horai, T. Iwanaga, H. Taniguchi, T. Kabuto, M. Sano, S. Ishiguro, and A. Wada: Argyrophil cell carcinoma (apudoma) of the esophagus. A histopathologic entity. Virchows Archiv der Allgemeinen Pathologie, Anatomie und Histologie. *371* (1976) 283-294.

[28] Voss, A.-C., und H.-C. Seeliger: Das inoperable Oesophaguskarzinom. Ergebnisse der Strahlentherapie und Folgerungen für die Bestrahlungsplanung. Strahlentherapie *155* (1979) 230-236.

[29] Wieland, C., und U. Hymmen: Strahlentherapie und Behandlungsergebnisse des Ösophaguskarzinoms. Strahlentherapie *153* (1977) 719-725.

5 Tumors of the stomach

1. The frequency of carcinoma of the stomach is decreasing. This has been reported from different countries. This observation has not yet been explained.
2. To cure cancer of the stomach one must detect this tumor in its early stages of development.
   Gastric biopsies should be fully used.
3. Polyps of the gastric mucosa often include precancerous lesions and are sometimes associated with fully developed cancer at other sites in the gastric mucosa.
4. It is important to perform frozen sections of the proximal surgical margins in cancer of the esophagus and stomach. Cancer of the esophagus often reaches up to 5 cm above (or distal to) the border of the tumor.

T – primary tumor

Tis = preinvasive carcinoma (carcinoma in situ)

T 0 – no evidence of primary tumor

T 1 = tumor limited to the mucosa or mucosa and submucosa, regardless of its extent or location

T 2 = tumor with deep infiltration occupying not more than half of one region

T 3 = tumor with deep infiltration occupying more than half but not more than one region

T 4 = tumor with deep infiltration occupying more than one region or extending to neighboring structures

T x = the minimal requirements to assess the primary tumor cannot be met (clinical examination including laparotomy, radiography, and endoscopy)

N – regional lymph nodes

(perigastric nodes, nodes along the left gastric, celiac, and splenic arteries, nodes along the hepatoduodenal ligament, paraaortic and other intraabdominal nodes)

N 0 = no evidence of regional lymph node involvement

N 1 = evidence of lymph node involvement within 3 cm of the primary tumor along the lesser or greater curvatures

N 2 = evidence of lymph node involvement more than 3 cm from the primary tumor, including those along the left gastric, splenic, celiac, and common hepatic arteries

N 3 = evidence of involvement of the paraaortic and hepatoduodenal lymph nodes and/or other intraabdominal lymph nodes

N x = the minimal requirements to assess the regional lymph nodes cannot be met (clinical examination including laparotomy and radiography)

M – distant metastases

M 0 = no evidence of distant metastases

M 1 = evidence of distant metastases

M x = the minimal requirements to assess the presence of distant metastases cannot be met (clinical examination including laparotomy and radiography)

pTNM – postsurgical histopathological classification

pT – primary tumor

pTis = preinvasive carcinoma (carcinoma in situ)

pT 0 = no evidence of tumor found on histological examination of specimen

pT 1 = tumor with invasion of the mucosa or submucosa but not the muscularis propria

pT 2 = tumor with invasion of the muscularis propria or the subserosa

pT 3 = tumor with invasion of the serosa without invasion of contiguous structures

pT 4 = tumor with invasion of contiguous structures

pT x = the extent of invasion cannot be assessed

G – histopathological grading

G 1 = high degree of differentiation

G 2 = medium degree of differentiation

G 3 = low degree of differentiation or undifferentiated

G x = grade cannot be assessed

pN – regional lymph nodes
the pN categories correspond to the N categories

pM – distant metastases
the pM categories correspond to the M categories

Stage grouping-TNM

Stage I	T 1	N 0	M 0
Stage II	T 2	N 0	M 0
	T 3	N 0	M 0
Stage III	T 1, T 2, T 3	N 1, N 2	M 0
	T 1, T 2, T 3 (resectable for cure)	N 3	M 0
	T 4 (resectable for cure)	any N	M 0
Stage IV	T 1, T 2, T 3 (not resectable for cure)	N 3	M 0
	T 4 (not resectable for cure)	any N	M 0
	any T	any N	M 1

Stage grouping-pTNM

Stage I	pT 1	pN 0	pM 0
Stage II	pT 2	pN 0	pM 0
	pT 3	pN 0	pM 0
Stage III	pT 1, pT 2, pT 3	pN 1, pN 2	pM 0
	pT 1, pT 2, pT 3 (resected for cure)	pN 3	pM 0
	pT 4 (resected for cure)	any pN	pM 0
Stage IV	pT 1, pT 2, pT 3 (not resected for cure)	pN 3	pM 0
	pT 4 (not resected for cure)	any pN	pM 0
	any pT	any pN	pM 1

M-8140/3
T 151.9

1. Adenocarcinoma of the stomach (WHO)

**General
Remarks**

Incidence: One of the very common malignant tumors; in some countries this is the most common tumor.

In the last 20 years this tumor has become increasingly less frequent.

Age: The peak age is the 6th to 8th decades; however, patients younger than 40 years can be affected. This tumor is very rare in patients under 30 and is observed only exceptionally in patients under 20 years [29]. Carcinoma of the stomach in children is exceedingly rare. One mucinous adenocarcinoma in a 20-month-old girl has been reported [42].

Sex: Men are more frequently affected than women.

Site: The main site is the antrum and pylorus on the lesser curve, followed by the cardia and fornix.

Further notes: About 3% of cancers of the stomach occur after partial gastrectomy for a benign ulcer [20], often many years after the operation [36].

Macroscopy
M-8260/3

a) **Ulcerating cancer** with infiltration of the wall and overhanging edges.

b) **Polypoid (nodular) carcinoma** (papillary carcinoma – well differentiated and moderately differentiated) (WHO).

c) **Linitis plastica** with extensive tumor infiltration of the stomach (leather bottle stomach).

d) **Superficial spreading carcinoma:** This tumor might have only a discretely thickened mucosa; therefore it is barely detectable and can easily be overlooked by the operating doctor.

Histology

According to growth pattern a variety of subclassifications are possible:

M-8211/3

a) **Adenocarcinoma, nonspecific type, gastric epithelial pattern**
(tubular adenocarcinoma – WHO)
The tumor cells grow in papillary, glandular, and/or tubular formations. The lumina of the glands are of different sizes (Figs. 198 to 202).
Different amounts of mucin are produced by the cells.
If mucin dominates the histological and gross picture, this cancer can be called

M-8480/3

b) **Colloid carcinoma**
(mucinous adenocarcinoma, well differentiated or poorly differentiated – WHO).

M-8144/3

c) **Adenocarcinoma with intestinal epithelial pattern**
(carcinoma of the stomach, intestinal type – WHO)
The tumor cells are arranged mainly in glandular structures (Figs. 203 to 206); numerous papillary formations and occasionally solid complexes of tumor cells are observed.
Often the connective tissue reaction is marked.
In this tumor the gastric mucosa, surrounding the tumor, shows extensive intestinal metaplasia (Fig. 207).

---

[20] Kienzle 1977.
[29] Moritz and Wense 1974.
[36] Pygott and Shah 1968.
[42] Siegel et al. 1976.

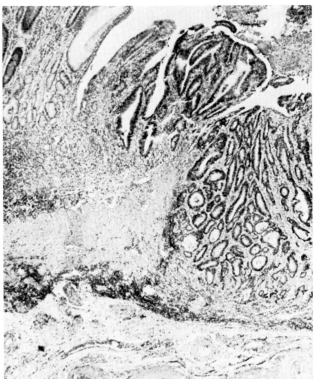

Fig. 198. Tubular adenocarcinoma of the stomach, nonspecific type, infiltrating the inner muscle layer (77-year-old female, × 40).

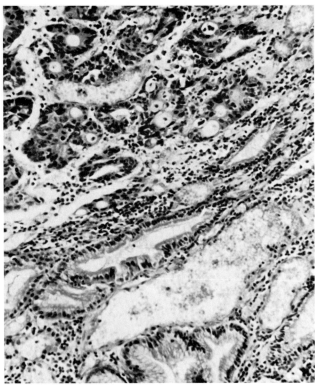

Fig. 199. Tubular adenocarcinoma of the stomach, nonspecific type (62-year-old male, × 125).

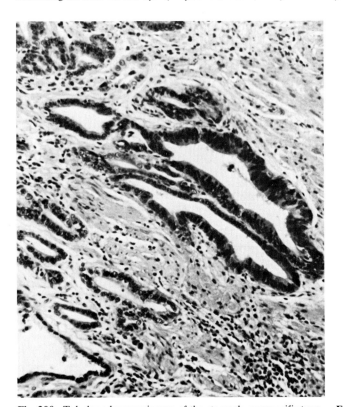

Fig. 200. Tubular adenocarcinoma of the stomach, nonspecific type (75-year-old male, × 200).

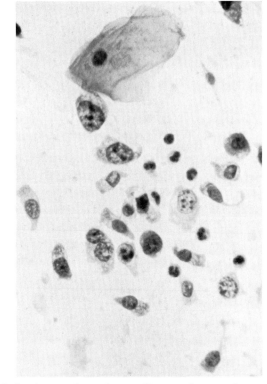

Fig. 201. Cells of a gastric carcinoma: Sharp nuclear membrane, pleomorphic cell size and shape, prominent nucleoli (× 400).

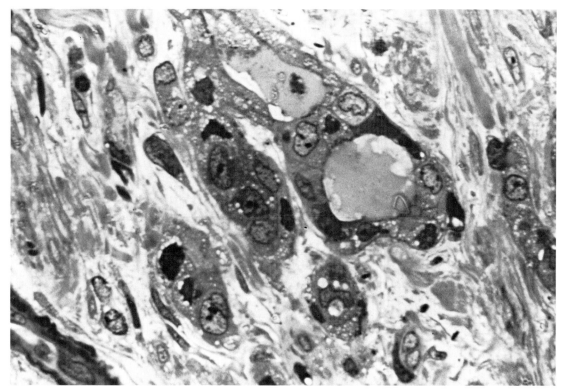

Fig. 202. Tumor cells in a poorly differentiated adenocarcinoma of the stomach (67-year-old female, × 600).

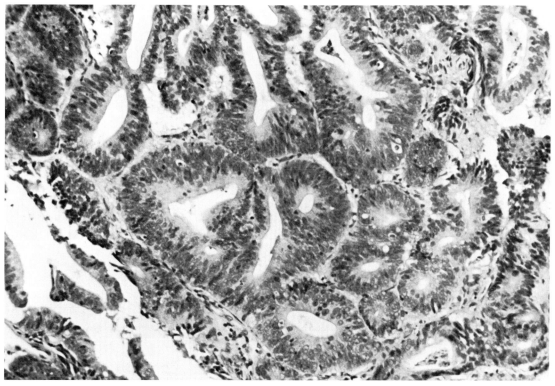

Fig. 203. Adenocarcinoma of the stomach, intestinal type (83-year-old female, × 200).

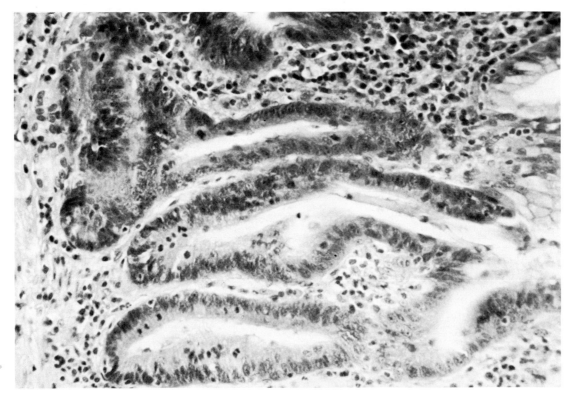

Fig. 204. Adenocarcinoma of the stomach, intestinal type (55-year-old male, × 200).

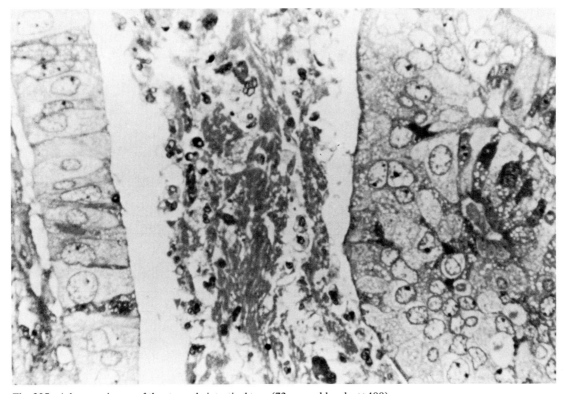

Fig. 205. Adenocarcinoma of the stomach, intestinal type (72-year-old male, × 400).

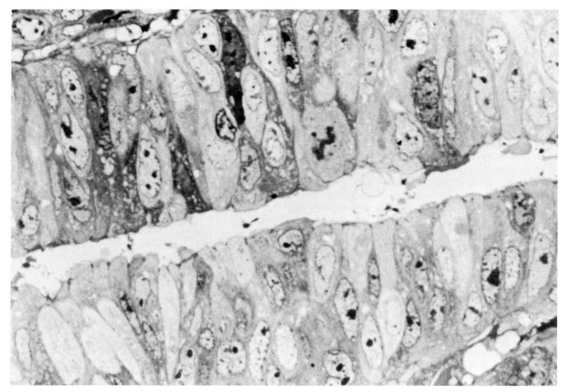

Fig. 206. Adenocarcinoma of the stomach, intestinal type (72-year-old female, × 600).

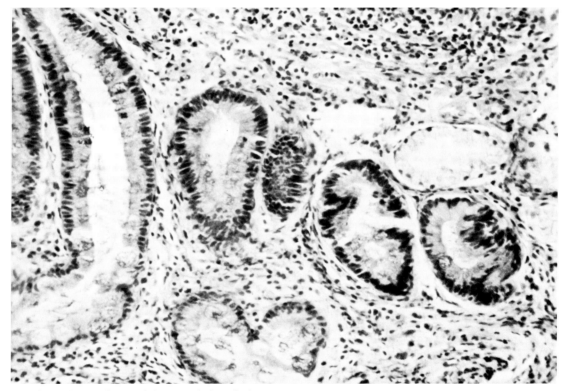

Fig. 207. Adenocarcinoma of the stomach, intestinal type: Dysplasia and intestinal metaplasia in the surrounding noncarcinomatous infiltrated mucosa (59-year-old male, × 200).

213

Adenocarcinoma

M-8145/3

d) Diffuse adenocarcinoma
(carcinoma of the stomach, diffuse type – WHO; or tubular adenocarcinoma, poorly differentiated – WHO)
This carcinoma is composed of undifferentiated cells. They form large or small complexes with discrete or without organoid glandular or tubular structures (Figs. 208 to 214). Intestinal metaplasia in the surrounding mucosa of the stomach is observed rarely. The reaction of the connective tissue might be moderately strong or weak; the inflammatory cell infiltration surrounding or in the tumor is very poor.

e) Adenocarcinoma with peptic ulcer (ulcer cancer)
This carcinoma has at its margin intact gastric mucosa (Figs. 215 to 217). If the ulceration is surrounded by tumor cells, the lesion should be labeled as ulcerating carcinoma (see Possible precarcinomatous lesions in the stomach, page 225).

M-8142/3

f) Linitis plastica
The tumor cells are very poorly differentiated, and they do not show any tendency to form organoid tubular or glandular patterns. The tumor cells are disseminated throughout the wall of the stomach, with infiltration of the lymphatics and the surrounding tissue.
The tumor cells induce a strong connective tissue reaction.

M-8490/3

g) Signet ring cell carcinoma (WHO)
The tumor cells of this cancer are characterized by a strong mucin-positive reaction in their large cytoplasm with the nucleus in a signet ring-similar position (Figs. 218 to 221). The tumor cells can form an organoid pattern with a tubular, papillary, or glandular structure, or they may grow diffusely.

M-8143/3

h) Superficial carcinoma
(superficial spreading carcinoma, "early epithelial cancer") (WHO)
This cancer is characterized by tumor cells that grow in the lamina propria and do not extend beyond the muscularis mucosae (Figs. 222 and 223).
Many cases show a multifocal origin of the tumor. The main site is the antrum.
The tumor can grow in any pattern (Fig. 224).

Electron Microscopy

In poorly differentiated adenocarcinoma of the stomach the tumor cells might show primitive lumina and microvilli. Mucin vacuoles may not be present.

Immunohisto-chemistry

In well-differentiated adenocarcinoma, carcinoembryonic antigen (CEA) can be found on the surface of the tumor cells by immunofluorescence [11].

Differential Diagnosis

1. Undifferentiated carcinoma (WHO) **with malignant lymphoma.**
2. Undifferentiated carcinoma and linitis plastica **with inflammatory cell infiltration:**
   The differential diagnosis is often decided by mucin stain.
3. Special attention must be paid to **precancerous lesions** observed in gastric biopsies (see also page 225).
4. Adenocarcinoma **with gastritis cystica profunda** (Figs. 225 to 227).

Staging

5. Adenocarcinoma **with heterotopic pancreatic tissue** (Fig. 228), see page 208.

---

[11] Denk et al 1973.

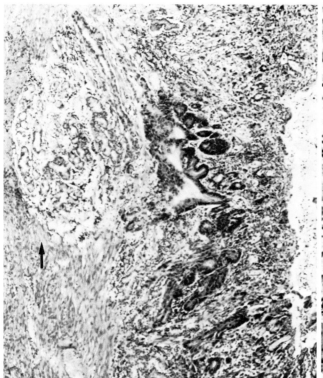

Fig. 208. Adenocarcinoma of the stomach, poorly differentiated, with beginning infiltration into the muscle layer (arrow and Fig. 209) (33-year-old female, × 50).

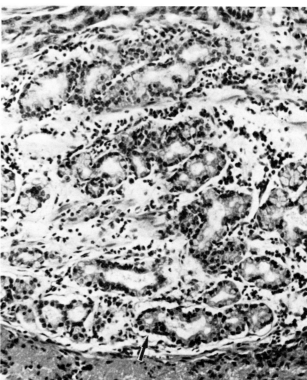

Fig. 209. Poorly differentiated (partly tubular) adenocarcinoma of the stomach, reaching the muscle layer (arrow, see Fig. 208) (33-year-old female, × 125).

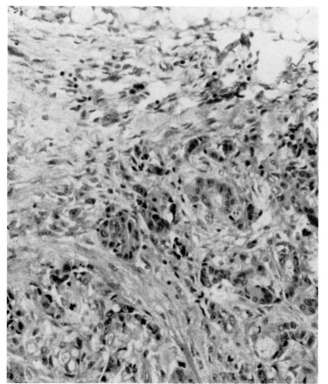

Fig. 210. Poorly differentiated adenocarcinoma of the stomach infiltrating the fat tissue (73-year-old female, × 125).

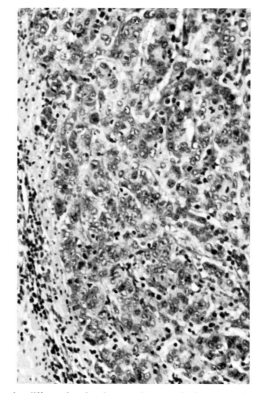

Fig. 211. Poorly differentiated adenocarcinoma of the stomach (71-year-old female, × 125).

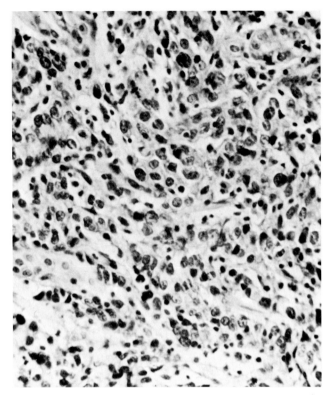

Fig. 212. Poorly differentiated adenocarcinoma of the stomach (58-year-old male, × 200).

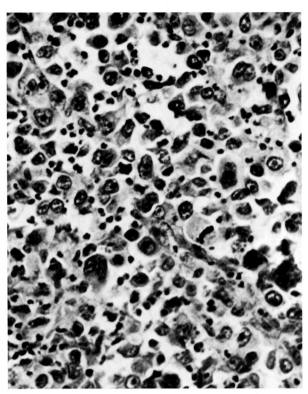

Fig. 214. Undifferentiated adenocarcinoma of the stomach with giant cells (× 200).

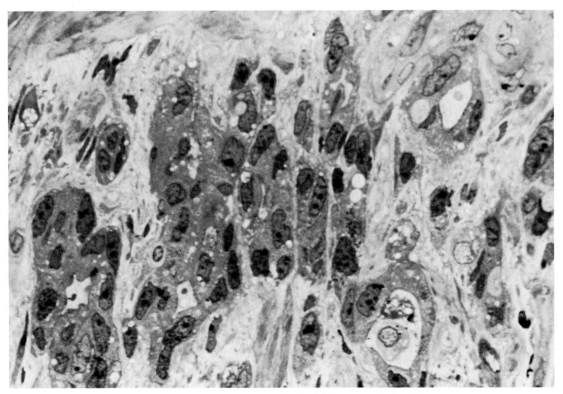

Fig. 213. Poorly differentiated adenocarcinoma of the stomach: Nuclei of tumor cells (× 600).

216

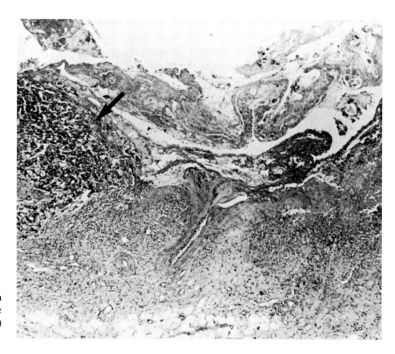

Fig. 215. Peptic ulcer of the stomach with developing carcinoma in one margin (arrow, see Fig. 216) (58-year-old male, × 40).

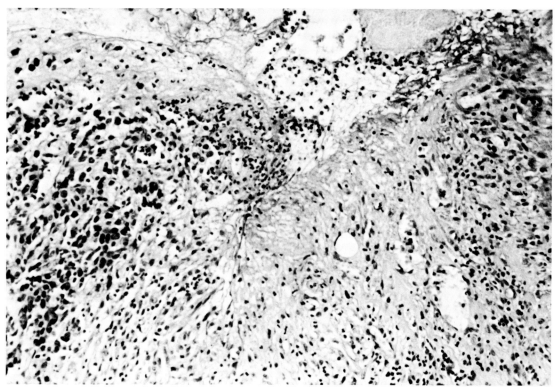

Fig. 216. Ulcer carcinoma of the stomach (poorly differentiated) arising in one margin (see Fig. 215) (58-year-old male, × 125).

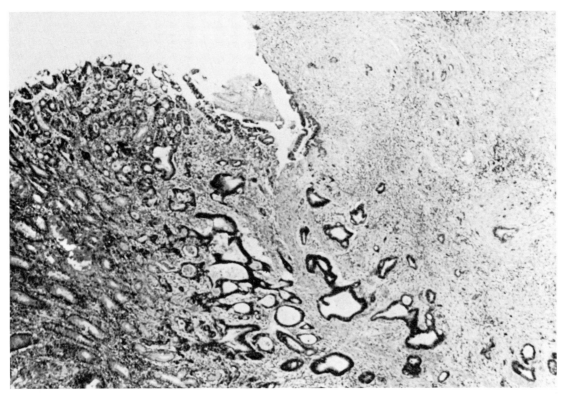

Fig. 217. Ulcer carcinoma (nonspecific adenocarcinoma) (62-year-old male, × 40).

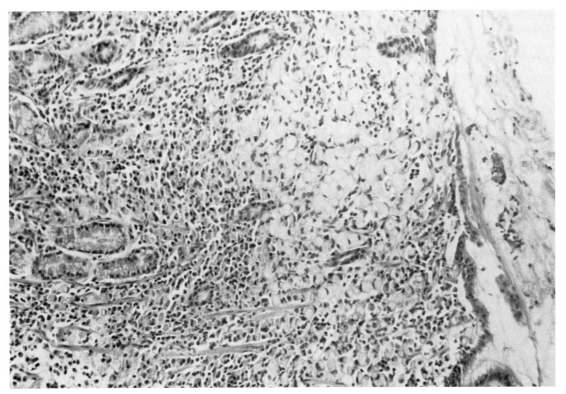

Fig. 218. Signet ring cell carcinoma of the stomach (62-year-old female, × 125).

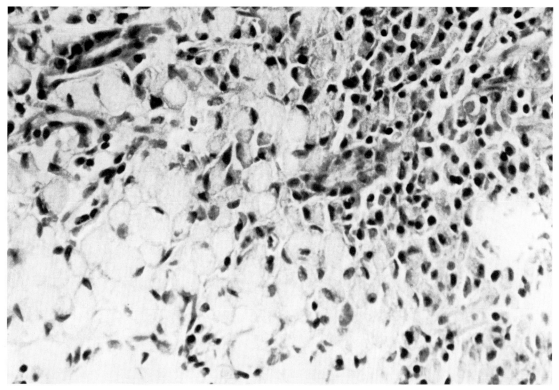

Fig. 219. Signet ring cell carcinoma of the stomach (62-year-old female, × 310).

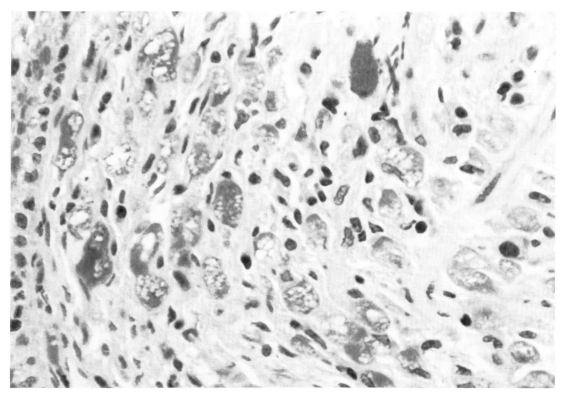

Fig. 220. Signet ring cell carcinoma (early cancer) of the stomach (PAS stain, × 400).

Adenocarcinoma

Spread

1. Tumors of the cardia extend frequently into the esophagus. Tumors of the pylorus rarely involve the duodenum.
2. At the time of operation, in many instances the tumor has spread into the subserosa.
3. Invasion of the lymphatics and blood vessels is frequent.
4. Metastases into regional lymph nodes occur in 40 to 80% of the cases, depending on the size and depth of infiltration of the tumor.
5. Hematogenous metastases are often observed and involve the liver or lung, followed by the adrenal, pancreas, ovary, bone, kidney, spleen, or any other organ.
6. At autopsy a disseminated carcinomatous involvement of the peritoneum is observed in about 40% of the cases.

Clinical Findings

- Discomfort, epigastric pain, anorexia, slight nausea, dysphagia (tumors of the cardia).
- 25% of the patients show symptoms of an ulcer.
- In about 50% of the patients, weight loss is stated.
- Occult blood in the feces.
- The tumor cells produce carcinoembryogenic antigen (CEA).
- The usual duration of symptoms before the patient seeks medical care is 6 months to several years.
- Early detection by biopsy, especially for cases of superficial spreading carcinoma, is possible [38].

Treatment

Surgery:
- The first approach to treat cancer of the stomach is surgery.
- About 50% of gastric carcinomas cannot be treated by surgery because of a late diagnosis.
- The extent of surgery depends on the localization and size of the tumor: Subtotal gastrectomy for cancer of the distal and midstomach; proximal gastrectomy and distal esophagectomy for tumors of the proximal stomach. Total gastrectomy should be performed only occasionally.
- The resection site should be about 4 cm proximal and distal to the tumor and should be controlled by frozen section.
- The operation includes resection of the regional lymph nodes (resection of the greater and lesser omentum, if necessary).
- Operative mortality: Higher than 10%.

Radiation therapy:
No cure; occasionally indicated for palliative purposes.

Chemotherapy:
- Chemotherapy gives only a poor possibility of response and improvement; its efficiency is still debated.
- In advanced gastric carcinoma chemotherapy with 5-fluorouracil in combination with nitrosourea (for instance, methyl-BCNU) has been proposed [8, 28].

---

[8] Davis Jr. et al. 1978.
[28] Moertel et al. 1976.
[38] Rösch and Thoma 1974.

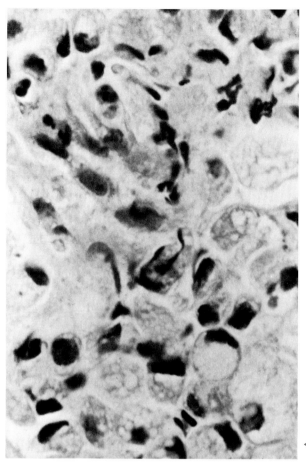

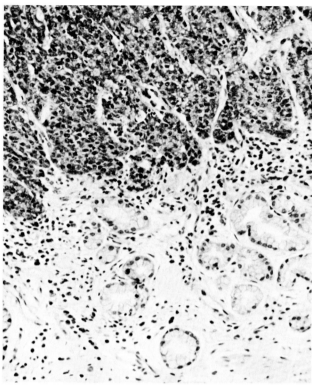

Fig. 222. Superficial spreading carcinoma of the stomach, poorly differentiated (63-year-old male, × 50).

◁ **Fig. 221.** Adenocarcinoma of the stomach: Signet ring cells (× 800).

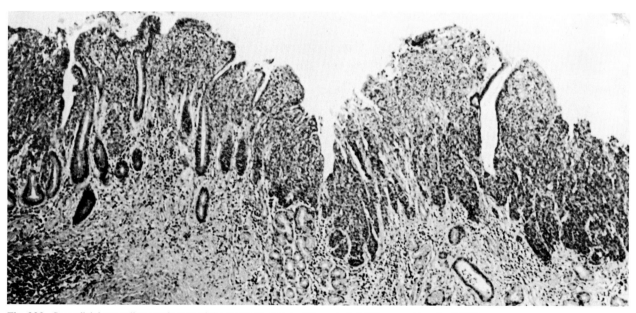

Fig. 223. Superficial spreading carcinoma of the stomach, poorly differentiated (63-year-old male, × 125).

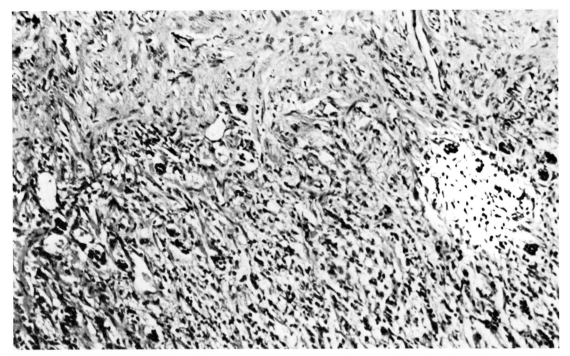

Fig. 224. Superficial spreading carcinoma of the stomach, undifferentiated (anaplastic) type (73-year-old female, × 125).

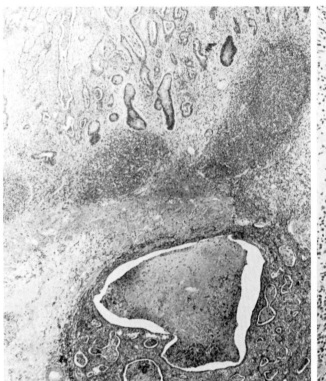

Fig. 225. Gastritis cystica profunda (68-year-old male, × 40).

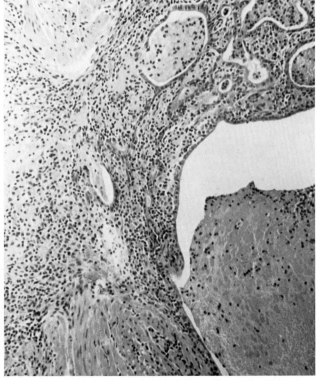

Fig. 226. Gastritis cystica profunda (68-year-old male, × 125).

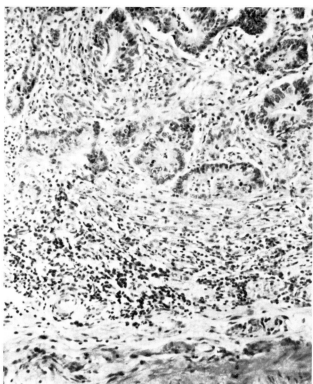

Fig. 227. Infiltrating adenocarcinoma of the stomach (nonspecific type) almost reaching the muscle layer (77-year-old female, × 125).

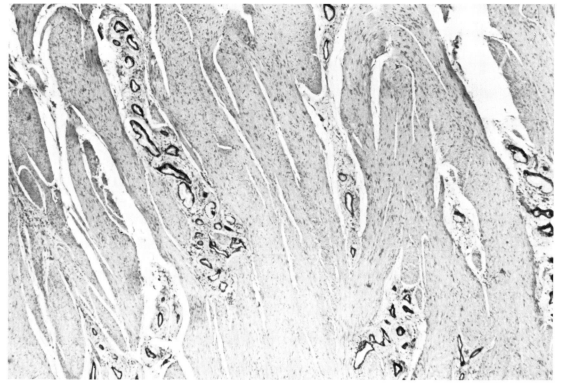

Fig. 228. Heterotopic pancreatic tissue in the gastric wall, mimicking infiltrating carcinoma (36-year-old male, × 40).

Adenocarcinoma

Treatment

– The combination of chemotherapy and radiation therapy has been recommended [15]. However, the usefulness of this combined therapy has not yet been evaluated clearly.

Prognosis

1. Incurable, untreated cancer of the stomach:
   Survival after 1 year, 10%.
   Survival after 5 years, 2%.
   Survival after 10 years, 1% [27].
2. Overall survival rate for gastric carcinoma, 5%.
   Overall 5-year survival rate after diagnosis, 10%.
   The 5-year survival rate for resected patients, 25% [34].
3. In individual cases the following factors are important for prognosis:
   a) Extension of the tumor:
      – Superficial carcinomas have an excellent prognosis (tumor confined to the mucosa or submucosa [12, 40].
        The 5-year survival rate is 66 to 95% [31, 35].
      – There is a 50% 5-year survival rate if the lymph nodes are not involved.
      – There is a 10 to 20% 5-year survival rate if the tumor extends through the serosa.
   b) The histological appearance seems to have little significance for the prognosis; however, the intestinal pattern of stomach cancer has perhaps a better prognosis than does the diffuse carcinoma.
      The histological extension of the tumor is important for the prognosis: The deeper the tumor cells infiltrate the wall, the worse the prognosis.
      A lymphocytic reaction in or surrounding the tumor is claimed to be favorable for the prognosis [18, 49].
   c) Tumors smaller than 2 cm in diameter have a better prognosis than do larger tumors.
   d) Lymph node metastases worsen the prognosis:
      – the 5-year survival rate without lymph node metastases is 50%.
      – the 5-year survival rate with lymph node metastases is less than 10% (the 1-year survival rate is about 50%).

Further Information

1. In Japan mass screening has increased the incidence of detection of early superficial carcinoma to 35% [35].
2. Attention should be paid to the fact that superficial spreading carcinoma often is of a multifocal origin.
3. Very rarely in undifferentiated carcinomas of the stomach, granules of the neurosecretory type have been observed in tumor cells:
   Malignant gastric neuroendocrinomas [6].
4. The simultaneous occurrence of a squamous cell carcinoma of the esophagus infiltrating an adenocarcinoma of the cardia has been reported exceptionally **(collision tumor)** [48].

[6] Chejfec and Gould 1977.
[12] Elster and Thomasko 1978.
[15] Hartmann and Obrecht 1978.
[18] Inokuchi et al. 1967.
[27] Moertel 1975.
[31] Nakamura et al. 1968.
[34] Perrotta 1977.
[35] Prolla et al. 1969.
[40] Schlag et al. 1979.
[48] Wanke 1972.
[49] Watanabe et al. 1976.

2. Possible precarcinomatous lesions in the stomach

M-8140/2
T 151.9

a) Carcinoma in situ (WHO)
(intraglandular carcinoma)
In this lesion the atypical cells forming glandular structures are limited to the mucosa; the lamina propria is not invaded (Figs. 229 to 232).
This distinguishes the intraglandular carcinoma from the superficial spreading carcinoma.

M-7400/0
T 151.9

b) Dysplasia of the glandular and surface epithelium
Dysplastic cells proliferate in a papillary pattern into the lumen of the foveolae gastricae:. The cells have hyperchromatic nuclei and little mucin. Multiple mitotic figures can be observed.

M-7300/0
T 151.9

c) Intestinal metaplasia
This lesion must be considered precancerous, especially for the development of carcinoma of the intestinal epithelial pattern (Fig. 207).
Intestinal metaplasia has its main location in the lesser curve of the antrum and the pyloric region.

d) Gastric adenomatous polyp, covered by intestinal epithelium
These polyps should be considered precancerous lesions [3].

e) Chronic peptic ulcer
The incidence of ulcer-carcinoma is still uncertain. Probably considerably less than 1% of all gastric chronic ulcers develop into a cancer [1, 25, 30].

[1] Ackerman and Rosai 1974.
[3] Bötticher et al. 1975.
[25] Ming 1973.
[30] Morson and Dawson 1974.

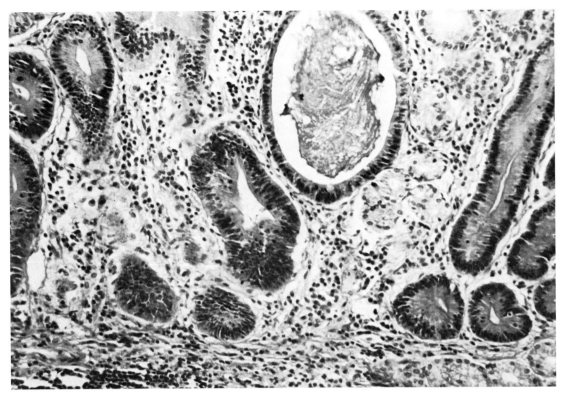

Fig. 229. Intrafoveolar foci of carcinoma in situ of the stomach (77-year-old female, × 200).

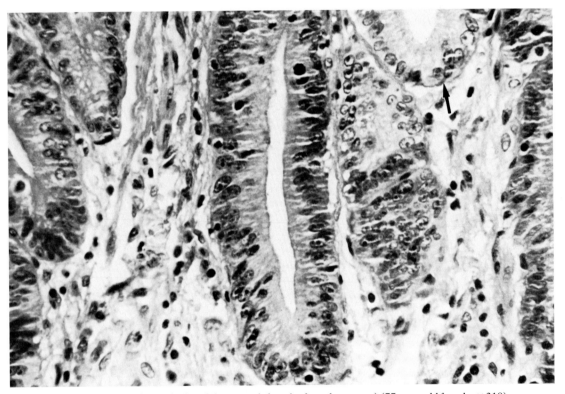

Fig. 230. Intraglandular carcinoma in situ of the stomach (regular foveolae, arrow) (77-year-old female, × 310).

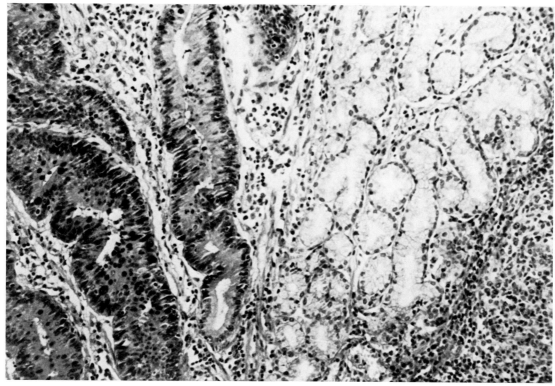

Fig. 231. Multifocal carcinoma in situ of the stomach (77-year-old female, × 125).

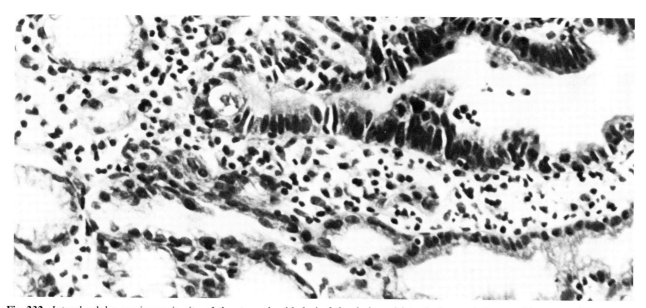

Fig. 232. Intraglandular carcinoma in situ of the stomach with foci of dysplasia and intestinal metaplasia, atrophic mucosa (52-year-old male, × 200).

3. Gastric polyps

M-8210/0

a) Adenomatous polyp
(tubular adenoma, papillotubular adenoma-WHO)

M-8261/1
T 151.9

b) Villous polyp
(papillary adenoma – WHO)
These tumors correspond to polyps of the large bowel.
The polyps are composed of glands lined by atypical cells or regular cells (Figs. 233 to 235).
The polyps may contain foci of intestinal metaplasia and areas of inflammation.
These polyps should be considered premalignant: There is not only an increased frequency of carcinoma in the polyps (Figs. 236 to 239), but also an increased frequency of carcinoma in the mucosa other than in the polyp [26].

M-7563/0
T 151.9

c) Benign epithelial polyp
(Peutz-Jeghers polyp – WHO) (hamartoma – WHO)
This hamartomatous (**hyperplastic** – WHO) lesion is composed of pyloric mucosa. The foveolae gastricae are occasionally dilated. This polyp is infiltrated by inflammatory cells (Figs. 315 to 317).
The cells lining the glands are regular (**inflammatory fibroid polyp** – WHO). These hamartomatous polyps also occur in familial polyposis and Gardner's syndrome. These polyps are not precancerous lesions.

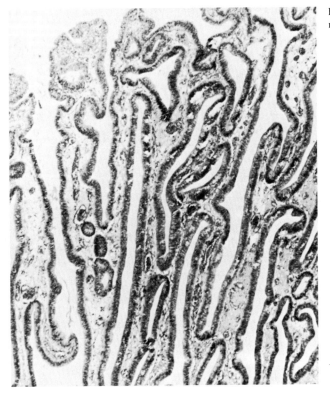

Fig. 233. Adenomatous polyp of the stomach (papillotubular adenoma): Foci of dysplasia and carcinoma in situ (see Fig. 235) (× 40).

[26] Ming 1976.

228

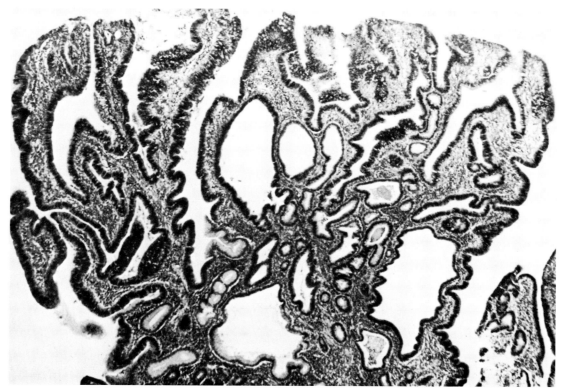

Fig. 234. Villous polyp of the stomach (papillary adenoma) (66-year-old female, × 40).

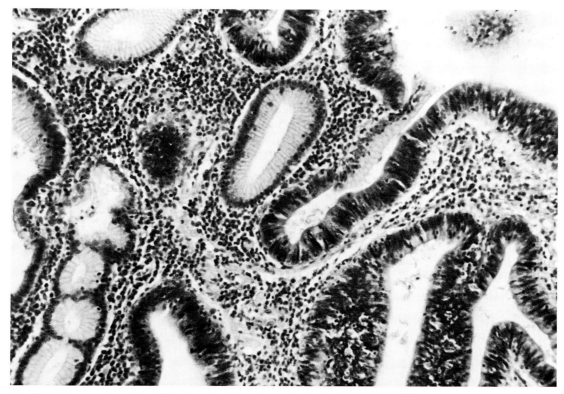

Fig. 235. Adenomatous polyp of the stomach with carcinoma in situ (see Fig. 233) (× 200).

229

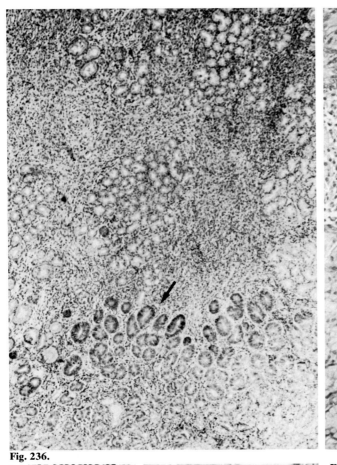

Fig. 236.

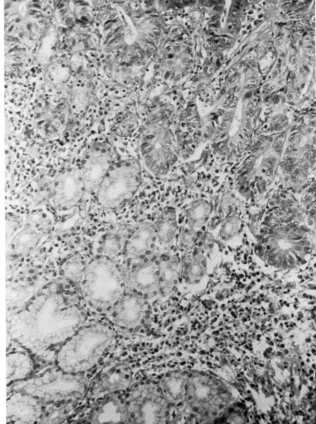

Fig. 237.

Fig. 238.

Fig. 236. Part of large adenomatous polyp of the stomach with superficial carcinoma (arrow, see Fig. 237) (79-year-old female, × 40).

Fig. 237. Adenomatous polyp of the stomach with superficial carcinoma (79-year-old female, × 125).

Fig. 238. Villous polyp of the stomach with beginning infiltrating carcinoma (see inset and Fig. 239) (66-year-old female, × 40; inset, × 200).

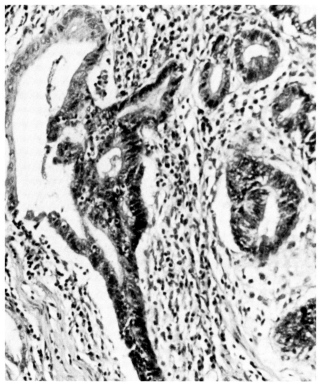

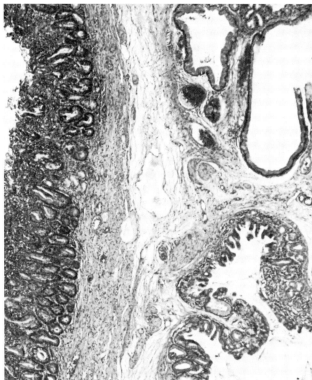

Fig. 239. Part of a villous polyp of the stomach: Multifocal origin of carcinoma (66-year-old female, × 125).

Fig. 240. Polypous lesion of the stomach due to heterotopic intestinal mucosa in the wall of the stomach (64-year-old male, × 40).

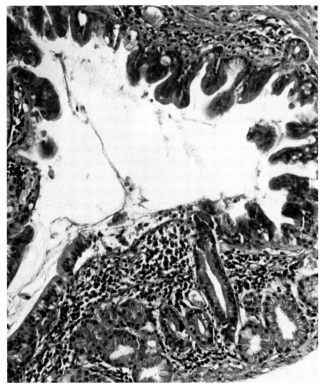

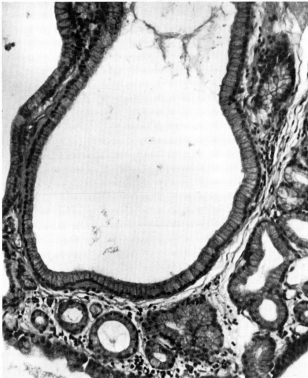

Fig. 241. Heterotopic intestinal tissue in the wall of the stomach (64-year-old male, × 125).

Fig. 242. Heterotopic intestinal mucosa in the wall of the stomach (64-year-old male, × 125).

231

M-2600/0
d) Heterotopic adenomatous polyp
(heterotopias – WHO)
These polyps of the stomach contain heterotopic pancreatic tissue and duodenal or gastric tissue. This lesion is not precancerous (Figs. 240 to 242).

4. Carcinoid (WHO) (Figs. 321 to 328)

M-8240/1
T 151.9

This is a rare, mostly circumscribed, solitary tumor. Its growth is slow.

Differential Diagnosis
1. Occasionally it is difficult to separate the carcinoid tumor from an **islet cell tumor.**
2. It is often impossible on histological grounds to predict the **benign or malignant behavior** of the carcinoid.

Treatment
In cases of large or multiple tumors: subtotal gastrectomy.

Prognosis
Good, even if metastases have developed [21].
Metastases develop in about 30 % of the cases.
In cases of liver metastases the removal of tumor tissue should be attempted.

M-8242/3, 1
T 151.9
This tumor is argentaffin-negative.
Very rarely, ACTH production by carcinoid tumors in the stomach has been observed [17].

5. Adenoacanthoma (WHO)

M-8570/3
T 151.9

This rare tumor is characterized by foci of squamous cell metaplasia in an adenocarcinoma. It is observed in less than 1 % of gastric carcinomas [44].

M-8070/3
T 151.9
Very rarely a malignant tumor of the stomach is entirely composed of cells of a **squamous cell carcinoma** (WHO).
In most instances a "squamous cell carcinoma" is an **adenoacanthoma** with predominance of the squamous cell metaplasia (Fig. 243).
Exceedingly rare are carcinomas composed of malignant squamous cells and malignant glandular epithelial cells:
M-8560/3
T 151.9
Adenosquamous carcinoma (WHO).

---

[17] Imura et al. 1975.
[21] Lattes and Grossi 1956.
[44] Straus et al. 1969.

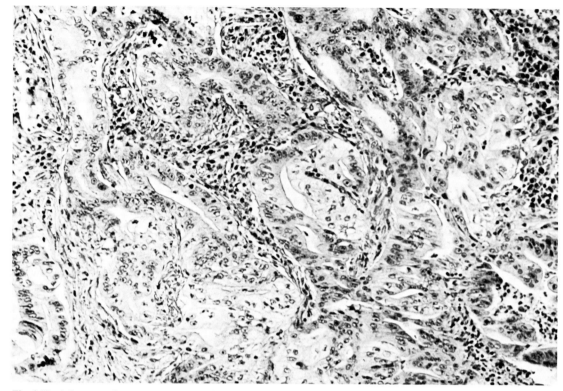

Fig. 243. Adenoacanthoma of the stomach (73-year-old male, × 125).

T 151.9

6. Vascular tumors

M-8711/0

a) Glomus tumor
This tumor develops mostly in the distal part of the stomach and may occur at any age [50] (Fig. 95).

M-9120/0

b) Hemangioma (Fig. 71)

M-9150/0

c) Hemangiopericytoma [24] (Fig. 89)

M-9170/0

d) Lymphangioma (Fig. 96)

M-9140/3

e) Kaposi's sarcoma
Kaposi's sarcoma might involve the stomach in cases of dissemination (Figs. 84 to 88).

[24] Marangos 1965.
[50] Weitzner 1969.

M-9590/3
T 151.9

7. Malignant lymphoma of the stomach
(lymphosarcoma – WHO; reticulosarcoma – WHO)

General Remarks

Incidence: 2 to 5% of all gastric malignancies are malignant lymphomas.
Age: The peak age is the 5th to 7th decades.
Sex: Men and women are affected equally.
Site: Main site is the antrum and pylorus.

Macroscopy

Malignant lymphoma presents as an ulcerating tumor or polypoid mass.
Malignant lymphoma is clinically, radiographically, and grossly indistinguishable from carcinoma of the stomach.

Histology

All types of malignant lymphoma including Hodgkin's lymphoma can occur in the stomach.
This malignant tumor begins to develop in the lamina propria and the submucosal tissue (Figs. 244 to 246).

Differential Diagnosis

1. Malignant lymphoma **with undifferentiated carcinoma:**
   In malignant lymphoma tumor cells do not form organoid structures, and there are no mucin-producing cells. There are no precancerous lesions in the glandular epithelium of the mucosa.
   According to the nature of the lymphoma, the cytological features and PAS reactions usually indicate malignant lymphoma.
2. Non-Hodgkin's lymphoma **with Hodgkin's disease** (WHO).

M-7229/0

3. Malignant lymphoma **with pseudolymphoma** (lymphoid hyperplasia) (WHO):
   Indicators of pseudolymphoma are the appearance of follicles in the lymphoid tissue (Figs. 247 and 248), the presence of inflammatory cells (plasma cells and neutrophils), and a chronic lymphadenitis [32].

Spread

1. The majority of malignant lymphomas of the stomach are part of a systemic disease.
2. In cases of malignant lymphoma restricted to the stomach, about 23 to 62% have lymph node involvement [25].

Clinical Findings

Epigastric pain, discomfort, good physical condition without weight loss.

Treatment

Surgery:
Local radical treatment by partial gastrectomy has been recommended in cases of restricted lymphoma of the stomach.
This tumor seems to behave in many instances as an unifocal tumor [39].
Combination of surgery and radiotherapy of up to 40 to 60 Gy [19].
Radiation therapy:
Radiation therapy alone should be used in cases of nonresectable tumor.

[19] Joseph and Lattes 1966.
[25] Ming 1973.
[32] Naqvi et al. 1969.
[39] Rudders et al. 1978.

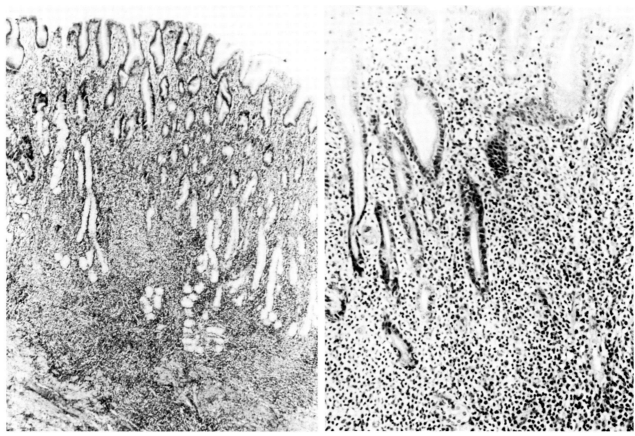

Fig. 244. Malignant lymphoma of the stomach (note intestinal metaplasia) (63-year-old male, × 50).

Fig. 245. Malignant lymphoma of the stomach (63-year-old male, × 125).

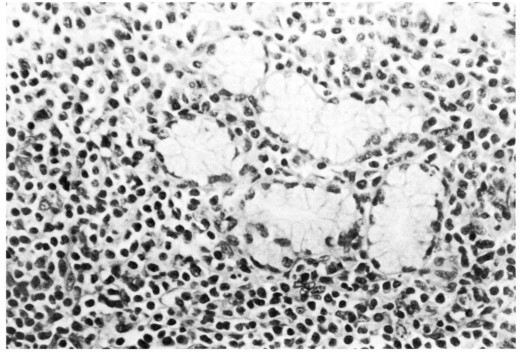

Fig. 246. Malignant lymphoma of the stomach (63-year-old male, × 310).

Malignant lymphoma

Prognosis

1. The prognosis is better than that for gastric carcinoma.
2. The prognosis is correlated with the stage of the disease and not with the histological type of the lymphoma [22].
3. The 5-year survival rate for lymphoma T 1 (limited to the mucosa and submucosa), independent of its size: 88%.
4. The 5-year survival rate for T 2 lymphoma (infiltration of about half the thickness of the gastric wall): 65%.
5. The 5-year survival rate of malignant lymphoma with involvement of the regional lymph nodes (N 1): 32%.
6. Nonresectable tumor with radiation therapy alone: only occasionally do patients survive for 5 years.
7. The overall 5-year survival rate is between 29 and 67% [32, 43].
8. The better prognosis for malignant lymphomas compared with that for gastric carcinoma is due to the lesser degree of infiltration of the malignant cells at the time of diagnosis and start of treatment [23].

Further Information

Occasionally a gastric adenocarcinoma can develop after a successfully treated gastric lymphoma [41].

[22] Lewin et al. 1978.
[23] Lim et al. 1977.
[32] Naqvi et al. 1969.
[41] Shani et al. 1978.
[43] Stobbe et al. 1966.

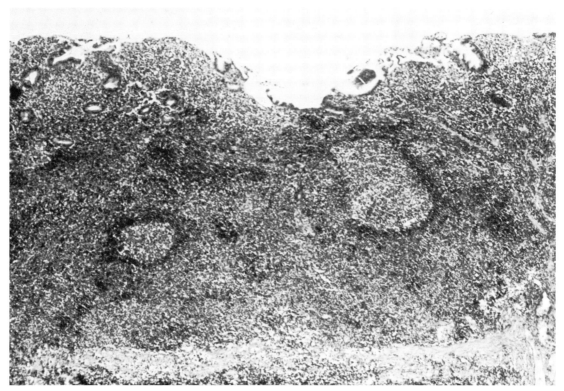

Fig. 247. Pseudolymphoma (lymphoid hyperplasia) of the stomach (64-year-old male, × 50).

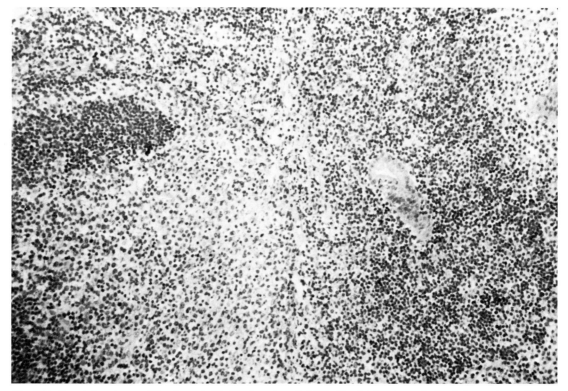

Fig. 248. Pseudolymphoma of the stomach: Besides lymphocytic infiltration, histiocytes and other inflammatory cells (64-year-old male, × 125).

M-8890/0
T 151.9

8. Leiomyoma (WHO)

M-8890/3
T 151.9

9. Leiomyosarcoma (WHO)

General Remarks

Incidence: Leiomyoma is the most common benign tumor of the stomach.
Age and Sex: Middle-aged men are affected most often.
Site: The main site of development is the lower half of the stomach.

Macroscopy

Leiomyoma and leiomyosarcoma can present as solitary or multiple nodular tumors. The mucosa covering the tumor is often ulcerated and shows signs of bleeding.
Leiomyomas can develop also at the serosa.

Histology

Interlacing smooth muscle fibers with regular nuclei (Fig. 249) or nuclei atypia and mitotic figures (see Differential diagnosis of leiomyoma with leiomyosarcoma).
Leiomyoma can be subclassified according to its growth and cellular particularities:
a) Some leiomyomas show extreme hyperchromatic nuclei and cellularity:

M-8893/0
    Bizarre leiomyoma (leiomyoblastoma – WHO).
b) Other leiomyomas have tumor cells with nuclei similar to those of epithelioid cells (Fig. 250):

M-8891/1
    Epithelioid leiomyoma (leiomyoblastoma – WHO).
c) Occasionally the leiomyoma contains numerous blood vessels:

M-8894/0
    Vascular leiomyoblastoma.

Electron Microscopy

The tumor cells contain microtubules and 50- to 90-Å-thick microfilaments [33].

Differential Diagnosis

Leiomyoma with leiomyosarcoma:
It is often difficult to distinguish leiomyomas from leiomyosarcomas, especially if the benign tumor presents as a bizarre leiomyoma (leiomyoblastoma) (Figs. 253 to 255).
Generally, the leiomyosarcoma cells are smaller than those in leiomyomas and the number of mitoses is occasionally elevated. Sometimes only the appearance of metastases decides for leiomyosarcoma [2, 13].

Clinical Findings

1. Leiomyomas often are discovered accidentally.
2. Leiomyosarcomas: Loss of weight and epigastric pain.

Spread

Main site for metastases: lung and liver (about 25% of the cases).
Regional lymph nodes are less frequently involved.
About 60% of the patients with leiomyosarcoma develop metastases [2].

---

[2] Appelman and Helwig 1976.
[13] Giberson et al. 1954.
[33] Nevalainen and Linna 1978.

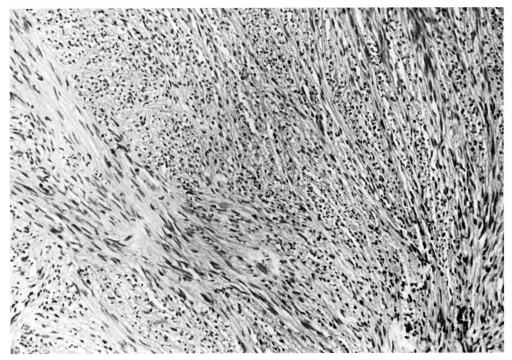

Fig. 249. Leiomyoma of the stomach: Regular nuclei, no mitoses (74-year-old male, × 125).

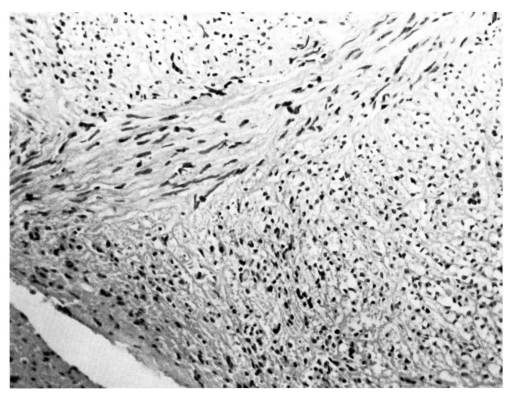

Fig. 250. Leiomyoma of the stomach: Areas of epithelioid leiomyoma (74-year-old male, × 200).

Leiomyoblastoma

Fig. 251. Vascular leiomyoblastoma of the stomach causing severe intestinal bleeding (74-year-old male, × 40).

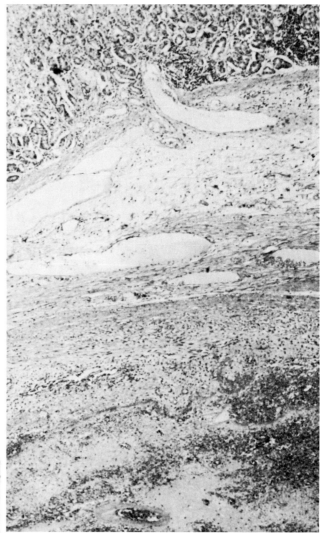

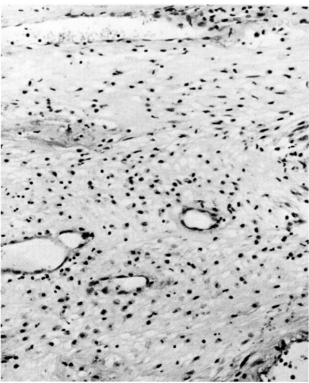

Fig. 252. Vascular leiomyoblastoma of the stomach (74-year-old male, × 125).

240

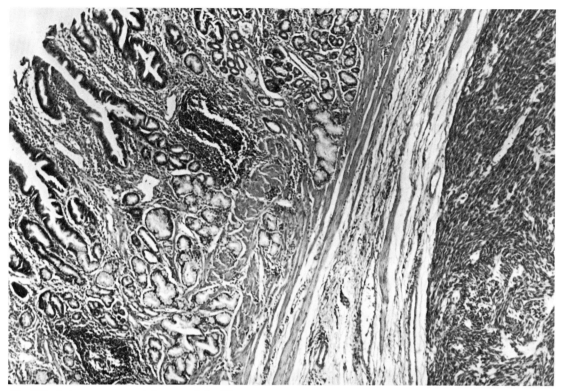

Fig. 253. Leiomyosarcoma of the stomach (× 50).

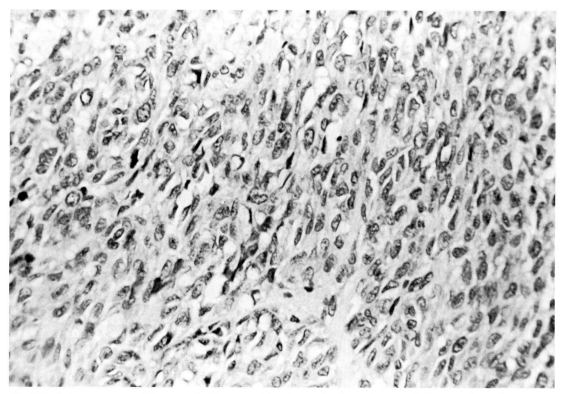

Fig. 254. Leiomyosarcoma of the stomach: Bizarre nuclei with vacuolated cytoplasm, atypical mitotic figures (× 200).

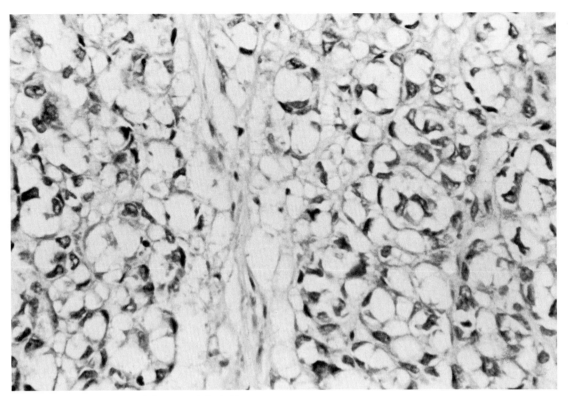

Fig. 255. Leiomyosarcoma of the stomach (×310).

Treatment	**Surgery:**
	Surgery alone for leiomyoma and leiomyosarcoma.
	Radiotherapy and **chemotherapy:**
	Radiotherapy and chemotherapy seem to be without benefit.

Prognosis

1. Leiomyoma: cure after surgical removal.
2. Leiomyosarcoma: the 5-year survival rate is about 50%.
   Cure after operation: about 40%.

Further Information

1. A multitumoral syndrome consisting of a combination of gastric leiomyosarcoma and functioning extraadrenal paraganglioma and pulmonary chondroma has been observed [4, 5].

M-8891/3

2. There is a report of a recurrent and metastasizing gastric **epithelioid leiomyosarcoma.** This sarcoma was associated with multiple pulmonary chondrohamartomas [46].

[4] Carney 1979.
[5] Carney et al. 1977.
[46] Tisell et al. 1978.

M-8980/3
T 151.9

10. Carcinosarcoma

This tumor consists of a combination of malignant epithelial and mesenchymal tissue [45] (Figs. 1361 to 1364).

11. Collision tumor

This name indicates the rare combination of an admixture of adenocarcinoma of the stomach with malignant lymphoma [1].
Occasionally these two different tumors can follow each other [41].

M-9730/3
T 151.9

12. Primary gastric plasmacytoma (WHO)

Primary gastric plasmacytoma is very rare. This tumor is treated by surgery and irradiation.
The prognosis is very poor [37].

M-9100/3
T 151.9

13. Choriocarcinoma (WHO)

Choriocarcinomas occur exceedingly rarely in the stomach.

[1] Ackerman and Rosai 1974.
[37] Remigio and Klaum 1971.
[41] Shani et al. 1978.
[45] Tanimura and Furuta 1967.

M-9080/0
T 151.9

14. Benign teratoma

Benign teratomas are very rare in the stomach and are observed in male infants and young children [10].

M-8000/6
T 151.9

15. Metastatic lesions

Metastatic lesions in the stomach are rarely observed [9]. The primary tumors in these instances are malignant melanomas and tumors of the pancreas, the breast, and the lung.

M-9800/3
T 151.9

16. Leukemic infiltration of the stomach

Leukemic infiltration of the stomach is observed in about 5% of leukemias [7, 30].

T 151.9

17. Soft tissue tumors
(non-epithelial tumors – WHO) (see Soft tissue tumors, page 7).

M-8810/0 **a) Fibroma**

M-8850/0 **b) Lipoma** [16]

M-8850/3 **c) Liposarcoma** [16]

M-9560/0 **d) Neurilemoma** [30] (Fig. 256)

M-9550/0 **e) Neurofibroma**

M-8852/0 **f) Myxolipoma**

M-9580/0 **g) Granular cell tumor** [14].

---

[7] Cornes and Jones 1962.
[9] Davis and Zollinger 1960.
[10] DeAngelis 1969.
[14] Goodman et al. 1962.
[16] Hawkins and Terrell 1965.
[30] Morson and Dawson 1974 (further references)

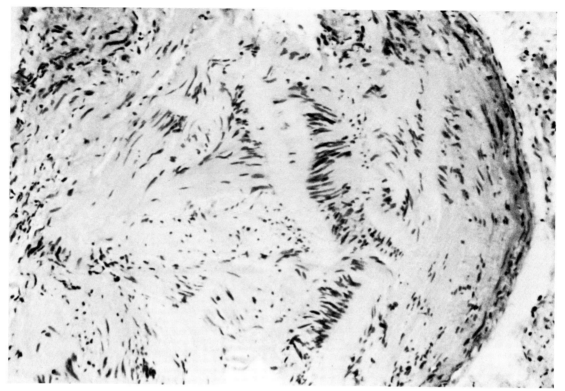

Fig. 256. Neurilemoma of the stomach in von Recklinghausen's disease (29-year-old male, ×125).

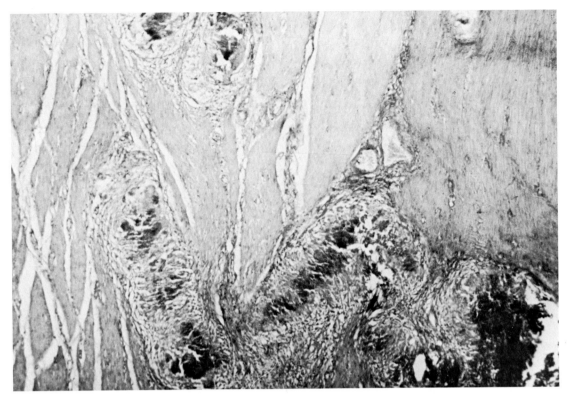

Fig. 257. Parasitic granuloma in the wall of the stomach (× 40).

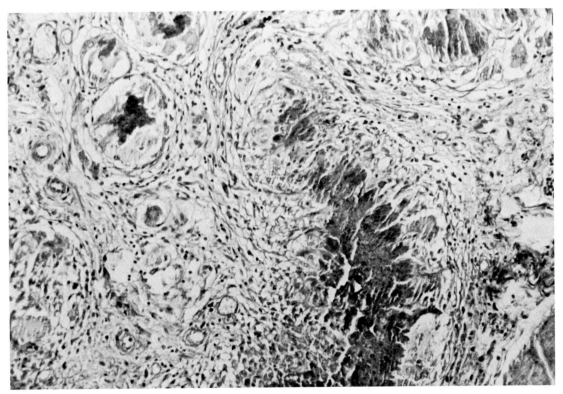

Fig. 258. Parasitic granuloma in the wall of the stomach (× 125).

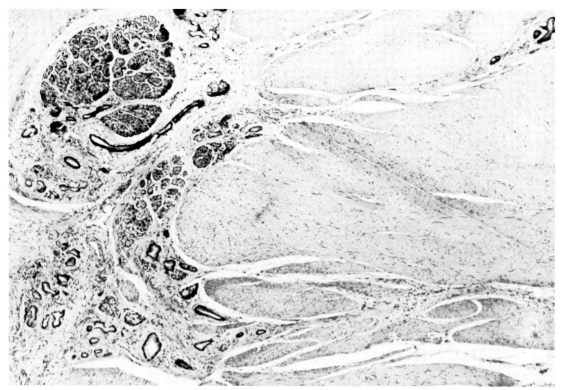

Fig. 259. Heterotopic pancreatic tissue in the gastric wall (36-year-old male, × 50).

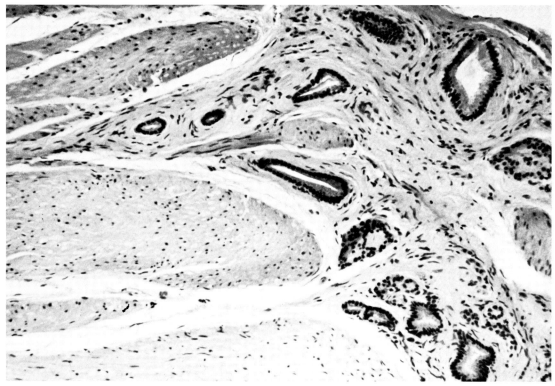

Fig. 260. Heterotopic pancreatic tissue in the gastric wall (36-year-old male, × 125).

18. Tumor-like lesions of the stomach

a) Parasitic granuloma (Figs. 257 and 258)

b) Pancreatic heterotopia (WHO) (Figs. 259 and 260)

M-4318/0
T 151.9

c) Malakoplakia (Figs. 1397 and 1398) [47].

M-8153/1, 3
T 151.9

19. Gastrinoma

Gastrinomas can occur in the antropyloric mucosa [20 a] (see page 422).

M-8000/3
T 151.9

20. Unclassified tumors (WHO)

[20a] Larsson et al. 1973.
[47] Wanke 1971.

Recommendations for differential diagnosis in tumors of the stomach

undifferentiated adenocarcinoma (diffuse adenocarcinoma)	with	– malignant lymphoma – chronic inflammation
carcinoma in situ (intraglandular carcinoma)	with	– superficial spreading carcinoma
adenocarcinoma, nonspecific type	with	– adenocarcinoma of an intestinal epithelial pattern
chronic inflammation	with	– malignant lymphoma – leukemic infiltration – extramedullary plasmacytoma – linitis plastica – undifferentiated carcinoma
non-Hodgkin's lymphoma	with	– Hodgkin's lymphoma – undifferentiated carcinoma – leukemic infiltration – pseudolymphoma (lymphoid hyperplasia with chronic inflammation)
adenomatous-villous polyp	with	– carcinoma developing in the polyp – carcinoma developing outside the polypous mucosa
leiomyoma (especially the bizarre type)	with	– leiomyosarcoma
adenocarcinoma	with	– gastritis chronica profunda – tumor-like lesions: heterotopic pancreatic tissue, parasitic granuloma
malakoplakia	with	– diffusely growing malignant tumor

References

[1] Ackerman, L.V., and J. Rosai: Surgical pathology. Fifth ed., C.V. Mosby Comp. 1974.

[2] Appelman, H.D., and E.B. Helwig: Gastric epithelioid leiomyoma and leiomyosarcoma (leiomyoblastoma). Cancer *38* (1976) 708-728.

[3] Bötticher, R., H. Bünte, P. Hermanek und W. Rösch: Magenpolypen. Prognose und Therapie. Dtsch. Med. Wschr. *100* (1975) 167-170.

[4] Carney, J.A.: The triad of gastric epithelioid leiomyosarcoma, functioning extra-adrenal paraganglioma, and pulmonary chondroma. Cancer *43* (1979) 374-382.

[5] Carney, J.A., S.G. Sheps, V.L.W. Go, and H. Gordon: The triad of gastric leiomyosarcoma, functioning extra-adrenal paraganglioma, and pulmonary chondroma. N. Engl. J. Med. *296* (1977) 1517-1518.

[6] Chejfec, G., and V.E. Gould: Malignant gastric neuroendocrinomas: Ultrastructural and biochemical characterization of their secretory activity. Hum. Pathol. *8* (1977) 433-440.

[7] Cornes, J.S., and T.G. Jones: Leukaemic lesions of the gastrointestinal tract. J. Clin. Pathol. *15* (1962) 305-313.

[8] Davis, H.L., Jr., D.D. von Hoff, M. Rozencweig, H. Handelsman, W.T. Soper, and F.M. Muggia: Gastrointestinal cancer: Esophagus, stomach, small bowel, colorectum, pancreas, liver, gallbladder, and extrahepatic ducts. In: Randomized trials in cancer: A critical review by sites. Edited by M.J. Staquet, Raven Press, New York, 1978.

[9] Davis, G.H., and R.W. Zollinger: Metastatic melanoma of the stomach. Am. J. Surg. *99* (1960) 94-96.

[10] DeAngelis, V.R.: Gastric teratoma in a newborn infant: Total gastrectomy with survival. Surgery *66* (1969) 794-797.

[11] Denk, H., G. Tappeiner, A. Davidovits, and J.H. Holzner: The carcinoembryonic antigen (CEA) in carcinomata of the stomach. Virchows Arch. A Path. Anat. and Histol. *360* (1973) 339-347.

[12] Elster, K., und A. Thomasko: Klinische Wertung der histologischen Typen des Magenfrühkarzinoms. Eine Analyse von 300 Fällen. Leber, Magen, Darm *8* (1978) 319-327.

[13] Giberson, R.G., N.D. Dockerty, and H.K. Gray: Leiomyosarcoma of the stomach. Clinicopathologic study of 40 cases. Surg. Gynec. Obstet. *98* (1954) 186-196.

[14] Goodman, M.L., L.S. Gottlieb, and M. Zamcheck: Granular-cell myoblastoma of stomach and colon. Am. J. Dig. Dis. *7* (1962) 432-441.

[15] Hartmann, D., und J.P. Obrecht: Stand der Therapie bei gastrointestinalen Tumoren. Schweiz. Med. Wschr. *108* (1978) 1373-1377.

[16] Hawkins, P.E., and G.K. Terrell: Liposarcoma of the stomach: A case report. JAMA *191* (1965) 758-759.

[17] Imura, H., S. Matsukura, H. Yamamoto, Y. Hirata, Y. Nakai, J. Endo, A. Tanaka, and M. Nakamura: Studies on ectopic ACTH-producing tumors. II. Clinical and biochemical features of 30 cases. Cancer *35* (1975) 1430-1437.

[18] Inokuchi, K., S. Inutsuka, M. Furusawa, K. Soejima, and T. Ikeda: Stromal reaction around tumor and metastasis and prognosis after curative gastrectomy for carcinoma of the stomach. Cancer *20* (1967) 1924-1929.

[19] Joseph, J.I., and R. Lattes: Gastric lymphosarcoma. Clinicopathologic analysis of 71 cases and its relation to disseminated lymphosarcoma. Am. J. Clin. Pathol. *45* (1966) 653-669.

[20] Kienzle, H.-F.: Das Magenstumpfkarzinom, klinische Erfahrung und Beobachtung aus 15 Jahren. Med. Klin. *72* (1977) 399-405.

[20a] Larsson, L.I., O. Ljungberg, F. Sundler, R. Håkanson, S.O. Svensson, J. Rehfeld, F. Stadil, and J. Holst: Antro-pyloric gastrinoma associated with pancreatic nesidioblastosis and proliferation of islets. Virchows Arch. A Path. Anat. and Histol. *360* (1973) 305-314.

[21] Lattes, R., and C. Grossi: Carcinoid tumors of the stomach. Cancer *9* (1956) 698-711.

[22] Lewin, K.J., M. Ranchod, and R.F. Dorfman: Lymphomas of the gastrointestinal tract. A study of 117 cases presenting with gastrointestinal disease. Cancer *42* (1978) 693-707.

[23] Lim, F.E., A.S. Hartman, E.G.C. Tan, B. Cady, and W.A. Meissner: Factors in the prognosis of gastric lymphoma. Cancer *39* (1977) 1715-1720.

[24] Marangos, G.N.: Hemangiopericytoma of the stomach. Gut *6* (1965) 77-79.

[25] Ming, S.C.: Tumors of the esophagus and stomach. Atlas of tumor pathology, A.F.I.P., Washington, D.C. 1973.

[26] Ming, S.C.: The adenoma-carcinoma sequence in the stomach and colon. II. Malignant potential of gastric polyps. Gastrointest. Radiol. *1* (1976) 121-125.

[27] Moertel, C.G.: Carcinoma of the stomach: Prognostic factors and criteria of response to therapy. In: Cancer therapy: Prognostic factors and criteria of response; edited by M.J. Staquet, Raven Press, New York 1975.

[28] Moertel, C.G., J.A. Mittelman, R.F. Bakemeier, P. Engstrom, and J. Hanley: Sequential and combination chemotherapy of advanced gastric cancer. Cancer *38* (1976) 678-682.

[29] Moritz, E., und G. Wense: Das Magenkarzinom im jugendlichen Alter. Dtsch. Med. Wschr. *99* (1974) 180-181.

[30] Morson, B.C., and I.M.P. Dawson: Gastrointestinal pathology. Blackwell Scientific Publication, Oxford–London–Edinburgh–Melbourne 1974.

[31] Nakamura, K., H. Sugano, and K. Takagi: Carcinoma of the stomach in incipient phase: Its histogenesis and histological appearances. Gann *59* (1968) 251-258.

[32] Naqvi, M.S., L. Burrows, and A.E. Kark: Lymphoma of the gastrointestinal tract: Prognostic guides based on 162 cases. Ann. Surg. *170* (1969) 221-231.

[33] Nevalainen, T.J., and M.I. Linna: Ultrastructure of gastric leiomyosarcoma. Virchows Arch. A Path. Anat. and Histol. *379* (1978) 25-33.

[34] Perrotta, R.C.: Gastric carcinoma: Six years' experience with radical gastric resection. J. Am. Osteopath. Assoc. *76* (1977) 326-334.

[35] Prolla, J.C., S. Kobayashi, and J.B. Kirsner: Gastric cancer. Some recent improvements in diagnosis based on the Japanese experience. Arch. Int. Med. *124* (1969) 238-246.

[36] Pygott, F., and V.L. Shah: Gastric cancer, associated with gastroenterostomy and partial gastrectomy. Gut *9* (1968) 117-124.

[37] Remigio, P.A., and A. Klaum: Extramedullary plasmocytoma of the stomach. Cancer *27* (1971) 562-568.

[38] Rösch, W., und R. Thoma: Anamnese beim Frühkarzinom des Magens. Med. Klin. *69* (1974) 2063-2066.

[39] Rudders, R.A., M.E. Ross, and R.A. DeLellis: Primary extranodal lymphoma. Response to treatment and factors influencing prognosis. Cancer *42* (1978) 406-416.

[40] Schlag, P., H. Meister, P. Merkle, O. Haferkamp und C. Herfarth: Prognostische Aspekte des Magenfrühkarzinoms. Dtsch. Med. Wschr. *104* (1979) 659-662.

[41] Shani, A., A.J. Schutt, and L.H. Weiland: Primary gastric malignant lymphoma followed by gastric adenocarcinoma. Report of 4 cases and review of the literature. Cancer *42* (1978) 2039-2044.

[42] Siegel, S.E., D.M. Hays, S. Romansky, and H. Isaacs: Carcinoma of the stomach in childhood. Cancer *38* (1976) 1781-1784.

[43] Stobbe, J.A., M.B. Dockerty, and P.E. Bernatz: Primary gastric lymphoma and its grades of malignancy. Am. J. Surg. *112* (1966) 10-19.

[44] Straus, R., S. Heschel, and D.J. Fortmann: Primary adenosquamous carcinoma of the stomach. A case report and review. Cancer *24* (1969) 985-995.

[45] Tanimura, H., and M. Furuta: Carcinosarcoma of the stomach. Am. J. Surg. *113* (1967) 702-709.

[46] Tisell, L.-E., L. Angervall, I. Dahl, C. Merck, and B.F. Zachrisson: Recurrent and metastasizing gastric leiomyoblastoma (epithelioid leiomyosarcoma) associated with multiple pulmonary chondrohamartomas. Long survival of a patient treated with repeated operations. Cancer *41* (1978) 259-265.

[47] Wanke, M.: Magen. In: Spezielle pathologische Anatomie. Band II, Teil 1. Hrsg.: W. Doerr, G. Seifert, E. Uehlinger. Springer, Berlin–Heidelberg–New York 1971.

[48] Wanke, M.: Case report. – Collision-tumour of the cardia. Virchows Arch. A Path. Anat. and Histol. *357* (1972) 81-86.

[49] Watanabe, H., M. Enjoji, and T. Imai: Gastric carcinoma with lymphoid stroma. Its morphologic characteristics and prognostic correlations. Cancer *38* (1976) 232-243.

[50] Weitzner, S.: Glomus tumor of the stomach. Report of a case and review of the literature. Am. J. Gastroent. *51* (1969) 322-328.

6 Tumors of the small bowel

M-8140/3
T 152.9

1. Adenocarcinoma (WHO) [9]
(no TNM classification)

**General
Remarks**

Incidence: A rare tumor.

Macroscopy

In most instances this is an ulcerated, stenosing tumor.
Occasionally the tumor is polypoid and large (up to 10 cm in diameter).

Histology

In most instances this is a well-differentiated or moderately differentiated adenocarcinoma. Occasionally undifferentiated carcinomas with no signs of glandular structures are found (Fig. 261).

Spread

Regional lymph node metastases.

**Clinical
Findings**

In most instances there are signs of intestinal obstruction.

Treatment

Surgery:
Resection of the tumor.
Radiotherapy and **chemotherapy:**
Radiotherapy or chemotherapy are probably of low or no efficiency.

Prognosis

Poor.

**Further
Information**

Occasionally, adenocarcinoma of the small bowel is associated with regional enteritis (Crohn's disease) [18].

M-8140/3
T 152.0

2. Primary adenocarcinoma of the duodenum

Adenocarcinoma of the duodenum is very rare.
The tumor can be detected by fiberoptic esophagogastroduodenoscopy.
Adenocarcinoma of the ampulla of Vater arises only occasionally from the mucosa of the duodenum (see page 398).

Treatment

In resectable tumors, pancreaticoduodenectomy should be attempted [16].

[9] Morson 1976.
[16] Spira et al. 1977.
[18] Valdes-Dapena et al. 1976.

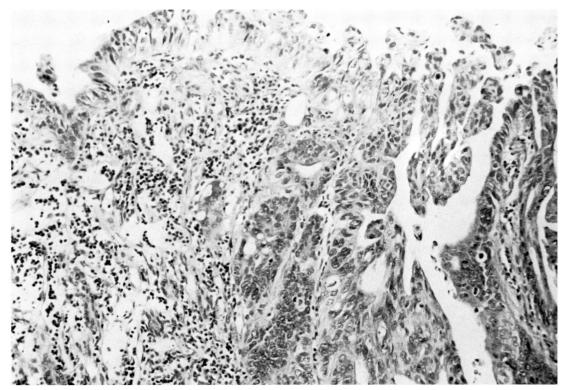

Fig. 261. Adenocarcinoma of the jejunum (51-year-old male, × 200).

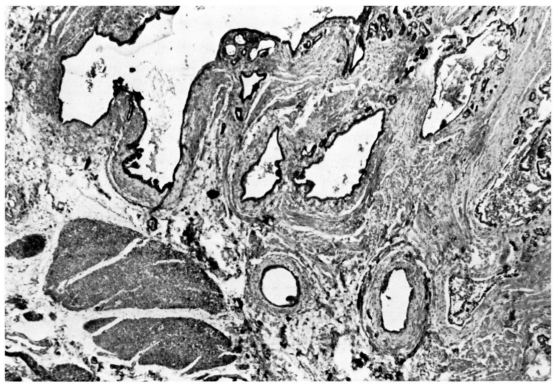

Fig. 262. Heterotopic pancreatic tissue in the wall of the small intestine (50-year-old male, × 40).

M-8000/6
T 152.9

3. Metastatic carcinoma

Solitary or multiple metastases into the small bowel wall can occur. However, this is a rare event.

The primary tumor can be in any organ; in most instances it is located in

the stomach,

the lung, or

the large bowel

or the tumor is disseminated from a malignant melanoma.

M-7650/0
T 152.9

4. Endometriosis in the wall of the small bowel (WHO)

Endometriosis in the wall of the small bowel can mimic a metastatic lesion, clinically and on gross and even on histological examination (Figs. 274 and 275).

This is particularly true if a decidual reaction of the stromal cells occurs.

M-2600/0
T 152.9

5. Pancreatic heterotopia (WHO)

Heterotopic pancreatic tissue in the wall of the small bowel should not be mistaken for carcinoma (Figs. 262 to 264).

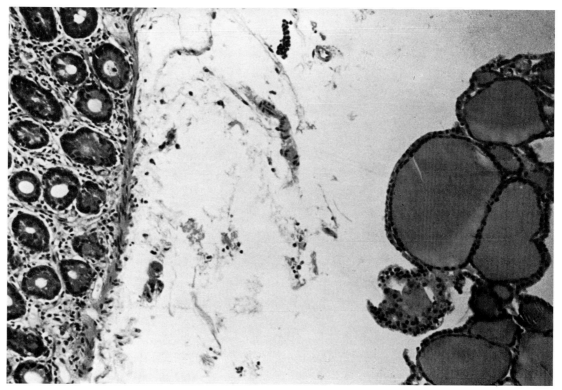

Fig. 263. Heterotopic thyroid-like tissue in the wall of the small intestine (62-year-old male, × 125).

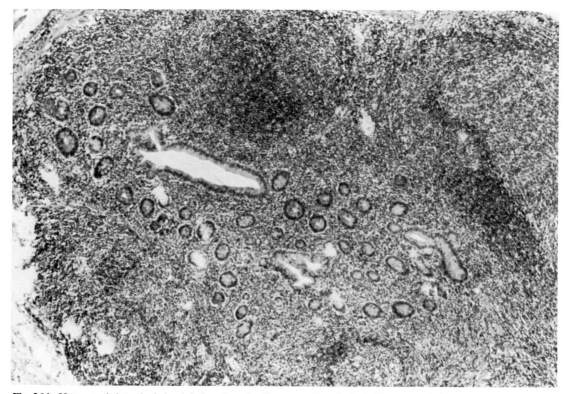

Fig. 264. Heterotopic intestinal glands in lymph node adherent to diverticulosis. No metastasis (65-year-old male, × 50).

M-8241/1, 3
T 152.9

6. Carcinoid

**General
Remarks**

Incidence: These are relatively rare tumors.
Age: The peak age is the 6th and 7th decades.
Sex: Men are affected more frequently than women.
Site: Mainly the ileum, also the jejunum and duodenum.

Macroscopy

Solitary or very often multiple tumors (occasionally more than 100) of different sizes.
The cut surface is yellowish.
The tumors are covered by mucosa, which only occasionally is ulcerated.
Some tumors are pedunculated.

Histology

Uniform-looking tumor cells grow in nests (Fig. 268).
The tumors of the proximal duodenal region occasionally show a tubular or trabecular arrangement.
The tumor cells infiltrate the wall, are found in the lymphatics, and reach the serosa.
The nuclei are round or oval. The chromatin is regularly distributed.
Mitotic figures are very rare.
The tumor cell nests may be similar to basaloid growth structures.
(Subclasses of carcinoids and distribution of the tumors, see under Further information, page 259).

**Electron
Microscopy**

(See Fig. 271) [3].

**Histochemistry
M-8241/1, 3**

Carcinoid tumors of the ileum and jejunum show an argentaffin-positive reaction:
Argentaffin-positive carcinoids (WHO).
Carcinoids of the proximal duodenal region are argentaffin-negative:

M-8242/1, 3

Nonargentaffin carcinoids (WHO) (Figs. 321 to 323).

**Differential
Diagnosis**

Carcinoid **with other endocrine tumors, especially islet cell tumor:**
Occasionally only immunohistochemical or histochemical findings solve the diagnostic problem (see Histochemistry and Immunochemistry in islet cell tumors, page 420).

Spread

Carcinoids are tumors that grow very slowly.
Although the development of metastases into the liver and lymph nodes occurs late in the course of the disease, most of these metastases are already present at the time of diagnosis.
Liver metastases have a whitish (not yellowish) cut surface.

**Clinical
Findings**

Symptoms are caused by the secretion of serotonin and/or kinins and histamine:
Watery feces, patchy flushing of the face, palpitations, cyanosis, signs of tricuspidal and pulmonary stenosis.
Signs of intestinal ischemia can develop due to arterial and venous sclerosis in the neighborhood of the tumor or even some distance from the tumor.

---

[3] Gyorkey et al. 1975.

Treatment	**Surgery:** Resection of localized tumors. Surgical removal of hepatic metastases should be attempted because amelioration of the carcinoid syndrome can be expected. **Radiation therapy:** Radiation therapy is without effect. **Chemotherapy:** Chemotherapy with 5-fluorouracil or streptozotocin can be attempted. An overall response rate of 15 to 35% has been reported [2, 12].
Prognosis	The tumor is slow-growing with late metastases; survival for many years can be expected.
Further Information	Two subgroups of carcinoid tumor can be distinguished and their distribution is as follows (Figs. 268, 269, 271 and 321 to 328):
M-8242/1, 3	**a) APUD cell tumor** (**a**mine **p**recursor **u**ptake **d**ecarboxylation) (argyrophil tumors; non-argentaffin tumors – WHO) **Histology:** The tumor cells grow as solid nests, forming ribbons and festoons. Rosette formations and acinar arrangements are observed. **Histochemistry:** The tumor cells show a negative argentaffin reaction (silver salts are not reduced to metallic silver). The tumor cells become silver-positive when external reducing agents are used (argyrophil). These carcinoid tumors are mainly observed in lung, rectum, stomach, and duodenum [9, 10, 19].
M-8241/0, 3	**b) Argentaffin-positive tumors** (WHO) (argentaffinoma; enterochromaffin cell tumors) These tumor cells contain granules with 5-hydroxytryptamine and secrete serotonin. **Histology:** This carcinoid forms tumor cells arranged in nests, clusters, and sheets with little tendency to imitate acinous structures. **Histochemistry:** These tumor cells reduce silver salt to metallic silver without the use of external reducing agents (Fontana reaction, argentaffin reaction). This type of carcinoid occurs mainly in the duodenum, small bowel, appendix, and colon. **c) Composite carcinoid** (WHO) contains cells with argentaffin properties and the growth pattern of nonargentaffin carcinoid [9].

---

[2] De Vita Jr. 1977.
[9] Morson 1976.
[10] Morson and Dawson 1974.
[12] Oates 1977.
[19] Williams and Sandler 1963.

M-9590/3
T 152.9

7. Malignant intestinal lymphoma
(No TNM classification)
(WHO: Hodgkin's disease; lymphosarcoma; Burkitt's lymphoma; reticulosarcoma)

**General
Remarks**

Incidence: Low incidence in Western countries; high incidence in Mediterranean countries (see Further information).
Age: Any age group can be affected by this tumor, including children.
Sex: Males are more often affected than females.
Site: Main site is the terminal ileum and the cecum.
Malignant lymphomas are also encountered in the upper small intestine and duodenum.

Macroscopy

The intestinal wall shows a patchy or diffuse thickening. The lumen is narrowed. The mucosa can be ulcerated.
The tumor can form polypoid masses; it can be sessile or pedunculated.

Histology

Any type of malignant lymphoma can occur; however, Hodgkin's lymphoma is rare (see Malignant lymphomas, page 1247).
The tumor starts growing in the lamina propria and gradually extends throughout the wall.

**Differential
Diagnosis
M-7229/0
T 152.9**

1. Malignant intestinal lymphoma **with benign lymphoid hyperplasia** (WHO):
   Lymphoid hyperplasia shows a follicular pattern and follicles (Fig. 247). Benign lymphoid hyperplasia is observed mainly in the terminal ileum. This disease affects males more often than females.
   Although the lumen of the intestine is narrowed by lymphoid hyperplasia, the mucosa is ulcerated very rarely.

**M-7682/0
T 152.9**

2. Early stages of malignant lymphoma **with inflammatory fibroid polyp** (WHO):
   This polypous lesion is covered by occasionally ulcerated mucosa. The stroma is densely infiltrated by inflammatory cells (lymphocytes and also granular leukocytes and plasma cells).
3. Primary localized malignant intestinal lymphoma **with malignant intestinal lymphoma as one of multiple foci in systemic disease.**
4. Non-Hodgkin's lymphoma **with Hodgkin's lymphoma.**

**Clinical
Findings**

Intestinal malabsorption. Signs of abnormalities of the globulins: Alpha-chain disease, Waldenström macroglobulinemia.
Intestinal obstruction.

Treatment

1. **Localized Malignant lymphoma:**
   Combination of surgical resection of the tumor, followed by radiation therapy (whole abdominal irradiation) and chemotherapy (multiple agent chemotherapy) [11].
2. **Nonlocalized lymphoma:**
   Systemic treatment (chemotherapy) or, according to the extent of the disease, radiation therapy (see Malignant lymphomas, page 1247).

---

[11] Nelson et al. 1977.

Prognosis

The prognosis is correlated with the stage of the disease and not with the histological type of the lymphoma [6].

The overall prognosis is poor, especially in children.

Further Information

1. Because intestinal lymphomas occur more often in Mediterranean countries, attempts were made to separate a "Western" from a "Mediterranean" type:

   a) **Western type of lymphoma:**

   Monomorphic lymphocytic or histiocytic cell infiltration in the distal small bowel.

   b) **Mediterranean type of lymphoma:**

   Pleomorphic (lymphocytic-histiocytic type) malignant lymphoma cell infiltration in the duodenum and jejunum [5].

   The Mediterranean type of lymphoma shows alpha-chain disease [13] and malabsorption [14].

2. The gastrointestinal tract is involved in 15% of the leukemias [10].

3. Involvement of the intestinal wall by Hodgkin's disease and extramedullary plasmacytoma is very rare.

[5] Lewin et al. 1976.
[6] Lewin et al. 1978.
[10] Morson and Dawson 1974.
[13] Seligmann 1975.
[14] Shahid et al. 1975.

M-8210/0
M-8261/1
T 152.9

8. Benign adenoma (WHO)

These benign adenomas can occur as solitary or multiple lesions.
Adenomas or papillomas are sessile or pedunculated.
The latter tumors can cause intestinal bleeding by hemorrhagic necroses.
A number of the polyps in the small intestine are hamartomatous lesions as part of the
Peutz-Jeghers syndrome [8, 10].

M-7563/0

One duodenal adenoma composed entirely of Paneth's cells with signs of malignant
change has been observed [7].

M-8890/0
M-8890/3
T 152.9

9. Leiomyoma and leiomyosarcoma (WHO)

**General
Remarks**

Incidence: About 20% of all benign tumors of the small bowel are leiomyomas.
Age: Average age is about 50 years.
Site: 80% grow in the jejunum and ileum; 20% grow in the duodenum.

Macroscopy

The leiomyoma and leiomyosarcoma present as circumscribed tumors with a yellowish or
whitish cut surface, which contains cysts and shows a whorling pattern.
The covering mucosa in most instances is ulcerated.
The tumor might protrude into the lumen.

Histology

The tumor is composed of interlacing bundles of smooth muscle fibers. The leiomyoma
has regular nuclei.
Varieties with high cellularity and hyperchromatic bizarre nuclei are called

M-8893/0

bizarre leiomyomas (leiomyoblastomas – WHO) (Figs. 265 and 266).

**Differential
Diagnosis**

Benign leiomyoma with leiomyosarcoma:
A high number of mitoses (in high power fields), high cellularity, and many atypical cells
indicate leiomyosarcoma.
The distinction between benign and malignant tumors can be very difficult because giant
cells and atypical cells can occur in benign leiomyomas, as can high cellularity.
The most important sign is the number of mitoses.
Even without signs of malignancy the behavior of leiomyomas cannot always be pre-
dicted on the basis of histological observations!

**Clinical
Findings**

Intestinal bleeding and signs of intestinal obstruction.

[7] Miyajima and Takeuchi 1976.
[8] Morson 1962.
[10] Morson and Dawson 1974.

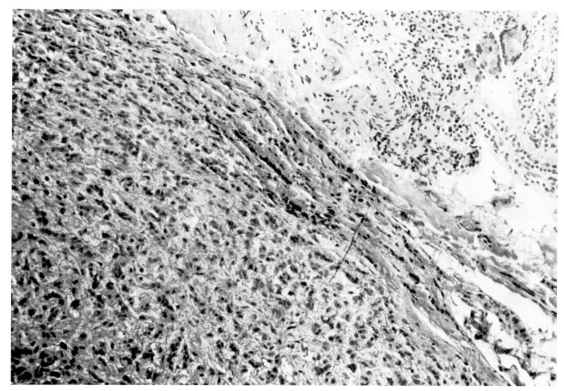

Fig. 265. Epithelioid leiomyoma of the small intestine (86-year-old female, × 125).

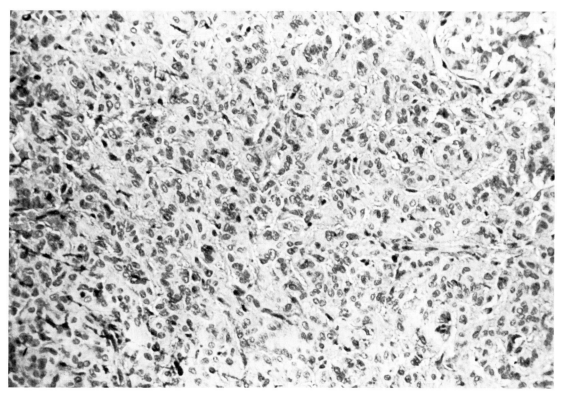

Fig. 266. Epithelioid leiomyoma of the small intestine (86-year-old female, × 200).

Treatment	For leiomyoma and leiomyosarcoma: Resection of the tumor. Irradiation and chemotherapy are not effective.
Prognosis	1. For leiomyoma: After resection, excellent. 2. For leiomyosarcoma: Depending on the extent of the tumor. A 5-year survival can be expected for 50% of the patients.

T 152.9

10. Soft tissue tumors of the small intestine
(non-epithelial tumors – WHO)
(See Soft tissue tumors, page 7).

M-8850/0

a) Lipoma

Lipomas are rare and do not cause symptoms. There are no reports of liposarcoma of the intestine.

T 153.4

Localized hyperplasia of the fat tissue at the region of the **ileocecal valve** is called: **Lipohyperplasia** (WHO).

M-9540/1
(M-9550/1)

b) Neurofibromatosis

Solitary or multiple tumors occur as part of the systemic von Recklinghausen's disease.

Occasionally, the tumors cause intestinal bleeding.

M-9560/0

c) Neurilemoma (WHO)

Neurilemoma is rare in the small bowel.

M-9120/0

d) Hemangioma (WHO)

Hemangiomas grow in most instances as the cavernous type. These hemangiomas can ulcerate and cause major intestinal bleeding [15].

A particular variety of hemangiomas occurs in the hereditary telangiectasia (Rendu-Osler-Weber's disease). This lesion also can cause major intestinal bleeding. These hemangiomas are often barely visible at gross inspection.

---

[15] Smith Jr. et al. 1963.

M-8680/0, 1
T 152.0

e) Gangliocytic paraganglioma [4]

This tumor grows in the duodenum.

The tumor is small and pedunculated and is covered by an occasionally ulcerated mucosa.

The tumor is composed of large or spindle-shaped cells, which grow beside other cells of an epithelioid shape. The large cells occasionally resemble gangliocytes [17].

It is supposed that this tumor is a combination of a chemodectoma, ganglioneuroma, and carcinoid tumor [1].

11. Somatostatinoma

Recently a malignant tumor composed of somatostatin-containing cells was investigated. The tumor was localized in the jejunum [1 a].

M-8000/3
T 152.9

12. Unclassified tumors (WHO)

[1]   Ackerman and Rosai 1974.
[1a] Alumets et al. 1978.
[4]   Kepes and Zacharias 1971.
[17] Taylor and Helwig 1962.

Recommendations for differential diagnosis in tumors of the small bowel and duodenum

primary adenocarcinoma	with	– metastatic adenocarcinoma – carcinoid – heterotopic gastric or pancreatic tissue – endometriosis – enteritis chronica profunda
adenocarcinoma of the papilla Vateri	with	– noninfiltrating mucosal polyp of the duodenal mucosa with chronic inflammation – chronic inflammation in the bile duct
carcinoid	with	– islet cell tumor – adenocarcinoma
non-Hodgkin's lymphoma	with	– Hodgkin's lymphoma – chronic inflammation – plasmacytoma – benign lymphoid hyperplasia – undifferentiated carcinoma
leiomyoma	with	– leiomyosarcoma

References

[1] Ackerman, L.V., and J. Rosai: Surgical pathology. Fifth ed., C.V. Mosby Company 1974.

[1a] Alumets, J., G. Ekelund, R. Håkanson, O. Ljungberg, U. Ljungqvist, F. Sundler, and S. Tibblin: Jejunal endocrine tumour composed of somatostatin and gastrin cells and associated with duodenal ulcer disease. Virchows Arch. A Path. Anat. and Histol. *378* (1978) 17-22.

[2] DeVita, V.T., Jr.: In: Harrison's Principles of internal medicine. Eighth edition. McGraw-Hill Book Company, New York–Düsseldorf etc. 1977.

[3] Gyorkey, F., K.-W. Min, J. Krisko, and P. Gyorkey: The usefulness of electron microscopy in the diagnosis of human tumours. Hum. Pathol. *6* (1975) 421-441.

[4] Kepes, J.J., and D.L. Zacharias: Gangliocytic paragangliomas of the duodenum: A report of two cases with light and electron microscopic examination. Cancer *27* (1971) 61-70.

[5] Lewin, K.J., L.B. Kahn, and B.H. Novis: Primary intestinal lymphoma of "western" and "Mediterranean" type, alpha chain disease and massive plasma cell infiltration. A comparative study of 37 cases. Cancer *38* (1976) 2511-2528.

[6] Lewin, K.J., M. Ranchod, and R.F. Dorfman: Lymphomas of the gastrointestinal tract. A study of 117 cases presenting with gastrointestinal disease. Cancer *42* (1978) 693-707.

[7] Miyajima, H., and T. Takeuchi: Paneth cell tumor. An additional case of duodenal adenoma with malignant change. Beitr. Path. *157* (1976) 419-425.

[8] Morson, B.C.: Some peculiarities in the histology of intestinal polyps. Dis. Col. Rect. *5* (1962) 337-344.

[9] Morson, B.C.: Histological typing of intestinal tumours. WHO, Geneva 1976.

[10] Morson, B.C., and I.M.P. Dawson: Gastrointestinal pathology. Blackwell Scientific Public. Oxford–London–Edinburgh–Melbourne 1974.

[11] Nelson, D.F., J.R. Cassady, D. Traggis, A. Baez-Giangreco, G.F. Vawter, N. Jaffe, and R.M. Filler: The role of radiation therapy in localized resectable intestinal non-Hodgkin's lymphoma in children. Cancer *39* (1977) 89-97.

[12] Oates, J.A.: In: Harrison's Principles of internal medicine. Eighth edition. McGraw-Hill Book Company, New York–Düsseldorf etc. 1977.

[13] Seligmann, M.: Alpha chain disease – immunoglobulin abnormalities, pathogenesis and current concepts. Br. J. Cancer *31,* Suppl. II (1975) 356-361.

[14] Shahid, M.J., S.Y. Alami, V.H. Nassar, J.B. Balikian, and A.A. Salem: Primary intestinal lymphoma with paraproteinemia. Cancer *35* (1975) 848-858.

[15] Smith, C.R., Jr., L.G. Bartholomew, and J.C. Cain: Hereditary hemorrhagic telangiectasia and gastrointestinal hemorrhage. Gastroenterology *44* (1963) 1-6.

[16] Spira, I.A., A. Ghazi, and W.I. Wolff: Primary adenocarcinoma of the duodenum. Cancer *39* (1977) 1721-1726.

[17] Taylor, H.B., and E.B. Helwig: Benign non chromaffin paragangliomas of the duodenum. Virchows Arch. Pathol. Anat. *335* (1962) 356-366.

[18] Valdes-Dapena, A., I. Rudolph, A. Hidayat, J.L.A. Roth, and R.B. Laucks: Adenocarcinoma of the small bowel in association with regional enteritis. Four new cases. Cancer *37* (1976) 2938-2947.

[19] Williams, E.D., and M. Sandler: The classification of carcinoid tumours. Lancet *1* (1963) 238-239.

7 Tumors of the appendix

M-8240/0, 1
T 153.5

1. Carcinoid (WHO)

**General
Remarks**

Incidence: Carcinoids are the most common tumors in the appendix: 0.1 to 0.3% of all appendixes contain a carcinoid.
Age: The peak age is the 3rd and 4th decades.
Site: 70% are located in the tip of the appendix.
Further notes: Both argentaffin and argyrophil carcinoids occur in the appendix.

Macroscopy

A yellowish, small lesion, which is usually less than 1 cm.
This tumor is often detected only on histological analysis.

Histology

The tumor is composed of nests of regular tumor cells forming strands (Figs. 267 to 269).
The tumor cells can also form tubular or adenoid-like structures.
The tumor cells are found in the muscle and the lymphatics (Fig. 270).
They can reach the surrounding fat tissue and even be observed on the peritoneal surface [3].

**Electron
Microscopy**

Polymorphic intracytoplasmatic granules (Fig. 271).

**Differential
Diagnosis**

In cases of carcinoid with a tubular or adenoid growth pattern **with primary or metastatic adenocarcinoma:**
Mucin stain will allow diagnosis.

Spread

Metastases are very rare and usually do not appear beyond the regional lymph nodes.

**Clinical
Findings**

Signs of acute appendicitis.

Treatment

Appendectomy.

Prognosis

Excellent.

---

[3] Warkel et al. 1978.

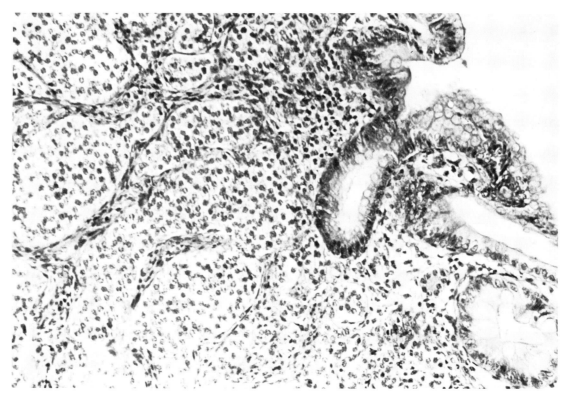

Fig. 267. Carcinoid tumor of the appendix: Nests of tumor cells (10-year-old female, symptoms of acute appendicitis, ×125).

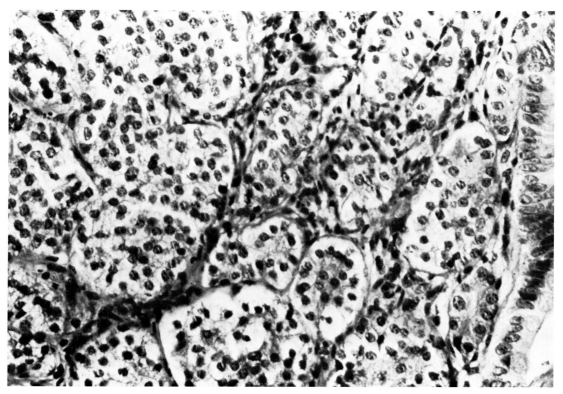

Fig. 268. Carcinoid tumor of the appendix: Solid nests (argentaffinoma) (10-year-old female, ×200).

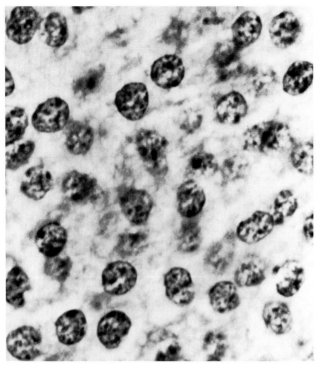

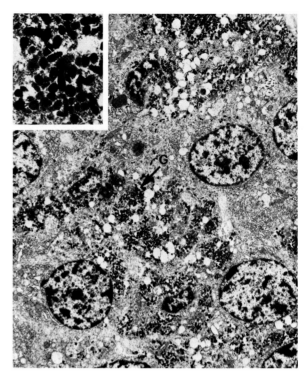

Fig. 269. Carcinoid tumor of the appendix: Round or oval nuclei (10-year-old female, ×800).

Fig. 271. Carcinoid tumor of appendix: Polymorphic dense granules (×3,750; inset, ×15,000) (Gyorkey et al., Hum. Pathol. *6* (1975) 421-441).

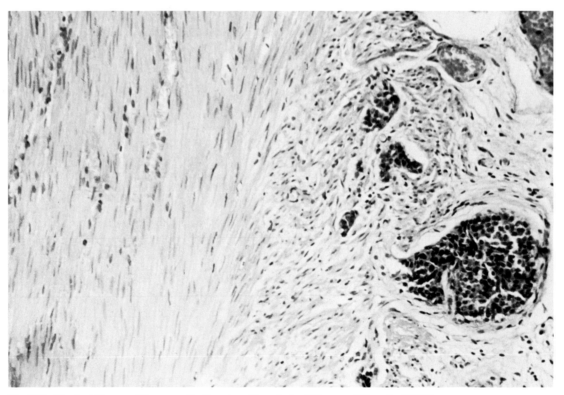

Fig. 270. Carcinoid tumor of the appendix: Invasion of lymphatics (10-year-old female, ×125).

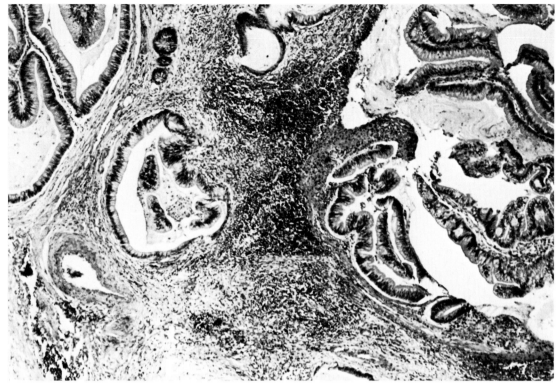

Fig. 272. Adenocarcinoma of the appendix: Papillary and invasive growth (68-year-old male, × 60).

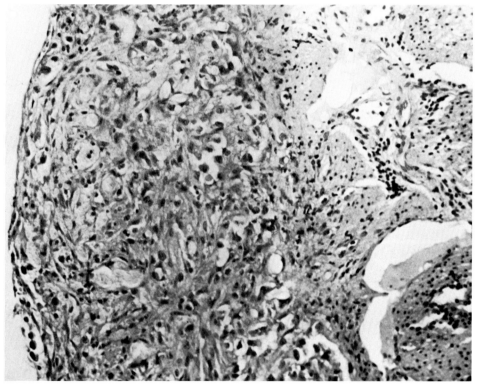

Fig. 273. Peritoneal metastatic tumor, appendix (68-year-old male, × 125).

M-8140/3
T 153.5

2. Adenocarcinoma (WHO)

**General
Remarks**

Incidence: Adenocarcinomas of the appendix are very rare (probably 0.01 % or less of all operated appendixes).

Macroscopy

Sometimes they are not detectable.

**Electron
Microscopy**

The tumor cells of adenocarcinoma of the appendix (adenocancroid) of the goblet cell type often contain electron-dense pleomorphic enterochromaffin granules of different sizes. The remaining cytoplasm is often electron-lucent [2].

**Differential
Diagnosis**

Endometriosis or **diverticulosis** in the wall of the appendix should not be mistaken for infiltrating carcinoma (Figs. 272 to 275).

Spread

The carcinoma spreads into the regional lymph nodes.
Adenocarcinoma of the appendix can invade the cecum; however, more often a tumor of the cecum invades the appendix.

Prognosis

The extent of the tumor determines the prognosis (see Dukes classification and Prognosis in colonic tumor, page 301).

---

[2] Cooper and Warkel 1978.

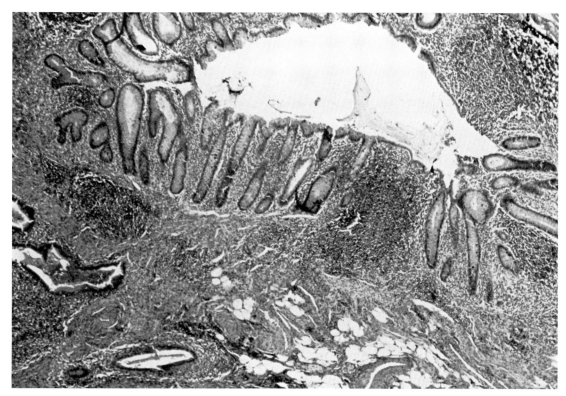

Fig. 274. Endometriosis in the wall of the appendix, no adenocarcinoma (32-year-old female, × 50).

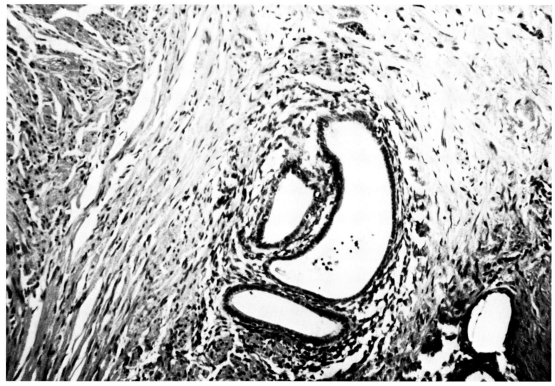

Fig. 275. Endometriosis in the wall of the appendix (32-year-old female, × 125).

M-8260/0

3. Adenomatous polyp
(tubular adenoma – WHO)

M-8261/1
T-153.5

4. Villous polyp
(villous adenoma – WHO)

Adenomatous and villous polyps may occur in the appendix; however, they are rare in this location.

Carcinomatous changes in polyps of the appendix are very rare.

Histology

The appearance of these polyps can be determined by the mucus production of the tumor cells (Figs. 276 and 277). The mucus can dilate the appendix, especially the distal part (see Mucocele, page 278).

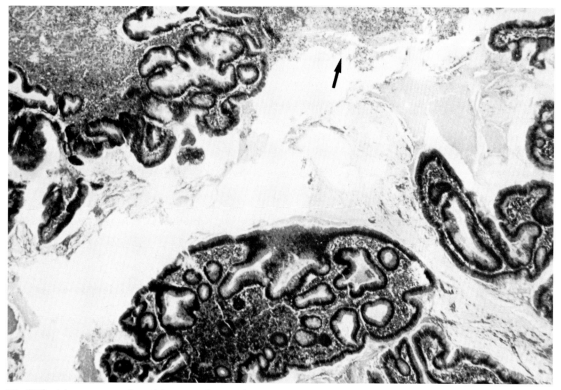

Fig. 276. Adenomatous polyp of the appendix combined with ulcerative appendicitis (arrow) (68-year-old male, × 40).

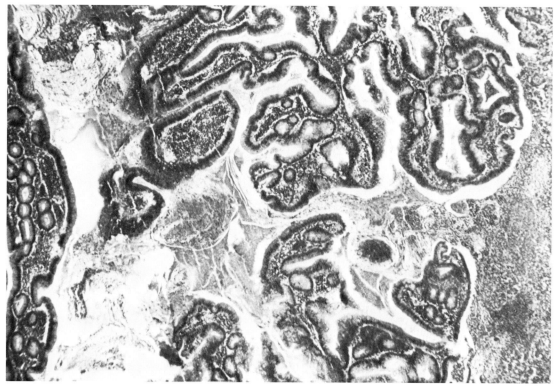

Fig. 277. Adenomatous polyp of the appendix (68-year-old male, × 70).

5. Mucocele

**General
Remarks**

M-8470/0, 1

M-8470/3

M-8210/0

T 153.5

The appearance of mucinous material in the lumen of the appendix (mucocele) can be caused by

– **mucinous cystadenoma** (WHO)

– **mucinous cystadenocarcinoma** (WHO), **mucinous adenocarcinoma** (WHO)

– **mucin-producing polyp**

Macroscopy

The appendix is dilated. The dilatation occurs mostly in a particular segment.

The cut surface shows a lumen, which is filled with mucinous material.

Histology

The mucinous material is sometimes limited to the lumen; however, it can be found in different areas of the wall und may reach the surrounding tissue.

The lining epithelium can be flattened, columnar, or cuboidal.

The nuclei are sometimes hyperchromatic.

The epithelium lines cysts or occasionally forms papillary structures (Fig. 278).

**Differential
Diagnosis**

Mucocele of benign origin with malignant origin:

Indicating a malignant origin:

Signs of less well-differentiated lining cells with only a discrete adenoid growth pattern and a reduced mucin production (also the colonic type of mucocele).

Spread

M-8480/6

T 158.9

1. Lymph node metastases develop rarely.

2. **Pseudomyxoma peritonei:**

   This disease is identified only if the abdominal mucinous material contains mucin-producing cells (Fig. 279).

**Clinical
Findings**

In most instances there are signs of acute appendicitis.

Treatment

1. Benign mucocele: Appendectomy.

2. Malignant mucocele:

   – If the tumor is limited to the tip of the appendix:
   Appendectomy.

   – If the tumor grows at other sites of the appendix or if the lining epithelium shows a papillary colonic type, a right hemicolectomy has been recommended [1].

Prognosis

1. This adenocarcinoma has a prognosis like that of adenocarcinoma of the colon, which is according to Dukes classification (that is, the extent of the disease) (see Colonic tumor, page 301).

2. Pseudomyxoma peritonei:

   The main prognostic indication is the number of mucin-producing cells in the mucinous material of the abdominal cavity:

   – few cells predict a good prognosis;

   – high cellularity indicates a doubtful prognosis.

---

[1] Andersson et al. 1976.

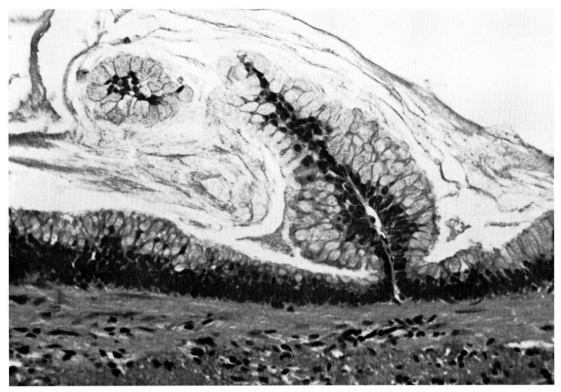

Fig. 278. Mucocele of the appendix, due to benign mucinous cystadenoma: Papillary formation of mucin-producing cuboidal cells in the lumen of the appendix (76-year-old female, × 200).

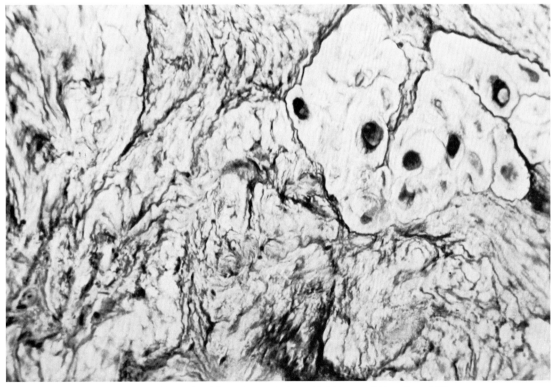

Fig. 279. Pseudomyxoma peritonei: Mucin with mucin-producing cells (74-year-old female, × 200).

6. Unclassified tumors (WHO)

Recommendations for differential diagnosis in tumors of the appendix

primary adenocarcinoma of the appendix	with	– metastatic adenocarcinoma into the appendix – infiltration of adenocarcinoma of the cecum into the appendix – endometriosis
benign mucocele	with	– malignant mucocele
pseudomyxoma peritonei of low grade malignancy	with	– pseudomyxoma peritonei of high grade malignancy
benign polyps	with	– polyps with foci of carcinoma
adenocarcinoma associated with mucocele	with	– adenocarcinoma of the colonic type

References

[1] Andersson, Å., L. Bergdahl, and L. Boquist: Primary carcinoma of the appendix. Ann. Surg. *183* (1976) 53-57.
[2] Cooper, P.H., and R.L. Warkel: Ultrastructure of the goblet cell type of adenocarcinoid of the appendix. Cancer *42* (1978) 2687-2695.
[3] Warkel, R.L., P.H. Cooper, and E.B. Helwig: Adenocarcinoid, a mucin-producing carcinoid tumor of the appendix. Cancer *42* (1978) 2781-2793.

8 Tumors of the large bowel and the anorectal region

Large bowel and anorectal region

1. For cancer of the bowel and rectum, early detection means a very good prognosis. However, more than 50% of the intestinal cancers are Dukes C tumors at the time of diagnosis!
2. Improvement in surgical techniques has brought progress in the treatment of intestinal cancer.
3. Few compounds have been investigated for chemotherapeutic treatment of disseminated disease.
   There is no chemotherapeutic approach to gastrointestinal carcinoma that is valuable enough to justify its application as a standard clinical treatment.
4. There is a good correlation between the behavior of the tumor and the CEA level.
   The level of CEA can also be elevated in benign lesions (for instance, colitis ulcerosa).
5. Cancer of the rectum shows earlier symptoms and is detected earlier than is colonic cancer.
   About 80% of these tumors are operable.
6. The most successful application of radiation therapy for intestinal tumors is for the superficial carcinoma of the anorectal region.

Tumors of the colon

T – primary tumor

Tis = preinvasive carcinoma (carcinoma in situ)

T 0 = no evidence of primary tumor

T 1 = tumor limited to the mucosa or mucosa and submucosa

T 2 = tumor with extension to muscle or muscle and serosa

T 3 = tumor with extension beyond the colon to immediately contiguous structures

    T 3 a = tumor without fistula formation

    T 3 b = tumor with fistula formation

T 4 = tumor extending beyond the immediately adjacent organs or tissues

T x = the minimal requirements to assess the primary tumor cannot be met (clinical examination including laparotomy, radiography, and endoscopy), (pericolic nodes and nodes along the ileocolic, right colic, middle colic, and inferior mesenteric arteries, paraaortic, and other intraabdominal nodes)

N – regional and juxtaregional lymph nodes

N 0 = no evidence of regional lymph node involvement

N 1 = evidence of involvement of the regional lymph nodes

N 4 = evidence of involvement of the juxtaregional lymph nodes

N x = the minimal requirements to assess the regional and/or juxtaregional lymph nodes cannot be met (clinical examination including laparotomy and radiography)

M – distant metastases

M 0 = no evidence of distant metastases

M 1 = evidence of distant metastases

M x = the minimal requirements to assess the presence of distant metastases cannot be met (clinical examination including laparotomy and radiography)

pTNM – postsurgical histopathological classification

pT – primary tumor

the pT categories correspond to the T categories

G – histopathological grading

G 1 = high degree of differentiation

G 2 = medium degree of differentiation

G 3 = low degree of differentiation or undifferentiated

G x = grade cannot be assessed

pN – regional lymph nodes

the pN categories correspond to the N categories

pM – distant metastases

the pM categories correspond to the M categories

Stage grouping

Stage I a	T 1	N 0	M 0
Stage 1 b	T 2	N 0	M 0
Stage II	T 3, T 4	N 0	M 0
Stage III	any T	N 1	M 0
Stage IV	any T	N 4	M 0
	any T	any N	M 1

Tumors of the rectum

T – primary tumor

Tis = preinvasive carcinoma (carcinoma in situ)

T 0 = no evidence of primary tumor

T 1 = tumor limited to the mucosa or mucosa and submucosa

T 2 = tumor with extension to muscle or muscle and serosa

T 3 = tumor with extension beyond the rectum to immediately contiguous structures

    T 3 a = tumor without fistula formation

    T 3 b = tumor with fistula formation

T 4 = tumor extending beyond the immediately adjacent organs or tissues

T x = the minimal requirements to assess the primary tumor cannot be met (clinical examination, radiography, and endoscopy)

N – regional and juxtaregional lymph nodes

(perirectal nodes, nodes distal to the origin of the inferior mesenteric artery, paraaortic and other intraabdominal nodes)

N 0 = no evidence of regional lymph node involvement

N 1 = evidence of involvement of the regional lymph nodes

N 4 = evidence of involvement of the juxtaregional lymph nodes

N x = the minimal requirements to assess the regional and/or the juxtaregional lymph nodes cannot be met (clinical examination and radiography)

M – distant metastases

M 0 = no evidence of distant metastases

M 1 = evidence of distant metastases

M x = the minimal requirements to assess the presence of distant metastases cannot be met (clinical examination and radiography)

pTNM – postsurgical histopathological classification
pT – primary tumor

    the pT categories correspond to the T categories

G – histopathological grading

G 1 = high degree of differentiation

G 2 = medium degree of differentiation

G 3 = low degree of differentiation or undifferentiated

pN – regional and juxtaregional lymph nodes

the pN categories correspond to the N categories

pM – distant metastases

the pM categories correspond to the M categories

Stage grouping

Stage I a	T 1	N 0	M 0
Stage I b	T 2	N 0	M 0
Stage II	T 3, T 4	N 0	M 0
Stage III	any T	N 1	M 0
Stage IV	any T	N 4	M 0
	any T	any N	M 1

M-8140/3
T 153.9

1. Adenocarcinoma of the large bowel (WHO)

**General
Remarks**

Incidence: Carcinomas of the large bowel are frequently observed tumors:
– About 10% of all malignant tumors grow in the large bowel.
– Cancer of the colon is the second leading cause of death from cancer for both sexes.
– Cancer of the colon has the highest incidence of malignant tumor for both sexes.
Age: The peak age is about 60 years; in the older age groups, colonic carcinoma is the most frequent cancer [49].
The tumor can also be observed in young patients, especially in cases of familial incidence.
Sex: Females are affected more often than males.
Site: Rectosigmoid region and rectum: more than 50%.
     Sigmoid: about 25%.
     Remaining intestine: 25%.
Further notes: There is a high familial incidence of colonic carcinoma [41].

Macroscopy

In most instances, the tumor constricts the lumen by circumferential growth. Intestinal obstruction can also occur by polypoid tumor masses growing into the lumen.
The tumor is in almost all cases ulcerated.
The size of this carcinoma is variable, but small tumors are more frequent than large ones.
The cut surface permits evaluation of the depth of infiltration of the tumor into the wall and the surrounding fat tissue. Occasionally growth similar to the linitis plastica type of carcinoma is encountered [5].

Histology

The malignant cells form an adenoid pattern as observed in typical adenocarcinoma.
The tumor shows different degrees of differentiation, evaluated by the extent of the adenoid growth pattern and the degree of cellular atypias (Figs. 280 to 285).
Occasionally (about 10%) the adenocarcinoma is dominated in its macroscopic and histological appearance by mucin production:

M-8480/3
Mucinous adenocarcinoma (WHO), **colloid adenocarcinoma** (Figs. 286 to 291).
If discrete mucin production is observed and organoid structures are barely visible, the tumor is called

M-8020/3
Undifferentiated carcinoma (WHO) (Figs. 292 to 294).

**Electron
Microscopy**

In well-differentiated adenocarcinoma of the large bowel the tumor cells contain mucin vacuoles with different structures and density. The mucin is surrounded by membranes (Fig. 295).

**Immunohisto-
chemistry**

It has been recommended that immunohistochemical staining for CEA be used. The histological findings and the blood CEA values may reflect the activity of the disease (not only for carcinoma of the large bowel, but also for other cancers) [21, 40, 43].

Fig. 282. Adenocarcinoma of the rectum (42-year-old female, × 160). ▷

[5] Amorn and Knigth Jr. 1978.
[21] Goldenberg et al. 1978.
[40] Loewenstein and Zamcheck 1978.
[41] Lynch et al. 1977.
[43] Martin et al. 1976.
[49] Noltenius et al. 1977.

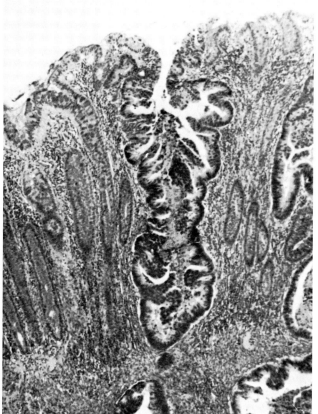

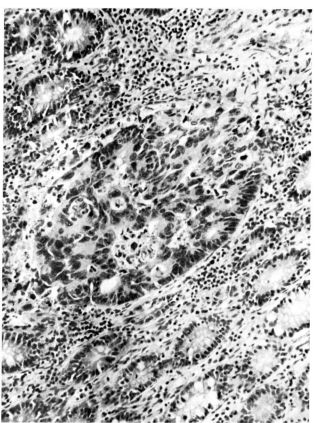

Fig. 280. Adenocarcinoma of the colon (42-year-old female, intestinal bleeding, ×60).

Fig. 281. Adenocarcinoma of the colon (×200).

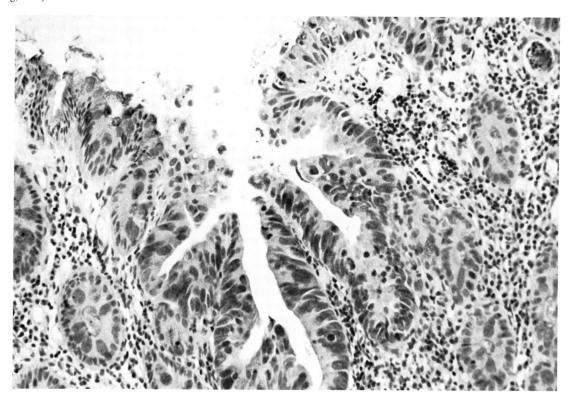

Fig. 282.

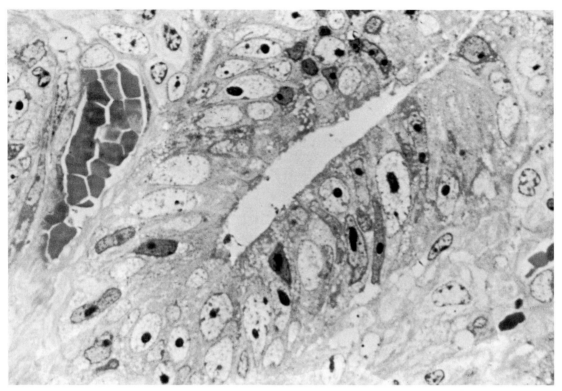

Fig. 283. Adenocarcinoma of the colon: Almost no mucin production by tumor cells (75-year-old female, × 800).

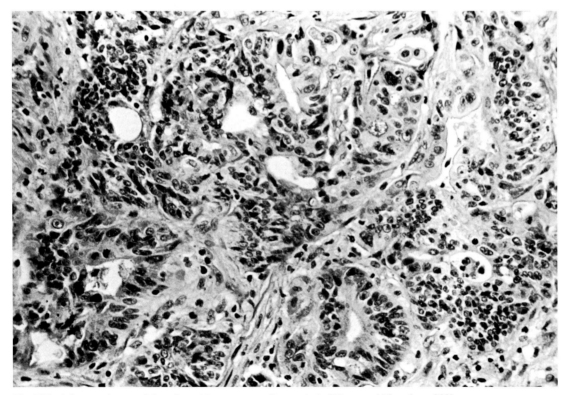

Fig. 284. Adenocarcinoma of the colon with squamous cell metaplasia (48-year-old female, × 200).

288

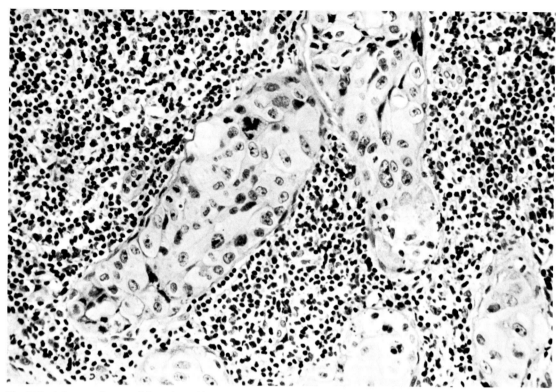

Fig. 285. Adenocarcinoma of the colon with squamous cell metaplasia: Mimicking squamous cell carcinoma (48-year-old female, × 200).

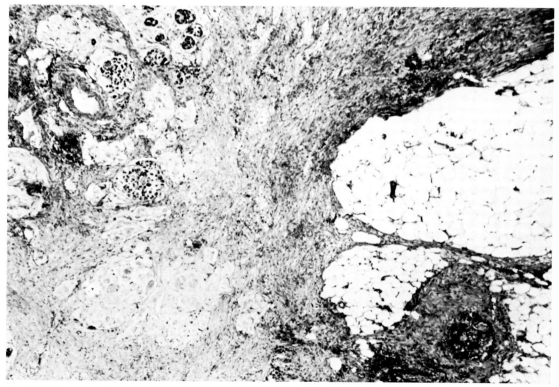

Fig. 286. Mucinous adenocarcinoma of the colon (74-year-old male, × 40).

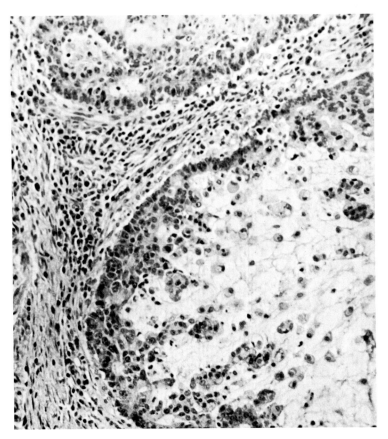

Fig. 287. Mucinous adenocarcinoma of the colon: Mucinous material with tumor cells (74-year-old male, × 125).

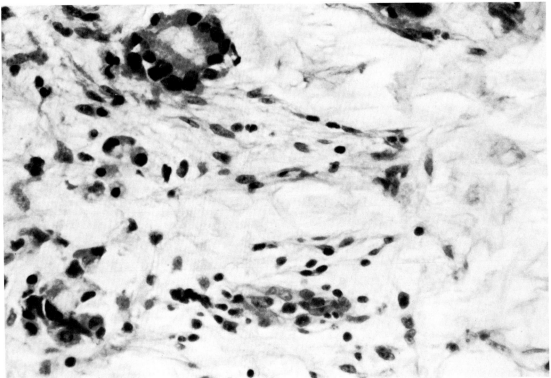

Fig. 288. Mucinous adenocarcinoma of the colon: Mucinous material with tumor cells (74-year-old male, × 310).

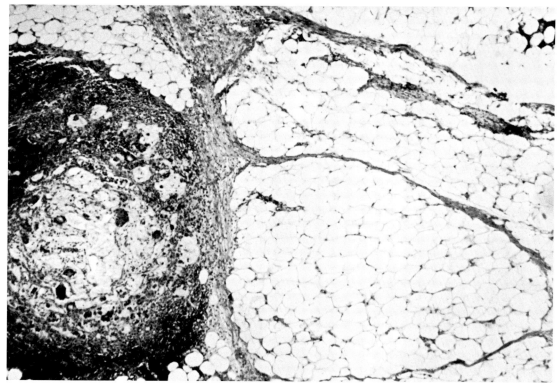

Fig. 289. Mucinous adenocarcinoma of the colon, lymph node metastasis (Dukes C) (74-year-old male, × 40).

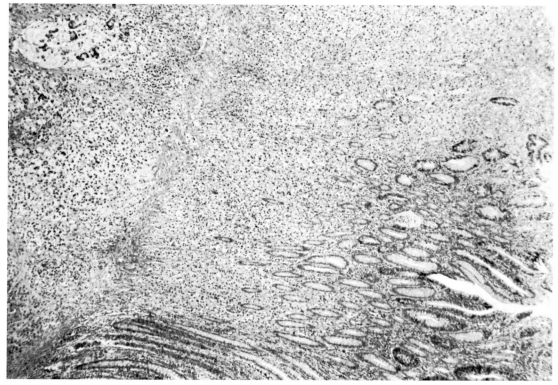

Fig. 290. Mucinous adenocarcinoma of the colon, signet ring cell type (74-year-old male, × 40).

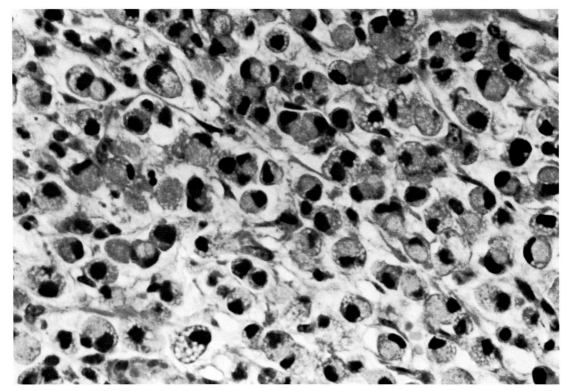

Fig. 291. Mucinous adenocarcinoma of the colon, signet ring cell type (74-year-old male, × 400).

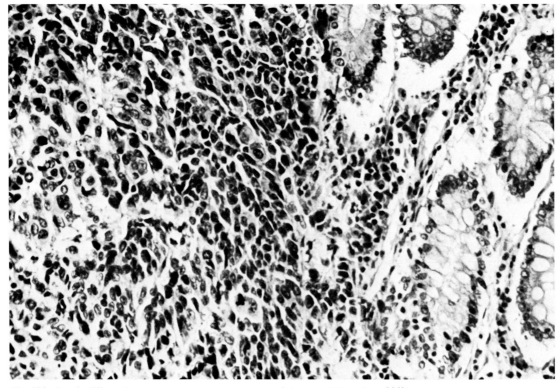

Fig. 292. Poorly differentiated adenocarcinoma of the colon (79-year-old female, × 200).

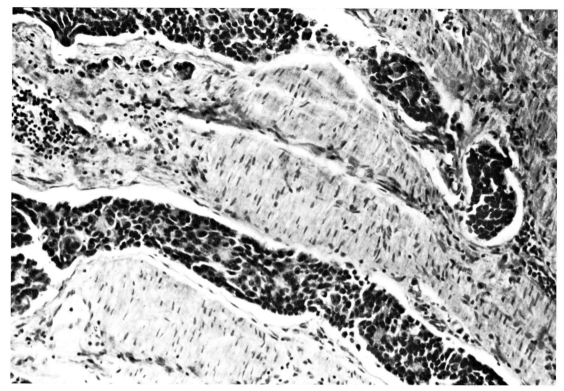

Fig. 293. Poorly differentiated adenocarcinoma of the colon: Lymphatic invasion (79-year-old female, × 125).

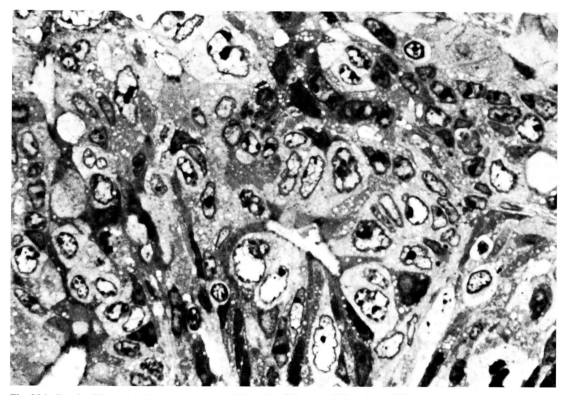

Fig. 294. Poorly differentiated adenocarcinoma of the colon (48-year-old female, × 600).

Adenocarcinoma

Differential Diagnosis

1. Colloid carcinoma **with colitis cystica profunda** [51] (Figs. 225 and 226).
2. **Irradiation** of the colon might induce cytological abnormalities in the colonic mucosa, which are localized in the crypts.
   Normally the differential diagnosis with malignant cells is possible, even without clinical information (Fig. 535) [69].
3. Adenocarcinoma **with intestinal polyps.**
4. Adenocarcinoma **with endometriosis** (Fig. 296).

Staging

Dukes A:
The tumor does not infiltrate the wall beyond the muscularis propria; that is, the tumor is limited to the mucosa and submucosa (Figs. 297 to 299).
This situation is encountered in about 15% of the operated cases.

Dukes B I:
Tumor infiltration of the muscularis propria (Fig. 300).

Dukes B II:
Tumor infiltration reaching the surrounding fat tissue (Figs. 301 and 302).
No lymph node metastases.
The situation of Dukes B I and B II is encountered in about 35% of the operated cases.

Dukes C:
Tumor infiltration of the wall and the surrounding tissue and lymph node metastases.
Dukes C is encountered in about 50% of the operated cases [13 to 15, 25, 71].

Grading

There is a good correlation between the degree of differentiation and the prognosis because tumors with high grade malignancy have a high tendency for lymphatic and hematogenous spread [15].

The grading is determined by the degree of formation of adenomatous growth patterns, the number of mitotic figures, and the amount of nuclear atypias.

High grade malignancy is encountered in about 20% of the cases, low grade malignancy in about 20%, and the majority of adenocarcinomas show an average grade of malignancy (about 60%).

Spread

1. Local spread: Extension through the wall into the surrounding fat tissue.
2. Lymphatic spread into the regional lymph nodes.
   Lymphatic spread occurs in about 20% of tumors of low grade malignancy.
   In tumors of an average grade of malignancy lymphatic spread occurs in about 35%, and in high grade malignancy it occurs in about 80% [15].
3. Hematogenous spread into the liver, lung, bone, brain, and other organs.

Fig. 295. Undifferentiated adenocarcinoma of the colon: Slit-like space surrounded by tumor cells and ▷ containing microvilli of the tumor cells (× 11,000).

Fig. 296. Endometriosis in the wall of the colon (× 125).

[13] Dukes 1937.
[14] Dukes 1946.
[15] Dukes 1949.
[25] Hermanek 1978.
[51] Otto et al. 1976.
[69] Weisbrot et al. 1975.
[71] Wood et al. 1979.

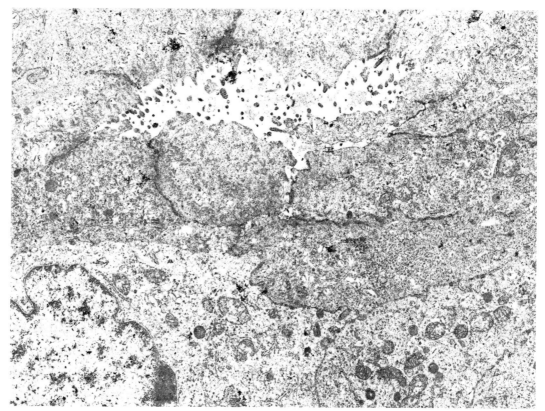

Fig. 295.

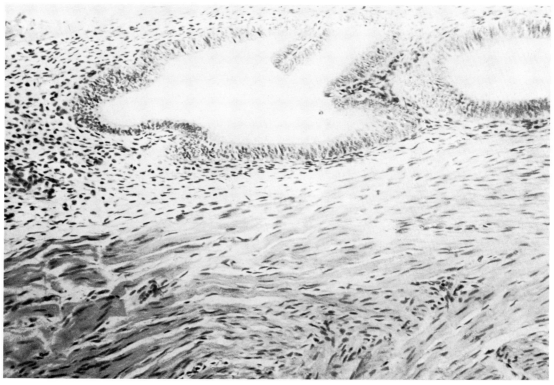

Fig. 296.

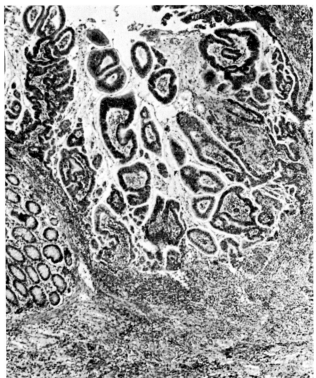

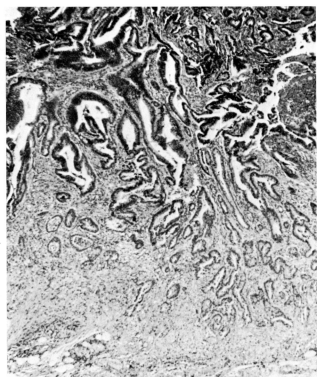

Fig. 297. Adenocarcinoma of the colon, Dukes A (71-year-old male, one of four small adenocarcinomas in Stages A and B I, × 40).

Fig. 298. Adenocarcinoma of the colon, Dukes A (see Fig. 299) (69-year-old female, × 40).

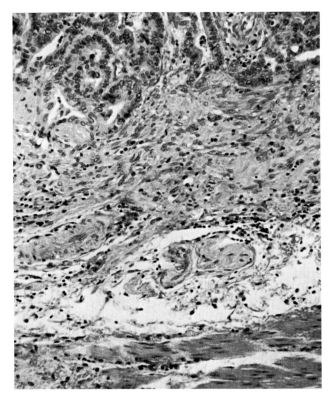

Fig. 299. Adenocarcinoma of the colon, Dukes A (muscularis propria not infiltrated) (69-year-old female, × 125).

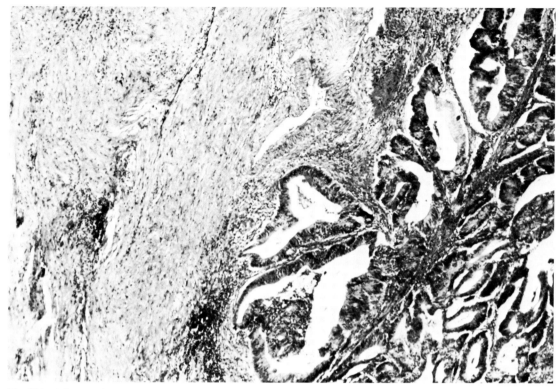

Fig. 300. Adenocarcinoma of the colon: Infiltration of the inner muscle layer (Dukes B I) (× 125).

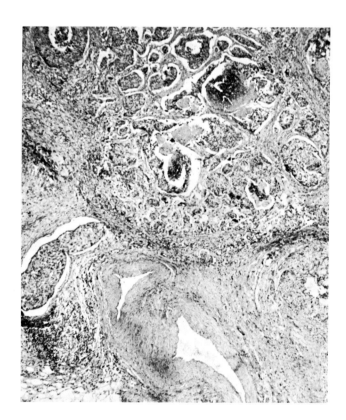

Fig. 301. Adenocarcinoma of the colon, Dukes B II (including lymphatic invasion) (70-year-old female, × 40).

Adenocarcinoma

Clinical Findings

The symptoms are determined by the size and the growth pattern of the tumor:
- signs of intestinal obstruction
- bleeding
- diarrhea alternating with obstipation (changes in bowel habits are often a warning signal for early cancer!)
- anemia, loss of weight
- no symptoms
- carcinoembryonic antigen can be detected in 27 to 97% of the cases [72, 73]; occasionally steroid hormone receptors [3].

Treatment

Surgery:
- Removal of the tumor by the no-touch isolation technique [66].
- Resection of regional lymph nodes.
- 75 to 90% of the patients can be operated upon either for exstirpation of the tumor or for palliation.
- Operative mortality: less than 5%.

Radiation therapy:
- Radiation therapy alone is only indicated if no surgical intervention is possible.
- There is no final demonstration that preoperative irradiation (up to 45 Gy) improves the surgical survival results.
- Postoperative radiation therapy can be tried in cases of incomplete removal of the tumor.

Chemotherapy:
- Chemotherapy is still being clinically investigated and seems to have a poor response potential.
- Combinations of 5-fluorouracil and me-CCNU have been tried.
  Occasionally there is an improvement of symptoms, especially in cases of liver metastases.
  Prolongation of survival has not been demonstrated [2, 10, 12, 23, 27, 54, 55].

[2] Alberto et al. 1978.
[3] Alford et al. 1979.
[10] De Vita Jr. 1977.
[12] Douglass et al. 1978.
[23] Gropp and Havemann 1978.
[27] Higgins Jr. et al. 1976.
[54] Presant et al. 1978.
[55] Presant et al. 1978.
[66] Turnbull Jr. et al. 1967.
[72] Zamcheck 1975.
[73] Zamcheck et al. 1972.

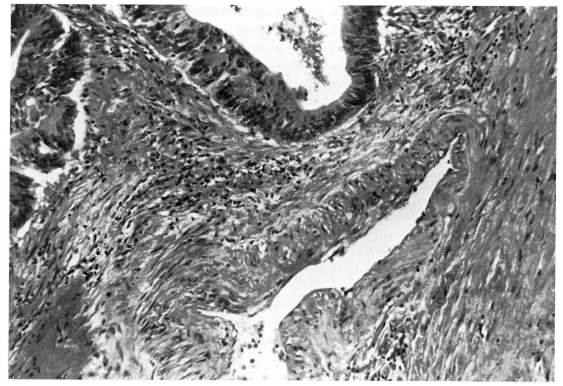

Fig. 302. Adenocarcinoma of the colon: Infiltration of the outer muscle layer close to a large artery (Dukes B II) (×200).

Treatment for adenocarcinoma of the rectum:

Surgery:
– The abdominoperineal resection is considered to be the treatment of choice [34, 39].

Radiation therapy:
– Radiotherapy alone can be tried in small superficial tumors.
– Endocavitary irradiation has yielded remarkable results: The overall dose for very small lesions by contact irradiation is 100 to 150 Gy in 4 weeks [53].
– Radiation therapy may be tried not only for palliation, but also for definitive treatment of operable disease [32, 58] (50 to 70 Gy in 4 to 6 weeks).
– The combination of radiation therapy and surgery can be used for extensive tumors.
– For adenocarcinoma of the rectum, preoperative irradiation can be tried [60, 61] (about 20 to 50 Gy in 4 to 6 weeks).
– It is undecided whether the surgery should be completed by radiation therapy, chemotherapy, anticoagulation therapy, or immunotherapy [30].

Chemotherapy:
– It is still not decided if adjuvant chemotherapy improves the prognosis [27].
– Encouraging results have been reported with the use of adjuvant immunotherapy (FAC-BCG) and chemotherapy in carcinoma Dukes C after potentially curative surgery [44, 45].
– Immunotherapy alone did not show responses [47].
– Combination chemotherapy (5-fluorouracil and 5-fluorodeoxyuridine, or 5-fluorouracil in combination with me-CCNU) can show a response [46]. The combination of 5-fluorouracil, me-CCNU, and vincristine has also been used [47].

[27] Higgins Jr. et al. 1976.
[30] Jackson 1977.
[32] Kligerman 1975.
[34] Langer and Buss 1979.
[39] Localio and Eng 1979.
[44] Mavligit et al. 1975.
[45] Mavligit et al. 1978.
[46] Mayer et al. 1978.
[47] Moertel et al. 1978.
[53] Papillon 1975.
[58] Rider 1975.
[60] Sack 1975.
[61] Scherer and Sack 1979.

Prognosis

For colorectal adenocarcinoma:

1. The overall 5-year survival rate for all intestinal carcinomas is about 25 to 30%.
2. The overall 5-year survival rate for operated patients is about 50%.
3. The prognosis for the individual case is influenced by:

   a) The site of the tumor:
   - Tumors of the cecum and the colon ascendens have a better prognosis than carcinomas of the rectum and rectosigmoid.

   b) The type of operation:
   - 5-year survival, no-touch isolation technique: 68.8%
   - 5-year survival, conventional surgery: 52.1%
   - 5-year survival, no-touch isolation technique, Dukes C: 57.8%
   - 5-year survival, conventional surgery Dukes C: 28.0%.
   - Abdominoperineal resection for adenocarcinoma of the rectum:
     - 5-year survival, Dukes A: 91%
       - Dukes B: 59%
       - Dukes C: 25% [42].

   c) Age of the patient:
   - Young patients have a less favorable prognosis than older patients. In younger age groups the tumor has a higher tendency to metastasize [18].

   d) The preoperative level of carcinoembryonic antigen seems to provide prognostic information:
   - Patients with a high CEA level are in high risk groups.
   - A low preoperative CEA level indicates low risk in cases of resectable Dukes B and C adenocarcinoma [68].

   e) Pathological findings:
   - Dukes A – about 100% chance of cure.
   - Dukes B – 5-year survival rate, about 50%.
   - Dukes C – 5-year survival rate, about 15 to 30%.

Grading
   - small carcinomas with high grade malignancy have a poor prognosis, large tumors with low grade malignancy have a better prognosis [62].
   - Lymph node involvement:
   - The more lymph nodes that are involved and the greater the distance of the involved lymph nodes from the primary tumor, the poorer the prognosis [63].
   - Vascular invasion by tumor cells in Dukes B has no prognostic significance [31].
4. The 5-year survival rate after resection of the tumor without lymph node metastases: about 80%.
   with lymph node metastases: about 20%.

[18] Gérard 1975.
[31] Khankhanian et al. 1977.
[42] MacLennan et al. 1976.
[62] Spjut et al. 1979.
[63] Spratt Jr. and Spjut 1967.
[68] Wanebo et al. 1978.

1. It has been proposed that the reaction of regional lymph nodes in cases of carcinoma (not only carcinoma of the colon) should be evaluated by a standardized system [8]. However, caution should be applied when interpreting these morphological lymph node changes as prognostic features or immunological reactions of the organism to tumor cell growth [67].

2. It is noteworthy that well-differentiated carcinomas very often have a marked lymphocytic infiltration.

3. There are reports of the familial occurrence of colonic carcinoma associated with uterine carcinoma and malignant lymphoma [35, 36].

4. Carcinoembryonic antigen has been found by immunochemistry not only in carcinomatous tissue, but also in intestinal polyps and normal mucosa surrounding carcinoma [64].

5. There is a very low incidence of colorectal carcinomas in Africa.

[8] Cottier et al. 1972.
[35] Law et al. 1977.
[36] Law et al. 1977.
[64] Tappeiner et al. 1973.
[67] van de Velde et al. 1978.

2. Intestinal polyps

M-8210/0
T 153.9

a) Adenomatous polyp
(tubular adenoma – WHO)

General Remarks

Incidence: This is a frequently observed lesion.
Age: The tumor can occur at any age.
Site: 80% occur in the colon ascendens and descendens; about 20% occur in the rectum.

Macroscopy

The tumors occur as multiple or solitary lesions. They are pedunculated or sessile and are of various sizes.
The surface is smooth; occasionally ulcerations are observed.

Histology

This tumor is composed of glandular structures, which are packed closely together (Fig. 303). The epithelial cells that line these structures can show normal nuclei; however, hyperchromasia and numerous mitotic figures are frequently encountered (Figs. 304 and 305). The mucin production is discrete.
Occasionally the surface can show a villous structure (Fig. 306), and foci of mucin production are observed.
These polyps are called:

M-8263/0

b) Adenomatous-villous polyps
(tubulovillous adenoma – WHO) [70].

M-8261/1
T 153.9

c) Villous polyp
(villous adenoma – WHO)

General Remarks

Incidence: The villous polyp occurs less frequently than adenomatous polyps or adenomatous-villous polyps.
Age: Elderly patients are mainly affected.
Site: Villous polyps develop preferentially in the rectum and rectosigmoid.

Macroscopy

The size of these mostly sessile tumors differs. The tumor is soft, and the surface is covered by papillary formations. The mucosa is often ulcerated.
In cases of pronounced pedunculated tumors, hemorrhagic infarction with bleeding can be observed.

Histology

This tumor is characterized by a surface that shows a villous-papillary pattern (Fig. 307). These processes are covered by epithelium, which is supported by smooth connective tissue (lamina propria). These processes reach the muscularis mucosae (Fig. 308).
The covering epithelial cells are often double-layered, and hyperchromatic nuclei and mitotic figures can be observed (Fig. 309).
Usually the mucin production is discrete; however, foci of major deposits of mucin can be observed.

---

[70] Wiebecke et al. 1974.

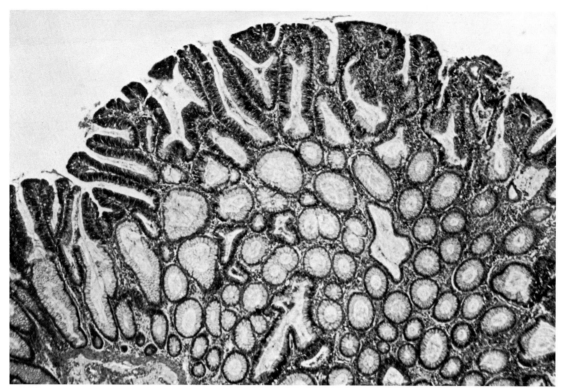

Fig. 303. Adenomatous polyp of the colon with foci of carcinoma in situ (see Fig. 304) (66-year-old female, × 40).

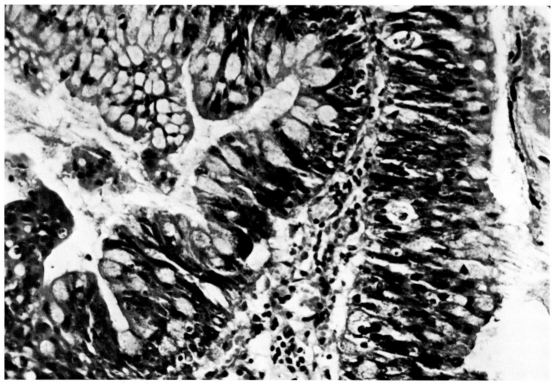

Fig. 304. Foci of carcinoma in situ in adenomatous polyp of the colon (66-year-old female, × 200).

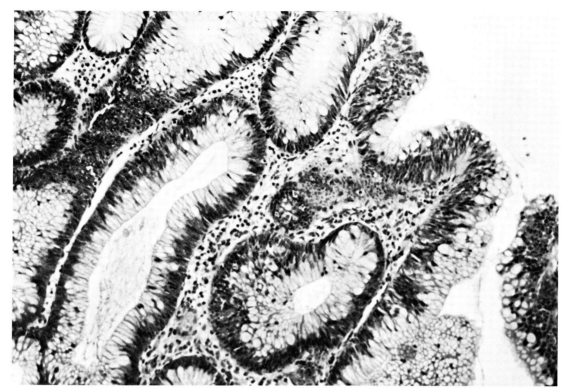

Fig. 305. Adenomatous polyp of the rectum: Multilayered, partly mucin-producing cells with hyperchromatic nuclei (61-year-old male, × 125).

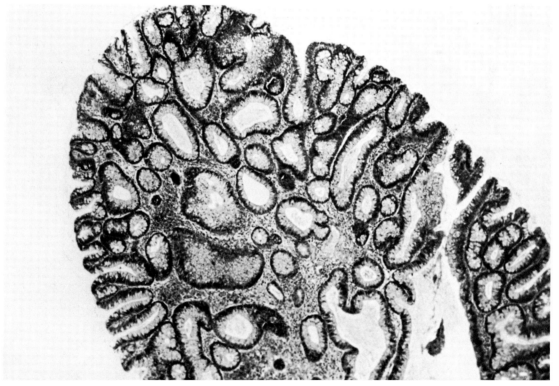

Fig. 306. Adenomatous polyp of the rectum (61-year-old male, × 40).

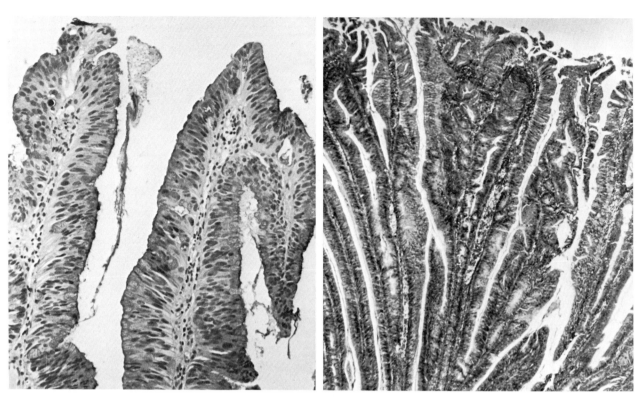

Fig. 307. Villous polyp of the colon: Surface covered by two and more cell rows (80-year-old female, × 125).

Fig. 308. Villous polyp of the colon (68-year-old male, × 40).

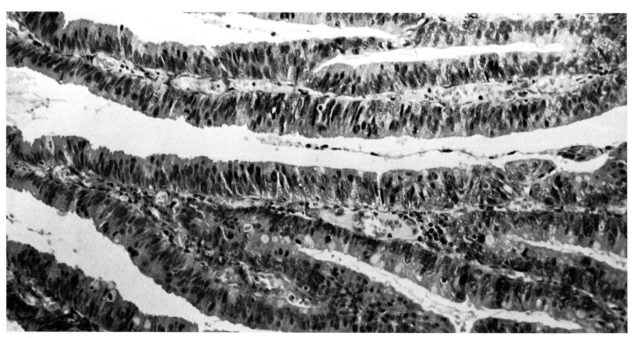

Fig. 309. Villous polyp of the colon: Numerous hyperchromatic nuclei (× 125).

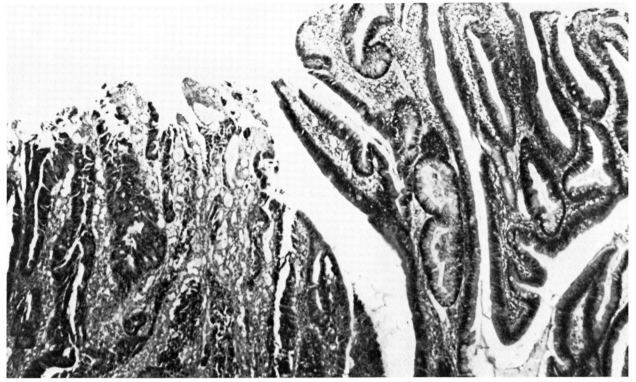

Fig. 310. Villous polyp of the colon: Segment of infiltration carcinoma (71-year-old female, × 40).

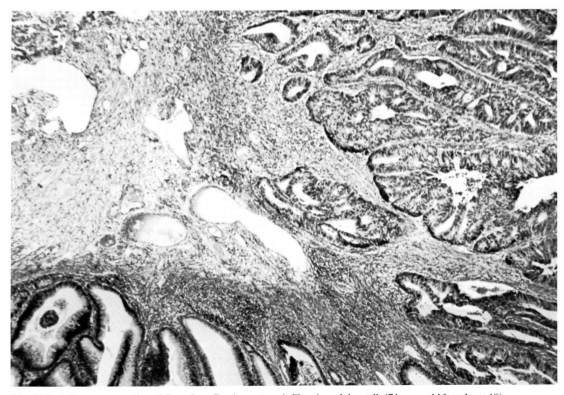

Fig. 311. Adenomatous polyp of the colon: Carcinomatous infiltration of the stalk (71-year-old female, × 40).

Polyps of the colon

Differential Diagnosis

M-8261/3

Intestinal polyp (adenomatous, adenomatous-villous, and villous polyps) **with adenocarcinoma:**

– Infiltration of tumor cells into the stalk, the submucosa, or the muscularis mucosae is evidence for adenocarcinoma in a polyp (Figs. 310 to 313).

– It has been reported that the presence of carcinoembryonic antigen (CEA) (immunoperoxidase technique) indicated malignant changes in the colonic mucosa [29].

– Occasionally in polyps one observes foci of atypical cells confined to the mucosa. These are foci of carcinoma in situ: They are not invasive carcinomas (Fig. 314).

Clinical Findings

Occasionally bleeding with blood in the feces (occult blood).

Treatment

For adenomatous, villous, and adenomatous-villous polyps:

1. a) Polyps larger than 1 cm should be removed.

   b) In cases of resected villous polyps a follow-up examination should be done.

   c) In cases of adenomatous polyps, no new polyps are observed during the following 10 years in about 50% of the patients.

2. In cases of carcinomatous polyps a local removal is permitted if the pathologist can show that the entire tumor has been removed, if the infiltration of tumor cells does not extend beyond the muscularis mucosae, and if the surgical margins in the surrounding mucosa are free of tumor cells.

3. In cases of poorly differentiated carcinoma in a polyp, local removal is not sufficient, even when the infiltration did not reach the muscularis mucosae [48].

Prognosis

1. Benign polyps: Excellent; however, follow-up examination for recurrences in cases of villous polyps is recommended.

2. The probability of developing cancer increases with the size of the polyp:

– Polyps less than 1 cm in diameter only rarely show invasive cancer.

– The carcinomatous development in a polyp can occur in very small areas. Therefore, it is recommended that the pathologist do multiple sections.

– The development of cancer occurs more frequently in a villous polyp than in an adenomatous polyp.

3. Metastases from a carcinomatous polyp occur usually only if the tumor has overgrown the muscularis mucosae. In these cases the prognosis follows Dukes classification.

M-8220/0
T 153.9
M-8210/3

d) Adenomatous polyposis coli

(adenomatosis – WHO; familial polyposis)

This disease is characterized by multiple polyps in the colon. These polyps can be adenomatous (tubular), adenomatous-villous (tubulovillous), or villous.

Treatment

Prophylactic colectomy has been recommended, since about 100% of the patients develop cancer of the colon. It is debated whether this colectomy should also include the rectum. About 60% of the patients with polyposis have a carcinoma at the time of presentation (in most instances at the age of about 40 years).

---

[29] Isaacson and Le Vann 1976.
[48] Morson and Dawson 1974.

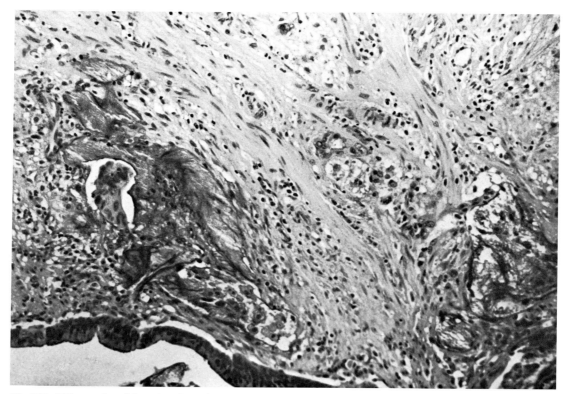

Fig. 312. Villous polyp of the colon: Part of a beginning carcinomatous infiltration (× 125).

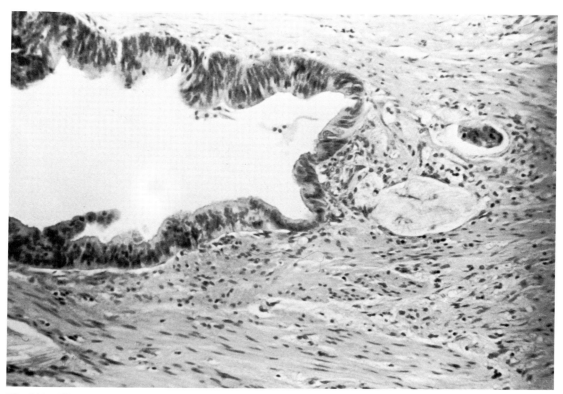

Fig. 313. Villous polyp of the colon: Beginning carcinomatous infiltration (× 125).

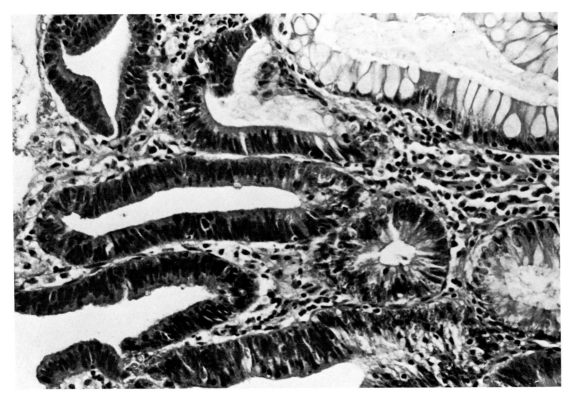

Fig. 314. Carcinoma in situ of the colon (×310).

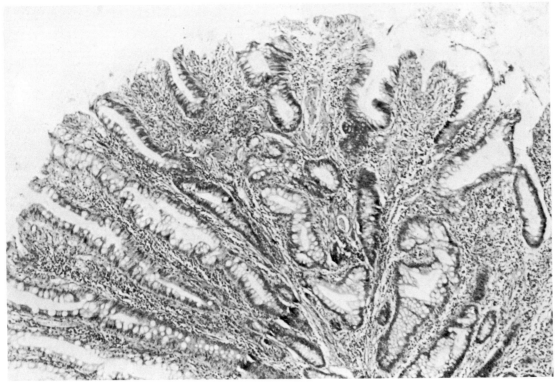

Fig. 315. Peutz-Jeghers polyp of the colon (21-year-old male, ×50).

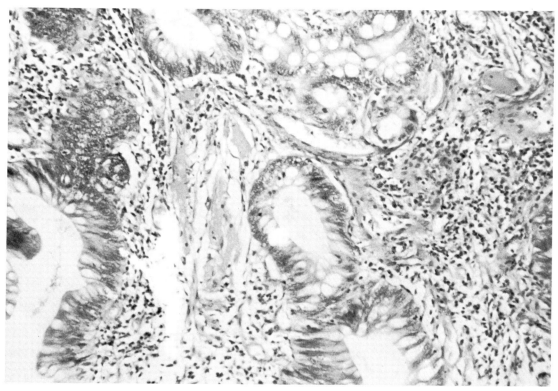

Fig. 316. Peutz-Jeghers polyp of the colon: Glands and smooth muscle fibers, foci of inflammation (21-year-old male, ×125).

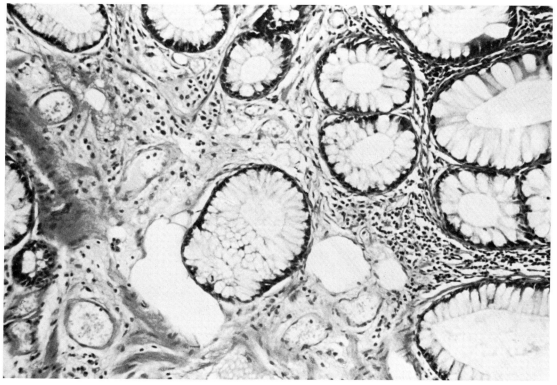

Fig. 317. Peutz-Jeghers polyp of the colon: Smooth muscle fibers supporting the stroma (21-year-old male, ×125).

Polyps of the colon

Further Information

There is a report of a family in which colonic polyps were associated with a high incidence of gastric cancer [4].

M-7563/0
T 153.9

e) Peutz-Jeghers polyp (WHO)
(hamartoma – WHO)

This is a hamartomatous lesion, which is benign.
The cells form glands, often extended to cysts. The cells are without atypias (Fig. 315).
The polyp is supported by smooth muscle fibers (Fig. 316 and 317).
Peutz-Jeghers polyps are often multiple (Peutz-Jeghers syndrome, Peutz-Jeghers polyposis).

M-7204/0
T 153.9

f) Hyperplastic polyp (WHO)
(metaplastic polyp)

These polyps never become malignant.
They are multiple, small, and sessile, and are frequently observed in the rectum and rectosigmoid region.
However, all parts of the large bowel can be affected by these polyps.

Histology

The tumor contains glands, which can have a cystic or tubular pattern (Fig. 318).
The lining cells have regular nuclei which are in a basic position in the cell.
The cytoplasm contains mucin. The cell resembles the small intestinal epithelium.

M-7688/0
T 153.9

g) Benign lymphoid polyp (WHO)

The peak age for this lesion is the 3rd to 4th decade; men are more frequently affected than women.
Multiple benign lymphoid polyps can occur (benign lymphoid polyposis).

Histology

The tumor is composed of hyperplastic lymphoid tissue with multiple follicles [57].

Differential Diagnosis

The differential diagnosis **with malignant lymphoma** might be necessary.
The appearance of follicles indicates benign lymphoid polyp (benign lymphoma).

---

[4] Ammann et al. 1976.
[57] Ranchod et al. 1978.

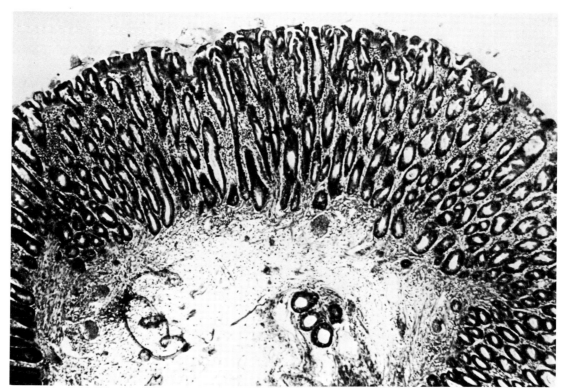

Fig. 318. Hyperplastic polyp of the colon: Tubular pattern of the glands (40-year-old male, ×40).

M-7410/0
T 153.9

h) Lipomatous polyposis

In this lesion the polyps are formed by lipoma-like tissue, which elevates the intact mucosa into the lumen of the colon.

M-7564/0
T 153.9

i) Juvenile polyp (WHO)
(retention polyp)

This hamartomatous lesion contains numerous cysts, which are embedded in a connective tissue stroma (lamina propria) (Figs. 319 and 320).
The cysts and the tubules, which are often close to the surface, are lined by a regular mucin-producing epithelium.
Bleeding due to ulcerations can occur.
These juvenile polyps can be multiple: **juvenile polyposis.**

M-7682/0
T 153.9

k) Inflammatory polyp (WHO)
(inflammatory polyposis)

This lesion is characterized by an elevation of the mucosa due to underlying inflammatory changes, with granulation tissue and dense inflammatory cell infiltration.
This lesion can show, besides regular epithelium, zones with large dark nuclei (regeneration).
Inflammatory polyps occur in association with colitis (Crohn's disease, ulcerative colitis, or fibrinous colitis).

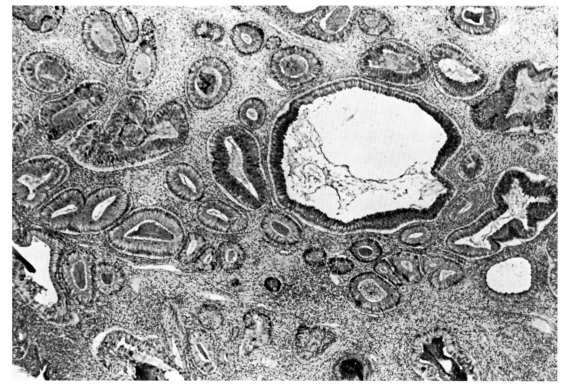

Fig. 319. Juvenile polyp (4-year-old female, × 40).

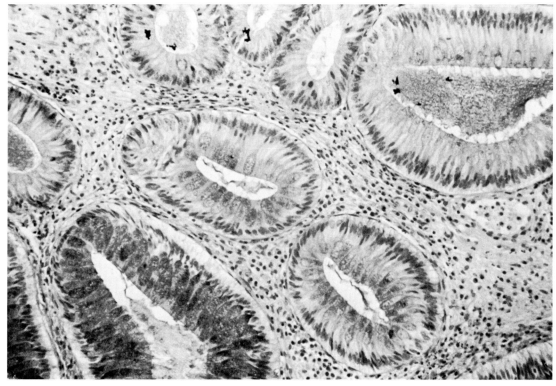

Fig. 320. Juvenile polyp: Hamartomatous lesion, no malignancy (4-year-old female, × 125).

315

M-8240/1, 3
T 153.9

3. Carcinoid (WHO)

General Remarks

Incidence: Carcinoids of the colon are very rare and they only occasionally metastasize. Carcinoids of the rectum are rare tumors.

Macroscopy

These are usually small tumors, rarely more than 2 cm in diameter.
The solitary lesion is hard and covered by an intact mucosa.
Carcinoids in the rectum that are larger than 1 cm must be considered malignant.

Histology

Most of the carcinoids in the rectum are

M-8242/1

a) Argentaffin-negative carcinoid
(nonargentaffin carcinoid – WHO) (see page 258):
The tumor cells are arranged in a tubular or adenoid pattern; occasionally they form solid complexes (Figs. 321 to 324). The nuclei are regular and usually round; there are practically no mitotic figures (Figs. 325 to 327).
The tumor grows in the submucosa and occasionally infiltrates the mucosa or the surrounding submucosal tissue.

M-8241/0, 3

b) Argentaffin-positive carcinoid (WHO):
These tumors are very rare in the rectum.
The growth of the tumor cells is similar to the growth of basaloid carcinoma, with palisading of tumor cells at the periphery of the tumor cell nests (Fig. 328).

Spread

Very rarely, lymph node metastases are observed [38].

Treatment

Local excision in almost all instances is possible for tumors that are smaller than 2 cm.
Tumors larger than 2 cm require radical surgery.

Prognosis

The prognosis is determined by the size of the carcinoid.
Larger carcinoids (more than 2 cm) can disseminate into the lymph nodes.
On histological examination, the appearance of atypical nuclei, mitotic figures, and infiltration into the lymphatics indicates malignant growth.
Rectal carcinoids can be very malignant, and early metastases into lymph nodes and visceral organs must be expected.

Further Information

1. Other than in the small bowel, carcinoids in the rectum are almost always solitary tumors.
2. The carcinoid of the rectum almost never produces a carcinoid syndrome.
3. There have been observations of an adenocarcinoma growing with a carcinoid [26].

[26] Hernandez and Reid 1969.
[38] Lemozy 1973.

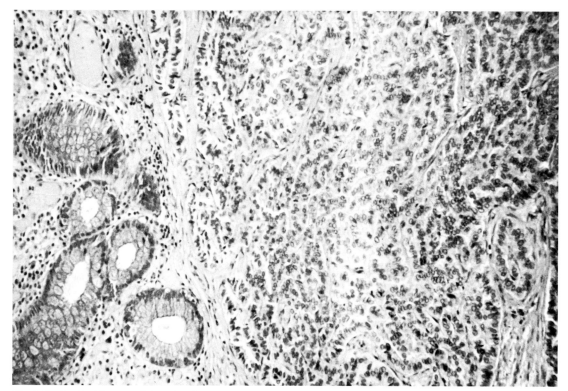

Fig. 321. Carcinoid tumor of the colon (nonargentaffin type) (60-year-old male, ×125).

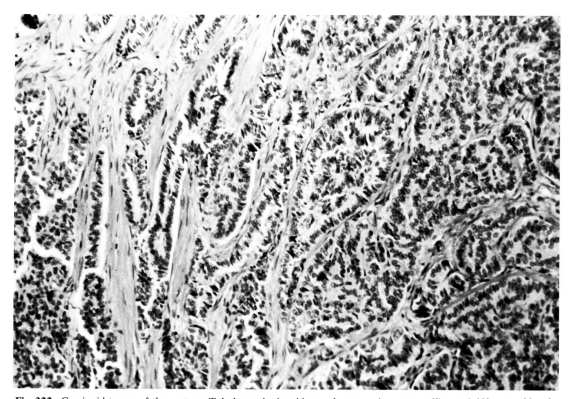

Fig. 322. Carcinoid tumor of the rectum: Tubular and adenoid growth pattern (nonargentaffin type) (60-year-old male, ×125).

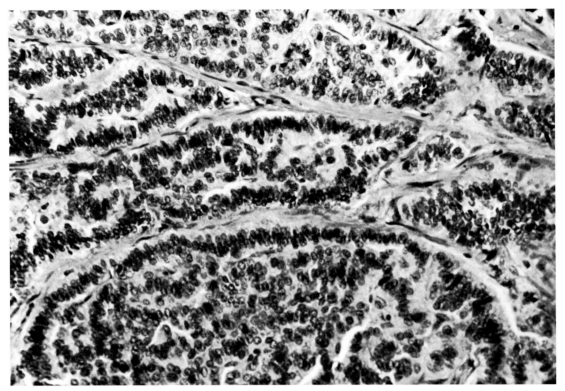

Fig. 323. Carcinoid tumor of the rectum (nonargentaffin type): Formation of ribbons and tubules (60-year-old male, ×200).

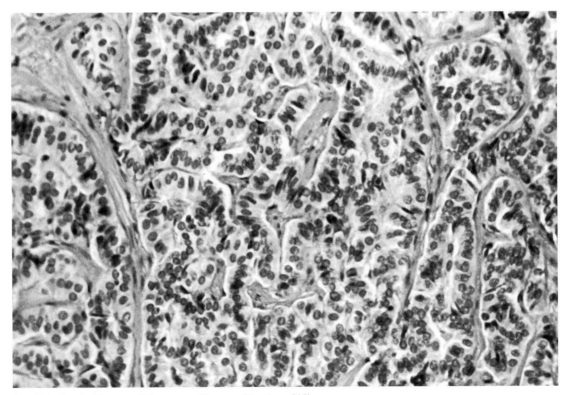

Fig. 324. Carcinoid tumor of the rectum (60-year-old male, ×200).

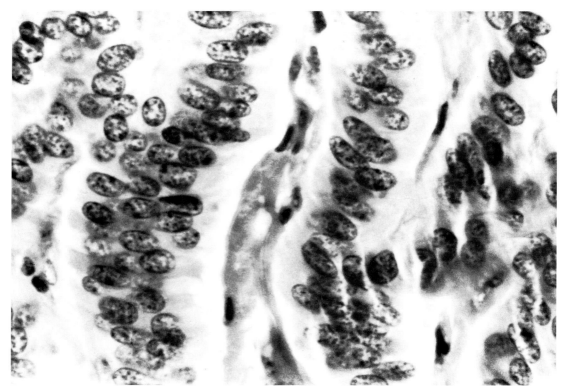

Fig. 325. Oval, regular nuclei in nonargentaffin carcinoid tumor of the rectum (60-year-old male, × 800).

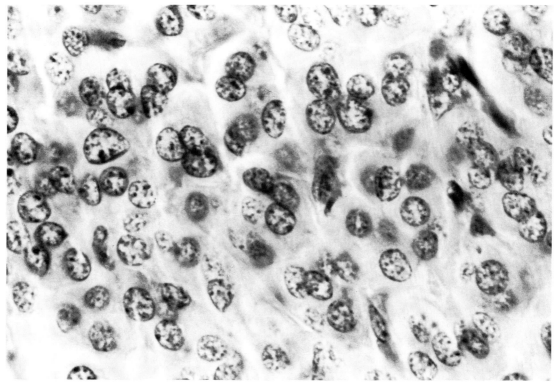

Fig. 326. Round, regular nuclei in nonargentaffin carcinoid tumor of the rectum (60-year-old male, × 800).

M-8070/3
T 153.4
T 153.9
T 154.1

4. Squamous cell carcinoma of the large bowel (WHO)

Squamous cell carcinomas of the cecum, colon, and rectum are exceedingly rare [9, 28], as are **adenosquamous carcinomas** (WHO).

5. Neuroendocrine carcinoma

This type of tumor in the colon has been reported. Histologically it appears as a "small cell, undifferentiated carcinoma" [22].

[9] Crissman 1978.
[22] Gould and Chejfec 1978.
[28] Horne and McCulloch 1978.

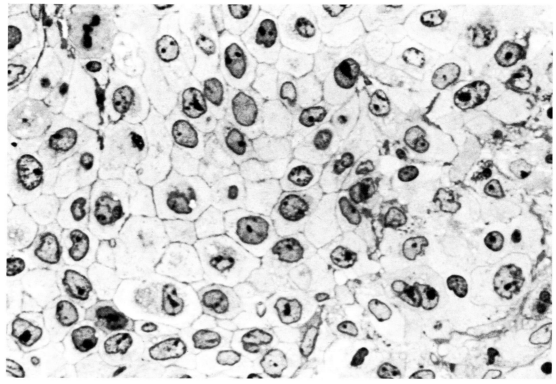

Fig. 327. Carcinoid tumor of the rectum: Well-delineated tumor cells (× 600).

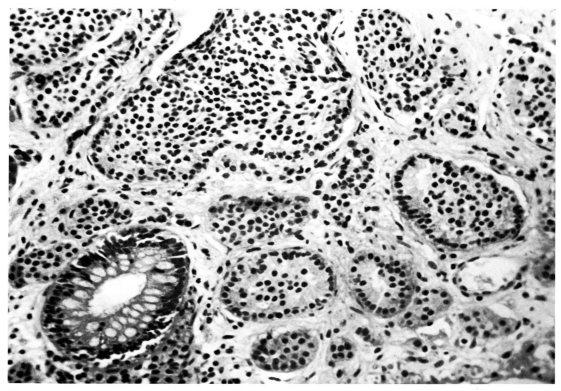

Fig. 328. Carcinoid tumor of the rectum (argentaffin-positive type): Formation of solid tumor nests, palisading of cells at the periphery (63-year-old male, × 200).

M-8890/0, 3
T 153.9

6. Leiomyoma and leiomyosarcoma (WHO)

This soft tissue tumor is very rare in the colon and rectum.

As elsewhere, nuclear atypia and, in particular, the appearance of mitotic figures are signs of malignancy. The indicators of malignancy may be lacking, and benign-looking tumors may behave as sarcomas (of low grade malignancy) (Fig. 329) [48, 56].

There is a report of a leiomyomatosis in the colon [17].

Treatment   Surgical resection and, for leiomyosarcoma, chemotherapy have been proposed [59].

M-8850/0
M-9120/0
T 153.9

7. Lipoma and hemangioma (WHO)

These tumors are very rare in the colon and rectum (Fig. 330) (see pages 57 and 72).

M-9550/1
M-9560/0

8. Neurogenic tumors

Neurilemoma (WHO) as part of von Recklinghausen's disease can occur in the colon and rectum; however, the incidence is very low.

[17] Freni and Keeman 1977.
[48] Morson and Dawson 1974.
[56] Ranchod and Kempson 1977.
[59] Rückert et al. 1977.

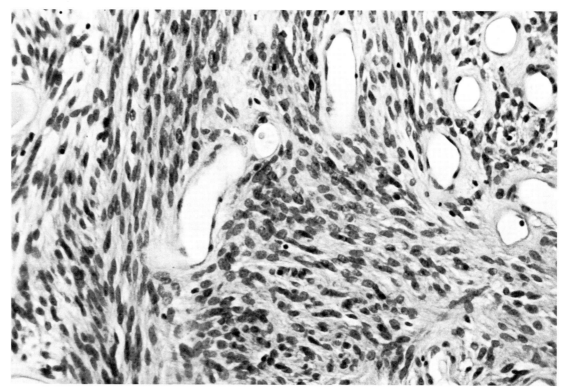

Fig. 329. Leiomyoma of the colon: Discrete atypia and no mitotic figures. One year later, numerous recurrences and metastases (70-year-old female, × 200).

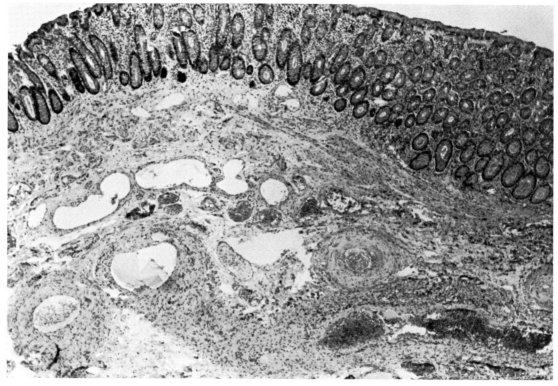

Fig. 330. Cavernous hemangioma of the colon, causing intestinal bleeding (54-year-old female, × 30).

323

M-9590/3
T 153.9

9. Malignant lymphoma

Malignant lymphoma of any type and leukemias [7] can occur in any part of the large bowel (Figs. 331 to 333).
The incidence, however, is relatively low.

10. Tumor-like lesions of the colon and rectum (WHO)

M-4318/0
T 153.9

a) Malakoplakia

This tumor-like lesion is composed of large histiocytes [37].
These histiocytes grow underneath the mucosa. They have an abundant cytoplasm and regular nuclei. The cytoplasm is acidophilic and granular.
Small inclusion granules in the cytoplasm give a positive calcium stain and iron stain reaction and are called Michaelis-Gutmann bodies (Figs. 1397 and 1398).
These solid nests of histiocytes can elevate the mucosa and form polypoid elevations. This lesion is relatively seldom observed in the colon [65].
Malakoplakia can also occur elsewhere (see chapters on the kidney, urinary bladder, prostate, small intestine, and stomach).
It is possible that this disease reflects a defective bactericidal response of histiocytes to phagocytozed E. coli [1].
Due to the dense cell proliferation, this malakoplakia enters into the differential diagnosis with malignant tumors.

M-4380/0
T 153.9

b) Colitis cystica profunda (WHO)

This disease is characterized by cysts and mucin deposits found in the wall (submucosa) of the large bowel.
The lining epithelial cells do not reveal atypias.
However, this lesion (probably due to inflammation with displacement of epithelium into the wall) can be mistaken for an infiltrating carcinoma.

---

[1] Abdou et al. 1977.
[7] Cornes and Jones 1962.
[37] Le Charpentier et al. 1973.
[65] Terner and Lattes 1965.

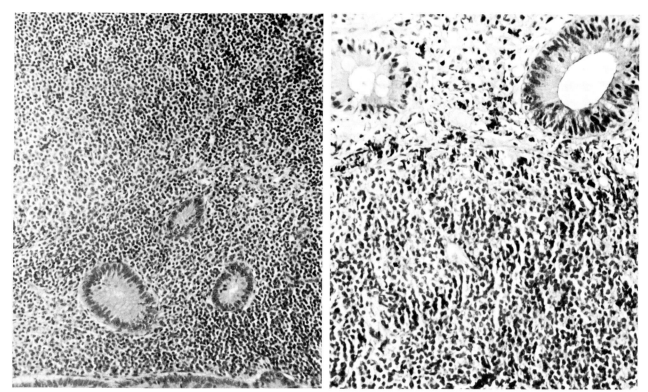

Fig. 331. Malignant lymphoma (appendix) (79-year-old female, ×60).

Fig. 332. Malignant lymphoma of the rectum (66-year-old male, ×200).

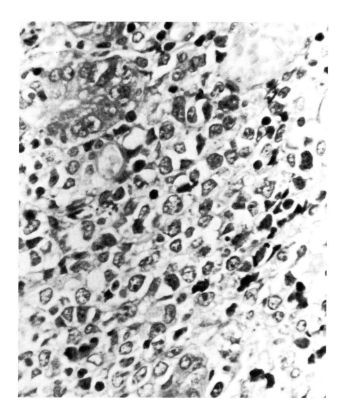

Fig. 333. Malignant lymphoma of the rectum (65-year-old male, ×400).

c) Solitary ulcer of the colon and rectum

Due to the misplacement of epithelial cells into the wall, this lesion can be mistaken for an infiltrating carcinoma (especially in biopsy material).
This solitary ulcer can be caused by a colitis cystica profunda, an inflammation in diverticulosis, or ischemia.
In a number of cases the cause of this ulcer is unclear.
It seems that particularly the solitary ulcer of the rectum may be confused with carcinoma [48].

M-7650/0
T 153.9

d) Endometriosis (WHO) (Figs. 274 and 275)

Very occasionally the differential diagnosis with carcinoma in cases of endometriosis is necessary especially if glands and endometrial stroma are separated from each other (by biopsy) or if a decidual reaction modifies the histological picture.
Clinically the endometriosis can cause intestinal obstruction since this lesion can reach a considerable size (diameter, up to 5 cm).

---

[48] Morson and Dawson 1974.

Tumors of the anal canal and anal orifice

T – primary tumor – anal canal

Tis = preinvasive carcinoma (carcinoma in situ)

T0 = no evidence of primary tumor

T1 = tumor occupying not more than one-third of the circumference or length of the canal and not infiltrating the external sphincter muscle

T2 = tumor occupying more than one-third of the circumference or length of the canal or tumor infiltrating the external sphincter muscle

T3 = tumor with extension to the rectum or skin but not to other neighboring structures

T4 = tumor with extension to neighboring structures

Tx = the minimal requirements to assess the primary tumor can not be met (clinical examination, radiography, and endoscopy)

N – regional lymph nodes – anal canal

(perirectal nodes and nodes distal to the origin of the inferior mesenteric artery)

N0 = no evidence of regional lymph node involvement

N1 = evidence of involvement of regional lymph nodes

Nx = the minimal requirements to assess the regional lymph nodes cannot be met (clinical examination and radiography)

T – primary tumor – anal orifice

Tis = preinvasive carcinoma (carcinoma in situ)

T0 = no evidence of primary tumor

T1 = tumor 2 cm or less in its greatest dimension, strictly superficial or exophytic

T2 = tumor more than 2 cm but not more than 5 cm in its greatest dimension or tumor with minimal infiltration of the dermis

T3 = tumor more than 5 cm in its greatest dimension or tumor with deep infiltration of the dermis

T4 = tumor with extension to muscle, bone, etc.

Tx = the minimal requirements to assess the primary tumor cannot be met (clinical examination, radiography, and endoscopy)

N – regional lymph node – anal orifice

(inguinal nodes)

N0 = no evidence of regional lymph node involvement

N1 = evidence of involvement of the movable unilateral regional lymph nodes

N2 = evidence of involvement of the movable bilateral regional lymph nodes

N3 = evidence of involvement of the fixed regional lymph nodes

Nx = the minimal requirements to assess the regional lymph nodes cannot be met (clinical examination and radiography)

M – distant metastases – anal canal and anal orifice

M0 = no evidence of distant metastases

M1 = evidence of distant metastases

Mx = the minimal requirements to assess the presence of distant metastases cannot be met (clinical examination and radiography)

pTNM – postsurgical histopathological classification
the pTNM categories correspond to the respective TNM categories for the two regions

Stage grouping
No stage grouping is at present recommended

M-8070/3
T 154.2

11. Squamous cell carcinoma (WHO)

**General
Remarks**

Incidence: About 80% of the cancers in the anorectal region are squamous cell carcinomas.
The overall incidence, however, is low.
Age: The peak age is about the 7th decade.
Sex: Women are more frequently affected than men.

Macroscopy

Hard, ulcerating tumor, which infiltrates the rectum and the surrounding tissue.

Histology

Squamous cell carcinoma with different degrees of keratinization and differentiation.

Spread

1. Local spread into the surrounding tissue and the lower part of the rectum.
2. Lymph node metastases: Inguinal region, superior hemorrhoidal region, lateral wall of the pelvis.

Treatment

Surgery:
Radical operation is indicated in cases of superficial carcinoma or large tumors (possibly preceded by irradiation).
Radiation therapy:
Radiation therapy can be used in superficial and small carcinomas (recommended dose, up to 60 to 90 Gy in 6 to 8 weeks) [11, 20].
Surgery and radiation therapy can be combined (especially for preoperative irradiation).

Prognosis

The prognosis is determined individually by the degree of infiltration and the degree of differentiation:
– Small tumors without or with beginning infiltration show a 5-year survival rate of 70 to 90%.
– The 5-year survival rate for well-differentiated carcinoma: More than 80%.
– For moderately differentiated carcinoma, 50%.
– For poorly differentiated carcinoma, 30% [48].

[11] Dold and Sack 1976.
[20] Glanzmann 1978.
[48] Morson and Dawson 1974.

M-8124/3
T 154.2

12. Cloacogenic carcinoma
(carcinoma, basaloid [anal canal] – WHO)

**General
Remarks**

Incidence: About 20% of the tumors in that region are cloacogenic carcinomas.
Age: The peak age is about the 7th decade.
Sex: Women are more frequently affected than men.
Site: The tumor arises in the transitional zone between the mucosa of the rectum and the squamous cell layer of the anus [19].

Macroscopy

This is an ulcerated lesion with often circumferential growth.
The tumor is hard.
The tumor infiltrates the rectum and the surrounding perirectal tissue.
The tumor narrows the lumen of the anal canal.

Histology

This carcinoma is composed of cells, which show different degrees of differentiation.
Their growth pattern can be basaloid; the individual complexes in these cases are surrounded by palisading of the peripheral tumor cells (Figs. 334 to 337).
The tumor cells occasionally have the arrangement of the transitional cell carcinoma of the urinary bladder:

M-8130/3
T 154.2

Transitional cell carcinoma.
Occasionally areas of squamous cell differentiation occur [33] (Fig. 338).
In most instances an infiltration of the tumor into the surrounding tissue and the lymphatics can be shown [50].

**Differential
Diagnosis**

1. Cloacogenic carcinoma **with squamous cell carcinoma** of the anal margin.
2. Cloacogenic carcinoma **with basal cell carcinoma** (WHO) of the anal margin (Fig. 343):
   In most instances the differential diagnosis is difficult; the detection of the origin of the tumor is helpful in these instances.
3. Undifferentiated cloacogenic carcinoma (Fig. 339) **with undifferentiated adenocarcinoma** of the lower rectum:
   The detection of mucin indicates adenocarcinoma.
4. Cloacogenic carcinoma **with carcinoid of the rectum** (Figs. 321 to 328).

Grading

It has been reported that the degree of differentiation is related to the prognosis [52]. Therefore, the tumor should be graded as
well-differentiated
moderately differentiated
poorly differentiated carcinoma according to the degree of mitotic figures and nuclear atypias and the preservation of a basaloid (or transitional) growth pattern.

Spread

1. Local spread into the lower rectum or into the skin.
2. Infiltration of the lymphatics with dissemination into the regional lymph nodes.
   This event has occurred in about 20% of the cases at the time of operation.

---

[19] Gillespie and MacKay 1978.
[33] Klotz et al. 1967.
[50] Otto et al. 1979.
[52] Pang and Morson 1967.

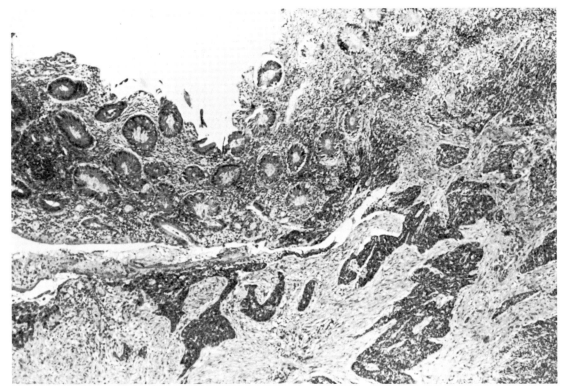

Fig. 334. Cloacogenic carcinoma (64-year-old female, × 50).

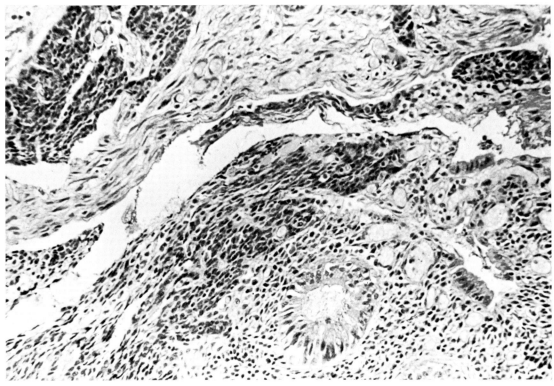

Fig. 335. Cloacogenic carcinoma (64-year-old female, × 125).

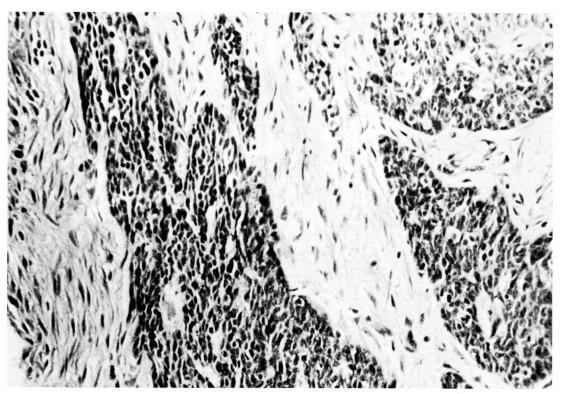

Fig. 336. Cloacogenic carcinoma: Poorly differentiated cells. Remnants of the basaloid pattern are still recognizable (64-year-old female, × 200).

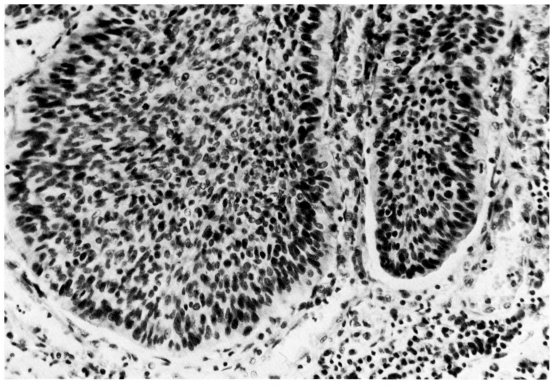

Fig. 337. Cloacogenic carcinoma: Basaloid growth pattern (79-year-old female, × 200).

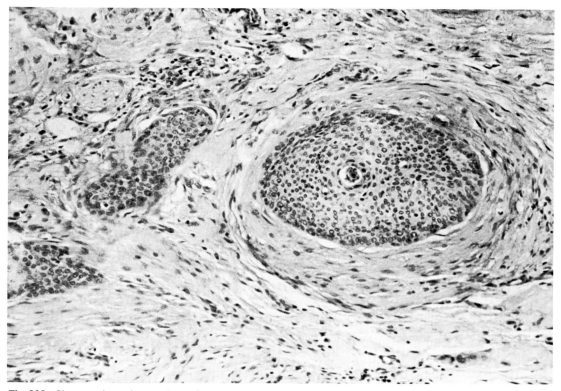

Fig. 338. Cloacogenic carcinoma: Area of squamous cell differentiation; invasion of lymphatics and blood vessel (46-year-old female, × 125).

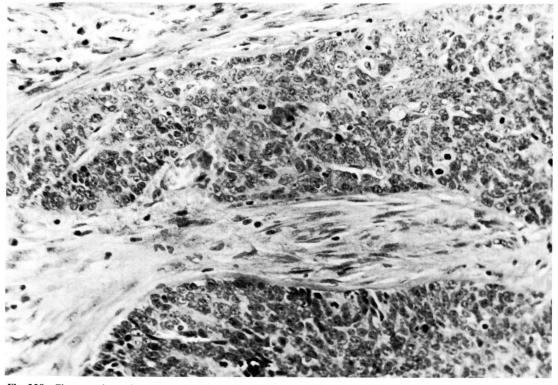

Fig. 339. Cloacogenic carcinoma, poorly differentiated (64-year-old female, × 200).

333

Clinical Findings	Signs of obstruction. Bleeding.
Treatment	**Surgery:** Wide abdominoperineal resection. Lymph node metastases should be resected. **Irradiation:** Irradiation, especially for small tumors (50 to 60 Gy in about 5 weeks). **Chemotherapy:** Adriamycin and cis-platinum [16].

Prognosis	1. In cases of lymph node involvement, the prognosis is poor.
	2. The prognosis correlates with the degree of differentiation:
	   – the 5-year survival rate for highly differentiated carcinoma, 90%
	   – for moderately differentiated carcinoma, 60%,
	   – for poorly differentiated carcinoma, 0%.

Further Information	1. In the transitional zone of the anorectal canal, very rarely **carcinoma in situ** (WHO) might be observed. On histological analysis these carcinomas in situ are similar to those of the cervix. 2. Very rarely **leukoplakia** will develop not only at the region of squamous cells of the anal canal but also in the anorectal canal. These lesions are not precancerous.

M-8140/3
T 154.2

13. Adenocarcinoma of the anorectal region
(adenocarcinoma of anal glands – WHO)

Adenocarcinoma originating from the anal glands is very rare.
This tumor can appear as colloid carcinoma, arising from the glands in an anorectal fistula.

---

[16] Fisher et al. 1978.

M-8720/3
T 154.2

14. Malignant melanoma of the anal canal (WHO)

General Remarks

Incidence: Malignant melanoma in the anorectal canal is a rare tumor.
Age: The peak age is the 7th decade.
Sex: Males are affected slightly more frequently than females.
Site: Anal canal at the transitional zone.

Macroscopy

The tumor is large, soft, and polypoid and narrows the lumen of the anus. The tumor is ulcerated and infiltrates the surrounding tissue.

Histology

Pigmented tumor cells with the usual grade of variety in cytological and histological appcarance, typical for this tumor (Figs. 340 to 342) (see Malignant melanoma, page 1222).

Spread

This is a very malignant tumor, with early spread into lymph nodes and distant metastases.

Clinical Findings

Rectal bleeding.

Treatment

According to the extent of the disease, **surgery** or **chemotherapy** can be attempted. Postoperative irradiation of up to 40 to 50 Gy in 5 weeks (see pages 1230, 1236, 1242).

Prognosis

Very poor.

M-8430/3
T 154.2

15. Mucoepidermoid carcinoma of the anal canal (WHO)

This carcinoma is composed of tumor cells that exhibit the features of mucin-producing adenocarcinoma cells and squamous cells.
This tumor resembles, however, an adenocarcinoma with squamous cell metaplasia more than mucoepidermoid carcinoma of the salivary glands (Figs. 582 to 587).

Malignant melanoma

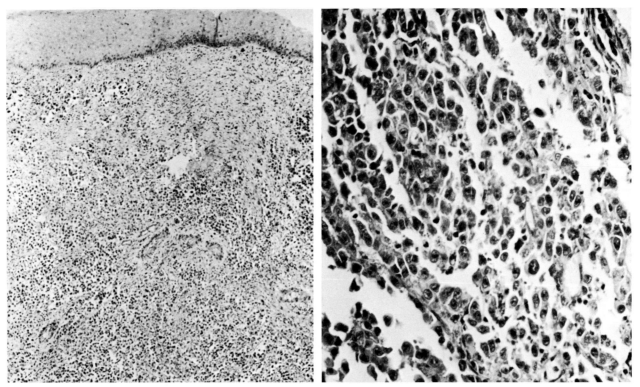

Fig. 340. Malignant melanoma of the anus (70-year-old female, ×40).

Fig. 341. Malignant melanoma of the anus (70-year-old female, ×200).

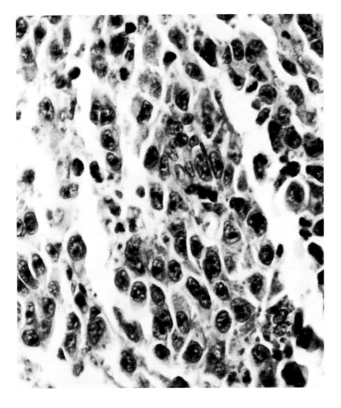

Fig. 342. Malignant melanoma of the anus (70-year-old female, ×400).

Tumors of the anal skin

16. Basal cell carcinoma (WHO)
(basaloid carcinoma – WHO)

This skin tumor has its peak age around the 6th to 7th decades.
Men are more often affected than women.
Local excision and irradiation cures the tumor.
On histological analysis the differential diagnosis with well-differentiated cloacogenic carcinomas might be difficult (Figs. 337 to 343).

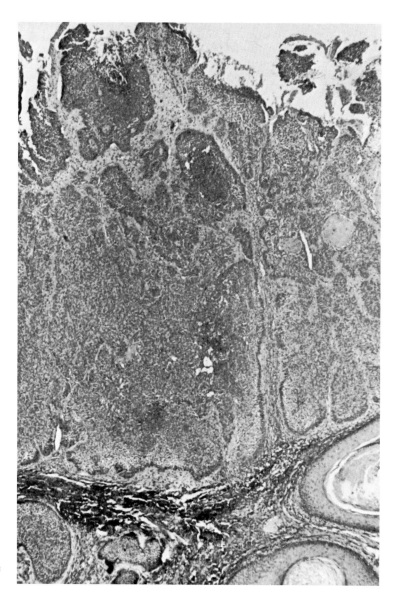

Fig. 343. Basal cell carcinoma of the anus (63-year-old male, × 40).

M-8081/2
T 173.5

17. Intraepithelial carcinoma
(Bowen's disease) (WHO)

This intraepithelial carcinoma is rare in the anal skin (Figs. 344 to 347) (for histology see page 1147).

M-7672/0
T 173.5

18. Condyloma acuminatum (WHO)
(Fig. 346) (for histology see page 1462).

M-7286/0
T 173.5

19. Keratoacanthoma
(Figs. 1102 and 1103).

M-8542/3
T 173.5

20. Extramammary Paget's disease (WHO)

General Remarks

Incidence: This is a very rare lesion.
Age: Elderly persons are affected.

Macroscopy

Reddish, ulcerated skin lesion.

Histology

The tumor corresponds to mammary Paget's disease:
The Paget's cells grow in an intradermal position. They originate from the apocrine glands.

Differential Diagnosis

1. Extramammary Paget's disease **with cells of malignant melanoma** (Figs. 919 to 922).
2. Extramammary Paget's disease **with Bowen's disease** (Figs. 1114 to 1117).
3. Extramammary Paget's disease **with infiltrating adenocarcinoma:**
   Paget's cells stain positive with PAS.

Spread

About 30% of the cases have regional lymph node metastases at the time of detection of the tumor [24].

Treatment

Local excision or radical surgery according to the extent of the tumor.
Without treatment it must be expected that the intraepidermal tumor will develop into an infiltrating adenocarcinoma.

---

[24] Helwig and Graham 1963.

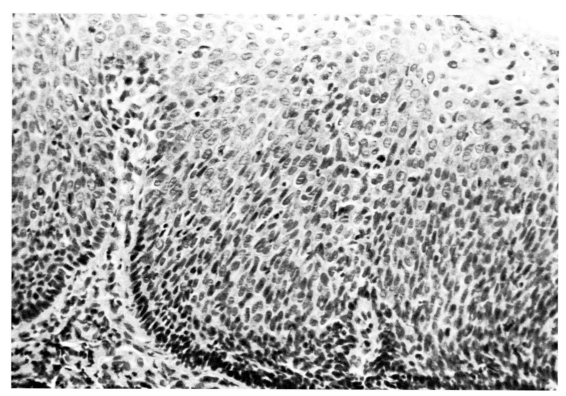

Fig. 344. Intraepithelial carcinoma combined with lichen sclerosus et atrophicus (see Fig. 345) (76-year-old female, ×200).

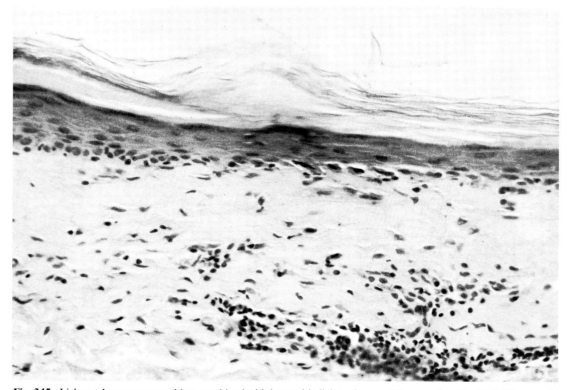

Fig. 345. Lichen sclerosus et atrophicus combined with intraepithelial carcinoma of the anus (see Fig. 344) (76-year-old female, ×200).

339

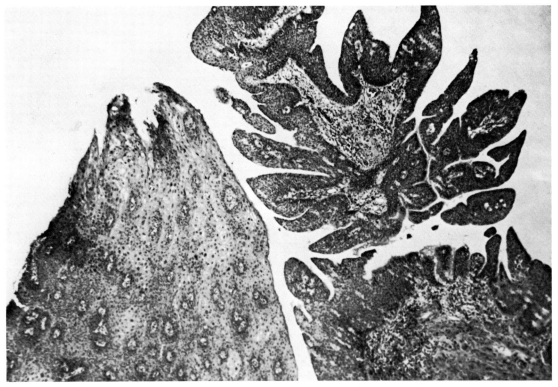

Fig. 346. Condyloma acuminatum, combined with intraepithelial carcinoma (× 40).

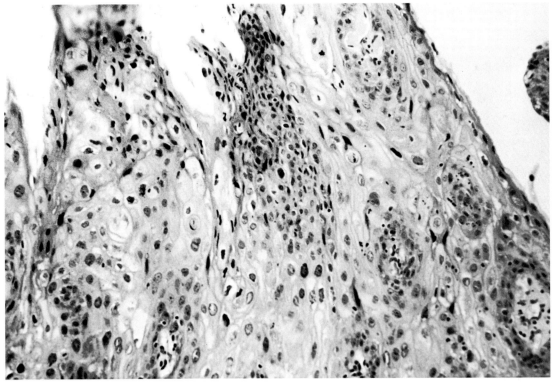

Fig. 347. Intraepithelial carcinoma of the anus (see Fig. 346) (× 200).

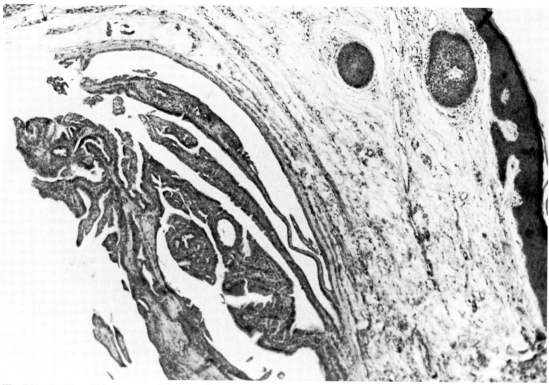

Fig. 348. Papillary hidradenoma of the anus (41-year-old female, × 50).

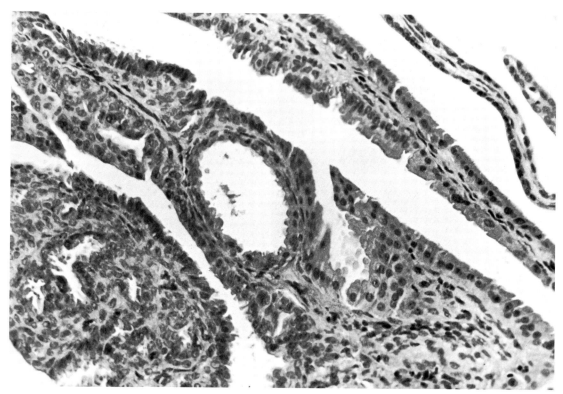

Fig. 349. Papillary hidradenoma of the anus (41-year-old female, × 200).

M-8400/0
T 173.5

21. Tumors of the sweat glands
(hidradenoma – WHO)
(Figs. 348 and 349) (see Tumors of the skin, page 1180).

M-7681/0
T 173.5

22. Fibrous polyp
(anal tag) (WHO)

This lesion is covered by a regular squamous cell layer, underneath which fibrous tissue has developed.
There are different degrees of chronic inflammation in the subepithelial position.

M-8140/6
T 154.2, 3
T 173.5

23. Metastatic adenocarcinoma into the anal region

The primary tumor in these instances is rather often located in the rectum.

M-4318/0
T 154.3

24. Malakoplakia [6]
(Figs. 1397 and 1398)

M-8000/3
T 153.9
T 154.2, 3

25. Unclassified tumors of the colon and anal canal (WHO)

---

[6] Colby 1978.

Recommendations for differential diagnosis in tumors of the large bowel

adenocarcinoma	with	– metastatic adenocarcinoma – heterotopic tissue – solitary ulcer – colitis chronica profunda – diverticulosis – endometriosis – regenerative epithelial cell changes (for instance, in Crohn's disease or ulcerative colitis) – epithelial cell changes following irradiation
poorly differentiated adenocarcinoma	with	– malignant lymphoma – malakoplakia
staging of adenocarcinoma	into	– Dukes classification
benign polyps	with	– polyps with foci of carcinoma in situ or foci of infiltrating carcinoma

Recommendations for differential diagnosis in tumors of the anorectal region

cloacogenic carcinoma (basaloid carcinoma, transitional cell carcinoma)	with	– basal cell carcinoma of the anal skin – undifferentiated adenocarcinoma – carcinoid
primary adenocarcinoma	with	– metastatic adenocarcinoma from the rectum
extramammary Paget's disease	with	– Bowen's disease – malignant melanoma – undifferentiated carcinoma

343

References

[1] Abdou, N.I., C.Na Pombejara, A. Sagawa, C. Ragland, D.J. Stechschulte, U. Nilsson, W. Gourley, I. Watanabe, N.J. Lindsey, and M.S. Allen: Malakoplakia: Evidence for monocyte lysosomal abnormality correctable by cholinergic agonist in vitro and in vivo. N. Engl. J. Med. *297* (1977) 1413-1419.

[2] Alberto, P., M. Rozencweig, D. Gangji, A. Brugarolas, F. Cavalli, P. Siegenthaler, and H.H. Hansen: Phase II study of anhydro-ara-5-fluorocytidine in adenocarcinoma of gastrointestinal tract, epidermoid carcinoma of lung, head and neck, breast carcinoma and small cell anaplastic carcinoma of lung. A study report of the E.O.R.T.C. early clinical trial cooperation group. Eur. J. Cancer *14* (1978) 195-201.

[3] Alford, T.C., H.-M. Do, G.W. Geelhoed, N.T. Tsangaris, and M.E. Lippman: Steroid hormone receptors in human colon cancers. Cancer *43* (1979) 980-984.

[4] Ammann, R., P. Deyhle und H. Sulser: Multiple adenomatöse papilläre Kolonpolypen in einer Familie mit gehäuftem Magenkarzinom, ein neuer Phänotyp der familiären Kolonpolypose? Schweiz. Med. Wschr. *106* (1976) 894-897.

[5] Amorn, Y., and W.A. Knight, Jr.: Primary linitis plastica of the colon. Report of two cases and review of the literature. Cancer *41* (1978) 2420-2425.

[6] Colby T.V.: Malakoplakia: Two unusual cases which presented diagnostic problems. Am. J. Surg. Path. *2* (1978) 377-382.

[7] Cornes, J.S., and T.G. Jones: Leukaemic lesions of the gastrointestinal tract. J. Clin. Pathol. *15* (1962) 305-313.

[8] Cottier, H., J. Turk, and L. Sobin: A proposal for a standardized system of reporting human lymph node morphology in relation to immunological function. Bull. WHO *47* (1972) 375-417.

[9] Crissman, J.D.: Adenosquamous and squamous cell carcinoma of the colon. Am. J. Surg. Path. *2* (1978) 47-54.

[10] DeVita, V.T. Jr.: In: Harrison's Principles of internal medicine. Eighth edition. McGraw-Hill Book Company, New York–Düsseldorf etc. 1977.

[11] Dold, N.W., und H. Sack: Praktische Tumortherapie. Die Behandlung maligner Organtumoren und Systemerkrankungen. Thieme, Stuttgart 1976.

[12] Douglass, H.O. Jr., P.T. Lavin, J. Woll, J.F. Conroy, and P. Carbone: Chemotherapy of advanced measurable colon and rectal carcinoma with oral 5-fluorouracil, alone or in combination with cyclophosphamide or 6-thioguanine, with intravenous 5-fluorouracil or beta-2′-deoxythioguanosine or with oral 3(4-methylcyclohexyl)-1(2-chlorethyl)-1-nitrosourea. A Phase II-III Study of the eastern cooperative oncology group (EST 4273). Cancer *42* (1978) 2538-2545.

[13] Dukes, C.E.: Histological grading of rectal cancer. Proc. R. Soc. Med. *30* (1937) 371-376.

[14] Dukes, C.E.: Peculiarities in the pathology of cancer of the ano-rectal region. Proc. R. Soc. Med. *39* (1946) 763-765.

[15] Dukes, C.E.: The surgical pathology of rectal cancer. J. Clin. Pathol. *2* (1949) 95-98.

[16] Fisher, W.B., K.D. Herbst, J.E. Sims, and C.F. Critchfield: Metastatic cloacogenic carcinoma of the anus: Sequential responses to adriamycin and cis-dichlorodiammineplatinum (II). Cancer Treat. Rep. *62* (1978) 91-97.

[17] Freni, S.C., and J.N. Keeman: Leiomyomatosis of the colon. Cancer *39* (1977) 263-266.

[18] Gérard, A.: Carcinoma of the colon and rectum: Prognostic factors and criteria of response. In: Cancer therapy: Prognostic factors and criteria of response, edited by M.J. Staquet, Raven Press, New York 1975.

[19] Gillespie, J.J., and B. MacKay: Histogenesis of cloacogenic carcinoma. Fine structure of anal transitional epithelium and cloacogenic carcinoma. Hum. Pathol. *9* (1978) 579-587.

[20] Glanzmann, Ch.: Radiotherapie in der Behandlung von Analkarzinomen. Erfahrungen an 28 Fällen aus dem Zeitraum 1950-1975 und Literaturergebnisse. Strahlentherapie *154* (1978) 174-178.

[21] Goldenberg, D.M., R.M. Sharkey, and F.J. Primus: Immunocytochemical detection of carcinoembryonic antigen in conventional histopathology specimens. Cancer *42* (1978) 1546-1553.

[22] Gould, V.E., and G. Chejfec: Neuroendocrine carcinomas of the colon. Ultrastructural and biochemical evidence of their secretory function. Am. J. Surg. Path. *2* (1978) 31-38.

[23] Gropp, C., und K. Havemann: Chemotherapie bei gastrointestinalen Tumoren. Zeitschrift für Gastroenterologie *16* (1978) 609-615.

[24] Helwig, E.B., and J.H. Graham: Anogenital (extramammary) Paget's disease; a clinicopathological study. Cancer *16* (1963) 387-403.

[25] Hermanek, P.: "Grading" und "Staging": Bedeutung für die klinische Onkologie. Fortschr. Med. *96* (1978) 520-524.

[26] Hernandez, F.J., and J.D. Reid: Mixed carcinoid and mucus-secreting intestinal tumours. Arch. Pathol. *88* (1969) 489-496.

[27] Higgins, G.A. Jr., E. Humphrey, G.L. Juler, H.H. LeVeen, J. McCaughan, and R.J. Keehn: Adjuvant chemotherapy in the surgical treatment of large bowel cancer. Cancer *38* (1976) 1461-1467.

[28] Horne, B.D., and C.F. McCulloch: Squamous cell carcinoma of the cecum. A case report. Cancer *42* (1978) 1879-1882.

[29] Isaacson, P., and H.P. Le Vann: The demonstration of carcinoembryonic antigen in colorectal carcinoma and colonic polyps using an immunoperoxydase technique. Cancer *38* (1976) 1348-1356.

[30] Jackson, B.R.: Contemporary management of rectal cancer. An overview. Cancer *40* (1977) 2365-2374.

[31] Khankhanian, N., G.M. Mavligit, W.O. Russell, and M. Schimek: Prognostic significance of vascular invasion in colorectal cancer of Dukes' B class. Cancer *39* (1977) 1195-1200.

[32] Kligerman, M.M.: Irradiation of the primary lesion of the rectum and rectosigmoid. JAMA *231* (1975) 1381-1384.

[33] Klotz, R.G., T. Pamukcoglu, and D.H. Souillard: Transitional cloacogenic carcinoma of the anal canal. Cancer *20* (1967) 1727-1745.

[34] Langer, S., und H. Buss: Der Mastdarmkrebs. Klinik und Morphologie der lokalen Kryotherapie. Dtsch. Med. Wschr. *104* (1979) 768-771.

[35] Law, I.P., R.B. Herberman, R.K. Oldham, J. Bouzoukis, S.M. Hanson, and M.C. Rhode: Familial occurrence of colon and uterine carcinoma and of lymphoproliferative malignancies. Clinical description. Cancer *39* (1977) 1224-1228.

[36] Law, I.P., A.C. Hollinshead, J. Whang-Peng, J.H. Dean, R.K. Oldham, R.B. Herberman, and M.C. Rhode: Familial occurrence of colon and uterine carcinoma and of lymphoproliferative malignancies. II. Chromosomal and immunologic abnormalities. Cancer *39* (1977) 1229-1236.

[37] Le Charpentier, Y., M. Le Charpentier, B. Franc. Ph. Galian, et R. Abelanet: Données fournies par l'etude ultrastructurale de deux observations de malakoplakie. Virchows Arch. A Path. Anat. and Histol. *359* (1973) 157-170.

[38] Lemozy, J.: Les tumeurs carcinoïdes du rectum. Arch. Fr. Mal. App. Dig. *62* (1973) 537-568.

[39] Localio, S.A., and K. Eng: Sphincter-saving operations for cancer of the rectum. N. Engl. J. Med. *300* (1979) 1028-1030.

[40] Loewenstein, M.S., and N. Zamcheck: Carcinoembryonic antigen (CEA) levels in benign gastrointestinal disease states. Cancer *42* (1978) 1412-1418.

[41] Lynch, P.M., H.T. Lynch, and R.E. Harris: Heraditary proximal colonic cancer. Dis. Col. Rect. *20* (1977) 661-668.

[42] MacLennan, G., R.D. Stogryn, and A.J. Voitk: Abdominoperineal resection. Treatment of choice for carcinoma of the rectum. Cancer *38* (1976) 953-956.

[43] Martin, F., M.S. Martin, and C. Bourgeaux: Perspectives in cancer research: Fetal antigens in human digestive tumors. Eur. J. Cancer *12* (1976) 165-175.

[44] Mavligit, G.M., J.U. Gutterman, M.A. Burgess, N. Khankhanian, G.B. Seibert, J.S. Speer, R.C. Reed, A.V. Jubert, R.C. Martin, C.M. McBride, E.M. Copeland, E.A. Gehan, and E.M. Hersh: Adjuvant immunotherapy and chemoimmunotherapy in colorectal cancer of Dukes' C classification. Preliminary clinical results. Cancer *36* (1975) 2421-2427.

[45] Mavligit. G.M., J.U. Gutterman, M.A. Malahy, M.A. Burgess, C.M. McBride, A. Jubert, and E.M. Hersh: Systemic adjuvant immunotherapy and chemoimmunotherapy in patients with colo-rectal cancer (Dukes' C class): Prolongation of disease-free interval and survival. In: Immunotherapy of cancer: Present status of trials in man, edited by W.D. Terry and D. Windhorst. Raven Press, New York 1978.

[46] Mayer, R.J., M.B. Garnick, G.D. Steele, and N. Zamcheck: Carcinoembryonic antigen (CEA) as a monitor of chemotherapy in disseminated colorectal cancer. Cancer *42* (1978) 1428-1433.

[47] Moertel, C.G., M.J. O'Connell, R.E. Ritts, Jr., A.J. Schutt, R.J. Reitemeier, R.G. Hahn, S.K. Frytak, and J. Rubin: A controlled evaluation of combined immunotherapy (MER-BCG) and chemotherapy for advanced colorectal cancer. In: Immunotherapy of cancer: Present status of trials in man, edited by W.D. Terry and D. Windhorst, Raven Press, New York 1978.

[48] Morson, B.C., and I.M.P. Dawson: Gastrointestinal pathology. Blackwell-Scientific Publication. Oxford–London–Edinburgh–Melbourne 1974.

[49] Noltenius, H., H. Giersch, A. Haake, H.-J. Raydt und M. Buchholz: Maligne Tumoren im Alter. Med. Klin. *72* (1977) 391-398.

[50] Otto, H.F., J.-O. Gebbers und R. Winkler: Untersuchungen zur Ultrastruktur der transitionalen cloacogenen Carcinome der recto-analen Grenzregion. Virchows Arch. A. Path. Anat. and Histol. *381* (1979) 223-239.

[51] Otto, H.F., M. Wanke und J. Zeitlhofer: Darm und Peritoneum. In: Spezielle pathologische Anatomie. Band II, Teil 2. Hrsg. W. Doerr, G. Seifert, E. Uehlinger. Springer, Berlin–Heidelberg–New York 1976.

[52] Pang, L.S.C., and B.C. Morson: Basaloid carcinoma of the anal canal. J. Clin. Pathol. *20* (1967) 128-135.

[53] Papillon, J.: Resectable rectal cancer: Treatment by curative endocavity irradiation. JAMA *231* (1975) 1385-1387.

[54] Presant, C.A., G. Ratkin, and C. Klahr: Phase II trial of 5-fluorouracil plus melphalan in colorectal carcinoma. Cancer Treat. Rep. *62* (1978) 461-462.

[55] Presant, C.A., G. Ratkin, and C. Klahr: Phase II study of mitamycin C, cyclophosphamide, and methotrexate in drug-resistant colorectal carcinoma. Cancer Treat. Rep. *62* (1978) 549-550.

[56] Ranchod, M., and R.L. Kempson: Smooth muscle tumors of the gastrointestinal tract and retroperitoneum. A pathologic analysis of 100 cases. Cancer *39* (1977) 255-262.

[57] Ranchod, M., K.J. Lewin, and R.F. Dorfman: Lymphoid hyperplasia of the gastrointestinal tract. A study of 26 cases and review of the literature. Am. J. Surg. Path. *2* (1978) 383-400.

[58] Rider, W.D.: Is the Miles operation really necessary for the treatment of rectal cancer? J. Can. Assoc. Radiol. *26* (1975) 167-175.

[59] Rückert, K., J. Grönniger und H. Brünner: Sarkome des Dünn- und Dickdarmes. Klinik, Therapie und Prognose. Dtsch. Med. Wschr. *102* (1977) 1631-1634.

[60] Sack, H.: Präoperative Strahlenbehandlung des

Rektum- und Rektosigmoidkarzinoms. Dtsch. Med. Wschr. *100* (1975) 2651-2653.

[61] Scherer, E., und H. Sack: Probleme der Strahlenbehandlung des Rektumkarzinoms. Strahlentherapie *155* (1979) 300-306.

[62] Spjut, H. J., N. B. Frankel, and M. F. Appel: The small carcinoma of the large bowel. Am. J. Surg. Path. *3* (1979) 39-46.

[63] Spratt, J. S. Jr., and H. J. Spjut: Prevalence and prognosis of individual clinical and pathologic variables associated with colorectal carcinoma. Cancer *20* (1967) 1976-1985.

[64] Tappeiner, G., H. Denk, R. Eckerstorfer und J. H. Holzner: Vergleichende Untersuchungen über Auftreten und Lokalisation des carcinoembryonalen Antigens (CEA) eines normalen perchlorsäureextrahierbaren Dickdarmschleimhaut-Antigens (NC) in Carcinomen und Polypen des Dickdarms. Virchows Arch. A Path. Anat. and Histol. *360* (1973) 129-140.

[65] Terner, J. Y., and R. Lattes: Malakoplakia of colon and retroperitoneum. Am. J. Clin. Path. *44* (1965) 20-31.

[66] Turnbull, R. B. Jr., K. Kyle, F. R. Watson, and J. Spratt: Cancer of the colon: The influence of the no-touch isolation technique on survival rates. Ann. Surg. *166* (1967) 420-427.

[67] Velde, van de, C. J. H., C. J. L. M. Meyer, C. J. Cornelisse, E. A. van der Velde, L. M. van Put-ten, and A. Zwaveling: A morphometrical analysis of lymph node responses to tumors of different immunogenicity. Cancer Res. *38* (1978) 661-667.

[68] Wanebo, H. J., B. Rao, C. M. Pinsky, R. G. Hoffman, M. Stearns, M. K. Schwartz, and H. F. Oettgen: Preoperative carcinoembryonic antigen level as a prognostic indicator in colorectal cancer. N. Engl. J. Med. *299* (1978) 448-451.

[69] Weisbrot, I. M., A. F. Liber, and B. S. Gordon: The effects of therapeutic radiation on colonic mucosa. Cancer *36* (1975) 931-940.

[70] Wiebecke, B., A. Brandts, and M. Eder: Epithelial proliferation and morphogenesis of hyperplastic adenomatous and villous polyps of the human colon. Virchows Arch. A Path. Anat. and Histol. *364* (1974) 35-49.

[71] Wood, D. A., G. F. Robbins, C. Zippin, D. Lum, and M. Stearns: Staging of cancer of the colon and cancer of the rectum. Cancer *43* (1979) 961-968.

[72] Zamcheck, N.: The present status of CEA in diagnosis, prognosis, and evaluation of therapy. Cancer *36* (1975) 2460-2468.

[73] Zamcheck, N., T. L. Moore, P. Dhar, and H. Kupchik: Immunologic diagnosis and prognosis of human digestive-tract cancer: Carcinoembryonic antigens. N. Engl. J. Med. *286* (1972) 83-86.

9 Tumors of the liver

Liver

1. Malignant tumors in this location do have a very poor prognosis due to late symptoms and early lymphatic spread. Only carcinomas growing in the ampulla of Vater have a slightly better prospect, since early obstruction and jaundice may lead to early treatment before lymph node metastases have developed.
2. The association between cirrhosis of the liver and carcinoma of the liver is well known. About 50% of carcinomas grow in a cirrhotic liver.
3. Well known is the possibility that environmental factors can induce malignant tumors in the liver: thorotrast, polyvinylchloride, aflatoxin. It is still debated whether anovulatory drugs can have this effect in certain cases.
4. The malignant cells of a liver cell carcinoma penetrate early into the blood vessels of the liver and cause liver cell necroses. Functional disturbances of the liver might therefore be expected earlier than in metastatic lesions in the liver, which only rarely occlude the portal or arterial blood vessels.

M-8170/3
T 155.0

1. Hepatocellular carcinoma (WHO)
(liver cell carcinoma; hepatoma)

General Remarks

Incidence: About 1% of all malignant tumors are liver cell carcinomas.
This tumor is common in Africa and Asia: about 20 to 30% of all malignant tumors.
Age: The peak age is the 6th decade.
Sex: Men are considerably more frequently affected than women (4 : 1).
Further notes: 50 to 75% of liver cell carcinomas are associated with cirrhosis of the liver.

Macroscopy

Diffuse infiltration, large tumors, or most often multiple nodules are seen at the surface and cut surface of the liver.
The portal veins are often occluded by tumor thrombi.

Histology

The tumor is composed of malignant liver cells: They exhibit different degrees of nuclei pleomorphism, different numbers of mitotic figures, and hyperchromasia (Figs. 350 to 355).
Even in tumor cells of poor differentiation, bile pigment can be detected in the cytoplasm, including metastatic tumor cells (Figs. 356 to 358).
Often the tumor cells mimic the pattern of normal liver architecture, and the tumor cell trabeculae are often lined by sinuses (Figs. 351 and 355).
In other instances the cell pattern is solid.
The tumor cells regularly infiltrate the blood vessels (Figs. 353 and 355).
Often more or less extensive ischemic necroses of the surrounding liver parenchyma result.

Electron Microscopy

In hepatocellular carcinoma the tumor cells contain endoplasmatic reticulum and mitochondria resembling the regular liver cell [19, 21] (Fig. 359).

Differential Diagnosis

1. Hepatocellular carcinoma **with cholangiocarcinoma** (Figs. 360 to 363).
2. Hepatocellular carcinoma **with metastatic tumors in the liver:**
   The liver-like trabecular arrangement of tumor cells and the finding of bile pigment in the tumor cells are helpful in recognizing the primary liver cell carcinoma.
3. Hepatocellular carcinoma **with benign adenoma of the liver** (see page 352).

Spread

1. Lymphatic spread into regional lymph nodes occurs frequently.
2. Hematogenous spread, especially to lung and bone, occurs early in the course of the disease.

Clinical Findings

1. The tumor might escape diagnosis because of the overlying liver cirrhosis.
2. Hepatomegaly with moderate pain, ascites, loss of weight, and jaundice.
3. In most cases (80 to 90%), the alpha-fetoprotein (AFP) content in the serum is highly elevated.
4. Production of gonadotropin (gynecomastia).
5. Insulin-like substances can be produced: hypoglycemia.

---

[19] Gyorkey et al. 1975.
[21] Hatzibujas et al. 1978.

Hepatocellular carcinoma

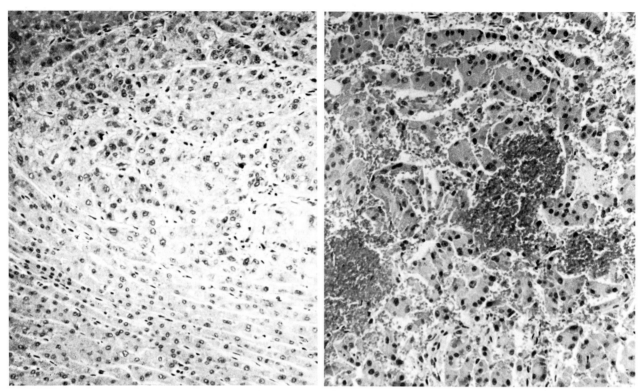

Fig. 350. Well-differentiated liver cell carcinoma (67-year-old male, × 125).

Fig. 351. Well-differentiated liver cell carcinoma (67-year-old female, × 125).

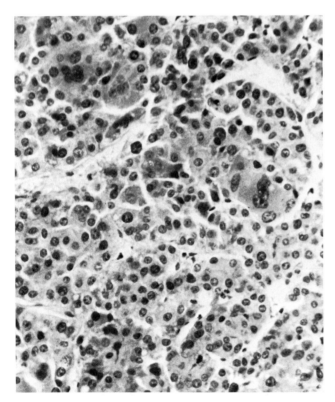

Fig. 352. Well to moderately differentiated liver cell carcinoma (× 200).

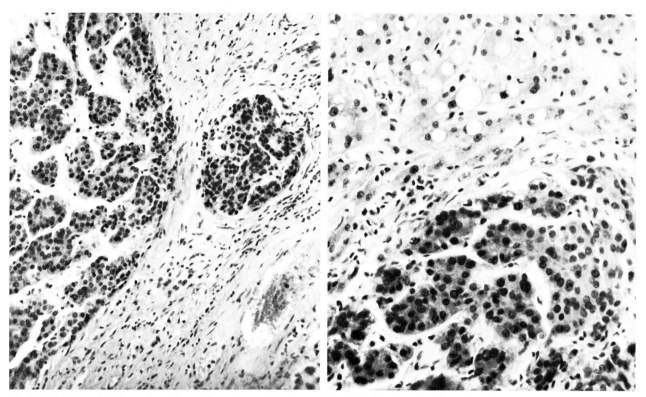

Fig. 353. Moderately differentiated liver cell carcinoma: Blood vessel invasion (× 125).

Fig. 354. Moderately differentiated liver cell carcinoma in liver cirrhosis (× 200).

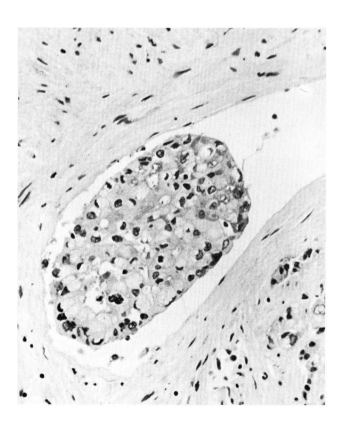

Fig. 355. Well-differentiated liver cell carcinoma: Blood vessel invasion (77-year-old female, × 200).

Hepatocellular carcinoma

Clinical Findings

6. Occasionally the carcinoid syndrome has been reported [33].
7. Occasionally erythropoietin can be produced: Erythrocytosis.
8. An essential tool for diagnosis is the liver biopsy [2].

Treatment

Surgery:
Occasionally resection of the tumor can be attempted in younger children.
No irradiation.
Chemotherapy:
5-Fluorouracil seems to be the best single agent (intravenous application) [14].
– A combination of 5-fluorouracil with BCNU has been recommended.
– Hepatic artery ligation combined with intraportal infusion therapy may be attempted [29, 30, 32].
– Quadruple chemotherapy did not show any benefit for the patient (5-fluorouracil, cyclophosphamide, methotrexate, and vincristine) [12].

Prognosis

Extremely poor.
Patients only rarely survive a few months after diagnosis.

Further Information
M-8170/0
T 155.0

1. **Liver cell adenoma** (WHO)
   (hepatocellular adenoma; benign hepatoma)
   Benign adenomas of the liver are exceedingly rare.
   Liver cell adenoma has no central vein or portal triads.
   There is no infiltration into the blood vessels by the adenoma cells.
   Liver cell adenomas do not have a capsule.
   Differential diagnosis:
   In cases of benign adenoma of the liver, the possibility of a very highly differentiated liver cell carcinoma should always be considered.
2. A strong association between hepatitis virus B and hepatocellular carcinoma has been reported [31].
3. There is no clinical or histological difference between liver cell carcinoma associated or not associated with HBS antigen [17].
4. Rarely the appearance of hepatic adenoma and/or hepatocellular carcinoma in association with the long-term use of female or male hormone has been reported [8, 25].
5. Very rarely hepatocellular carcinoma has been described following vinylchloride exposure [18].

[2] Alpert and Isselbacher 1977.
[8] Boyd and Mark 1977.
[12] Cochrane et al. 1977.
[14] Davis Jr. et al. 1978.
[17] Fisher et al. 1976.
[18] Gokel et al. 1976.
[25] Kay 1977.
[29] Nagasue et al. 1976.
[30] Nagasue et al. 1976.
[31] Nayak et al. 1977.
[32] Nilsson 1966.
[33] Primack et al 1971.

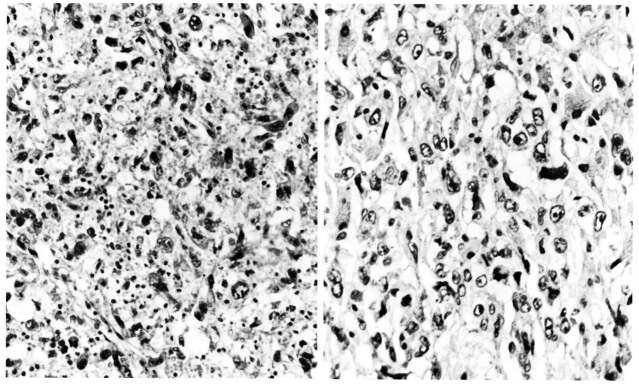

Fig. 356. Poorly differentiated liver cell carcinoma (70-year-old male, × 125).

Fig. 357. Poorly differentiated liver cell carcinoma (70-year-old male, × 200).

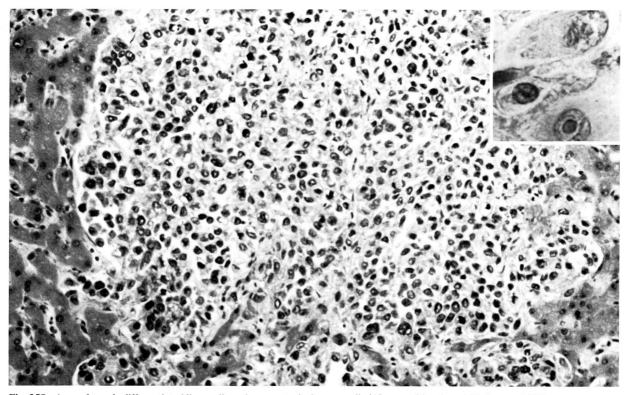

Fig. 358. Area of poorly differentiated liver cell carcinoma, atypical tumor cells (49-year-old male, × 125; inset, × 2000).

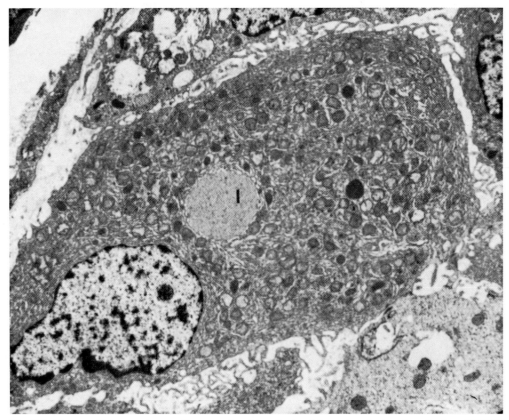

Fig. 359. Hepatocellular carcinoma: Tumor cells with mitochondria and endoplasmic reticulum (×6500) (Gyorkey et al., Hum. Pathol. *6*[1975] 421-441).

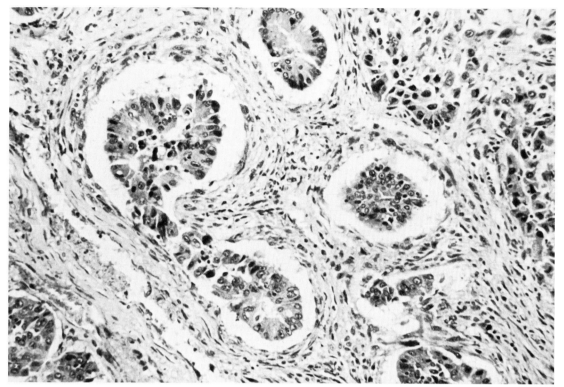

Fig. 360. Cholangiocarcinoma (×125).

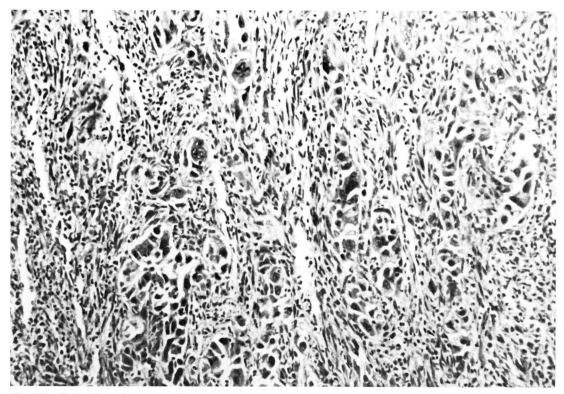

Fig. 361. Cholangiocarcinoma, poorly differentiated (×125).

M-8180/3
T 155.0

2. Cholangiocarcinoma (WHO)
(intrahepatic bile duct carcinoma)

General
Remarks

Incidence: About 10% of the malignant tumors of the liver are cholangiocarcinomas.
Age: The peak age is the 5th and 6th decades.
Sex: Men are more frequently affected than women.
Further notes: 20 to 40% of cholangiocarcinomas are associated with liver cirrhosis.

Macroscopy

These are multiple or solitary tumors disseminated in the liver. The tumors are of different sizes.

Histology

The tumor cells in cholangiocarcinoma form a glandular pattern, which mimics the lumen of the bile ducts. In these glandular patterns no bile pigment is found (Figs. 360 to 362). Usually these tumor cells are surrounded by abundant connective tissue.
Occasionally the tumor cells grow in a papillary fashion into the lumen of the pseudobile ducts (Fig. 363).

Differential
Diagnosis

1. Cholangiocarcinoma **with liver cell carcinoma** (hepatoma) (Figs. 350 to 358):
   In liver cell carcinoma there is considerably less connective tissue than in cholangiocarcinoma.
   The hepatoma cells do not attempt to imitate bile duct structures.

M-8180/3
T 155.0

However, a **combined tumor** containing structures of both cholangiocarcinoma and hepatoma can be found **(combined hepatocellular and cholangiocarcinoma – WHO).**

2. Cholangiocarcinoma **with metastatic tumor:**
   This differential diagnosis might be difficult in cases of less well-differentiated cholangiocarcinomas.

Spread

1. Early involvement of lymph nodes.
2. Hematogenous metastases into lung and bone and into other organs, also of early occurrence.

Clinical
Findings

1. The symptoms correspond to the symptoms of liver cell carcinoma.
2. In cholangiocarcinoma the alpha-fetoprotein serum level is also elevated in most cases.

Treatment
Prognosis

Treatment and prognosis are identical with those of liver cell carcinoma (see page 352).

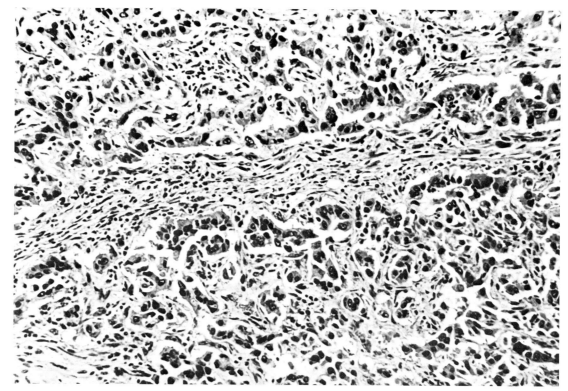

Fig. 362. Cholangiocarcinoma, poorly differentiated (× 125).

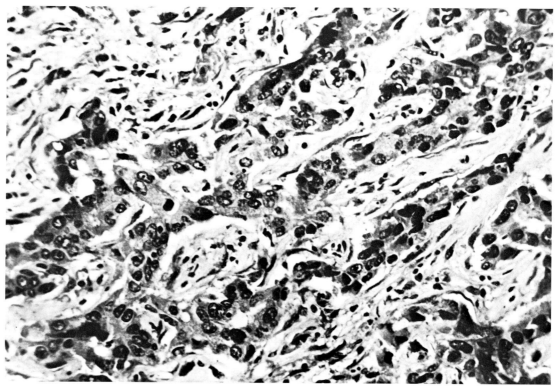

Fig. 363. Poorly differentiated cholangiocarcinoma (× 200).

357

M-8970/3
T 155.0

3. Hepatoblastoma (WHO)

(malignant hepatic mixed tumor) [7]
(embryonic hepatoma; embryonal mixed tumor)

**General
Remarks**

Age: This very malignant tumor occurs almost always in infants and children; very rare cases have been observed in adults [10, 22].
This tumor can be called **carcinosarcoma** (WHO).

Macroscopy

This is a soft tumor with multiple zones of hemorrhage and necrosis.
In most instances the tumor is very large and solitary.

Histology

The tumor is composed of malignant cells of an epithelial and mesenchymal origin. Each of these cell groups can have different degrees of differentiation and different growth patterns. The epithelial cells can form tubular structures or complexes or have papillary growth pattern (Figs. 364 to 366).
The malignant mesenchymal part can contain cartilage (Fig. 367), osteoid [36], or very rarely melanocytes (Fig. 368).
Occasionally hematopoiesis is found in the tumor [7].

Treatment

Surgery:
Partial hepatectomy with removal of the tumor can be attempted in young children.
Chemotherapy:
Chemotherapy (5-fluorouracil and methotrexate) can be tried, particularly by perfusion of the hepatic artery.
Relief of pain has occurred with this treatment [34].
In small localized tumors aggressive surgery or transplantation might be useful [2].

Prognosis

Very poor.

**Further
Information**

1. Hepatoblastoma can be entirely composed of malignant epithelial tumor cells.
   The arrangement resembles that observed in a fetal liver mimicking the arrangement of hepatocytes. Others show a papillary formation or a trabecular arrangement.

2. Hepatoblastoma can be entirely composed of mesenchymal malignant tissue:

M-8990/3
T 155.0

   Malignant mesenchymoma [38] **(embryonal sarcoma – WHO).**
   This is a very rare tumor.
   The tumor is multifocal and very large and occurs in infants and children.
   On histological analysis different mesenchymal structures can be observed, including rhabdomyosarcoma areas.

[2] Alpert and Isselbacher 1977.
[7] Bolck and Machnik 1978.
[10] Carter 1969.
[22] Imholz and Noltenius 1977.
[34] Shafer and Selinkoff 1977.
[36] Silverman et al 1975.
[38] Stanley et al. 1973.

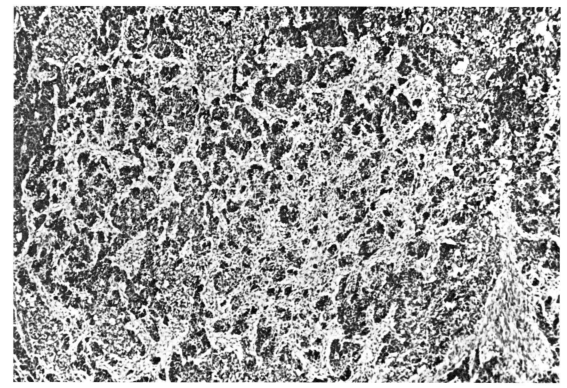

Fig. 364. Hepatoblastoma (2-year-old male, × 60).

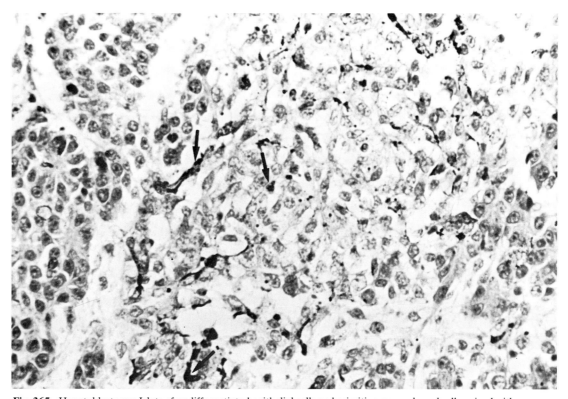

Fig. 365. Hepatoblastoma: Islets of undifferentiated epithelial cells and primitive mesenchymal cells, mixed with melanocytes (arrows) (× 200).

359

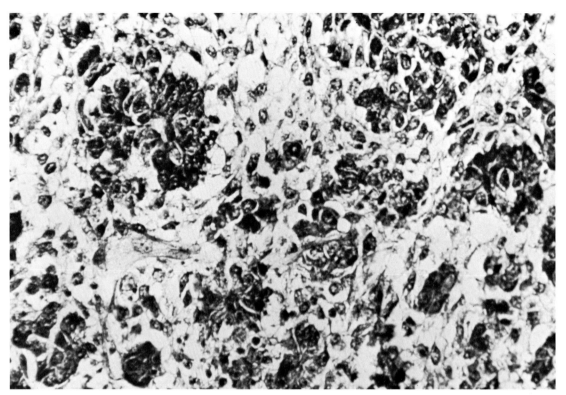

Fig. 366. Hepatoblastoma: Primitive mesenchyma, islets of undifferentiated embryonal epithelial cell nests (× 200).

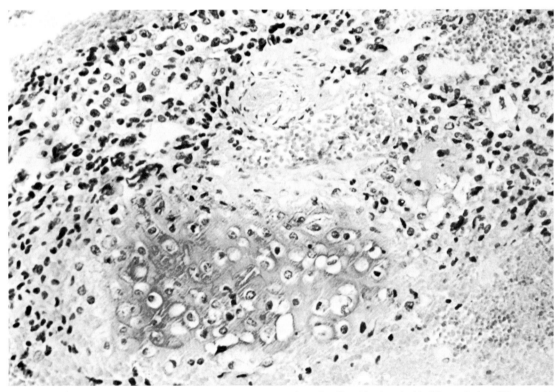

Fig. 367. Hepatoblastoma in adult: Islet of malignant mesenchymal cells with chondroid differentiation (58-year-old female, × 125).

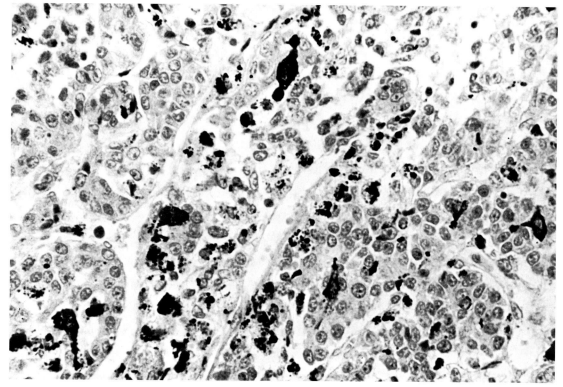

Fig. 368. Hepatoblastoma: Melanocytes (× 200).

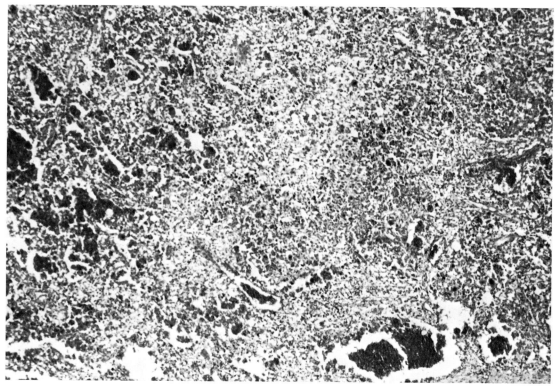

Fig. 369. Hemangiosarcoma of the liver (79-year-old female, × 40).

M-9130/3
T 155.0

4. Hemangiosarcoma (WHO)

**General
Remarks**

Incidence: This is a rare tumor.
Age: Most of the tumors occur in adults; very rarely children have been affected [5, 24].
Sex: Males are more frequently affected than females.
Further notes: A number of angiosarcomas are associated with thorotrast deposits, chronic arsenic intoxication, or exposure to vinylchloride [18, 26].

Macroscopy

Multiple tumors in the liver.
The tumors are red. Cysts and areas of necroses and hemorrhages are observed.

Histology

The tumor contains blood vessels of different sizes with multiple anastomoses. The endothelial cells are malignant: They grow in single or multiple layers, have numerous atypical mitotic figures, and are highly pleomorphic (Figs. 361 to 371).

**Differential
Diagnosis
M-9130/1**

The diagnosis of angiosarcoma usually is not difficult; however, occasionally benign-looking **hemangioendotheliomas** in infants have been shown to be malignant and aggressive [15, 16].

**Clinical
Findings**

The symptoms correspond to those of liver cell carcinoma.

Treatment

Surgical removal of the tumor can be attempted; usually no treatment is possible [29].

Prognosis

Very poor.

**Further
Information
M-9124/3
T 155.0**

As mentioned above, angiosarcomas can be induced by thorotrast. Since these particles are phagocytized by Kupffer's cells, this angiosarcoma can also be considered a **Kupffer cell sarcoma.**

[5] Baggenstoss 1970.
[15] Dehner and Ishak 1971.
[16] Edmondson 1958.
[18] Gokel et al. 1976.
[24] Kauffman and Stout 1961.
[26] Makk et al. 1976.
[29] Nagasue et al. 1976.

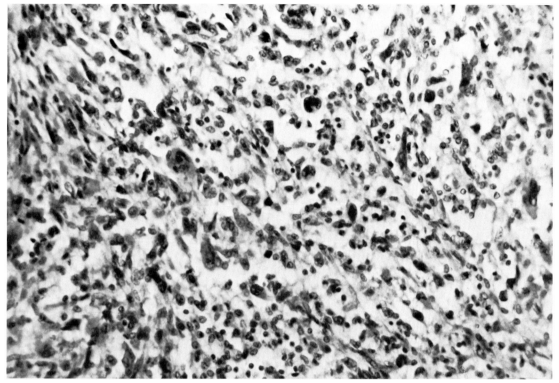

Fig. 370. Hemangiosarcoma of the liver (79-year-old female, × 200).

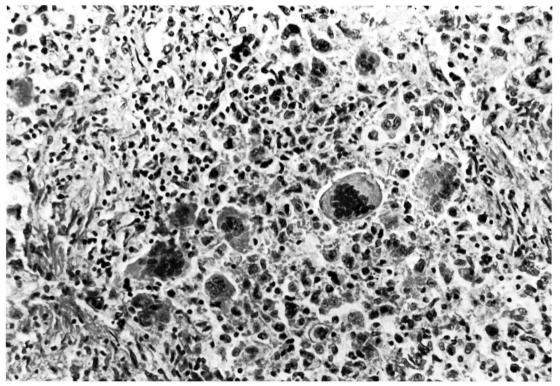

Fig. 371. Hemangiosarcoma of the liver: Numerous giant cells (79-year-old female, × 200).

M-9120/0
T 155.0

5. Hemangioma (WHO)

General
Remarks

Incidence: This is the most frequently observed benign liver tumor.
Age: All ages including infants and children can be affected.

Macroscopy

In most instances this is a solitary tumor.
The tumor is dark red and has a spongy cut surface.

Histology
M-9121/0

The tumor grows as a **cavernous type of hemangioma.**
The blood vessels are lined by regular endothelial cells. Often thrombi develop in these hemangiomas and total or partial sclerosis might occur due to organization of the thrombotic material (Figs. 372 and 373).

Differential
Diagnosis
M-9130/1

Hemangiomas in children **with infantile hemangioendothelioma** (WHO):
This tumor is often associated with angiomas of the skin and other organs [27].
These tumors have numerous endothelial cells lining the blood vessels.
The endothelial cells grow in multiple layers and might have hyperchromatic nuclei.

Clinical
Findings

Hemangiomas are almost always silent.
Occasionally bleeding has been observed.

Treatment

No treatment is required.

---

[27] McLean et al. 1972.

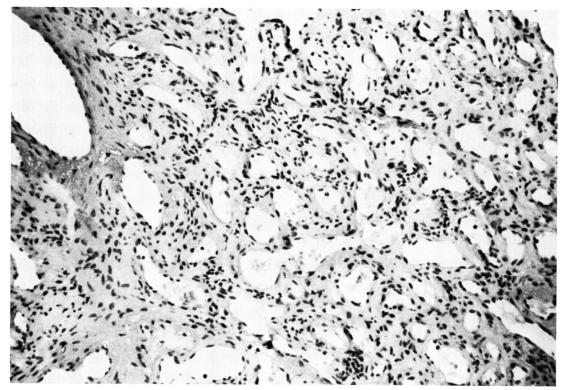

Fig. 372. Cavernous hemangioma of the liver (48-year-old male, × 125).

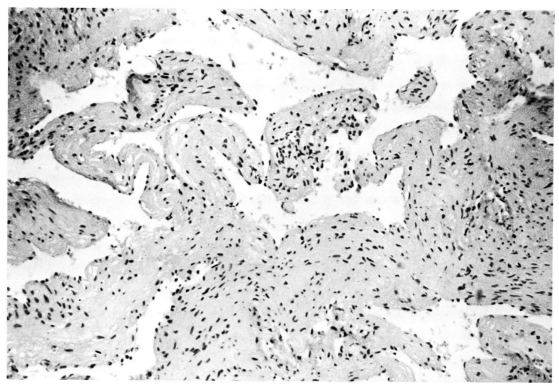

Fig. 373. Cavernous hemangioma of the liver: Regressive changes (48-year-old male, × 125).

365

M-8180/0
T 155.0

6. Intrahepatic bile duct adenoma (WHO)
(cholangioma)

**General
Remarks**

This bile duct adenoma is sometimes considered a hamartoma (**biliary hamartoma** – WHO) (M-9351/0) [9].

Macroscopy

These are solitary or multiple lesions that have a whitish cut surface [11].

Histology

This hamartoma is characterized by abundant connective tissue, in which tubules are embedded.
These tubules are lined by regular epithelial cells (Figs. 374 and 375). The lumen of the tubules does not contain bile pigment.

M-8161/0
T 155.0

7. Intrahepatic bile duct cystadenoma (WHO) [23]

This cystadenoma is not a hamartomatous lesion.
This very rare tumor occurs in middle-aged women.
The tumor contains tubules and cysts. The regular epithelium of the lining produces mucin.
Occasionally the epithelium forms papillary formations, which grow into the lumen.
There is only discrete connective tissue formation.

M-8161/3
T 155.0

8. Bile duct cystadenocarcinoma (WHO)

Very rarely the malignant variety is observed.
Males and females are affected about equally.

---

[9] Cain and Kraus 1977.
[11] Chung 1970.
[23] Ishak et al. 1977.

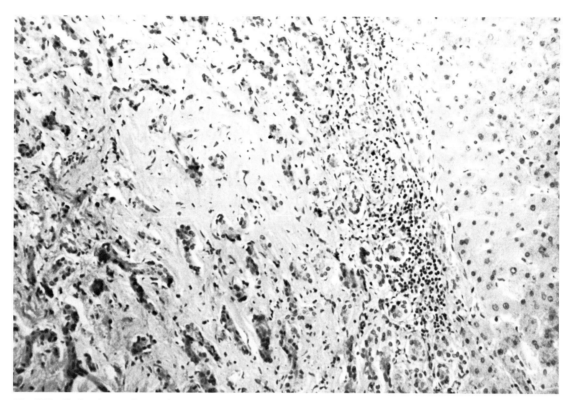

Fig. 374. Cholangioma: Connective tissue with tubular epithelial structures (80-year-old female, incidental finding at autopsy, × 125).

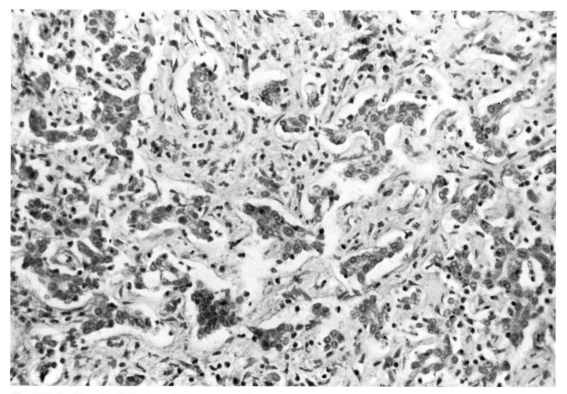

Fig. 375. Proliferating "bile ducts" in liver cirrhosis (× 200).

M-7550/0
T 155.0

9. Benign epithelial hamartoma
(focal nodular hyperplasia – WHO)

Grossly this lesion is a large nodule.
This lesion is occasionally associated with precocious puberty or hypertension [13].

Histology

The tumor contains epithelial cells, which do not form tubules, but mimic a regenerative nodule as observed in liver cirrhosis (Fig. 376).
The portal fields contain proliferating bile ducts.

M-9351/0
(M-7566/0)
T 155.0

10. Mesenchymal hamartoma (WHO)

This is a hamartomatous benign solitary lesion, containing connective tissue, blood vessels, and proliferated bile ducts (Figs. 377 to 381).
This lesion is mainly observed in infants [37].

M-8240/1, 3
T 155.0

11. Carcinoid (WHO)

Primary carcinoids in the liver are exceedingly rare. There is a report of a malignant primary **apudoma** in the liver with hypoglycemia [1].

[1] Ali et al. 1978.
[13] Cox et al. 1975.
[37] Srouji et al. 1978.

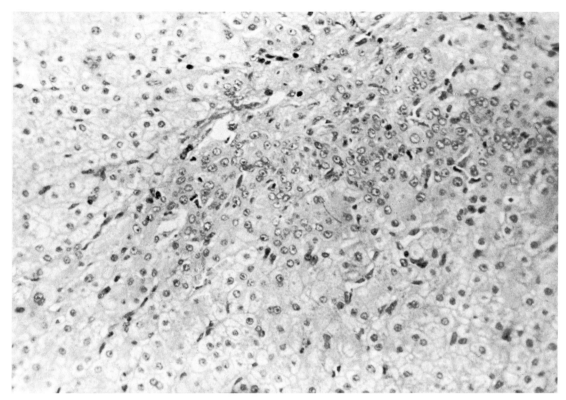

Fig. 376. Benign epithelial hamartoma in an otherwise normal liver (large white nodule, 22-year-old female, × 200).

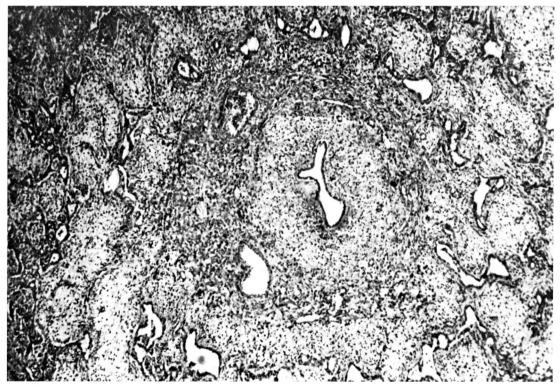

Fig. 377. Benign mesenchymal hamartoma of the liver: Proliferating bile ducts (× 40).

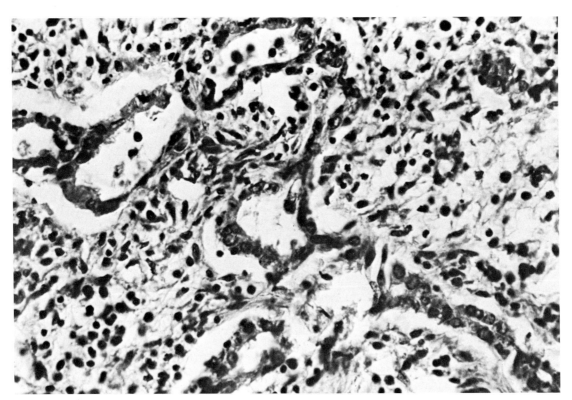

Fig. 378. Benign mesenchymal hamartoma of the liver: Proliferating bile ducts (× 200).

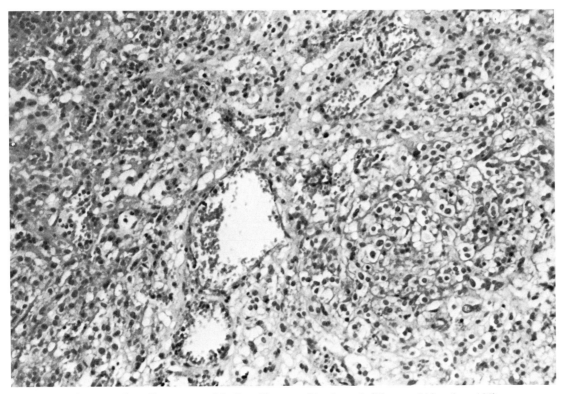

Fig. 379. Benign mesenchymal hamartoma of the liver: Numerous blood vessels (70-year-old female, × 125).

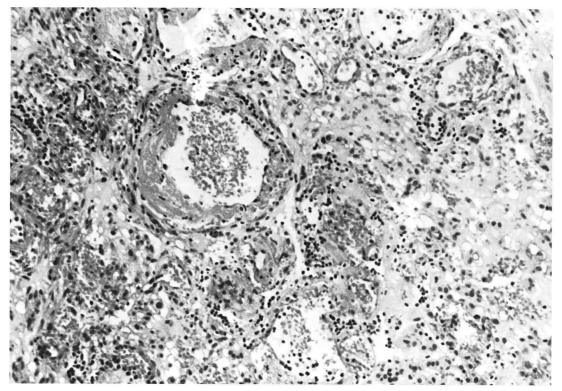

Fig. 380. Benign mesenchymal hamartoma of the liver: Besides connective tissue and some islets of fat tissue, numerous thick-walled blood vessels (70-year-old female, × 125).

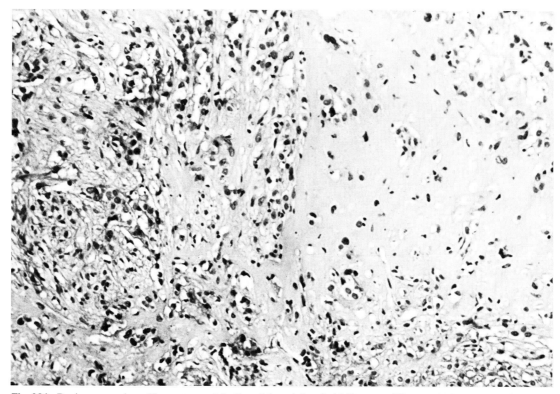

Fig. 381. Benign mesenchymal hamartoma of the liver: Islets of chondroid-like areas (70-year-old female, × 125).

M-8070/3
T 155.0

12. Squamous cell carcinoma originating from hepatic cysts

This epithelial malignant tumor is exceedingly rare [6].

M-9080/0, 3
T 155.0

13. Teratoma (WHO)

These teratomas are very rare; even more rare are malignant teratomas [28].

M-9071/3
T 155.0

14. Yolk sac tumor

One case of a yolk sac tumor in the liver has been reported [20].

T 155.0

15. Soft tissue tumors

These tumors occur rarely in the liver:

M-8850/0   **a) lipoma**

M-8840/0   **b) myxoma**

M-8900/3   **c) rhabdomyosarcoma** [16]

M-8810/3   **d) fibrosarcoma** [3, 35]

M-8890/3   **e) leiomyosarcoma.**

---

[3] Alrenga 1975.
[6] Bloustein and Silverberg 1976.
[16] Edmondson 1958.
[20] Hart 1975.
[28] Misugi and Reiner 1965.
[35] Shallow and Wagner Jr. 1947.

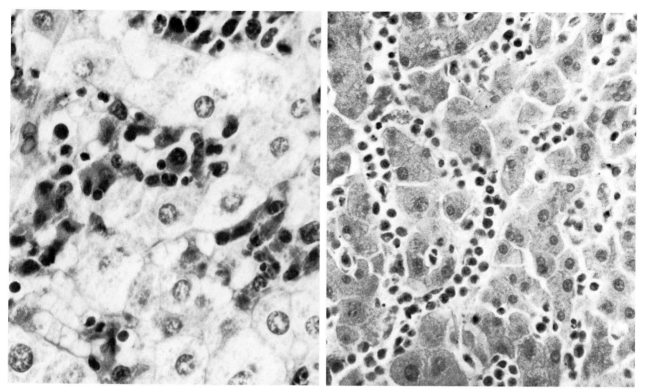

Fig. 382. Chronic myeloid leukemia in the liver (× 600).

Fig. 383. Myelomonocytic leukemia in the liver (× 200).

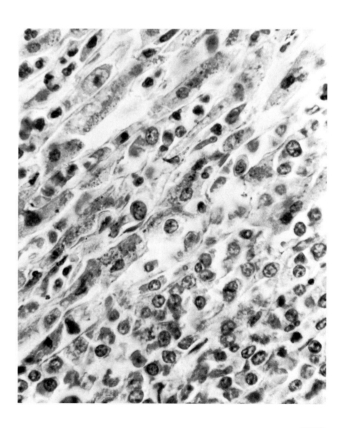

Fig. 384. Blast cells in the liver in the final stage of chronic myelocytic leukemia (66-year-old female, × 310).

M-8000/6
T 155.0

16. Metastatic tumors in the liver

General Remarks

1. The majority of malignant lesions in the liver are metastatic tumors.
2. Metastases are about 20 times as frequent as primary malignant liver tumors.
3. More than 50% of malignant tumors metastasize into the liver.
4. All tumors can grow in the liver.
   Primary tumors with a high frequency of metastatic lesions into the liver are tumors of the large bowel, pancreas, gall bladder, stomach, small intestine, breast, lung, and kidney; malignant lymphoma; leukemia; and Hodgkin's disease.

Macroscopy

Metastases usually elevate the surface in a nodular fashion; they can, however, be hidden in the interior of the liver.

Differential diagnostic problems on gross observation: with hepatic capsule scars; benign hamartomas; benign cysts; abscesses in inflammatory diseases, including tuberculosis; liver cirrhosis with discrete hyperplasia.

Histology

Usually the metastatic lesion can be separated from a primary liver tumor (Figs. 382 to 390).

Clinical Findings

Even intensive metastatic lesions in the liver might cause only very unspecific, discrete, or even no clinical symptoms.

Treatment

The majority of the cases offer no possibility of treatment.
Occasionally solitary metastases might be resected surgically [4].
This is especially valuable in cases of active endocrine tumors like **carcinoids** or metastasizing **insulinomas.**

---

[4] Attiyeh et al. 1978.

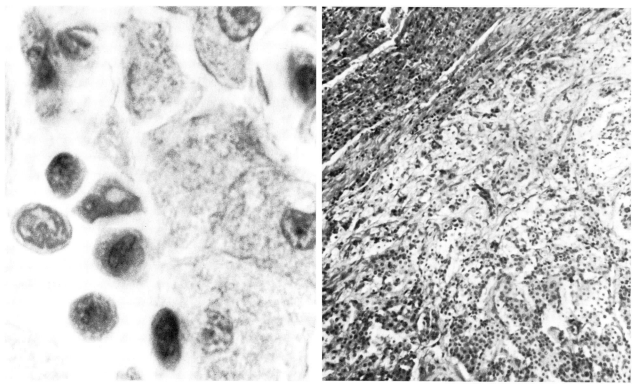

Fig. 385. Cell of a myelomonocytic leukemia in the liver (× 1250).

Fig. 386. Metastasis of islet cell carcinoma in the liver (61-year-old male, × 125).

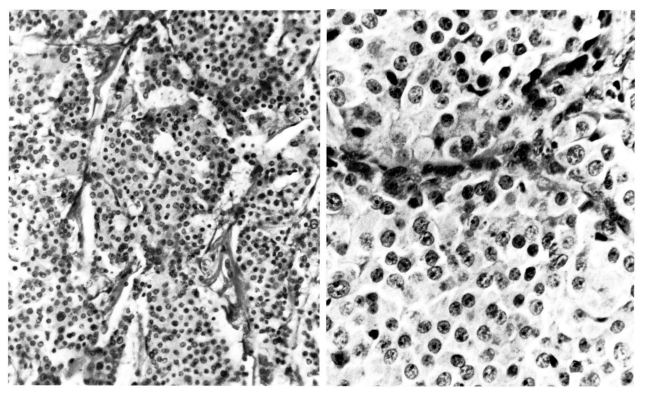

Fig. 387. Metastasis of islet cell carcinoma in the liver (61-year-old male, × 200).

Fig. 388. Metastasis of islet cell carcinoma in the liver (51-year-old female, × 400).

375

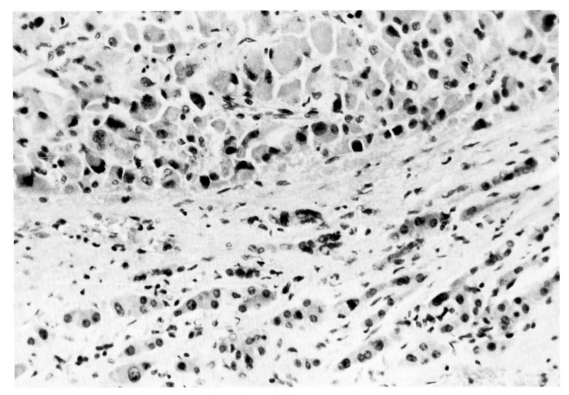

Fig. 389. Metastasis of pheochromocytoma in the liver (× 200).

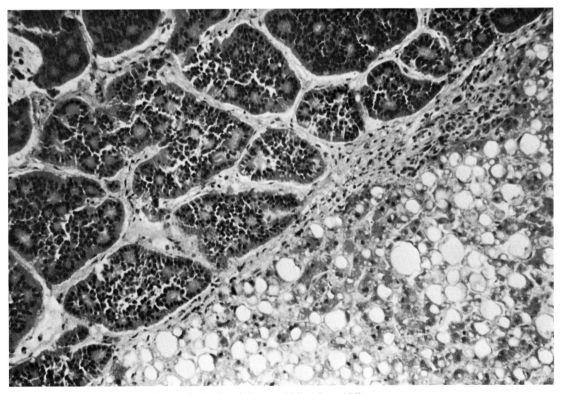

Fig. 390. Metastasis of carcinoid tumor in the liver (77-year-old female, × 125).

Recommendations for differential diagnosis in tumors of the liver

liver cell carcinoma	with	– cholangiocellular carcinoma – metastatic tumors – benign adenoma of the liver (with highly differentiated liver cell carcinoma)
hepatoblastoma	with	– metastatic carcinoma – angiosarcoma of the liver – metastatic sarcoma
cholangiocellular carcinoma	with	– liver cell carcinoma (see also combined tumors) – benign true cystadenoma of the bile duct – hamartomatous lesion of the bile duct (cholangioma)
primary sarcoma	with	– metastatic sarcoma
unspecific inflammation in the liver	with	– beginning leukemic infiltration – dissemination of the malignant lymphoma – dissemination of Hodgkin's disease (multiple sections are often required in liver biopsies)

References

[1] Ali, M., A.O. Fayemi, and E.V. Braun: Malignant apudoma of the liver with symptomatic intractable hypoglycemia. Cancer 42 (1978) 686-692.

[2] Alpert, E., and K.J. Isselbacher: In: Harrison's Principles of internal medicine. Eighth edition, McGrac-Hill Book Company, New York–Düsseldorf etc. 1977.

[3] Alrenga, D.P.: Primary fibrosarcoma of the liver. Case report and review of the literature. Cancer 36 (1975) 446-449.

[4] Attiyeh, F.F., H.J. Wanebo, and M.W. Stearns: Hepatic resection for metastasis from colorectal cancer. Dis. Col. Rect. 21 (1978) 160-162.

[5] Baggenstoss, A.H.: Pathology of tumors of liver in infancy and childhood. In: Pack, G.T., and A.H. Islami (Editors): Tumors of the liver. Vol. 26 of Recent results in cancer research. Springer Heidelberg–Berlin–New York 1970.

[6] Bloustein, P.A., and S.G. Silverberg: Squamous cell carcinoma originating in an hepatic cyst.

Case report with a review of the hepatic cyst-carcinoma association. Cancer 38 (1976) 2002-2005.

[7] Bolck, F., und G. Machnik: Leber und Gallenwege. In: Spezielle pathologische Anatomie. Band X. Hrsg. W. Doerr, G. Seifert, E. Uehlinger. Springer, Berlin–Heidelberg–New York 1978.

[8] Boyd, P.R., and O.J. Mark: Multiple hepatic adenomas and a hepatocellular carcinoma in a man of oral methyl testosterone for eleven years. Cancer 40 (1977) 1765-1770.

[9] Cain, H., und B. Kraus: Entwicklungsstörung der Leber und Leberkarzinom im Säuglings- und Kindesalter. Dtsch. Med. Wschr. 102 (1977) 505-509, 513-514.

[10] Carter, R.: Hepatoblastoma in the adult. Cancer 23 (1969) 191-197.

[11] Chung, E.B.: Multiple bile-duct hamartomas. Cancer 26 (1970) 287-296.

[12] Cochrane, A.M.G., I.M. Murray-Lyon, D.M.

Brinkley, and R. Williams: Quadruple chemotherapy versus radiotherapy in treatment of primary hepatocellular carcinoma. Cancer *40* (1977) 609-614.

[13] Cox, J.N., L. Paunier, M.B. Vallotton, J.R. Humbert, and A. Rohner: Epithelial liver hamartoma, systemic arterial hypertension and renin hypersecretion. Virchows Arch. A Path. Anat. and Histol. *366* (1975) 15-26.

[14] Davis, L. Jr., D.D. von Hoff, M. Rozencweig, H. Handelsman, W.T. Soper, and F.M. Muggia: Gastrointestinal Cancer: Esophagus, stomach, small bowel, colorectum, pancreas, liver, gallbladder, and extrahepatic ducts. In: Randomized trials in cancer: A critical review by sites. M.J. Staquet (Ed.) Raven Press, New York 1978.

[15] Dehner, L.P., and K.G. Ishak: Vascular tumors of the liver in infants and children; a study of 30 cases and review of the literature. Arch. Pathol. *92* (1971) 101-111.

[16] Edmondson, H.A.: Tumors of the liver and intrahepatic bile ducts. Atlas of tumor pathology, A.F.I.P.; Washington, D.C. 1958.

[17] Fisher, R.L., P.J. Scheuer, and S. Sherlock: Primary liver cell carcinoma in the presence or absence of hepatitis B antigen. Cancer *38* (1976) 901-905.

[18] Gokel, J.M., E. Liebezeit, and M. Eder: Hemangiosarcoma and hepatocellular carcinoma of the liver following vinyl chloride exposure. A report of two cases. Virchows Arch. A Path. Anat. and Histol. *372* (1976) 195-203.

[19] Gyorkey, F., K.-W. Min, J. Krisko, and P. Gyorkey: The usefulness of electron microscopy in the diagnosis of human tumours. Hum Pathol. *6* (1975) 421-441.

[20] Hart, W.R.: Primary endodermal sinus (yolk sac) tumor of the liver. First reported case. Cancer *35* (1975) 1453-1458.

[21] Hatzibujas, J., H. Ueberberg, R. Stoldt und H. Breining: Elektronenmikroskopische Befunde eines malignen Hepatoms nach oraler Kontrazeption. Zeitschrift für Gastroenterologie *16* (1978) 616-624.

[22] Imholz, H., und H. Noltenius: Maligner Mischtumor der Leber beim Erwachsenen. Zbl. Allg. Path. *121* (1977) 239-242.

[23] Ishak, K.G., G.W. Willis, S.D. Cummins, and A.A. Bullock: Biliary cystadenoma and cystadenocarcinoma. Report of 14 cases and review of the literature. Cancer *39* (1977) 322-338.

[24] Kauffman, S.L., and A.P. Stout: Malignant hemangioendothelioma in infants and children. Cancer *14* (1961) 1186-1196.

[25] Kay, S.: Nine year follow-up of a case of benign liver cell adenoma related to oral contraceptives. Cancer *40* (1977) 1759-1760.

[26] Makk, L., F. Delmore, J.L. Creech, Jr., L.L. Odgen, E.H. Fadell, C.L. Songster, J. Clanton, M.N. Johnson, and W.M. Christopherson: Clinical and morphologic features of hepatic angiosarcoma in vinyl chloride workers. Cancer *37* (1976) 149-163.

[27] McLean, R.H., J.H. Moller, W.J. Warwick, L. Satran, and R.V. Lucas Jr.: Multinodular hemangiomatosis of the liver in infancy. Pediatrics *49* (1972) 563-573.

[28] Misugi, K., and C.B. Reiner: A malignant true teratoma of liver in childhood. Arch. Pathol. *80* (1965) 409-412.

[29] Nagasue, N., Y. Ogawa, and K. Inokuchi: Hemangiosarcoma of liver and spleen treated with hepatic artery ligation, intraportal infusion chemotherapy and splenectomy. Cancer *38* (1976) 1386-1390.

[30] Nagasue, N., K. Inokuchi, M. Kobayashi, Y. Ogawa, A. Iwaki, and H. Yukaya: Hepatic dearterialization for nonresectable primary and secondary tumors of the liver. Cancer *38* (1976) 2593-2603.

[31] Nayak, N.C., A. Dhar, R. Sachdeva, A. Mittal, H.N. Seth, D. Sudarsanam, B. Reddy, U.L. Wagholikar, and C.R.R.M. Reddy: Association of human hepatocellular carcinoma and cirrhosis with hepatitis B virus surface and core antigens in the liver. Int. J. Cancer *20* (1977) 643-654.

[32] Nilsson, L.A.V.: Therapeutic hepatic artery ligation in patients with secondary liver tumours. Rev. Surg. *23* (1966) 374.

[33] Primack, A., J. Wilson, G.T. O'Connor, K. Engelman, and G.P. Canellos: Hepatocellular carcinoma with the carcinoid syndrome. Cancer *27* (1971) 1182-1189.

[34] Shafer, A.D., and P.M. Selinkoff: Preoperative irradiation and chemotherapy for initially unresectable hepatoblastoma. J. Pediatr. Surg. *12* (1977) 1001-1007.

[35] Shallow, T.A., and F.B. Wagner Jr.: Primary fibrosarcoma of the liver. Ann. Surg. *125* (1947) 439-446.

[36] Silverman, J.F. Y.S. Fu, N.B. McWilliams, and S. Kay: An ultrastructural study of mixed hepatoblastoma with osteoid elements. Cancer *36* (1975) 1436-1443.

[37] Srouji, M.N., J. Chatten, W.M. Schulman, M.M. Ziegler, and C.E. Koop: Mesenchymal hamartoma of the liver in infants. Cancer *42* (1978) 2483-2489.

[38] Stanley, R.J., L.P. Dehner, and A.E. Hesker: Primary malignant mesenchymal tumors (mesenchymoma) of the liver in childhood. An angiographic-pathologic study of three cases. Cancer *32* (1973) 973-984.

10. Tumors of the gallbladder and extrahepatic bile ducts

1. Carcinomas of the gallbladder, often related to chronic cholecystitis, usually do not cause any diagnostic problem for the pathologist. However, this carcinomatous lesion might be very discrete and difficult to differentiate from severe sclerosing inflammation.

2. The differential diagnosis of adenocarcinoma with sclerosing cholangitis must almost always be solved in cases of carcinoma of the extrahepatic bile ducts. One should attempt to solve this problem on frozen sections.

3. Early diagnosis and treatment in carcinoma of the ampulla of Vater are gratifying, since 20% of the patients reach treatment before they have lymph node metastases.
It should be remembered that there is a considerable difference in the cellular buildup between superficial parts of the carcinoma of the ampulla of Vater (highly differentiated) and the deep, infiltrating regions (poorly differentiated).

Tumors of the gallbladder

M-8140/3
T 156.0

1. Adenocarcinoma of the gallbladder (WHO)

General
Remarks

Incidence: About 5% of malignant tumors are adenocarcinomas of the gallbladder. About 0.2 to 5% of removed gallbladders are affected by carcinoma.
Age: The peak age is the 6th to 8th decades.
Sex: Females are considerably more often affected than males (5:1).
Further notes: 80 to 90% of cancers of the gallbladder are associated with gallstones and/ or chronic cholecystitis.

Macroscopy

In most instances the gallbladder wall is thickened by a chronic, recurrent cholecystitis. The carcinoma presents as a soft or firm tumor, which either is ulcerated or presents as a polypoid lesion.
The cut surface is yellowish or whitish (the scar tissue surrounding the carcinoma is grayish).
Often enough the carcinoma is detected only on histological analysis.

Histology

This adenocarcinoma presents with different degrees of differentiation:
The carcinomatous glands can be easily recognized or the tumor cells may form small nests of dispersed cells.
The tumor cells invade the lymphatics. This might be an important differential diagnostic sign, especially since this carcinoma often induces major connective tissue reaction.
According to the different growth patterns, different types of adenocarcinoma may be distinguished.

M-8260/3

a) Papillary adenocarcinoma:
This tumor shows malignant cells in papillary formations, which grow into the lumen of the gallbladder (Figs. 391 to 393).
The papillary growth pattern is also preserved at the infiltrating site of the tumor (Figs. 394 to 396).
This tumor has cells with only discrete signs of malignancy (Fig. 393).

M-8480/3

b) Mucinous adenocarcinoma (WHO):
This tumor contains cells with mucin production (Figs. 397 to 399).
Occasionally this carcinoma can be dominated by signet cells, which do not imitate an organoid growth pattern.

M-8560/3
M-8070/3
M-8570/3
M-8071/3

c) Squamous cell carcinoma (WHO); **adenosquamous carcinoma** (WHO):
Squamous cell carcinoma can show foci of keratinization (Figs. 400 to 402).
Adenosquamous cell carcinoma reveals areas of typical adenocarcinoma in which foci of squamous cell metaplasia have developed (Figs. 403 and 404).

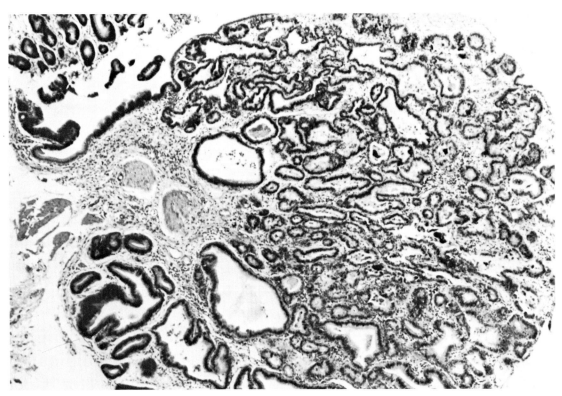

Fig. 391. Papillary adenocarcinoma of the gallbladder, highly differentiated (79-year-old female, × 40).

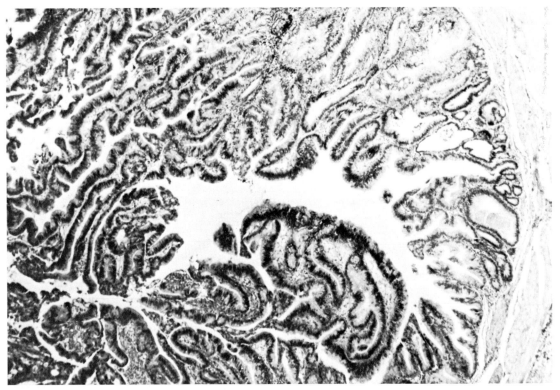

Fig. 392. Highly differentiated papillary adenocarcinoma of the gallbladder: Foci of numerous atypical cells (79-year-old female, × 40).

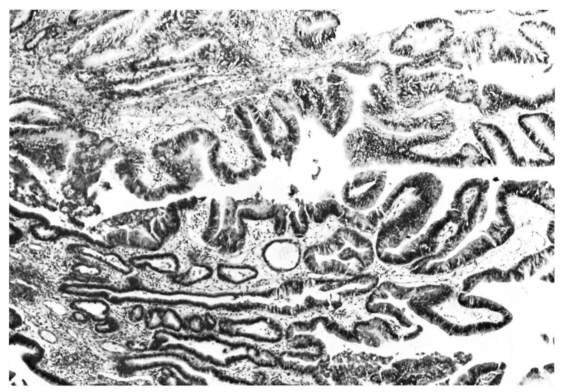

Fig. 393. Highly differentiated papillary adenocarcinoma of the gallbladder (79-year-old female, × 125).

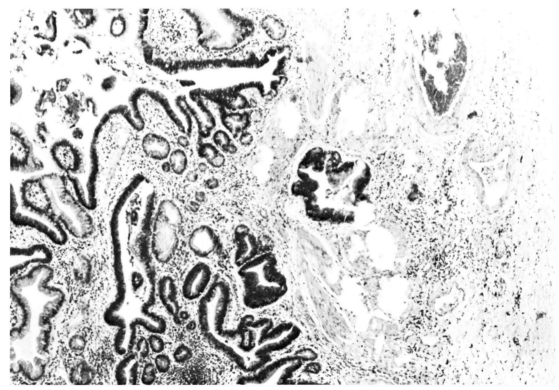

Fig. 394. Highly differentiated papillary adenocarcinoma of the gallbladder: Foci of infiltration (79-year-old female, × 60).

Adenocarcinoma

d) Ulcerating adenocarcinoma:

In this case the tumor can show different degrees of differentiation; poorly differentiated carcinomas are especially represented in this group.

The tumor cells in this case show early infiltration into the lymphatics. There is an intense reaction of the fibrous connective tissue (Figs. 405 and 406).

Differential Diagnosis

1. Papillary adenocarcinoma **with papillary adenoma** (Fig. 412):
   In papilloma there are no cellular atypias and no signs of infiltration into the wall or into the lymphatics.
2. Well-differentiated adenocarcinoma **with glandular diverticulosis** (WHO) (cholecystitis glandularis proliferans) of the gallbladder (Rokitansky-Aschoff sinuses and Luschka's crypts):
   In these cases the glands, usually observed as crypts, form diverticula. These structures are lined by regular epithelium. There is no sign of malignant infiltration (Fig. 407).

M-8140/2
T 156.0

3. Infiltrating adenocarcinoma with **adenocarcinoma in situ** (Fig. 411):
   There are two conditions in which a carcinoma in situ can be observed:
   a) in cases of chronic cholecystitis,
   b) in adenomas of the gallbladder.
   The atypical cells are confined to the mucosa, and there is no sign of infiltration into the wall or into the lymphatics.

Staging

A staging of adenocarcinoma has been attempted [7].

Stage I: The tumor grows in the mucosa.

Stage II: The tumor involves the mucosa and muscularis.

Stage III: All three layers of the wall are infiltrated by the tumor.

Stage IV: The gallbladder wall has been involved, and lymph node metastases are observed.

Stage V: The carcinoma of the gallbladder has extended into the liver and/or distant metastases are present.

Spread

1. Lymph node metastases develop early in the course of the disease.
2. There is an early dissemination into the liver.
3. In the course of the disease tumor dissemination into the peritoneal cavity can develop.
4. Other sites of metastases are lung, bone, kidney, adrenal, ovary, thyroid.

Clinical Findings

There is often a history of gallstone disease and cholecystitis.

Pain in the upper quadrant of the abdomen or in the epigastrium is often reported.

Anorrhexia, loss of weight.

Jaundice is often a terminal symptom.

[7] Nevin et al. 1976.

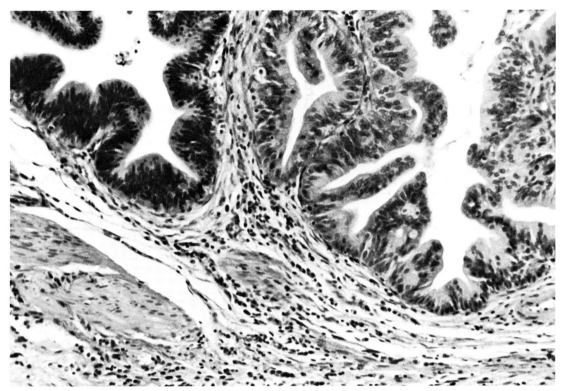

Fig. 395. Highly differentiated papillary adenocarcinoma of the gallbladder: Area of infiltration (detected after multiple sections, 79-year-old female, × 125).

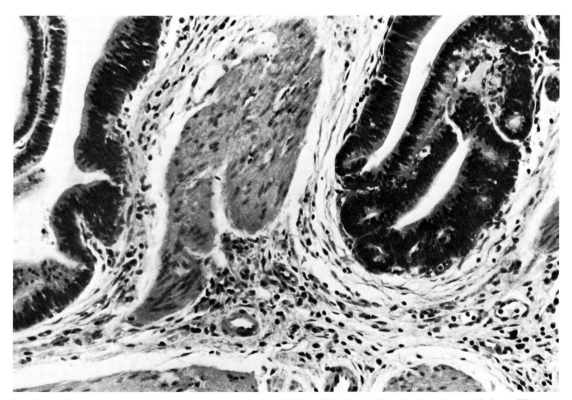

Fig. 396. Highly differentiated papillary adenocarcinoma of the gallbladder: Infiltration into the muscle layer (79-year-old female, × 125).

Adenocarcinoma

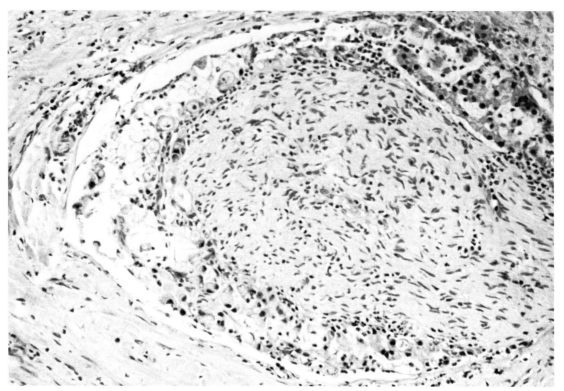

Fig. 397. Mucinous adenocarcinoma of the gallbladder: Tumor cells in perineural spaces (72-year-old female, × 125).

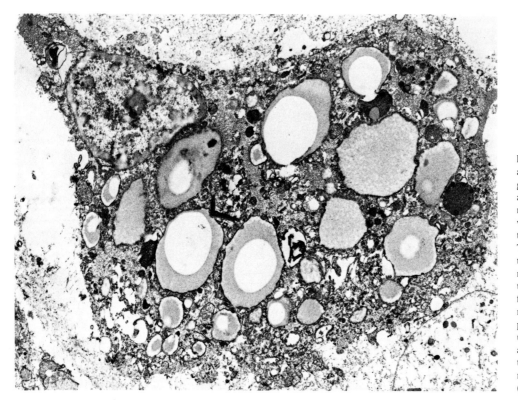

Fig. 398. Tumor cell of an adenocarcinoma of the gallbladder with peripherally located nucleus and numerous intracytoplasmic vacuoles (mucin production) of different sizes. Though the preservation of the tissue has been determined by the formalin-fixation procedure and is therefore not satisfactory for normal electron microscopy, the identification of vacuoles as mucin production and the identification of the tumor cells as adenocarcinoma cells is still possible (× 7000).

Fig. 399. Adenocarcinoma of the gallbladder. Poorly preserved tissue due to formalin fixation; however, vaguely recognizable ciliary rootlet (arrow) and cilium (arrow) at the surface of the tumor cell. This case demonstrates that exceptionally a formalin-prepared tissue can be studied by electron microscopy in order to solve differential diagnostic problems of the origin of an undifferentiated tumor (× 39,000).

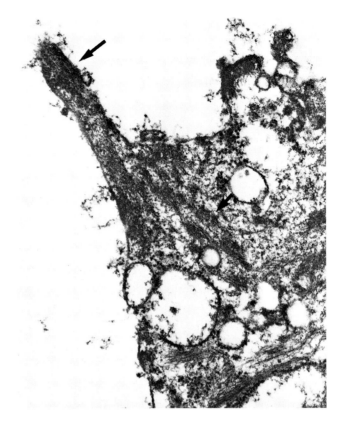

Fig. 400. Squamous cell carcinoma of the gallbladder (72-year-old female, × 40).

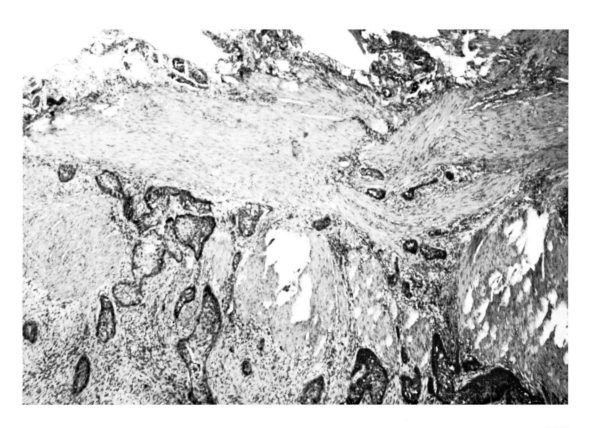

Fig. 400.

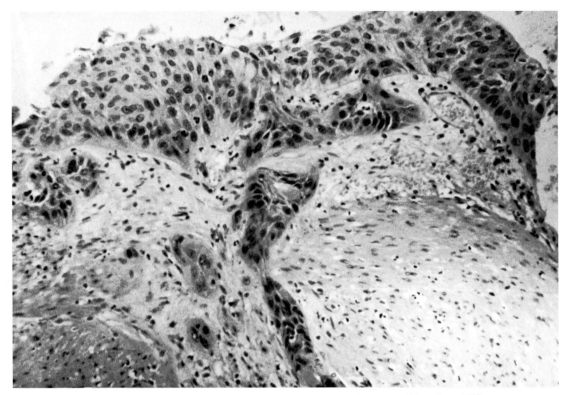

Fig. 401. Squamous cell carcinoma of the gallbladder in chronic cholecystitis (72-year-old female, × 125).

Treatment **Surgery:**
Cholecystectomy, attempted resection of the lymph node metastases [6].

Prognosis 1. Due to early metastases into lymph nodes and liver, the prognosis is very poor:
Overall 5-year survival rate is less than 3%.
2. The prognosis depends on the extent of the disease:
   – Early cancer in Stage I and II can be cured by surgery.
   – Stage III has a 3-year survival rate of 15% and a 4-year survival rate of 4%.
3. A better prognosis is reported for highly differentiated papillary adenocarcinoma [4].

[4] Edmondson 1967.
[6] Lund 1960.

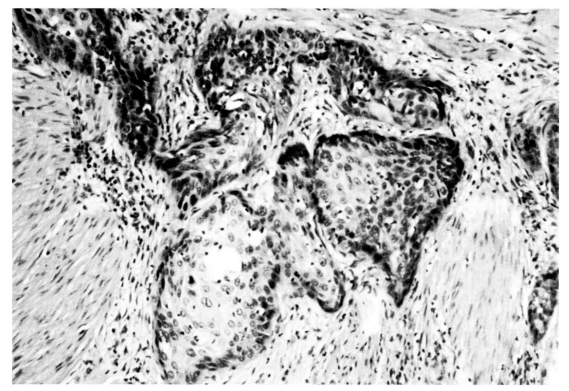

Fig. 402. Squamous cell carcinoma of the gallbladder: Infiltration of the muscle (72-year-old female, × 125).

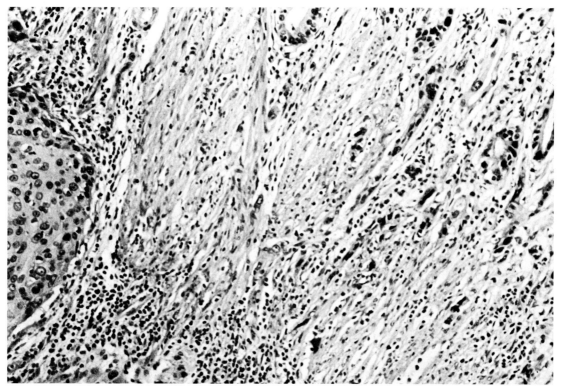

Fig. 403. Poorly differentiated adenocarcinoma of the gallbladder: Squamous cell metaplasia (69-year-old female, × 125).

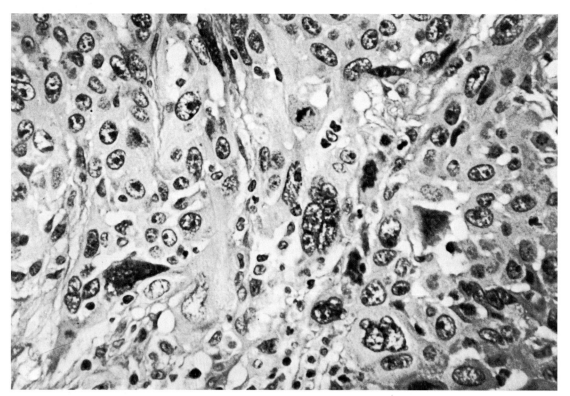

Fig. 404. Adenoacanthoma of the gallbladder: Foci of squamous cells and poorly differentiated adenocarcinoma cells (69-year-old female, × 310).

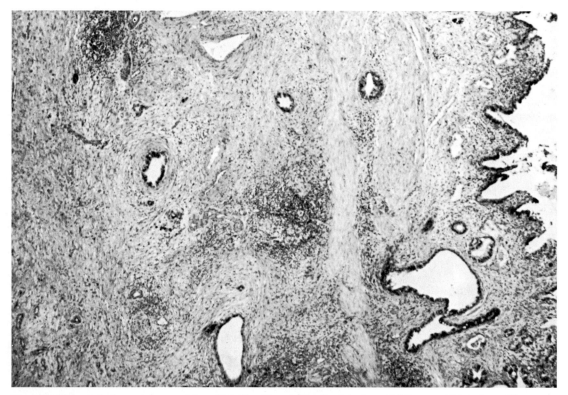

Fig. 405. Ulcerated adenocarcinoma of the gallbladder: Deep infiltration into the wall (66-year-old female, × 40).

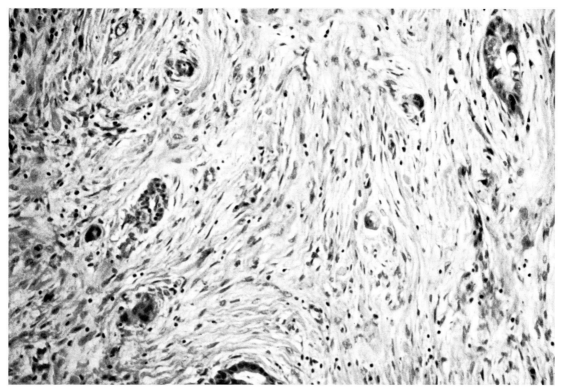

Fig. 406. Infiltrating, poorly differentiated adenocarcinoma of the gallbladder (66-year-old female, × 125).

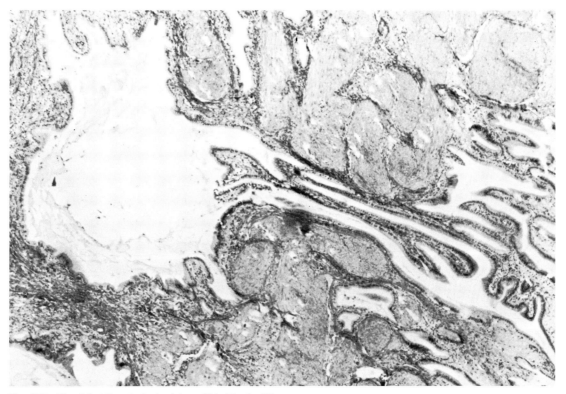

Fig. 407. Glandular diverticulosis of the gallbladder (× 50).

M-8140/0
T 156.0

2. Adenoma of the gallbladder (WHO)
(papillary adenoma)

General Remarks

Incidence: This is a rare tumor.

Macroscopy

The tumor is pedunculated with intraluminal growth or a sessile lesion of the gallbladder wall.
Adenomas of the gallbladder can be solitary or multiple.

Histology

Adenomas are composed of regular epithelial cells, covering a discrete connective tissue tree.
The adenoma may contain areas with a carcinoma in situ.

Differential Diagnosis

Carcinoma in situ in an adenoma **with highly differentiated papillary adenocarcinoma** (Fig. 391).

M-8240/1
T 156.0

3. Carcinoid of the gallbladder (WHO)

This tumor is very rare in the gallbladder [4].

M-8720/3
T 156.0

4. Malignant melanoma (WHO)

This tumor is exceedingly seldom encountered as a primary tumor of the gallbladder [10, 11].

---

[4] Edmondson 1967.
[10] Peison and Rabin 1976.
[11] Sierra-Callejas and Warecka 1976.

M-8800/3

5. Sarcoma (WHO)

M-8980/3

6. Carcinosarcoma (WHO) (Figs. 1361 to 1364)

T 156.0

Sarcomas and carcinosarcomas are very rarely encountered in the gallbladder [4].

7. Soft tissue tumors

Soft tissue tumors of the gallbladder are exceedingly rare (Figs. 408 and 409).

T 156.0

8. Tumor-like lesions of the gallbladder

M-7244/0

a) Adenomyomatous hyperplasia (WHO)
In this case multiple cystic glands are observed in the wall.
Differential diagnosis with highly differentiated, infiltrating adenocarcinoma may be necessary.

M-2600/0

b) Heterotopic gastric or pancreatic tissue (WHO) **in the gallbladder wall**
Usually these lesions are recognized; however, occasionally the differential diagnosis with a carcinoma must be solved.

c) Cholesterol polyp (WHO)
This polyp contains foamy histiocytes growing in the connective tissue. The lesion is covered by a regular epithelial layer.

---

[4] Edmondson 1967.

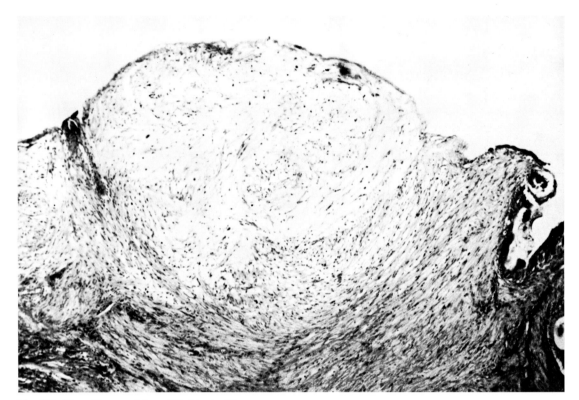

Fig. 408. Neurofibroma of the gallbladder (× 40).

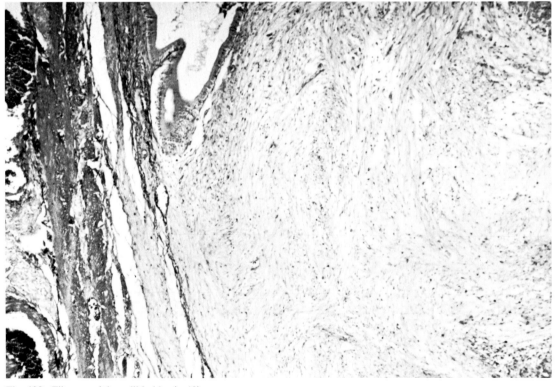

Fig. 409. Fibroma of the gallbladder (× 40).

Tumors of the extrahepatic bile ducts

M-8140/3
T 156.1

9. Adenocarcinoma of the extrahepatic bile ducts (WHO) [2]

General Remarks

Incidence: This carcinoma is rare; about 0.5% of all malignant tumors grow in the extrahepatic bile ducts.
Age: The peak age is the 6th to 7th decade.
Sex: Men are considerably more frequently affected than women.
Site: This carcinoma can appear in any part of the extrahepatic bile ducts.
The most frequently stated location is the common bile duct and the confluence of the extrahepatic bile ducts.

Macroscopy

This tumor presents as a circumscribed firmness in the wall of the extrahepatic bile duct. The wall at this site is thickened. Rarely the tumor grows in papillary formations into the lumen of the bile duct.

Histology

In light microscopy this tumor reveals itself as an adenocarcinoma, which might be well or poorly differentiated.
The tumor cells infiltrate the lymphatics.
The connective tissue reaction is often very marked and clusters the tumor cells.

Differential Diagnosis

1. Adenocarcinoma **with sclerosing cholangitis:**
   On gross and even on histological analysis, the differential diagnosis might be very difficult due to the extent of connective tissue reaction.
   The presence of tumor cells in perineural lymphatics is evidence for malignancy.
2. Well-differentiated papillary adenocarcinoma **with benign intraluminal papillary adenoma** (WHO):
   The papilloma does not show lymphatic invasion (Figs. 410 to 413).

Spread

1. The lymph nodes show relatively early involvement.
   The lymphatic spread reaches the other areas of the extrahepatic bile ducts and the gallbladder.
2. Metastases into the liver.

Clinical Findings

Loss of weight and signs of duct obstruction with jaundice.

Treatment

Surgery:
Surgical removal of the tumor.
In cases of intrahepatic bile duct carcinoma surgical removal should be attempted if the tumor is small [9].

Prognosis

Due to early lymphatic spread, the prognosis is poor.

---

[2] Bolck and Machnik 1978.
[9] Okuda et al. 1977.

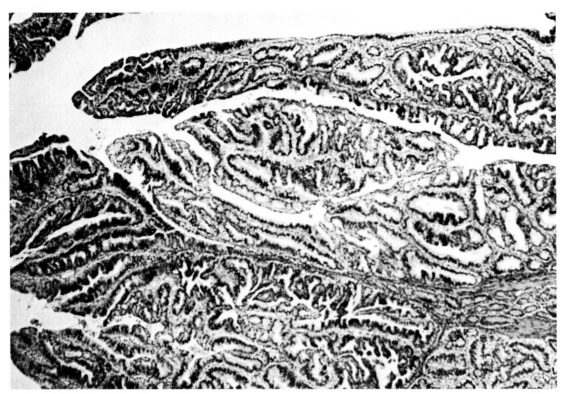

Fig. 410. Highly differentiated papillary intraluminal adenocarcinoma of extrahepatic bile duct (56-year-old male, × 40).

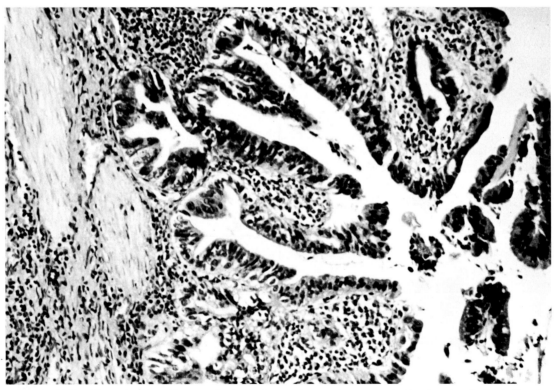

Fig. 411. Highly differentiated papillary intraluminal adenocarcinoma of extrahepatic bile duct: Beginning infiltration and foci of carcinoma in situ (56-year-old male, × 125).

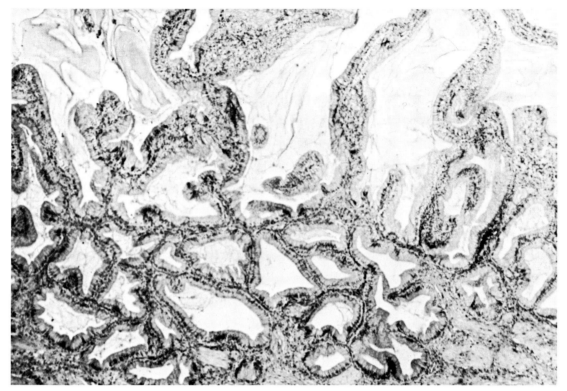

Fig. 412. Intraluminal adenoma of extrahepatic bile duct (× 40).

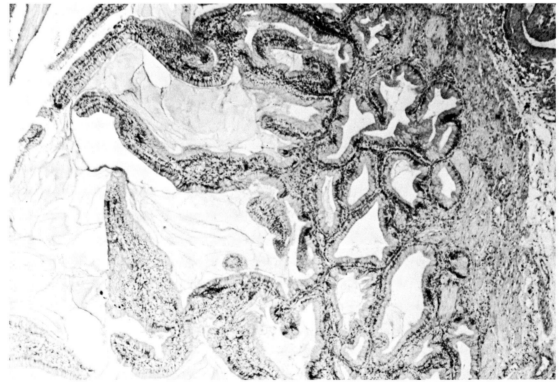

Fig. 413. Intraluminal papillary adenoma of extrahepatic bile duct: No infiltration into the muscle layer (× 40).

M-8140/3
T 156.2

10. Carcinoma of the ampulla of Vater

**General
Remarks**

Incidence: This is a very rare tumor.
Age: The peak age is the 7th decade.
Sex: Men and women are equally affected.
Further notes: This carcinoma can arise from the mucosa of the papilla of Vater, from the mucosa of the duodenum, or from glands of the pancreatic tissue [8].

Macroscopy

In most instances the tumor is a papillary carcinoma with intraluminal growth. The tumor is soft, with extension into the lumen of the duodenum.

Histology

In most instances the tumor is a highly differentiated papillary adenocarcinoma growing into the lumen and into the wall (Figs. 414 to 419).
The superficial part of the tumor is highly differentiated; the infiltrating areas are usually poorly differentiated.
Invasion of the lymphatics may be observed.

**Differential
Diagnosis**

1. Adenocarcinoma **with benign adenoma:**
   The adenoma does not show infiltrating malignant cells. In adenomas there are no cellular atypias.
   It is important to obtain for biopsy a specimen from the infiltrating part of the tumor, since the superficial part of a carcinoma may contain only highly differentiated cells, misleading one into the diagnosis of adenoma.
2. Adenocarcinoma **with chronic sclerosing inflammation of the papilla of Vater** (with obstruction):
   The inflammation of the papilla of Vater is often related to a chronic inflammation of the gallbladder and gallbladder stones, which is not often the case with carcinoma of the ampulla of Vater.
   Evidence of lymphatic infiltration by tumor cells will solve the problem of diagnosis.

Spread

Lymphatic spread into regional lymph nodes occurs.

**Clinical
Findings**

Signs of obstruction and jaundice are early symptoms in the disease due to the location of the tumor in the ampulla of Vater.

Treatment

Surgery:
Surgical radical resection (Whipple's operation).
If necessary, removal of metastatic lymph nodes.

Prognosis

Due to the early symptoms, a number of cases are detected before lymph node metastases develop. In these cases a very good chance for cure exists.
At the time of operation, however, 80% of the cases have associated regional lymph node metastases; the 5-year survival rate is 33% [1].

---

[1] Ackerman and Rosai 1974.
[8] Noltenius 1953.

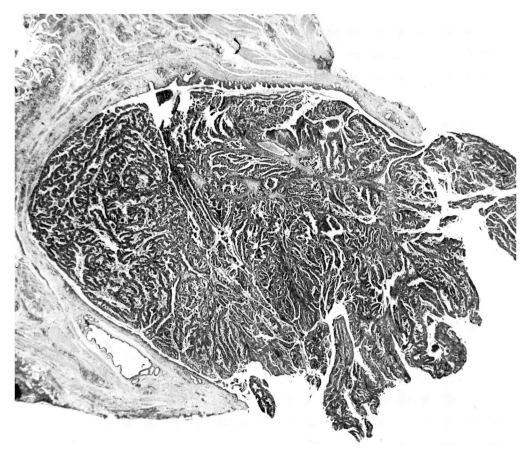

Fig. 414. Papillary carcinoma of the ampulla of Vater with occlusion of the lumen ($\times 30$) [8] (Noltenius, 1953).

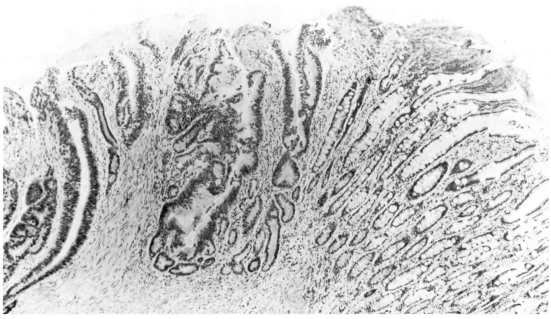

Fig. 415. Adenocarcinoma of the ampulla of Vater: Transition into the normal duodenal mucosa ($\times 40$).

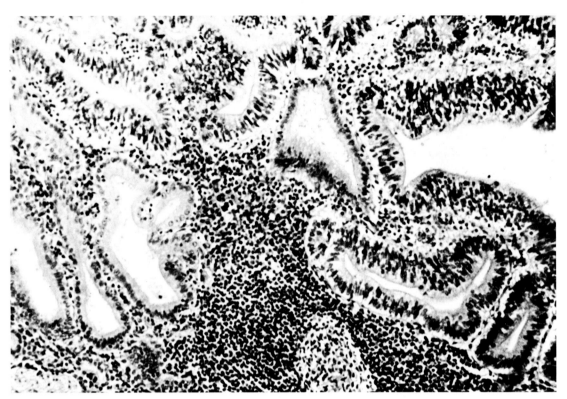

Fig. 416. Adenocarcinoma of the ampulla of Vater: Well-differentiated area in the superficial part of the tumor (56-year-old male, × 125).

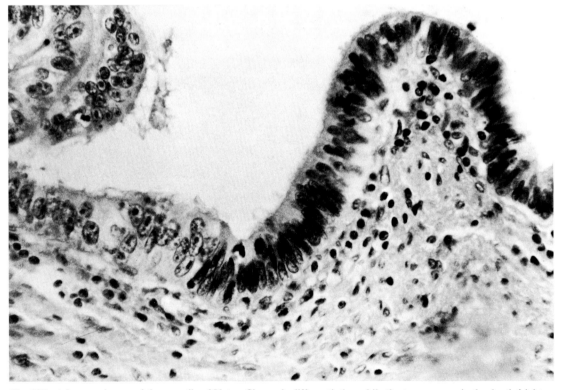

Fig. 417. Adenocarcinoma of the ampulla of Vater: Change in differentiation while the tumor grows in the depth (right = deeper part of the tumor) (× 200).

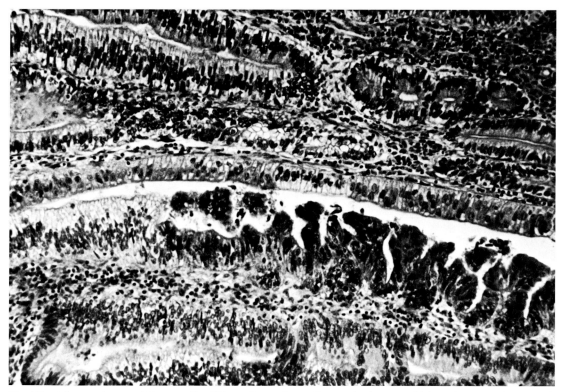

Fig. 418. Adenocarcinoma of the ampulla of Vater: Increasing malignancy in the tumor (right = downward infiltration) (56-year-old male, × 200).

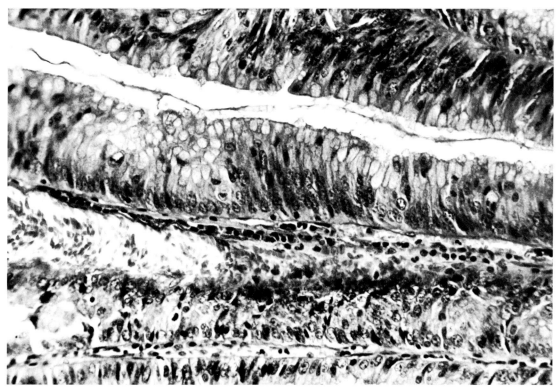

Fig. 419. Adenocarcinoma of the ampulla of Vater: Change of differentiation in the tumor (left = upper part of the tumor) (56-year-old male, × 310).

M-8240/1
T 156.1

11. Carcinoid

Primary carcinoids in the common bile ducts have been observed. They are rare [4].

M-9560/0
M-9571/0
T 156.1

12. Benign neurilemoma, amputation neuroma
(Figs. 180 and 181).

M-8890/0
T 156.1

13. Leiomyoma

Neurilemomas, amputation neuromas, and leiomyomas are rare.

M-8890/3
T 156.1

14. Leiomyosarcoma (Fig. 107)

This malignant soft tissue tumor occurring in the extrahepatic bile ducts is exceedingly rare [4].

---

[4] Edmondson 1967.

M-8910/3
T 156.1

15. Embryonal rhabdomyosarcoma (WHO)
(sarcoma botryoides) (Fig. 120)

This is a very malignant tumor of the extrahepatic bile ducts, which is observed in children [3, 5, 12].

M-9580/0
T 156.1

16. Granular cell tumor (WHO)
(myoblastoma) (Fig. 123)

This tumor is exceedingly rare [13].

[3] Davis et al. 1969.
[5] Isaacson 1978.
[12] Taira et al. 1976.
[13] Whitmore et al. 1969.

Recommendations for differential diagnosis
in tumors of the gallbladder and extrahepatic bile ducts

adenocarcinoma of the gallbladder	with	– chronic sclerosing inflammation – glandular diverticulosis – adenomyomatous hyperplasia – heterotopic tissue (gastric and pancreatic) – papillary adenoma
intraluminal papillary adenoma	with	– highly differentiated papillary adenocarcinoma
adenocarcinoma in situ	with	– infiltrating highly differentiated adenocarcinoma
primary squamous cell carcinoma	with	– metastatic squamous cell carcinoma
adenocarcinoma of the bile ducts	with	– sclerosing cholangitis – papillary adenoma
adenocarcinoma of the papilla of Vater	with	– papillary adenoma of the papilla of Vater

References

[1] Ackerman, L.V., and J. Rosai: Surgical pathology. Fifth edition, C.V. Mosby Company 1974.

[2] Bolck, F., und G. Machnik: Leber und Gallenwege. In: Spezielle pathologische Anatomie. Band X. Hrsg. W. Doerr, G. Seifert, E. Uehlinger. Springer, Berlin–Heidelberg–New York 1978.

[3] Davis, G.L., J.M. Kissane, and K.G. Ishak: Embryonal rhabdomyosarcoma (sarcoma botryoides) of the biliary tree; report of five cases and a review of the literature. Cancer 24 (1969) 333-342.

[4] Edmondson, H.A.: Tumors of the gall bladder and the extrahepatic bile ducts. Atlas of tumor pathology, A.F.I.P., Washington, D.C. 1967.

[5] Isaacson, C.: Embryonal rhabdomyosarcoma of the ampulla of Vater. Cancer 41 (1978) 365-368.

[6] Lund, J.: Surgical indication in cholelithiasis; prophylactic cholecystectomy elucidated on the basis of long-term follow-up on 526 nonoperated cases. Annals of Surgery 151 (1960) 153-162.

[7] Nevin, J.E., T.J. Moran, S. Kay, and R. King: Carcinoma of the gallbladder. Staging, treatment, and prognosis. Cancer 37 (1976) 141-148.

[8] Noltenius, H.: Ampoulome vatérien. Mémoire de la Faculté de Médecine de Paris (sponsored by Jacque de la Rue). 1953.

[9] Okuda, K., Y. Kubo, N. Okazaki, T. Arishima, M. Hashimoto, S. Jinnouchi, Y. Sawa, Y. Shimokawa, Y. Nakajima, T Noguchi, M. Nakano, M. Kojiro, and T. Nakashima: Clinical aspects of intrahepatic bile duct carcinoma including hilar carcinoma. A study of 57 autopsy-proven cases. Cancer 39 (1977) 232-246.

[10] Peison, B., and L. Rabin: Malignant melanoma of the gallbladder. Report of three cases and review of the literature. Cancer 37 (1976) 2448-2454.

[11] Sierra-Callejas, J.L., and K. Warecka: Primary malignant melanoma of the gallbladder. Virchows Arch. A Path. Anat. and Histol. 370 (1976) 233-238.

[12] Taira, Y., I. Nakayama, A. Moriuchi, O. Takahara, T. Ito, R. Tsuchiya, and T. Hirano et al.: Sarcoma botryoides arising from the biliary tract of children. A case report and review of the literature. Acta Path. Jap. 26 (1976) 709-718.

[13] Whitmore, J.T., J.P. Whitley, P. LaVerde, and J.J. Cerda: Granular cell myoblastoma of the common bile duct. Am. J. Dig. Dis. 14 (1969) 516-520.

11 Tumors of the pancreas

1. The malignant tumors of the exocrine tissue of the pancreas still have a very poor prognosis due to early metastases and often late symptoms. The signs of jaundice often occur late in the course of the disease, even with tumors located in the head of the pancreas.

   The incidence of these tumors is increasing.

2. The islet cell tumors are an example of how subclassification can be made by the use of ultrastructural methods and the application of immunochemistry and histochemistry.

   Besides surgery for treatment of these tumors, chemotherapy has an excellent field of action.

M-8140/3
T 157.9

1. Adenocarcinoma (WHO)

General
Remarks

Incidence: The incidence of this carcinoma has been increasing for the past several decades.

About 5% of malignant tumors are carcinomas of the pancreas.

Age: The peak age is the 7th and 8th decades.

This tumor is very rare in younger patients (under 40 years).

Sex: Men are more often affected than women (2:1).

157.0

Site: The majority of these carcinomas grow in the head (70 to 80%).

However, any other part of the pancreas can be affected.

Further notes: There is a particularly high incidence of this carcinoma in black patients.

Macroscopy

On palpation this tumor is ill-defined. The firm lesion has a yellowish to grayish cut surface, which occasionally shows discrete cysts. The pancreatic ducts proximal to the tumor are often dilated and the surrounding pancreatic tissue is reduced and hard because of the obstruction of the ducts.

On gross inspection, the differential diagnosis with chronic pancreatitis might be very difficult.

Histology

This tumor arises from epithelial cells of the acini or the ducts (Fig. 420). These tumor cells show different degrees of differentiation:

Poorly differentiated carcinomas (undifferentiated carcinoma – WHO) are composed of small nests and strands of highly atypical cells (Figs. 421 to 423), which can even show a sarcomatous arrangement [1, 32].

The tumor cells might be transformed into giant cells. Foci of squamous cell metaplasia can occur in areas with a discrete acinar or tubular pattern.

The tumor cells are surrounded by numerous collagen fibers.

The lymphatics are invaded by tumor cells in almost all cases [21] (Figs. 424 and 425).

Differential
Diagnosis

Adenocarcinoma **with sclerosing chronic pancreatitis** (WHO) (Figs. 426 and 427):

The carcinoma contains signs of malignant nuclear atypias.

The diagnosis is decided when invasion of lymphatics is evident.

The diagnosis of carcinoma might be difficult in frozen sections; caution should prevail. The mortality rate of surgical treatment in cases of carcinoma of the pancreas is 20 to 30%.

Spread

1. The tumor extends early into the surrounding tissue and the retroperitoneum.
2. There is early infiltration of the lymphatics with dissemination into the regional lymph nodes, the stomach, the duodenum, and the common bile duct.
3. Early metastases develop in the adrenal, liver, kidney, lung, bone marrow, and skin.

[1] Alguacil-Garcia and Weiland 1977.
[21] Kozuka et al. 1979.
[32] Tschang et al. 1977.

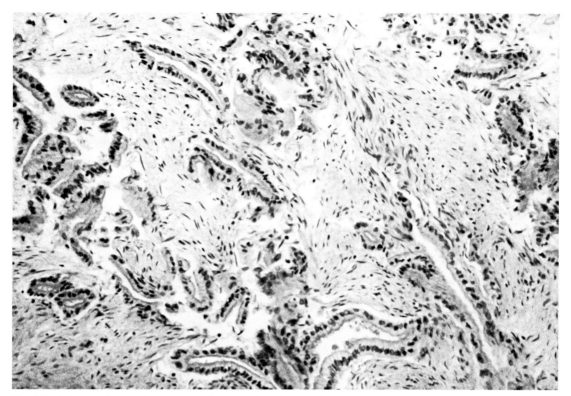

Fig. 420. Adenocarcinoma of the pancreas (78-year-old male, × 125).

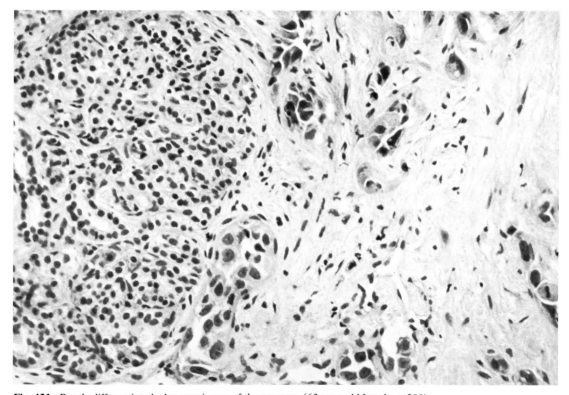

Fig. 421. Poorly differentiated adenocarcinoma of the pancreas (63-year-old female, × 200).

Adenocarcinoma

Clinical Findings

– Loss of weight, anorexia, nausea, obstipation, often severe abdominal pain, signs of psychological alterations (severe mental depression is rather often observed).
– Signs of obstruction with jaundice are observed when the tumor grows in the head of the pancreas, but often jaundice is a late or terminal symptom.
  For cancer in the tail or in the middle of the pancreas, these helpful obstructive signs are lacking.
– The CEA level in the serum might be elevated.
– Only 10% show abnormal serum amylase and lipase activities.

Treatment

Surgery:
Surgery is the primary approach of treatment.
– About 8 to 20% of the patients are eligible for duodenopancreatectomy (Whipple's technique) [18].
– A second-look operation is worthwhile [22].

Radiation therapy:
Radiation therapy seems to be ineffective. There is no indication that irradiation of up to 60 Gy adds to the patient's survival [10].
In cases of unresectable pancreatic adenocarcinoma, high dose, small volume irradiation might improve the palliation effect [12].
Postoperative irradiation has been recommended to reduce the frequency of local recurrences [31].

Chemotherapy:
This therapeutic possibility does not seem to have any value for patients with pancreatic carcinoma [27].
However, there is a report that single agent chemotherapy (adriamycin) gave a partial response in the treatment of an advanced pancreatic carcinoma [28].

Combination three-modality therapy:
Combination three-modality therapy with surgery, radiation therapy, and chemotherapy may be attempted [5].

Prognosis

The prognosis is poor:
– At the time of operation about 90% of the patients have lymph node metastases at the parapancreaticoduodenal area, at the superior head and the superior body of the pancreas [8].
– About 10 to 20% of the patients are operated upon at the time of diagnosis, less than 10% with curative intentions.
– The postoperative mortality rate is about 20 to 30% [13].

Further Information

1. There is one report of an adenocarcinoma of the pancreas associated with Zollinger-Ellison syndrome [26].
2. Adenocarcinomas of the pancreas very rarely occur in childhood [30].

[5] Carter and Comis 1975.
[8] Cubilla et al. 1978.
[10] Davis Jr. et al. 1978.
[12] Dobelbower Jr. et al. 1978.
[13] Dold and Sack 1976.
[18] Ihse et al. 1977.
[22] Kümmerle et al. 1976.
[26] Mihas et al. 1978.
[27] Moertel et al. 1977.
[28] Schein et al. 1978.
[30] Taxy 1976.
[31] Tepper et al. 1976.

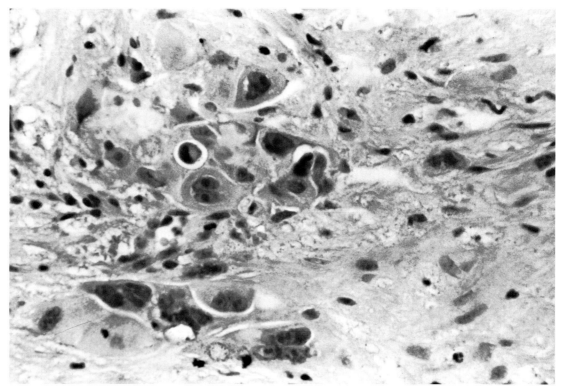

Fig. 422. Poorly differentiated adenocarcinoma of the pancreas (63-year-old male, × 310).

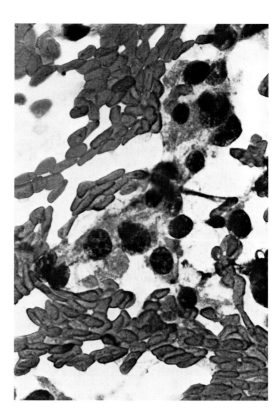

Fig. 423. Adenocarcinoma of the pancreas, poorly differentiated: Tumor cells with enlarged hyperchromatic nuclei, irregularly formed, coarse chromatin pattern, prominent nucleoli (needle biopsy, alcohol fixation, HE stain, × 630).

411

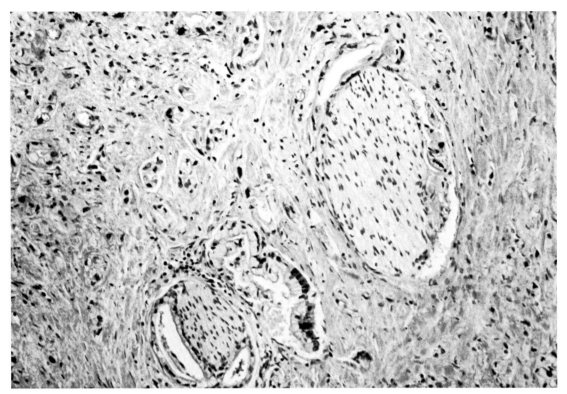

Fig. 424. Adenocarcinoma of the pancreas: Invasion of perineural spaces (× 125).

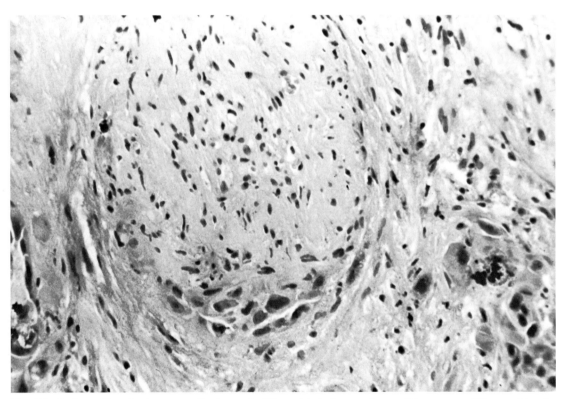

Fig. 425. Perineural invasion by tumor cells of a poorly differentiated adenocarcinoma of the pancreas (63-year-old male, × 200).

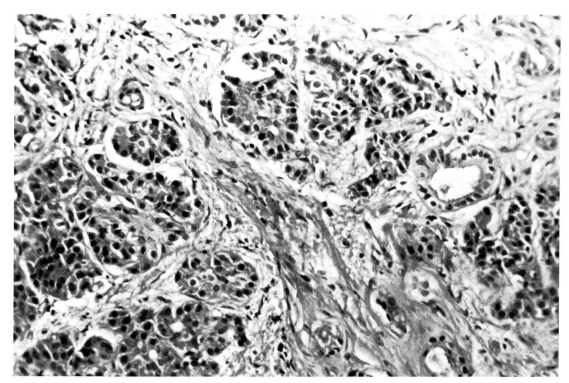

Fig. 426. Chronic pancreatitis (54-year-old male, × 200).

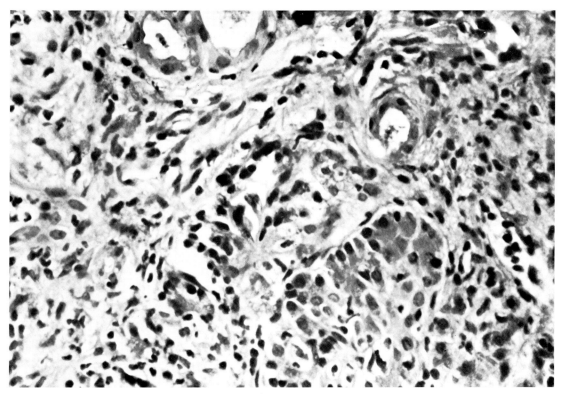

Fig. 427. Chronic pancreatitis (54-year-old male, × 200).

413

M-8440/0
T 157.9

2. Cystadenoma (WHO)

General
Remarks

Incidence: This benign tumor is rare.
Age: All ages can be affected.
Sex: This tumor is more frequently observed in women than in men.

T 157.1
T 157.2

Site: The tumor grows in the body and the tail of the pancreas and less frequently in the head.

Macroscopy

The tumor is lobulated and large (diameter, 2 to 20 cm).
The cut surface of this firm tumor contains cysts of different sizes. The cysts are filled with mucinous-gelatinous material and occasionally with clear yellowish fluid.

Histology

The tumor is composed of cysts. These cysts are lined by a monolayer of columnar epithelial cells. Occasionally these cells are cuboidal or flattened (Figs. 428 and 429).

M-8504/0
T 157.9

In some instances the lining cells form a papillary growth pattern in an intraluminal position (**papillary cystadenoma** – WHO), occasionally without cyst formation (**adenoma; papillary adenoma** – WHO).

Differential
Diagnosis
M-8504/3
T 157.9

Benign cystadenoma **with cystadenocarcinoma** (WHO) [3]:
This malignant variety is very rare. The malignancy is revealed by cytological abnormalities.

Clinical
Findings

1. The tumor can be accompanied by diabetes due to the destruction of the islet cells in the tail of the pancreas.
2. If the tumor grows in the head of the pancreas, signs of obstruction with jaundice develop.

Treatment

Surgery:
Surgical removal of the tumor should be attempted.

Prognosis

Good.

Further
Information

1. The origin of this cystadenoma is most probably the epithelial cells of pancreatic ducts [14, 16].

M-8550/0
T 157.9

2. Exceedingly rare are **adenomas of the acini.** They are without clinical significance (Figs. 430 and 431) [14].
   Equally rare are **acinar cell carcinomas** (WHO).

M-8070/3
T 157.9

3. **Squamous cell carcinoma** (WHO) rarely occurs in the pancreas.

---

[3] Becker 1973.
[14] Frantz 1959 (further references).
[16] Glenner and Mallory 1956.

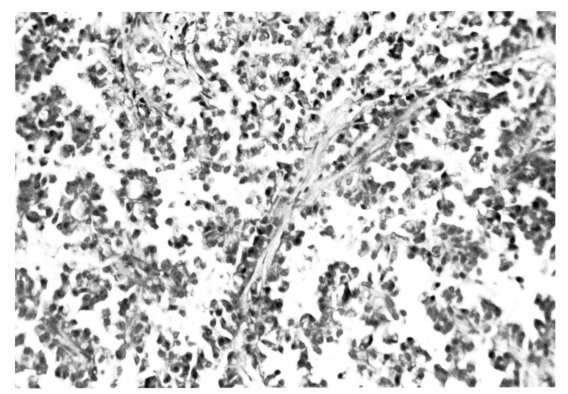

Fig. 428. Papillary cystadenoma of the pancreas (59-year-old male, × 200).

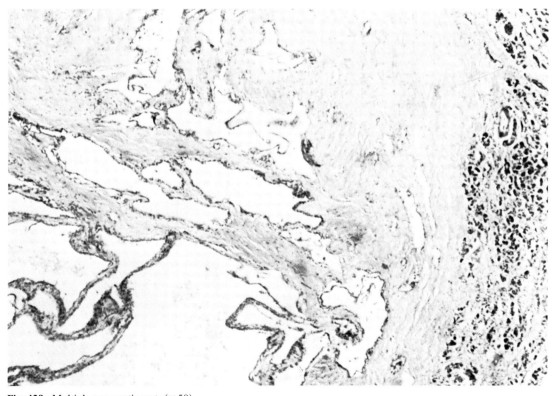

Fig. 429. Multiple pancreatic cysts (× 50).

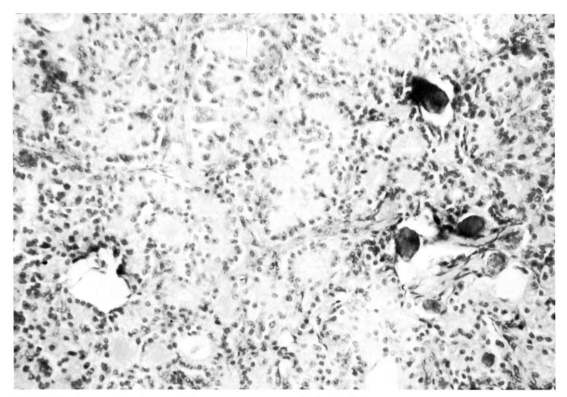

Fig. 430. Benign exocrine adenoma of the pancreas, psammoma bodies (× 125).

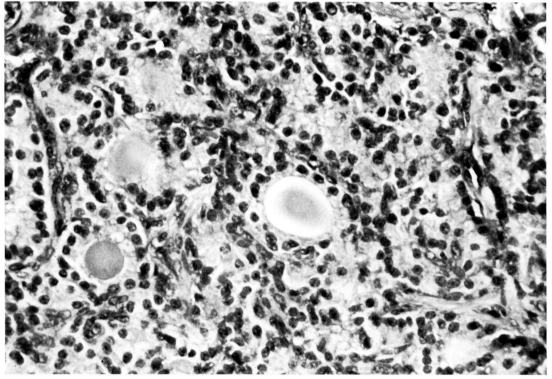

Fig. 431. Benign exocrine adenoma of the pancreas (× 200).

M-8150/0
M-8150/3
T 157.9

3. Islet cell tumors, benign and malignant
(islet cell adenoma, islet cell carcinoma)

**General
Remarks**

Incidence: Islet cell tumors are rare lesions.
Age: Any age can be affected. The 4th to 7th decades are the peak ages.
Sex: Males and females are equally affected.
Site: Islet cell tumors can grow in any part of the pancreas; however, the main sites are the tail and the body.
Further notes:
90% of islet cell tumors are solitary, 10% are multiple.
– The multiple islet cell tumors are rarely malignant.
– Of the functioning islet cell tumors 2% grow outside the pancreas (duodenum, stomach) [6, 11].
– About 60% of the gastrinomas are malignant [6].
– 90% of the functioning islet cell tumors are benign, 10% are malignant.

Macroscopy

Islet cell tumors are often small: diameter, 0.1 to 3 cm. Therefore, this lesion occasionally can be detected only by histological analysis.
On palpation the tumors are slightly firmer than the surrounding pancreatic tissue. The cut surface is reddish.
For the surgeon it is often difficult to find small islet cell adenomas.

Histology

The islet cells in this tumor grow in different patterns: Tubular formations, ribbon pattern, or solid complexes (Figs. 432 to 435).
The nuclei of the cells may be regular; however, hyperchromatic nuclei with atypias and mitotic figures are common (Figs. 435 to 437).
The tumor is very vascular (the tumor can be detected by angiography).

**Electron
Microscopy**

Different cells can be the origin of islet cell tumors. To some degree the different cells can be recognized by the size, shape, and density of the secretory granules.

M-8151/0, 3
T 157.9

a) **Beta cells:**
The granules are of different degrees of density, occasionally granular, occasionally containing crystaloid material. The size of these granules is uniform.
The granules are often concentrated at the Golgi area.
Often the granules are surrounded by a single membrane.
A dense core leaves a clear space underneath the membrane.
Amyloid-like microfilaments can occasionally be observed in fibroblast-like cells in this beta-cell insulinoma [25].
Amyloid-like stroma can also be recognized occasionally on light microscopy.

[6] Creutzfeldt et al. 1975.
[11] DeLellis et al. 1976.
[25] Le Charpentier et al. 1974.

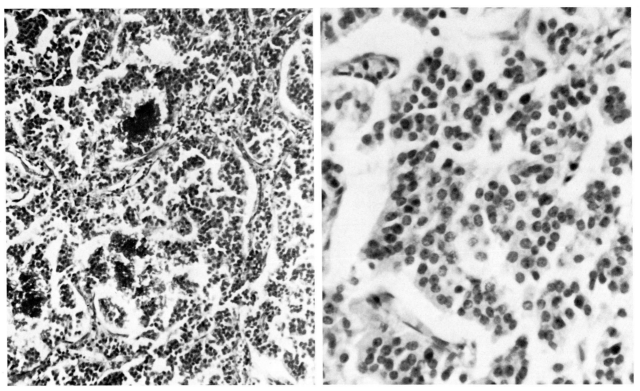

Fig. 432. Islet cell tumor (with metastases) of the pancreas (×125).   **Fig. 433.** Metastasizing islet cell carcinoma of the pancreas (×310).

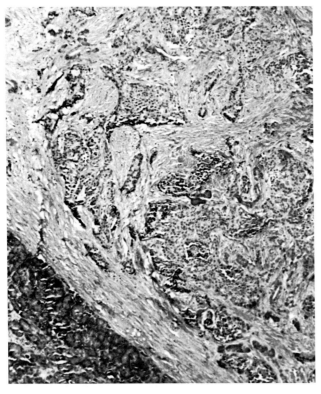

Fig. 434. Nests of an islet cell carcinoma of the pancreas (×60).

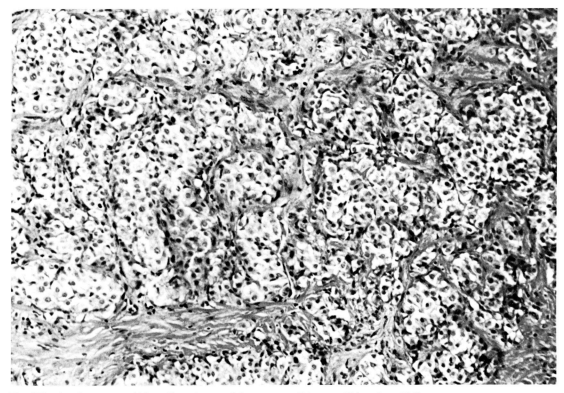

Fig. 435. Another aspect of islet cell carcinoma of the pancreas (51-year-old female, × 125).

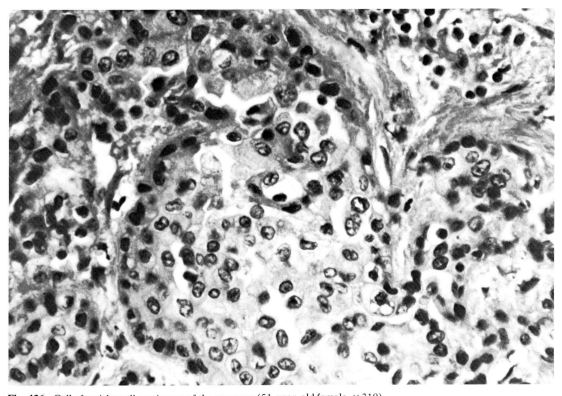

Fig. 436. Cell of an islet cell carcinoma of the pancreas (51-year-old female, × 310).

419

Islet cell tumors

M-8152/0, 3
T 157.9

b) **Alpha cells:**

These cells have granules with a dense content [4].

M-8153/1, 3
T 157.9

c) **Gastrinoma cells:**

Some of the cells do not contain granules; in other cells granules of different density (as in antral G cells, growing as gastrinomas in the antropyloric mucosa) are observed [24].

In some instances gastrinoma cells contain atypical granules and typical G-cell granules (Fig. 438) [6].

Histochemistry

There are some specific staining reactions for the different cells of origin of islet cell tumors:

– Aldehyde-theonin stain for beta cells – islet cell tumors.
– Davenport silver impregnation stains A_1-glucagon-alpha-cell tumor (or D cells).
– Grimelius silver technique impregnates islet A (or A_2) cells in antral G cells (gastrinomas).

Immunohisto-chemistry

These methods reveal by peroxidase-labeled antibodies against insulin or gastrin the product that is produced by the tumor. This is the most reliable technique for the diagnosis of gastrinomas [33].

Differential Diagnosis

1. Benign islet cell tumor **with malignant islet cell tumor:**
   – The cytological picture of the tumor cells does not indicate the benign or malignant biological behavior.
   – The malignancy of the tumor can be supposed by infiltration of the connective tissue; evidence is the invasion of veins and, of course, the appearance of metastases.
2. Islet cell tumor **with adenocarcinoma:**
   Occasionally the islet cell tumor can mimic glandular formations of an adenocarcinoma. Histochemical reactions will solve the problem of diagnosis.

Spread

1. Malignant islet cell tumors invade the lymphatics and spread into the lymph nodes.
2. The hematogenous spread goes into the liver.

Clinical Findings

The clinical symptoms are essentially determined by the hormone that is produced by the islet cell tumor:

M-8151/0, 3

a) **Beta-cell tumor:**

This is an insulin-producing tumor:

– fasting hypoglycemia (appearing especially in the morning hours),
– hypoglycemia after physical exercise,
– diffuse neurological and psychiatric symptoms,
– amelioration of the symptoms by the intravenous administration of glucose,
– due to prolonged episodes of hypoglycemia, convulsions may occur, the intellectual abilities can diminish, and the personality can change.

---

[4] Bretholz et Steiner 1973.
[6] Creutzfeldt et al. 1975.
[24] Larsson et al. 1973.
[33] Woodtli and Hedinger 1976.

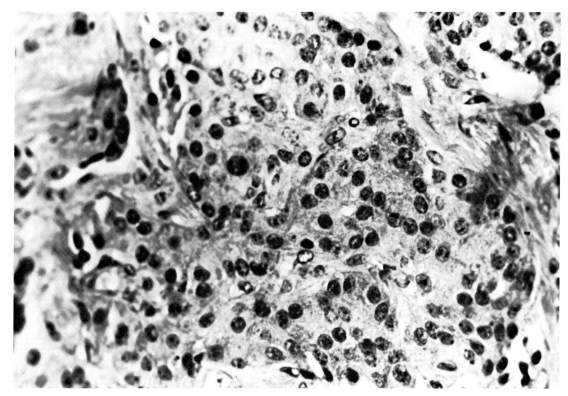

Fig. 437. Another variety of islet cell carcinoma of the pancreas (×310).

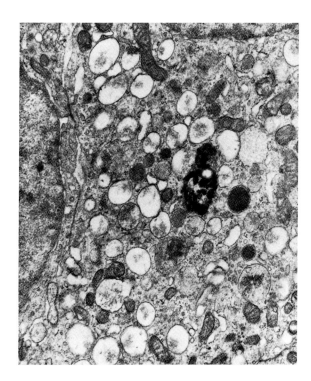

Fig. 438. Gastrinoma of the pancreas: Antral G cells with secretory granules (ultrastructural Type I) (×24,000) (Creutzfeldt et al., Hum Pathol. *6* [1975] 47-76).

M-8153/1, 3

b) Gastrinomas:
This tumor produces gastrin (Zollinger-Ellison syndrome).
The gastric hyperacidity is combined with peptic ulcers in the stomach, the duodenum, and jejunum.
Some patients have diarrhea.

c) Diarrhogenic islet cell tumor:
It is supposed that this tumor produces a secretin-like substance. It causes diarrhea.
There is no gastric hypersecretion.

d) Alpha-cell tumor producing glucagon:
These patients have an elevated plasma concentration of glucagon. They show signs of hyperglycemia.
This tumor is often malignant. It occurs predominantly in postmenopausal women.

e) Islet cell tumors producing serotonin:
The tumors can induce a carcinoid syndrome.

f) Islet cell tumors producing ACTH:
These tumors produce Cushing's syndrome.

g) A number of islet cell tumors can produce **HCG** and its subunits [20].
HCG elevation is not observed in benign islet cell neoplasms.

h) Islet cell tumors can also produce **cyclic AMP, ADH, and MSH.**

i) In most instances islet cell tumors are **uniendocrine tumors.** However **multiendocrine tumors** can occur. In most instances they are malignant.
The combination of hormones can be glucagon, insulin, and gastrin or insulin, glucagon, and ACTH [17, 23].

Treatment

Surgery:
– Resection of the tumor.
– The tumor can be localized by **celiac arteriography** (due to the numerous blood vessels in the tumor).
– The islet cell tumor can consist of multiple adenomas or diffuse hyperplasia of the islets (Figs. 439 to 441). In these cases the detection of the tumor at the time of operation is impossible. Subtotal pancreatectomy or resection at the level of the tail or body should be done.
– In cases of liver metastases, resection of these tumors should be attempted.

[17] Hammar and Sale 1975.
[20] Kahn et al. 1977.
[23] Larsson et al. 1976.

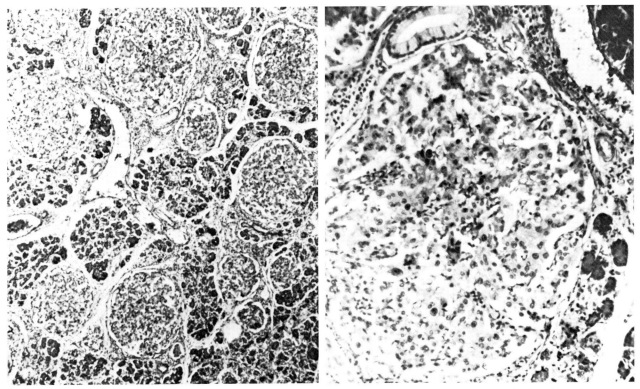

Fig. 439. Hyperplasia of pancreatic islets (1-day-old newborn, ×50).

Fig. 440. Hyperplasia of pancreatic islets (1-day-old newborn, ×125).

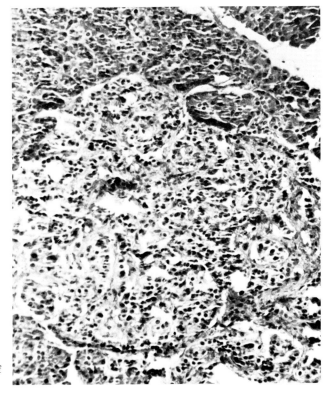

Fig. 441. Islet adenomatosis of the pancreas (insulinoma): One of the enlarged islets (×125).

Islet cell tumors

Treatment

Chemotherapy:

Chemotherapy with streptozotocin:
- The overall response rate is about 40%.
- Complete remissions are obtained with normal insulin levels lasting more than 1 year.
- Streptozotocin has been used also in case of Zollinger-Ellison syndrome [7] and in unresectable glucagon-secreting tumors [9].

Prognosis

Benign islet cell tumors:

When the tumor is removed, the patient is cured.

Malignant islet cell tumors:

When the tumor is entirely removed (recognized, for instance, by a decrease in the serum gastrin level to normal), the prognosis is good.
- In cases of nonresectable metastatic islet cell tumor, the prognosis is unpredictable and is determined by the degree of endocrine production and symptoms.
- After treatment with streptozotocin, regression of the tumor mass for years has been observed.

Further Information

Paraneoplastic syndromes:

1. Nonpancreatic tumors can produce **hypoglycemia:**
    - carcinoma of the adrenal cortex,
    - oat cell carcinoma of the bronchus,
    - hepatomas,
    - fibrosarcoma,
    - rhabdomyosarcoma,
    - liposarcoma,
    - malignant mesothelioma,
    - pseudomyxoma peritonei [14],
    - occasionally malignant lymphoma,
    - paraneoplastic syndromes of the central nervous system [34].
2. **ACTH-producing tumors:**

    Besides the pituitary and adrenal tumors, ACTH is particularly often produced by oat cell carcinomas; it has been observed in thymomas, oat cell carcinoma of the esophagus, and squamous cell carcinoma of the larynx [19].
3. There are a few reports of pancreatic **somatostatinomas** growing in the pancreas [15] and of its malignant variety in the jejunum [2].
4. Coexistence of bilateral pheochromocytomas and pancreatic islet cell tumors has been reported [29].

[2] Alumets et al. 1978.
[7] Cryer and Hill 1976.
[9] Danforth Jr. et al. 1976.
[14] Frantz 1959 (further references).
[15] Ganda et al. 1977.
[19] Imura et al. 1975.
[29] Tateishi et al. 1978.
[34] Zangemeister et al. 1978.

Recommendations for differential diagnosis in tumors of the pancreas

adenocarcinoma	with	– sclerosing chronic pancreatitis
cystadenoma, benign	with	– highly differentiated cystadenocarcinoma
islet cell tumor, benign	with	– islet cell tumor, malignant – well-differentiated adenocarcinoma – carcinoid

subclassification of the islet cell tumors by the use of histochemical reactions, immunohistochemistry, and electron microscopy.

References

[1] Alguacil-Garcia, A., and L.H. Weiland: The histologic spectrum, prognosis, and histogenesis of sarcomatoid carcinoma of the pancreas. Cancer *39* (1977) 1181-1189.

[2] Alumets, J., G. Ekelund, R. Håkanson, O. Ljungberg, U. Ljungqvist, F. Sundler, and S. Tibblin: Jejunal endocrine tumour composed of somatostatin and gastrin cells and associated with duodenal ulcer disease. Virchows Arch. A Path. Anat. and Histol. *378* (1978) 17-22.

[3] Becker, V.: Bauchspeicheldrüse. In: Spezielle pathologische Anatomie. Band VI. Hrsg. W. Doerr, G. Seifert, E. Uehlinger. Springer, Berlin–Heidelberg–New York 1973.

[4] Bretholz, A., et H. Steiner: Les insulomes. Intérêt d'un diagnostic morphologique précis. Virchows Arch. A Path. Anat. and Histol. *359* (1973) 49-66.

[5] Carter, S.K., and R.L. Comis: Adenocarcinoma of the pancreas: Current therapeutic approaches, prognostic variables, and criteria of response. In: Cancer therapy: Prognostic factors and criteria of response, edited by M.J. Staquet, Raven Press, New York 1975.

[6] Creutzfeldt, W., R. Arnold, C. Creutzfeldt, and N.S. Track: Pathomorphologic, biochemical, and diagnostic aspects of gastrinomas (Zollinger-Ellison syndrome). Hum. Pathol. *6* (1975) 47-76.

[7] Cryer, P.E., and G.J., Hill: Pancreatic islet cell carcinoma with hypercalcemia and hypergastrinemia. Response to streptozotocin. Cancer *38* (1976) 2217-2221.

[8] Cubilla, A.L., J. Fortner, and P.J. Fitzgerald: Lymph node involvement in carcinoma of the head of the pancreas area. Cancer *41* (1978) 880-887.

[9] Danforth, D.N Jr., T. Triche, J.L. Doppman, R.M. Beazley, P.V. Perrino, and L. Recant: Elevated plasma proglucagon-like component with a glucagon-secreting tumor. Effect of streptozotocin. N. Engl. J. Med. *295* (1976) 242-245.

[10] Davis, L. Jr., D.D. von Hoff, M. Rozencweig, H. Handelsman, W.T. Soper, and F.M. Muggia: Gastrointestinal cancer: Esophagus, stomach, small bowel, colorectum, pancreas, liver, gallbladder, and extrahepatic ducts. In: Randomized trials in cancer: A critical review by sites. Edited by Maurice J. Staquet, Raven Press, New York 1978.

[11] DeLellis, R.A., R.F. Gagel, M.M. Kaplan, and L.E. Curtis: Gastrinoma of duodenal G-cell origin. Cancer *38* (1976) 201-208.

[12] Dobelbower, R.R. Jr., B.B. Borgelt, N. Suntharalingam, and K.A. Strubler: Pancreatic carcinoma treated with high-dose, small-volume irradiation. Cancer *41* (1978) 1087-1092.

[13] Dold, U.W., und H. Sack: Praktische Tumortherapie. Die Behandlung maligner Organtumoren und Systemerkrankungen. Thieme, Stuttgart 1976.

[14] Frantz, V.K.: Tumors of the pancreas. Atlas of tumor pathology, A.F.I.P., Washington, D.C. 1959.

[15] Ganda, O.P., G.C. Weir, J.S. Soeldner, M.A. Legg, W.L. Chick, Y.C. Patel, A.M. Ebeid, K.H. Gabbay, and S. Reichlin; "Somatostatinoma": A somatostatin-containing tumor of the endocrine pancreas. N. Engl. J. Med. *296* (1977) 963-967.

[16] Glenner, G.G., and G.K. Mallory: The cystadenoma and related non-functional tumors of the pancreas; pathogenesis, classification, and significance. Cancer *9* (1956) 980-996.

[17] Hammar, S., and G. Sale: Multiple hormone producing islet cell carcinomas of the pancreas. A morphological and biochemical investigation. Hum. Pathol. *6* (1975) 349-362.

[18] Ihse, I., P. Lilja, B. Arnesjo, and S. Bengmark: Total pancreatectomy for cancer: An appraisal of 65 cases. Ann. Surg. *186* (1977) 675-680.

[19] Imura, H., S. Matsukura, H. Yamamoto, Y. Hirata, Y. Nakai, J. Endo, A. Tanaka, and M. Nakamura: Studies on ectopic ACTH-producing tumors. II. Clinical and biochemical features of 30 cases. Cancer *35* (1975) 1430-1437.

[20] Kahn, R.C., S.W. Rosen, B.D. Weintraub, S.S. Fajans, and P. Gorden: Ectopic production of chorionic gonadotropin and its subunits by isletcell tumors. A specific marker for malignancy. N. Engl. J. Med. *297* (1977) 565-569.

[21] Kozuka, S., R. Sassa, T. Taki, K. Masamoto, S. Nagasawa, S. Saga, K. Hasegawa, and M. Takeuchi: Relation of pancreatic duct hyperplasia to carcinoma. Cancer *43* (1979) 1418-1428.

[22] Kümmerle, F., P. Kirschner und G. Mangold: Zur Klinik und Chirurgie des Pankreaskarzinoms. Dtsch. Med. Wschr. *101* (1976) 729-734.

[23] Larsson, L.I., T. Schwartz, G. Lungqvist, R.E. Chance, F. Sundler, J.F. Rehfeld, L. Grimelius et al.: Occurrence of human pancreatic polypeptide in pancreatic endocrine tumors. Possible implication in the watery diarrhea syndrome. Am. J. Path. *85* (1976) 675-684.

[24] Larsson, L.I., O. Ljungberg, F. Sundler, R. Håkanson, S.O. Svensson, J. Rehfeld, F. Stadil, and J. Holst: Antro-pyloric gastrinoma associated with pancreatic nesidioblastosis and proliferation of islets. Virchows Arch. A Path. Anat. and Histol. *360* (1973) 305-314.

[25] Le Charpentier, Y., A. Louvel, P.P. de Saint-Maur, M. Daudet-Monsac, L. Léger, et R. Abelanet: Étude ultrastructurale d'un insulinome à stroma amyloïde. Discussion de l'histogénèse des amyloses localisées. Virchows Arch. A Path. Anat. and Histol. *362* (1974) 169-183.

[26] Mihas, A.A., R. Ceballos, A. Mihas, and R.G. Gibson: Zollinger-Ellison syndrome associated with ductal adenocarcinoma of the pancreas. N. Engl. J. Med. *298* (1978) 144-146.

[27] Moertel, C.G., H.O. Douglas Jr., J. Hanley, and P.P. Carbone: Treatment of advanced adenocarcinoma of the pancreas with combinations of streptozotocin plus 5-fluorouracil and strep-

tozotocin plus cyclophosphamide. Cancer *40* (1977) 605-608.

[28] Schein, P., S.P.T. Lavin, C.G. Moertel, S. Frytak, R.G. Hahn, M.J. O'Connell, R.J. Reitemeier, J. Rubin, A.J. Schutt, L.H. Weiland, M. Kalser, J. Barkin, H. Lessner, R. Mann-Kaplan, D. Redlhammer, M. Silverman, M. Troner, H.O. Douglass Jr., S. Milliron, J. Lokich, J. Brooks, J. Chaffe, A. Like, N. Zamcheck, K. Ramming, J. Bateman, H. Spiro, E. Livstone, and A. Knowlton: Randomized phase II clinical trial of adriamycin, methotrexate, and actinomycin – D in advanced measurable pancreatic carcinoma. A gastrointestinal tumor study group report. Cancer *42* (1978) 19-22.

[29] Tateishi, R., A. Wada, S. Ishiguro, M. Ehara, H. Sakamoto, T. Miki, Y. Mori, Y. Matsui, and O. Ishikawa: Coexistence of bilateral pheochromocytoma and pancreatic islet cell tumor. Report of a case and review of the literature. Cancer *42* (1978) 2928-2934.

[30] Taxy, J.B.: Adenocarcinoma of the pancreas in childhood. Report of a case and a review of the English language literature. Cancer *37* (1976) 1508-1518.

[31] Tepper, J., G. Nardi, and H. Suit: Carcinoma of the pancreas: Review of MGH experience from 1963 to 1973. Analysis of surgical failure and implications for radiation therapy. Cancer *37* (1976) 1519-1524.

[32] Tschang, T.-P., R. Garza-Garza, and J.M. Kissane: Pleomorphic carcinoma of the pancreas. An analysis of 15 cases. Cancer *39* (1977) 2114-2126.

[33] Woodtli, W., and C. Hedinger: Histologic characteristics of insulinomas and gastrinomas. Value of argyrophilia, metachromasia, immunohistology, and electron microscopy for the identification of gastrointestinal and pancreatic endocrine cells and their tumors. Virchows Arch. A Path. Anatomy and Histology *371* (1976) 331-350.

[34] Zangemeister, W.H., G. Schwendemann, and H.J. Colmant: Carcinomatous encephalomyelopathy in conjunction with encephalomyeloradiculitis. J. Neurol. *218* (1978) 63-71.

12 Tumors of the peritoneum

M-9050/0, 1, 3
T 158.9

1. Mesothelioma of the peritoneum
(peritoneal mesothelioma)

**General
Remarks**

Incidence: Mesotheliomas of the peritoneum are very rare tumors; they are associated with asbestosis.

**Macroscopy
M-9050/0**

a) The **benign mesothelioma** is a circumscribed papillary tumor of considerable firmness. Very rarely, circumscribed tumors can be malignant [4].

M-9050/3

b) The **malignant mesothelioma** covers the surface of the intestine and the mesentery and can finally obliterate the entire peritoneal cavity.

The tumor covers the surface of the peritoneal cavity in the form of small papillary lesions.

Histology

Both mesotheliomas (the solitary and the diffuse forms) have a similar growth pattern, which is composed of cells and connective tissue.

The strands of connective tissue are covered by cells that give a PAS-positive reaction in the cytoplasm. These cells grow in monolayers or multilayers.

The cells growing in the connective tissue form papillary or tubular formations (Figs. 442 and 443).

Cellular atypias and mitotic figures can be detected.

In most instances the tumor. is dominated by the growth of the cells. Very rarely the abundant production of collagen fibers can occur; this is the

M-9051/0, 3

fibrous type of peritoneal mesothelioma.

**Differential
Diagnosis**

1. Peritoneal mesothelioma, benign, **with malignant mesothelioma:**
   The benign mesothelioma in most instances is a solitary tumor; diffuse mesotheliomas are almost always malignant (Figs. 444 to 446).
2. Malignant mesothelioma **with metastatic adenocarcinoma:**
   This differential diagnosis might be difficult. The mucin stain, however, can give the solution (Fig. 447).
   In cases of assumed primary tumor in the ovary, one should look for psammoma bodies.
3. Mesothelioma **with granulomatous inflammation** (Fig. 448).

Treatment

Only chemotherapeutic treatment can be tried for palliation purposes [2, 3].

[2] Dold and Sack 1976.
[3] Kuguksu et al. 1976.
[4] Tang et al. 1976.

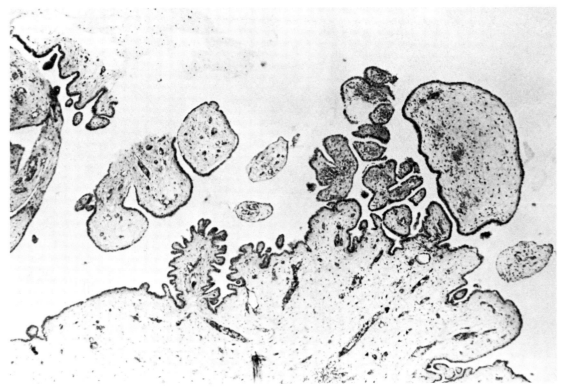

Fig. 442. Benign papillary mesothelioma of the peritoneum (45-year-old female, × 40).

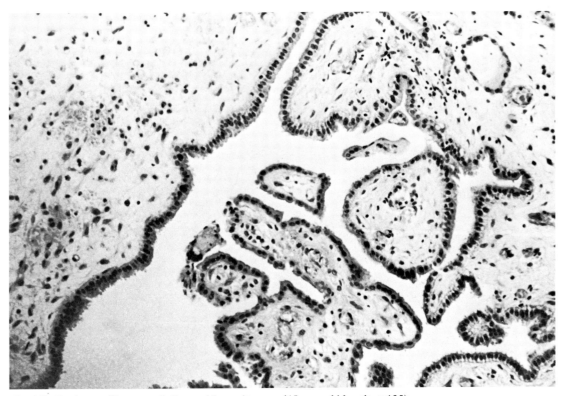

Fig. 443. Benign papillary mesothelioma of the peritoneum (45-year-old female, × 125).

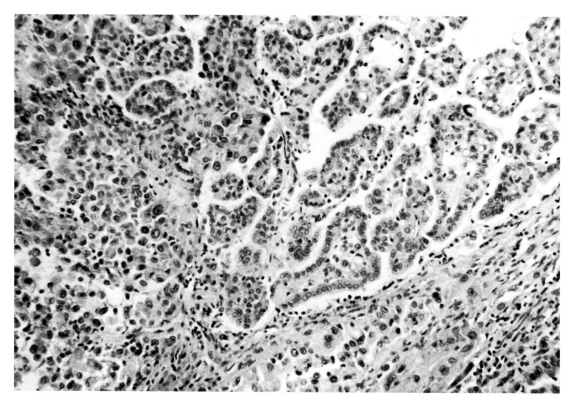

Fig. 444. Malignant mesothelioma of the peritoneum: Papillary and solid tumor cell growth (77-year-old male, × 125).

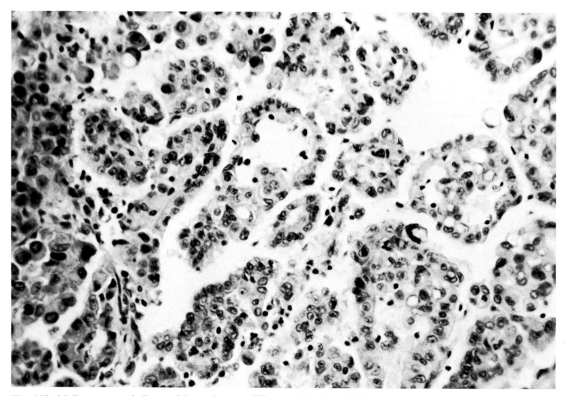

Fig. 445. Malignant mesothelioma of the peritoneum (77-year-old male, × 200).

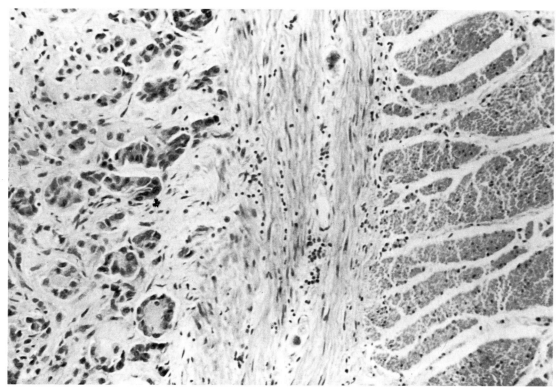

Fig. 446. Malignant mesothelioma of the peritoneum on the surface of the intestine (77-year-old male, × 125).

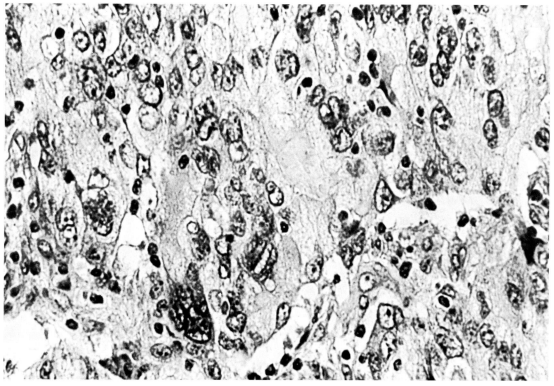

Fig. 447. Poorly differentiated adenocarcinoma growing in the peritoneum (mucicarmine, × 310).

433

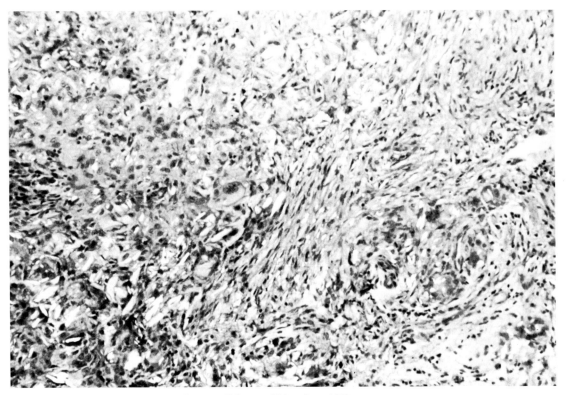

Fig. 448. Talcum granuloma in the peritoneum (36-year-old female, × 125).

M-8990/0
T 158.9

2. Benign mesenchymoma

This tumor is composed of cartilage, bone, and connective tissue (Figs. 136 and 137). This lesion represents a benign metaplasia, usually observed in the course of a chronic inflammation (for instance, postoperatively).

M-8000/6
T 158.9

3. Metastatic tumors

The majority of tumors of the peritoneum are metastatic lesions.
A particular variety is the **pseudomyxoma peritonei** (Fig. 279).

M-8480/6
T 158.9

434

4. Disseminated leiomyomas

Multiple leiomyomas on the peritoneum are a condition that is very rarely observed [1].

References

[1] Aterman, K., G.M. Fraser, and R.H. Lea: Disseminated peritoneal leiomyomatosis. Virchows Arch. A Path. Anat. and Histol. *374* (1977) 13-26.

[2] Dold, U.W., und H. Sack: Praktische Tumortherapie. Die Behandlung maligner Organtumoren und Systemerkrankungen. Thieme, Stuttgart 1976.

[3] Kuguksu, N., W. Thomas, and E.Z. Ezdinli: Chemotherapy of malignant diffuse mesothelioma. Cancer *37* (1976) 1265-1274.

[4] Tang, C.K., G.F. Gray, and J.G. Keuhnelian: Malignant peritoneal mesothelioma in an inguinal hernia sac. Cancer *37* (1976) 1887-1890.

---

[1] Aterman et al. 1977.

13 Tumors of the head and neck

1. Tumors of the oral cavity can arise from the buccal mucosa, the retromolar area, gingiva, hard palate, anterior two-thirds of the tongue affecting the inferior side and the lateral borders, the floor of the mouth, and the lips.
2. Two to 5% of all human cancers grow in the oral cavity.
   The great majority of these cancers are squamous cell carcinomas (up to 95%).
   The majority of these carcinomas grow in the lower lip, followed by the tongue [46].
3. Squamous cell carcinomas in this area are graded according to their differentiation.
   The biological behavior of these tumors, however, is more determined by their site of origin than by the histological appearance of the squamous cell carcinoma.
   The TNM classification respects this situation (see following pages).
4. Leukoplakias show clinically a great variety of histological pictures. Less than 5 to 10% of leukoplakias develop into squamous cell carcinoma.
5. Squamous cell carcinomas in the oral cavity are in most instances of a multifocal origin.
   Foci of squamous cell carcinoma can be surrounded by normal mucosa, by leukoplakias, or by carcinoma in situ.
   The multifocal origin is one of the reasons for the high recurrence rate.
6. Squamous cell carcinomas can grow in a papillary or ulcerating way.
7. There is a marked geographical difference in the incidence of carcinomas in the oral cavity according to environmental factors.

---

[46] Goldhaber 1977.

Tumors of the oral cavity

Buccal mucosa, upper alveolus and gingiva, lower alveolus and gingiva, hard palate, tongue, floor of the mouth.

T – primary tumor

Tis = preinvasive carcinoma (carcinoma in situ)
T 0 = no evidence of primary tumor
T 1 = tumor 2 cm or less in its greatest dimension
T 2 = tumor more than 2 cm but not more than 4 cm in its greatest dimension
T 3 = tumor more than 4 cm in its greatest dimension
T 4 = tumor with extension to bone, muscle, skin, antrum, neck, etc.
T x = the minimal requirements to assess the primary tumor cannot be met (clinical examination and radiography)

N – regional lymph nodes

(cervical nodes)
N 0 = no evidence of regional lymph node involvement
N 1 = evidence of involvement of the movable homolateral regional lymph nodes
N 2 = evidence of involvement of the movable contralateral or bilateral regional lymph nodes
N 3 = evidence of involvement of the fixed regional lymph nodes
N x = the minimal requirements to assess the regional lymph nodes cannot be met (clinical examination)

M – distant metastases

M 0 = no evidence of distant metastases
M 1 = evidence of distant metastases
M x = the minimal requirements to assess the presence of distant metastases cannot be met (clinical examination and radiography)

pTNM – postsurgical histopathological classification
pT – primary tumor

the pT categories correspond to the T categories

pN – regional lymph nodes

the pN categories correspond to the N categories

pM – distant metastases

the pM categories correspond to the M categories

Stage grouping

Stage I	T 1	N 0	M 0
Stage II	T 2	N 0	M 0
Stage III	T 3	N 0	M 0
	T 1, T 2, T 3	N 1	M 0
Stage IV	T 4	N 0, N 1	M 0
	any T	N 2, N 3	M 0
	any T	any N	M 1

M-8070/3

1. Squamous cell carcinoma (WHO)

Histology

Squamous cell carcinomas are composed of malignant cells that grow in large clusters and sheets. The tumor cells exhibit different degrees of differentiation, which is a basis for grading [120].

Grade I
The tumor contains numerous keratin pearls. There are clear intercellular bridges. There are less than 2 mitoses in a high power field ($\times 600$).
Multinucleated giant cells or atypical mitotic figures are rare.
The pleomorphism of the cells and nuclei is minimal (Fig. 449).
This squamous cell carcinoma is often observed in the buccal mucosa.

Grade II
There are few epithelial pearls or keratinization in the individual cells.
The number of mitotic figures increases (2 to 4 in a high power field, $\times 600$).
There are more atypical mitotic figures than in Grade I.
Although multinucleated giant cells are still infrequent, the pleomorphism of nuclei and cells is marked in comparison to Grade I (Fig. 450).

Grade III
Keratinization pearls are encountered very rarely or are absent.
There are no intercellular bridges.
There are more than 4 mitotic figures per high power field with frequent atypical mitoses.
There are numerous multinucleated giant cells and a considerable pleomorphism of cells and nuclei (Fig. 451).

M-8074/3

2. Squamous cell carcinoma, spindle cell type (WHO)

This variety of squamous cell carcinoma is composed of cells that are spindle-shaped and are similar to sarcoma cells. Foci of keratinization are rare.

---

[120] Wahi 1971.

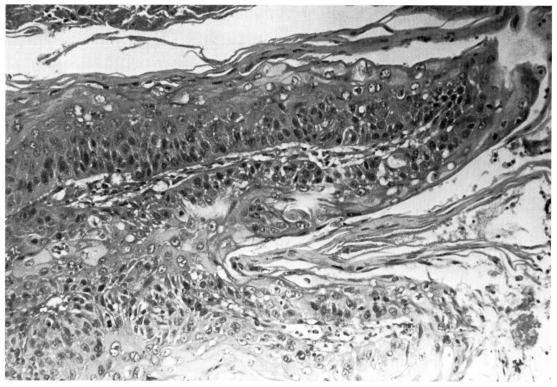

Fig. 449. Squamous cell carcinoma of the tonsil: Grade I in the upper part of the tumor (45-year-old male, × 200).

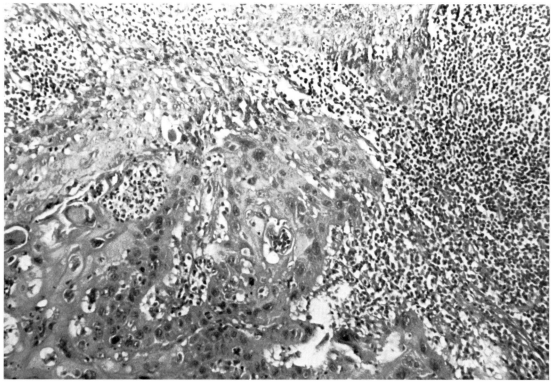

Fig. 450. Squamous cell carcinoma of the tonsil: Grade II in a lower part (45-year-old male, × 200).

M-8051/3

3. Squamous cell carcinoma, verrucous type (WHO)

This variety of squamous cell carcinoma grows over the surface (exophytic growth pattern), while the infiltration into the underlying connective tissue is very discrete (Fig. 520).

This is a highly differentiated tumor with intercellular bridges and abundant keratinization.

This tumor has a low degree of malignancy (Grade I).

Verrucous carcinomas are usually observed in the buccal mucosa of men who chew tobacco and in the gingiva.

M-8070/3
T 140.9

A. Carcinoma of the lip

**General
Remarks**

Incidence: Carcinoma of the lip is the most frequently observed carcinoma of the oral cavity.

Age: This tumor develops in elderly patients during the 6th to 7th decades.

Sex: Men are considerably more affected than women.

T 140.1
T 140.0

Site: The lower lip is about 10 times more frequently the site of carcinoma than the upper lip.

Further notes:

a) Farmers and sailors are often affected, perhaps due to exposure to the UV light of the sun [114].

b) Carcinoma of the lip can occasionally be of a multifocal origin.

c) The majority of squamous cell carcinomas of the lip are Grade I.

Macroscopy

Carcinoma of the lip is a firm lesion. Rarely the tumor is covered by keratosis; in most instances there is an ulceration.

Histology

Squamous cell carcinoma, often with keratinization and signs of Grade I.

Staging

T – primary tumor

Tis = preinvasive carcinoma (carcinoma in situ)

T 0 = no evidence for primary tumor

T 1 = tumor limited to the lip: 2 cm or less in its greatest dimension

T 2 = tumor limited to the lip: more than 2 cm but not more than 4 cm in its greatest dimension

T 3 = tumor limited to the lip: more than 4 cm in its greatest dimension

T 4 = tumor extending beyond lip to neighboring structures, e.g., bone, tongue, skin of neck.

T x = the minimal requirements to assess the primary tumor cannot be met (clinical examination)

---

[114] Szpak et al. 1977.

Staging

N – regional lymph nodes (cervical nodes)

N 0   = no evidence of regional lymph node involvement

N 1   = evidence of involvement of the movable homolateral regional lymph nodes

N 2   = evidence of involvement of the movable contralateral or bilateral regional lymph nodes

N 3   = evidence of involvement of the fixed regional lymph nodes

N x   = the minimal requirements to assess the regional lymph nodes cannot be met (clinical examination)

M – distant metastases

M 0   = no evidence of distant metastases

M 1   = evidence of distant metastases

M x   = the minimal requirements to assess the presence of distant metastases cannot be met (clinical examination and radiography)

pTNM – postsurgical histopathological classification

pT – primary tumor

the pT categories correspond to the T categories

pN – regional lymph nodes

the pN categories correspond to the N categories

pM – distant metastases

the pM categories correspond to the M categories

Stage grouping

Stage I	T 1	N 0	M 0
Stage II	T 2	N 0	M 0
Stage III	T 3	N 0	M 0
	T 1, T 2, T 3	N 1	M 0
Stage IV	T 4	N 0, N 1	M 0
	any T	N 2, N 3	M 0
	any T	any N	M 1

Spread

1. The tumor infiltrates the surrounding tissue.
2. Lymph node metastases develop late, only when the carcinoma infiltrates the middle portion of the lip.
3. Hematogenous distant metastases are late events.

Treatment

Surgery:
Removal of the tumor [51].
Radiation therapy [56, 87]:
40 to 70 Gy in 3 to 7 weeks, according to the size of the tumor.

Prognosis

Good chances for cure (see page 453).

---

[51] Hendricks et al. 1977.
[56] Hornback and Shidnia 1978.
[87] Pigneux et al. 1979.

M-8070/3
T 141.9

B. Carcinoma of the tongue

General Remarks

Incidence: The second most frequently observed carcinoma of the oral cavity is cancer of the tongue.

Age: The peak age is the 5th to 6th decades; younger persons, however, can be affected. The tumor is rare in patients less than 20 years old [85].

Sex: Men are affected considerably more often than women (about 7 : 1).

Site: The anterior two-thirds of the tongue is involved in about 75% of the cases; the remaining 25% develop at the base of the tongue.

The majority of carcinomas grow at the edge of the tongue; rarely or less frequently the tumor develops on the undersurface or the tip of the tongue.

Very rarely carcinomas are found in the midline of the tongue.

Further notes: Many patients are heavy smokers.

Macroscopy

The tumor presents as an ulceration with a firm infiltration into the underlying or surrounding tissue.

Histology

The tumor is composed of cells of a squamous cell carcinoma with different degrees of differentiation (Figs. 451 to 455). Occasionally foci of carcinoma in situ can be observed in the neighborhood; however, this is relatively rare.

Electron Microscopy

In poorly differentiated squamous cell carcinoma of the tongue, the tumor cells show evidence of desmosomes.

Spread

1. Early regional lymph node metastases.
2. Distant metastases into the lung, liver, kidney, and other organs.

Treatment

Surgery or **irradiation** [1]:

T 1-2: Radiation therapy alone can be recommended [45].

T 3:   Radiation therapy of up to 60 to 80 Gy in 5 to 8 weeks.

Radiation therapy can be combined with surgery according to the individual situation.

In advanced cases **chemotherapy** with bleomycin can be tried, combined with fast neutron beam teletherapy (Figs. 456 and 457) [48].

Prognosis

– The overall 5-year-survival rate is about 50%.
– Advanced disease with lymph node metastases: 5-year survival rate, less than 30%.
– In the early stages a 5-year survival rate of up to 70% can be obtained (further details, see page 453).

Further Information

1. Bleomycin alters endothelial cells in the blood vessels and induces ischemic necroses in the tumor tissue due to thrombotic occlusion of the blood vessels [17].
2. There is one report in which a squamous cell carcinoma of the tongue developed in a 26-year-old patient years after renal transplantation [68].

[1] Akanuma 1977.
[17] Burkhardt et al. 1976.
[45] Glanzmann 1978.
[48] Griffin et al. 1978.
[68] Lee and Gisser 1978.
[85] Patel and Dave 1976.

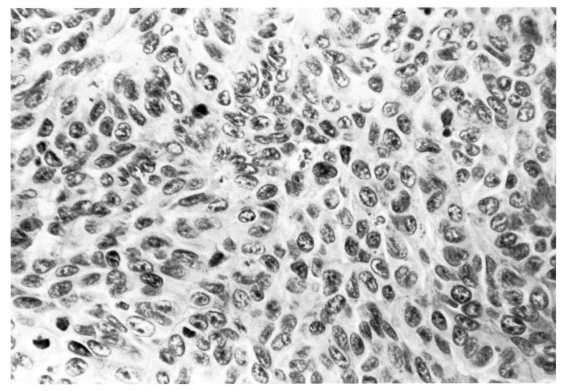

Fig. 451. Squamous cell carcinoma of the tongue, Grade III (×310).

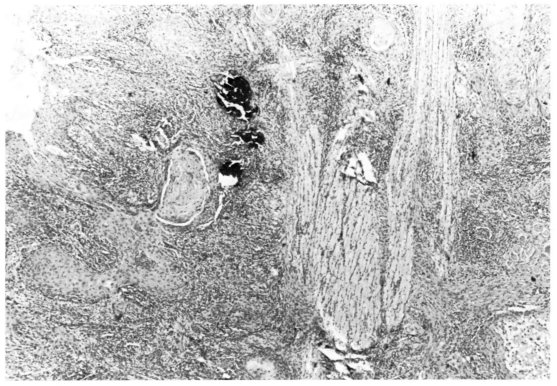

Fig. 452. Infiltrating squamous cell carcinoma of the tongue, ulcerating type (Grade I) (68-year-old female, ×40).

447

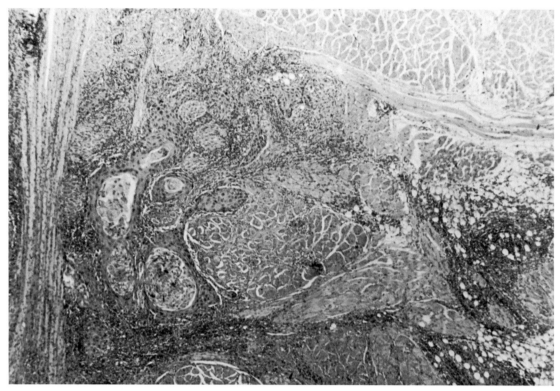

Fig. 453. Infiltrating squamous cell carcinoma of the tongue, well differentiated (68-year-old female, × 40).

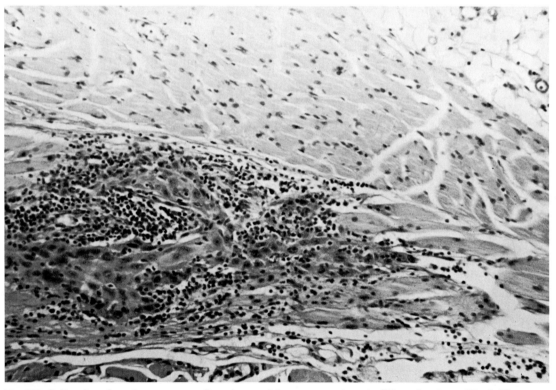

Fig. 454. Infiltrating, ulcerating squamous cell carcinoma of the tongue, moderately differentiated area (Grade II) (68-year-old female, × 125).

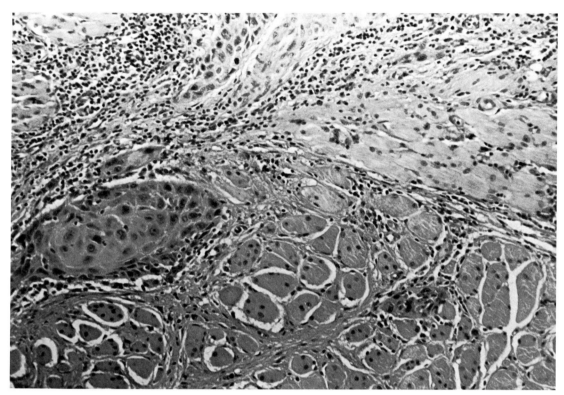

Fig. 455. Well-differentiated area of an infiltrating squamous cell carcinoma of the tongue, ulcerated type (Grade II) (68-year-old female, × 125).

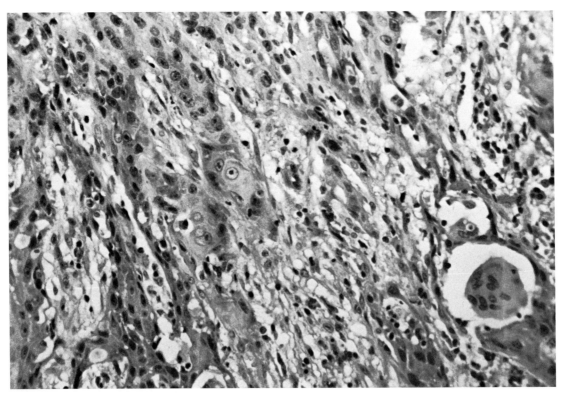

Fig. 456. Squamous cell carcinoma of the tongue, previous treatment with irradiation and bleomycin: Giant cells (85-year-old female, × 200).

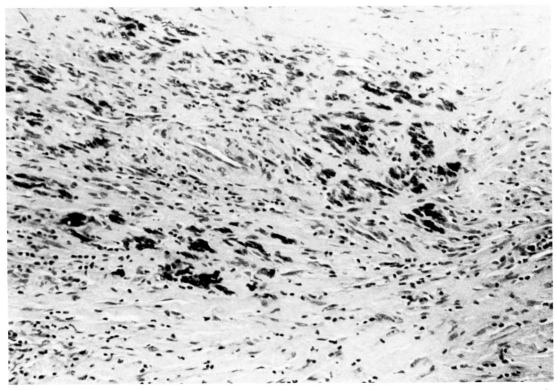

Fig. 457. Squamous cell carcinoma of the tongue: Biopsy following treatment with bleomycin and irradiation: Myogenic giant cells – no tumor cells (64-year-old male, × 125).

450

M-8070/3

C. Carcinoma of the base of the tongue
(posterior third)

T 141.0

These tumors are considered to be part of tumors of the oropharynx.

The separation of this carcinoma from the neoplasm developing in the anterior two-thirds is due to the poor survival in cancer in this location.

The poor prognosis of this tumor is due to

– late detection of the tumor
– poor differentiation of the carcinoma (Grade III)
– early infiltration into the underlying muscle and into the lymphatics with early regional lymph node metastases.

Treatment

Irradiation of up to 60 Gy [113].

Prognosis

The 5-year survival rate is about 30% (see page 453).

M-8070/3
T 145.0

D. Carcinoma of the cheek

**General
Remarks**

Incidence: Carcinomas of the cheek are less frequently observed than those of the tongue. They have about the same incidence as carcinomas of the floor of the mouth.

Age: The peak age is the 7th and 8th decades.

Sex: Men are more frequently affected than women.

Site: Carcinomas of the cheek can be of a multifocal origin. They are often associated with leukoplakia, which can occasionally be the origin of carcinoma.

Macroscopy

Carcinomas of the cheek can be of an ulcerating or a verrucous type. The ulcerating type causes infiltration into the underlying tissue; in these instances the tumor is firm.

Histology

Most of the carcinomas of the cheek are well-differentiated squamous cell carcinomas, Grade I or II.

Spread

1. Local infiltration into the surrounding tissue.
2. Lymphatic invasion with lymph node metastases.
3. Hematogenous metastases into distant organs (for instance, lung and brain).

Treatment

Surgery:
Resection of the tumor.
Radiation therapy:
Irradiation of up to 60 Gy in about 6 weeks.
Chemotherapy:
Application of bleomycin, combined with irradiation.

Prognosis

The 5-year survival rate for the early stages ist about 70%.

Advanced disease with metastases has a 5-year survival rate of about 30%.

The overall prognosis for this carcinoma is better than the prognosis for carcinoma of the base of the tongue (see also page 453).

Further Information

There are two cases reported of an adenoid squamous cell carcinoma of the oral mucosa [115].

M-8070/3
T 144.9

E. Carcinoma of the floor of the mouth

General Remarks

Incidence: Carcinomas of the floor of the mouth have about the same incidence as carcinomas in the cheek.

Age: The peak age is the 6th to 7th decades.

Sex: Males are more frequently affected than females.

Site: Carcinoma of the floor of the mouth develops usually close to the midline.

Macroscopy

In the majority of cases the carcinoma is of the ulcerated type, often small with a clear firmness due to tumor infiltration.

Histology

Carcinomas of the floor of the mouth are often poorly differentiated squamous cell carcinomas of Grade II and III.

Spread

1. Local infiltration into the tongue, the gingiva, the mandibula, and the sublingual and submandibular glands.
2. Lymphatic spread into the mandibular lymph nodes, often bilateral, later into the deep cervical lymph nodes.
3. Hematogenous spread.

Treatment

T 1   = Radiation therapy [11] of up to 80 Gy in about 8 weeks.

T 2-3 = Removal of the tumor following a preoperative irradiation of up to 50 Gy.

Details of therapy depend strongly on the individual situation [7, 103, 107].

Prognosis

– In early stages, the 5-year survival rate is around 70%.
– In advanced stages with lymph node metastases, the 5-year survival rate is about 30% (see also page 453).

[7] Barton and Ucmakli 1977.
[11] Berthelsen et al. 1977.
[103] Schulz et al. 1979.
[107] Shaw and Hardingham 1977.
[115] Takagi et al. 1977.

M-8070/3
T 145.2, 3
T 143.9

F. Carcinoma of the palate and gingiva

General Remarks

Incidence: Carcinomas in this location are rare.

Site:

a) Carcinomas of the lower gingiva are about three times as frequent as those of the upper gingiva.

b) Carcinomas of the palate usually originate in the soft palate.

Macroscopy

Usually ulcerating tumors with firmness of the infiltrated tissue.

Histology

Squamous cell carcinoma of various degrees of differentiation, Grades I and II, are found rather often.

Spread

1. Infiltration into the surrounding tissue.
2. Invasion of the lymphatics with regional lymph node metastases, first into the submandibular region and later into the deep cervical lymph nodes.
3. Hematogenous metastases into different organs (for instance, the lung and brain).

Treatment

Radical **surgery.**

Prognosis

Early stages, 5-year survival rate of 70%.

Advanced stages with lymph node metastases, 5-year survival rate 30%.

Prognosis for squamous cell carcinoma of the oral cavity:

a) The prognosis for these tumors depends in the individual case on the site of the tumor. For this reason, a classification has recently been proposed that includes in the existing TNM system the pathology (P) of the tumor and the site (S) of the tumor (STNMP) [91].

b) Well-differentiated squamous cell carcinoma (Grade I) dominates the tumors in the following locations:

Lip, anterior two-thirds of the tongue, buccal mucosa, palate.

c) Poorly differentiated squamous cell carcinomas (Grade III) dominate the cancers in the following locations:

– posterior pharyngeal wall,

– base of the tongue.

d) The differentiation of the tumor indicates to a certain degree the probability of future metastatic lesions [108].

e) Carcinomas of the tongue disseminate more frequently into regional lymph nodes than do carcinomas of the lip.

f) In all locations the T 1 carcinoma (measuring less than 2 cm in diameter) has a better prognosis than the carcinomas of T 2-4.

---

[91] Rapidis et al. 1977.
[108] Shear et al. 1976.

M-8070/2
T 145.9

4. Intraepithelial carcinoma
(carcinoma in situ – WHO)

Histology

Carcinoma in situ in the oral cavity can be of a multifocal origin and gives the clinical impression of a leukoplakia.

The tumor is characterized by atypical cells that grow in the epithelial layer without perforating the basement membrane and without infiltration of the underlying tissue (Fig. 462).

Carcinoma in situ can be a precursor of an infiltrating carcinoma. Carcinoma in situ can also be associated with an infiltrating carcinoma in the surrounding tissue.

Treatment

Carcinoma in situ should be treated by surgery or eventually by radiation therapy.

Due to the multifocal origin of this lesion, a follow-up examination is recommended.

M-7571/0
T 145.9

5. Epithelial lesions, clinically appearing as "leukoplakia" [104]

General Remarks

Incidence: Leukoplakias presenting as white plaques are rather common lesions.

Age: The patients are about 50 years old and older.

Site: Leukoplakias develop mainly in the tongue, buccal mucosa (molar region), lower lip, corner of the mouth, and palate.

Macroscopy

Leukoplakias are whitish plaques, which occasionally can have a papillary surface; more often they are ulcerated.

Histology

The histological lesion that causes the clinical leukoplakia can be of different natures:
- The epithelial layer can be hyperplastic and covered by keratin layers (keratosis) (Fig. 458). In these instances the underlying tissue contains inflammatory cells (mainly lymphocytes and plasma cells) (Fig. 459).
- In other leukoplakias the histological picture consists of an atrophic epithelial layer without keratin on the surface.
- A third possibility is that the covering epithelial layer is papillomatous and again is covered by abundant keratin layers. The rete is thickened and enlarged (Fig. 460).
- The histology of leukoplakia can also consist of dysplasias and carcinoma in situ (Figs. 461 and 462). This is the case in about 10% of the lesions [18].
- According to the geographical distribution, the leukoplakia can also contain or develop into a squamous cell carcinoma over a 10-year period. This is the case in about 2 to 5% of the leukoplakias [29, 88, 110].

[18] Burkhardt and Seifert 1977.   [104] Seifert 1966.
[29] Einhorn and Wersäll 1967.   [110] Silverman Jr. et al. 1976.
[88] Pindborg et al. 1968.

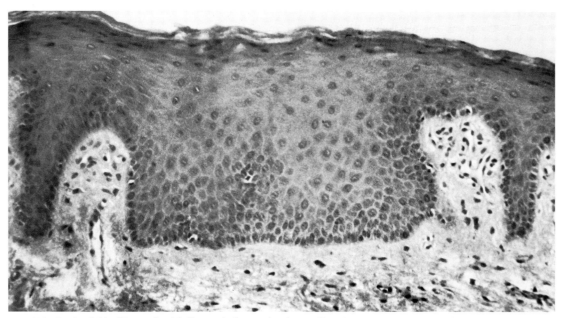

Fig. 458. Leukoplakia: Keratosis with discrete inflammation (upper lip, 50-year-old female, × 125).

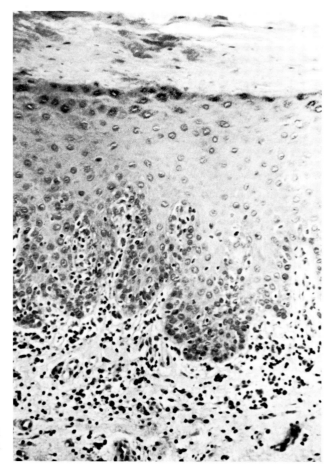

Fig. 459. Leukoplakia: Marked hyperplasia and keratosis, parakeratosis with major inflammation (tongue, 34-year-old female, × 125).

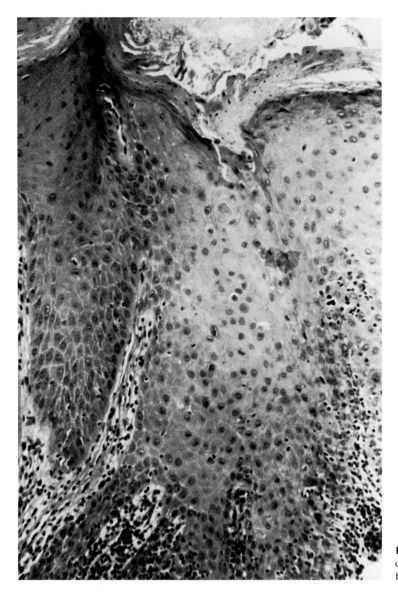

Fig. 460. Leukoplakia: Hyperplasia of the squamous cell layer, hyperparakaratosis (tongue, 34-year-old female, × 125).

Prognosis   The incidence of dysplasia and carcinoma developing in leukoplakias depends strongly on the site of this lesion.

Leukoplakias develop in dysplasias and carcinomas in the
- floor of the mouth, about 40%
- tongue, about 24%
- lips, 24%
- palate, 18%
- retromolar buccal mucosa, 11% [121].

[121] Waldron and Shafer 1975.

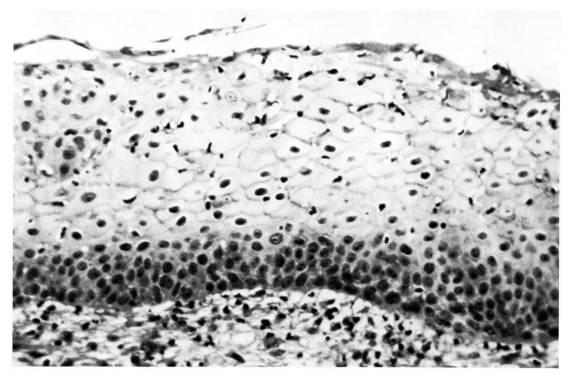

Fig. 461. Leukoplakia: Discrete dysplasia (× 200).

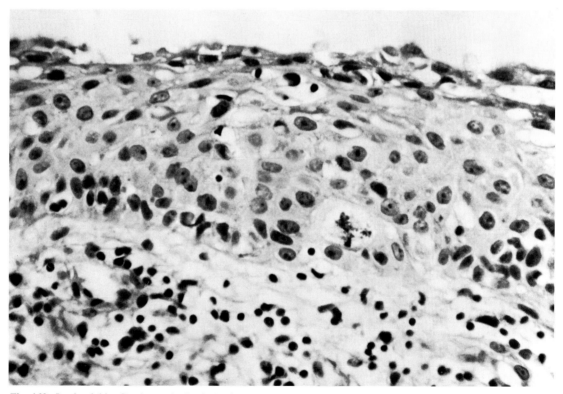

Fig. 462. Leukoplakia: Carcinoma in situ (× 310).

6. Erythroplakia

Erythroplakias are elevated and sometimes papillary or ulcerated lesions, which are reddish.

Histologically the lesion is mostly composed of severe epithelial dysplasia, carcinoma in situ, or invasive carcinoma [106].

For this reason it is very important to biopsy areas of erythroplakia [71].

M-8052/0
T 145.9

7. Squamous cell papilloma (WHO)

This is a benign lesion that can occur in the oral mucosa.

The tumor is composed of papillary formations of normal squamous epithelium. The squamous cell layer is thickened.

The papillary formations are covered by abundant amounts of keratin (Fig. 463).

This is a benign lesion that can be removed surgically.

---

[71] Mashberg and Meyers 1976.
[106] Shafer and Waldron 1975.

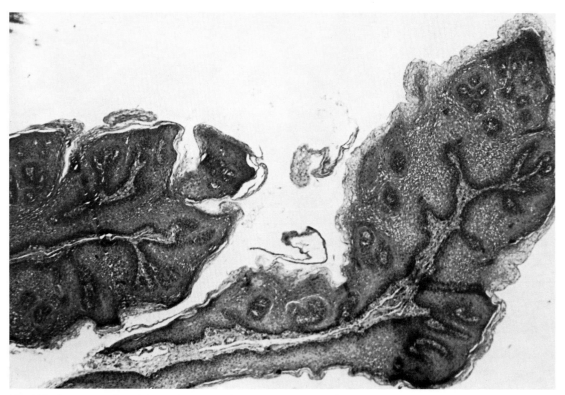

Fig. 463. Squamous cell papilloma of the tongue (71-year-old male, × 40).

M-9580/0

8. Granular cell tumor
(granular cell myoblastoma – WHO)

T 141.9

This soft tissue tumor (see page 116) is in the oral cavity, usually observed in the tongue. The tumor is composed of large cells with small regular nuclei. In the cells PAS-positive granules are deposited (Fig. 464).

The histology becomes important due to the fact that this tumor can induce an important hyperplasia of the covering squamous cell layer. This hyperplasia can be so major that it mimics an infiltrating squamous cell carcinoma (Fig. 465).

Treatment

Removal by surgery.

Prognosis

Excellent.

Further Information

Congenital "myoblastoma" (WHO)
Histologically this lesion corresponds to the granular cell tumor and develops in the gingiva.

This myoblastoma does not induce a pseudocarcinomatous hyperplasia in the squamous cell layer.

9. Tumors of the small salivary glands in the oral cavity

T 145.9

About 50% of tumors developing from the minor salivary glands are benign mixed tumors [30].

All types of salivary gland tumors can be observed, such as adenoid cystic carcinoma and mucoepidermoid carcinoma (see page 561).

---

[30] Eneroth 1970.

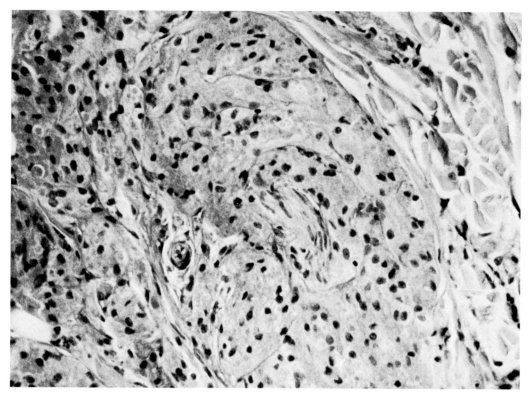

Fig. 464. Granular cell tumor of the tongue: Pale, granular cytoplasm of the large cells (32-year-old male, × 20).

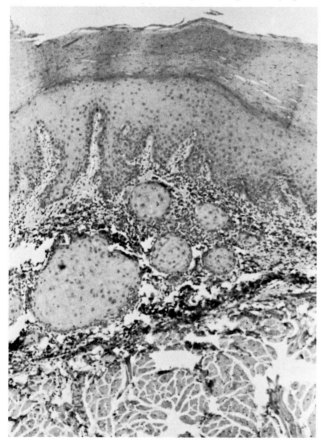

Fig. 465. Pseudoepitheliomatous hyperplasia in the neighborhood of granular cell tumor of the tongue (× 50).

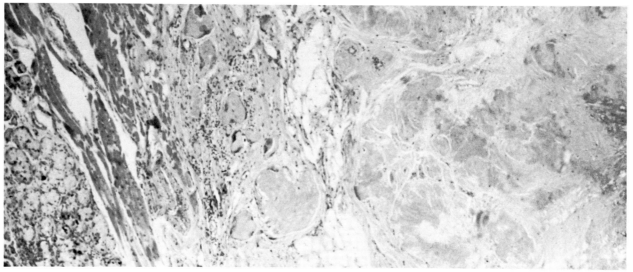

Fig. 466. "Mesenchymoma" of the tongue: Amyloid, giant cells, and metaplastic bone formation (60-year-old male, × 50).

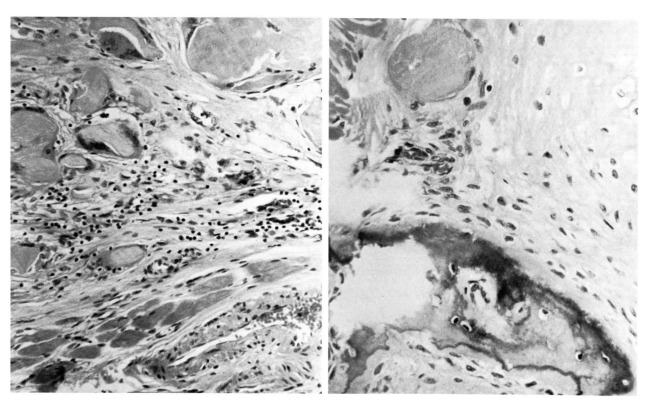

Fig. 467. "Mesenchymoma" of the tongue: Giant cells surrounding amyloid substance, connective tissue (× 125).

Fig. 468. "Mesenchymoma" of the tongue: Metaplastic bone formation, chondroid metaplasia, and amyloid (× 200).

461

10. Tumors of the melanogenic system (WHO)

M-8720/1
T 140.9

Benign and malignant lesions can develop in the oral cavity. The benign lesions (ephelis, lentigo, melanocytic nevi) develop mostly in the lips (see page 1205).

M-8720/3
T 143.9
T 145.2, 3

The malignant melanoma is mostly observed in the gingiva and palate.

11. Soft tissue tumors (WHO)

T 145.9

Occasionally the oral cavity can be occupied by soft tissue tumors, which correspond to the usual histological picture and behavior (Figs. 466 to 468) (see Soft tissue tumors, page 7).

M-9120/0
M-9170/0

Hemangiomas and **lymphangiomas** in the tongue or gingiva are occasionally observed in children and adolescents.

12. Metastatic tumors in the oral cavity

M-8000/6
T 145.9

All types of malignant tumors can disseminate into the oral cavity.
The incidence, however, is rather low.

T 145.9

13. Tumor-like lesions

M-3320/0

a) Mucocele (WHO)

Mucocele consists of mucinous material. This material is deposited in cysts, which can be lined by epithelium or simply surrounded by connective tissue.
The main site of mucocele is the lower lip.

M-4444/0

b) Pyogenic granuloma (WHO)

Pyogenic granuloma is a chronic granulomatous inflammation that develops under the squamous cell layer. The elevated cell layer can ulcerate (Figs. 80 and 81).
The pyogenic granuloma can heal and leave a scar. The overlying tissue in these instances might be hyperplastic.

M-7681/0

c) Fibroepithelial papilloma

A similar scar-like lesion can also be due to chronic irritation of the mucosa.

d) Chronic inflammation with numerous plasma cells

Occasionally the oral mucosa contains foci with numerous plasma cells. They are intermingled with lymphocytes.
However, this lesion occasionally must be separated from plasmacytomas.

M-7209/0

e) Pseudoepitheliomatous (pseudocarcinomatous) hyperplasia

In these instances the hyperplastic epithelium can mimic an infiltrating carcinoma (Figs. 465, 1106, and 1107).
This lesion is often observed in the surroundings of a chronic ulceration with granulomatous inflammatory lesions.

f) Chronic inflammation dominated by lymphocytes

Occasionally the oral cavity can contain numerous lymphocytes. The differential diagnosis with malignant lymphoma might be necessary.
The sign of germinal centers in these lymphocytic infiltrations indicates a benign behavior
M-7229/0
(pseudolymphoma).

463

M-4411/0
T 143.9

g) Giant cell epulis
(peripheral giant cell granuloma – WHO)

The giant cell epulis can develop at any age; it develops in the gingiva. In most instances the lesion is pedunculated; occasionally it is sessile.

Histologically the tumor contains numerous multinucleated giant cells. They grow in a connective tissue, which contains histiocytes, some of them loaded with hemosiderin, fibroblasts, and capillaries.

Recommendations for differential diagnosis in tumors of the oral cavity

squamous cell carcinoma	with	– pseudoepitheliomatous (pseudo-carcinomatous) hyperplasia in chronic inflammation – pseudoepitheliomatous lesion covering granular cell myoblastoma of the tongue – different gradings
pseudoepitheliomatous hyper-plasia in chronic inflammation	with	– squamous cell carcinoma, well differentiated
"leukoplakia"	with	– atrophic epithelium – keratosis and hyperplastic epithelium – dysplasia – carcinoma in situ – infiltrating carcinoma
"erythroplakia"	with	– infiltrating carcinoma – carcinoma in situ – dysplasia
primary tumors of the oral cavity	with	– metastatic lesions
malignant lymphoma	with	– pseudolymphoma
plasmacytoma	with	– chronic inflammation dominated by plasma cells

Tumors of the nasopharynx

Roof: extends from the level of the junction of the hard and soft palate to the base of the skull.

Lateral wall: including the fossa of Rosenmüller.

Inferior wall: consists of the superior surface of the soft palate.

T – primary tumor

Tis   = preinvasive carcinoma (carcinoma in situ)

T 0   = no evidence of primary tumor

T 1   = tumor confined to one site (including tumor identified from positive biopsy)

T 2   = tumor involving two sites

T 3   = tumor with extension to the nasal cavity and/or oropharynx

T 4   = tumor with extension to the base of the skull and/or involving the cranial nerves

T x   = the minimal requirements to assess the primary tumor cannot be met (clinical examination, endoscopy, and radiography)

N – regional lymph nodes

(cervival nodes)

N 0   = no evidence of regional lymph node involvement

N 1   = evidence of involvement of the movable homolateral regional lymph nodes

N 2   = evidence of involvement of the movable contralateral or bilateral regional lymph nodes

N 3   = evidence of involvement of the fixed regional lymph nodes

N x   = the minimal requirements to assess the regional lymph nodes cannot be met (clinical examination)

M – distant metastases

M 0   = no evidence of distant metastases

M 1   = evidence of distant metastases

M x   = the minimal requirements to assess the presence of distant metastases cannot be met (clinical examination and radiography)

pTNM – postsurgical histopathological classification

the pTNM categories correspond to the TNM categories

Stage grouping

Stage I	T 1	N 0	M 0
Stage II	T 2	N 0	M 0
Stage III	T 3	N 0	M 0
	T 1, T 2, T 3	N 0	M 0
Stage IV	T 4	N 0, N 1	M 0
	any T	N 2, N 3	M 0
	any T	any N	M 1

M-8070/3
M-8082/3
T 147.9

1. Nasopharyngeal carcinoma (WHO)

(squamous cell carcinoma; lymphoepithelial carcinoma; lymphoepithelioma; undifferentiated carcinoma of nasopharyngeal type – WHO)

General Remarks

Incidence: Lymphoepithelial carcinoma is the most frequent tumor of the lymphoepithelial mucosa.

About 30% of malignant tumors of the nasopharynx are lymphoepithelial carcinomas.

Age: This tumor affects younger patients more frequently than older patients: men in their 3rd decade are particularly often encountered.

Sex: Males are more frequently affected than females.

T 147.0
T 147.2

Site: Main sites of origin are the wall or the roof of the nasopharynx, the area of the fossa of Rosenmüller, and the region around the Eustachian tube.

Further notes: This tumor is rather frequently observed in the Chinese and Korean populations.

Macroscopy

The tumor is soft and has a grayish-whitish cut surface. The tumor can be small (Fig. 469) (and remain undetected clinically).

Histology

The lymphoepithelial carcinoma is composed of malignant epithelial cells, which are admixed with lymphocytes (Fig. 470).

The epithelial cells show the signs of an undifferentiated carcinoma with important pleomorphism of the cells, which can be spindle-shaped, polygonal, or round. The hyperchromasia of the pleomorphic nuclei is important. There are numerous atypical mitotic figures. The nuclei are often clear and have a centrally located prominent nucleolus (Fig. 471). The cell borders are indistinct (Fig. 472).

The tumor cells form large fascicles **(Régaud type)** or they form a diffuse growth pattern **(Schmincke type)** (Fig. 473).

The dense lymphocytic infiltration is an inflammatory reaction; the lymphocytic part is not malignant.

The tumor cells infiltrate into the lymphatics.

Electron Microscopy

The tumor cells show signs of epithelial cells with tonofibrils.

Differential Diagnosis

Lymphoepithelial carcinoma **with malignant lymphoma:**

This differential diagnosis is indicated by the aspect of the nuclei, which are vesicular and pale and contain a prominent nucleolis, therefore resembling the histiocytic type of malignant lymphoma.

Reticulin stain will show that in the carcinoma the tumor cells are grouped together by fibers, which is not the case in malignant lymphoma.

Cytological examination including PAS stain of the cells might show signs of malignant lymphoma (PAS-positive droplets in the cytoplasm in cases of immunoblastoma) (Fig. 1258).

However, it might be difficult to separate the carcinoma from the malignant lymphoma.

The use of electron microscopy might be helpful in recognizing epithelial structures in cases of carcinoma.

Lymphoepithelial carcinoma

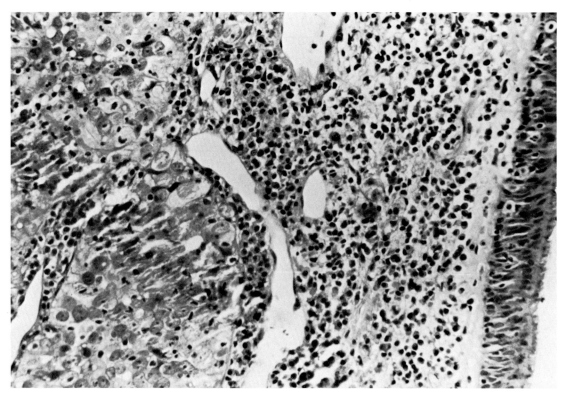

Fig. 469. Small nest of transitional cell carcinoma underneath the mucosa of the maxilla (73-year-old male, × 200).

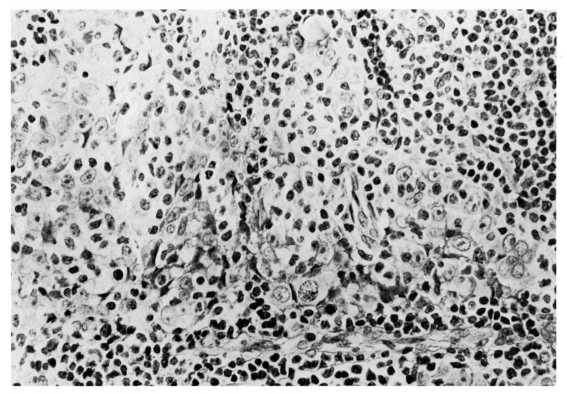

Fig. 470. Lymphoepithelial carcinoma of the epipharynx (× 200).

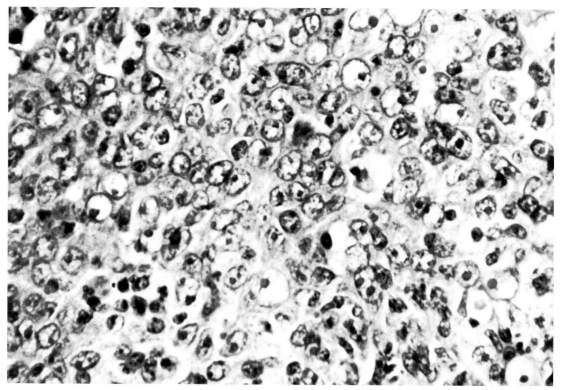

Fig. 471. Lymphoepithelial carcinoma: Vesicular nuclei with nucleoli (70-year-old female, × 310).

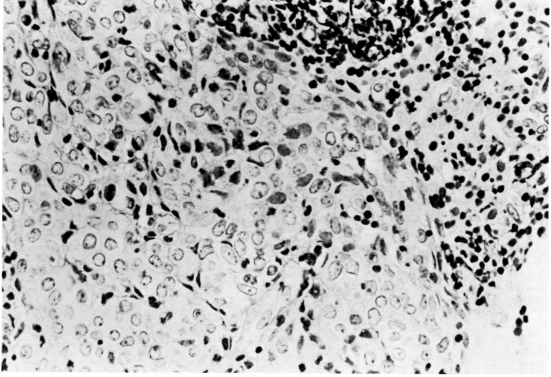

Fig. 472. Lymphoepithelial carcinoma: Indistinct cell borders and vesicular nuclei (× 200).

469

Spread

1. Early and rapid lymphatic spread into the regional cervical lymph nodes and further lymph nodes.
2. Hematogenous metastases into lung, bone, and other organs.

Clinical Findings

Lymphoepithelial carcinomas are often very small; the metastatic lesions might be, therefore, rather frequently the first sign of the tumor.

Lymphoepithelial carcinoma is associated with a high antibody titer to Epstein-Barr virus. This might be helpful in recognizing the lymphoepithelial carcinoma or detecting occult carcinomas [21, 101].

Treatment

Lymphoepithelial carcinomas are frequently disseminated at the time of diagnosis.

Therefore, the tumor should be treated by **radiation therapy.** The tumor cells are radiosensitive (recommended dose up to 60 Gy in about 6 weeks) [3].

Malignant lymphoepithelial carcinoma in children should also be treated by radiation therapy [25]. Prophylactic irradiation of the neck can be used to prevent lymph node metastases if the primary site of the tumor is under control [55].

Prognosis

The 5-year survival rate is about 40% [26].

M-9160/0
T 147.9

2. Nasopharyngeal (juvenile) angiofibroma (WHO)

General Remarks

Incidence: This is an uncommon tumor.

Age: The tumor affects young patients (young adults and adolescents) usually between 10 and 25 years old. Very rarely the tumor occurs in elderly patients [73].

Sex: Angiofibroma is almost always encountered in males [95].

Site: The majority of angiofibromas arise from the posterior nasal base and the wall of the nasopharyngeal cavity.

Further notes: It is debated whether myofibroblast is the cell of origin for angiofibromas [116].

Macroscopy

Angiofibromas are large tumors that have a reddish-whitish cut surface.

They are not encapsulated, smooth and lobulated, or nodular.

Some of the angiomas are pedunculated, and some are sessile. The tumor can occlude both posterior nasal orifices.

Histology

Angiofibromas are composed of numerous blood vessels. The blood vessel walls contain smooth muscle fibers. The lumen of the blood vessels is large. The blood vessels are surrounded by connective tissue (Fig. 474). Angiofibromas are covered by respiratory epithelium, which might show considerable squamous cell metaplasia.

---

[3] Ammon et al. 1978.
[21] Coates et al. 1978.
[25] Deutsch et al. 1978.
[26] Dold and Sack 1975.
[55] Hoppe et al. 1976.
[73] McGavran et al. 1969.
[95] Rominger and Santore 1968.
[101] Schmauz et al. 1975.
[116] Taxy 1977.

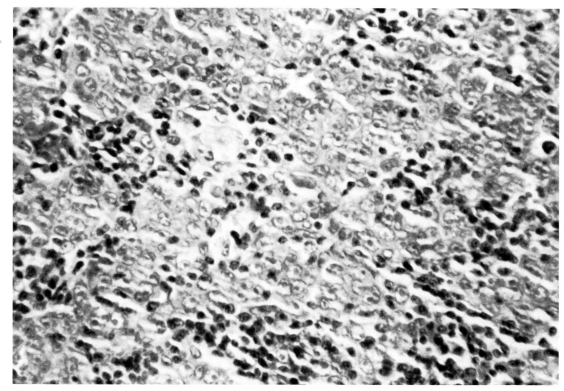

Fig. 473. Lymphoepithelial carcinoma: Diffuse growth pattern (Schmincke type) (×200).

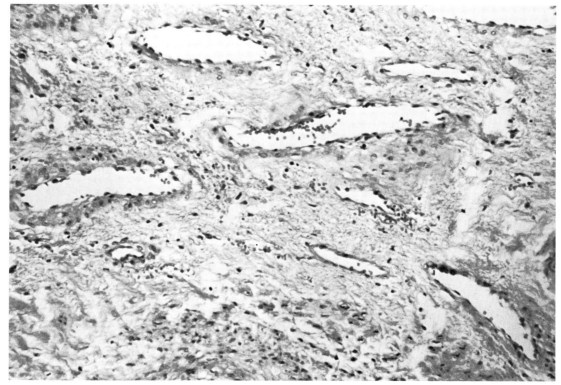

Fig. 474. Angiofibroma of the nose (×125).

Clinical Findings

Local symptoms due to the growth of the tumor, with nasal obstruction and deformation of the face or soft palate.

Treatment

Surgical removal of the tumor.
The surgical intervention can be complicated by severe hemorrhages.

Prognosis

Angiofibromas might recur or regress spontaneously (after puberty).

M-8140/3
T 147.9

3. Adenocarcinoma (WHO)

General Remarks

Incidence: Adenocarcinomas in the nasopharynx are rare tumors.
Site: The tumor grows in the nasopharynx or the paranasal sinuses and the nasal cavity.
Further notes: The tumor originates from the cells of the respiratory epithelium (Schneiderian mucosa).

Histology

The tumor is composed of malignant cells, which grow in a glandular pattern. The tumor cells produce mucin.
Occasionally this tumor is composed of clear cells, which are similar to renal cell carcinomas.
Besides the glandular structures the tumor cells often grow in a papillary fashion.

Spread

1. The tumor infiltrates the surrounding tissue.
2. Hematogenous and lymph node metastases occur late.

Treatment

Surgery.
Radiation therapy:
However, the tumor cells are not very sensitive to irradiation [3].

---

[3] Ammon et al. 1978.

M-8070/3
T 147.9

4. Squamous cell carcinoma (WHO)

**General
Remarks**

Incidence: About 40% of the tumors of the nasopharynx are squamous cell carcinomas.
Age: The majority of patients are in the 5th decade.
Sex: Males are more frequently affected than females.
Further notes: There is a strong geographic difference in the occurrence of this tumor.
Smoking habits or chronic inflammation of the nose and throat as well as exposure to
fumes and chemicals are considered to be risk factors.

Histology

The majority of the squamous cell carcinomas of the nasopharynx are poorly differentiated.

Spread

Early local infiltration and lymphatic spread into the regional lymph nodes.
The tumor might be undetected at its primary site while metastases dominate the clinical
picture.

Treatment

Surgery.
Radiation therapy:
Up to 60 Gy in 5 to 6 weeks.

Prognosis

The 5-year survival rate is about 40%.

T 147.9

5. Soft tissue tumors (WHO)

The different types of soft tissue tumors can rarely develop in the nasopharynx (see
page 7).

M-9730/3
M-9590/3
T 147.9

6. Plasmacytoma, malignant lymphoma (WHO)

Plasmacytomas and malignant lymphomas are also observed as primary tumors in the
nasopharynx (see page 1247).

Tumors of the oropharynx

T – primary tumor

Tis = preinvasive carcinoma (carcinoma in situ)

T 0 = no evidence of primary tumor

T 1 = tumor 2 cm or less in its greatest dimension

T 2 = tumor more than 2 cm but not more than 4 cm in its greatest dimension

T 3 = tumor more than 4 cm in its greatest dimension

T 4 = tumor with extension to bone, muscle, skin, antrum, neck, etc.

T x = the minimal requirements to assess the primary tumor cannot be met (clinical examination, endoscopy, and radiography)

N – regional lymph nodes

(cervical nodes)

N 0 = no evidence of regional lymph node involvement

N 1 = evidence of involvement of the movable homolateral regional lymph nodes

N 2 = evidence of involvement of the movable contralateral or bilateral regional lymph nodes

N 3 = evidence of involvement of the fixed regional lymph nodes

N x = the minimal requirements to assess the regional lymph nodes cannot be met (clinical examination)

M – distant metastases

M 0 = no evidence of distant metastases

M 1 = evidence of distant metastases

M x = the minimal requirements to assess the presence of distant metastases cannot be met (clinical examination and radiography)

pTNM – postsurgical histopathological classification

the pTNM categories correspond to the TNM categories

Stage grouping

Stage I	T 1	N 0	M 0
Stage II	T 2	N 0	M 0
Stage III	T 3	N 0	M 0
	T 1, T 2, T 3	N 1	M 0
Stage IV	T 4	N 0, N 1	M 0
	any T	N 2, N 3	M 0
	any T	any N	M 1

M-8070/3
T 146.0

1. Squamous cell carcinoma of the tonsil (WHO)

**General
Remarks**

Incidence: Carcinoma of the tonsil is a relatively uncommon tumor (about 1% of all malignant tumors). Carcinomas of the tonsils and of the larynx are the most common tumors in the head and neck.
Age: The peak age is the 5th to 7th decades.
Carcinomas at this location in patients under 40 years of age are rare.
Site: Squamous cell carcinomas are unilateral tumors.

Macroscopy

The tonsil is enlarged. The tumor can grow as a papillary lesion, or the surface is ulcerated.
The carcinoma is often surrounded by leukoplakia.
On touch the tumor bleeds easily.

Histology

The majority of squamous cell carcinomas of the tonsil are of the poorly differentiated type (Figs. 475 to 477). The tumor develops from the surface epithelium and infiltrates into the underlying tissue and the lateral wall of the oropharynx.
The degree of differentiation changes with the depth of infiltration:
Although at the surface the tumor might have signs of well-differentiated cells, the deeper tissue is involved by poorly differentiated carcinoma (Figs. 449 and 450).

Spread

1. Local infiltration of the surrounding tissue.
2. Lymph node metastases into the cervical lymph nodes and the lymph nodes underneath the mandibula.
3. Distant metastases are rare (occurring in about 5% of the cases).

**Clinical
Findings**

Persistent unilateral pain and dysphagia.

Treatment

Surgery and **irradiation:**
Surgical removal. Irradiation up to 80 Gy in 7 to 8 weeks.
The surgery can be preceded by irradiation.
The surgery can include neck dissection.
Since occult lymph node metastases are relatively frequent, irradiation of the regional lymph nodes (up to 70 Gy) is recommended [111].

Prognosis

The overall 5-year survival rate is about 40 to 50%.
In the individual case the prognosis depends on the extent of the tumor at the time of diagnosis and the existence of lymph node metastases [60, 69].
T 1, N 0 = 5-year survival, 100%
T 2, N 0 = 5-year survival, 60%
T 3, N 0 = 5-year survival, 37.5%
T 4, N 0 = 5-year survival, 25% [33].

---

[33] Fligiel and Kaneko 1975.
[60] Johnston and Byers 1977.
[69] Mantravadi et al. 1978.
[111] Snow et al. 1977.

Squamous cell carcinoma – tonsil

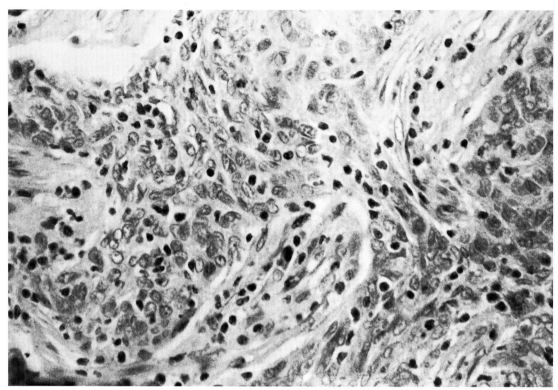

Fig. 475. Poorly differentiated squamous cell carcinoma (Grade III) of the tonsil (× 200).

Prognosis

The 5-year survival rate after radiation therapy alone:
42% without lymph node metastases
20% with lymph node metastases

Further Information

A small percentage of poorly differentiated carcinomas of the tonsils (about 5%) have the histological structure of lymphoepithelial carcinoma.
In these instances the differential diagnosis with malignant lymphoma of the tonsil might be difficult.

476

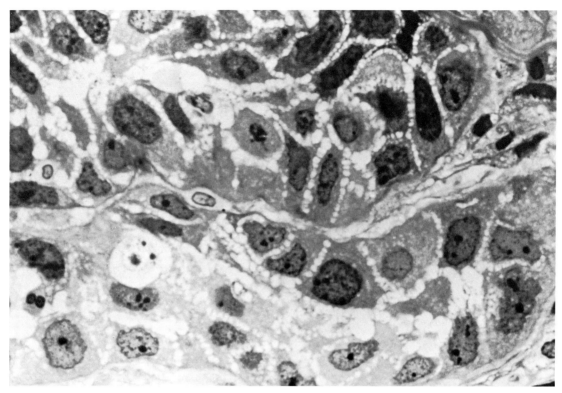

Fig. 476. Well-differentiated squamous cell carcinoma: Tonofibrils, moderate nuclear atypias (67-year-old male, × 600).

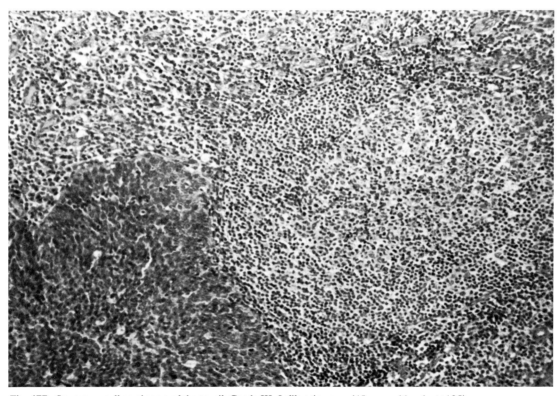

Fig. 477. Squamous cell carcinoma of the tonsil, Grade III: Infiltrating area (45-year-old male, × 125).

477

M-9590/3
T 146.0
T 149.1

2. Malignant lymphoma of the tonsil and Waldeyer's ring

The lymphoepithelial tissue of the oropharynx can be affected by all types of malignant non-Hodgkin's lymphomas (Figs. 478 to 480), including plasmacytomas.
The involvement of the tonsils is often unilateral.
Malignant lymphomas are observed in younger patients, including children.

Differential
Diagnosis

1. Malignant lymphoma **with mononucleosis** (Figs. 481 and 482).
2. Malignant lymphoma **with lymphoepithelial carcinoma** (Figs. 470 to 472).
3. **Hodgkin's disease** of the tonsils is exceedingly rare.

Treatment

1. Primary malignant lymphoma of the lymphoepithelial tissue: **Radiation therapy,** (up to 50 Gy) eventually followed by **surgery.**
2. In cases of disseminated tumor, **chemotherapy** (see page 1247).

M-8140/3
T 146.9

3. Adenocarcinoma

Adenocarcinoma in the oropharynx is rare.

M-8720/3
T 146.9

4. Malignant melanoma (WHO)

Malignant melanomas can be observed in the oropharynx, especially in the uvula [42].

M-9040/3
T 146.9

5. Synovial sarcoma (Figs. 129 to 132)

There is a report of a synovial sarcoma in the soft tissue of the pharyngeal region. These tumors are very rare [97].

---

[42] Gamel et al. 1978.
[97] Roth et al. 1975.

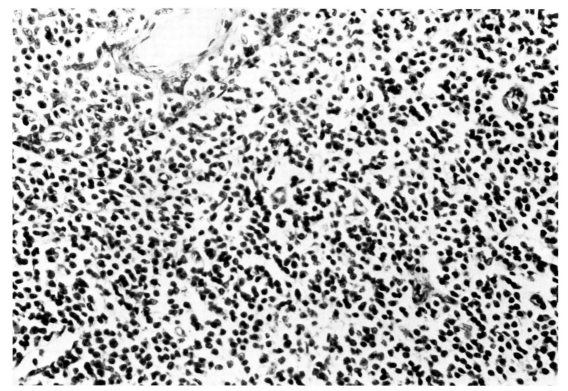

Fig. 478. Malignant lymphoma of the tonsil (66-year-old female, × 200).

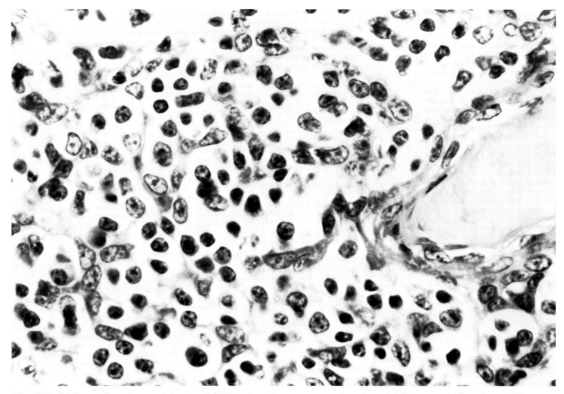

Fig. 479. Malignant lymphoma of the tonsil (diffuse lymphosarcoma, prolymphocytic) (66-year-old female, × 400).

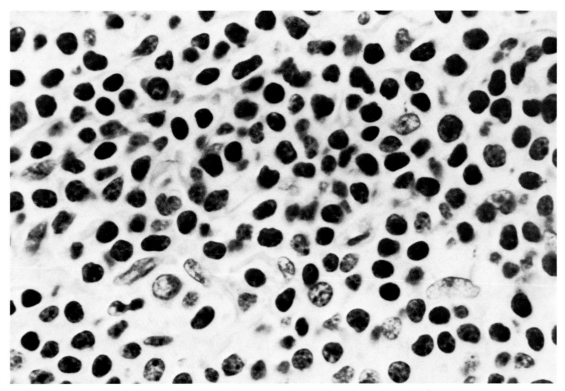

Fig. 480. Malignant lymphoma of the tonsil (diffuse lymphosarcoma, lymphoplasmacytic) (58-year-old male, × 800).

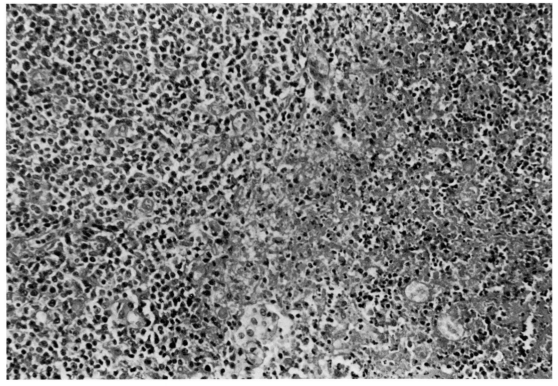

Fig. 481. Infectious mononucleosis of the tonsil: Area of necrosis (19-year-old female, × 125).

480

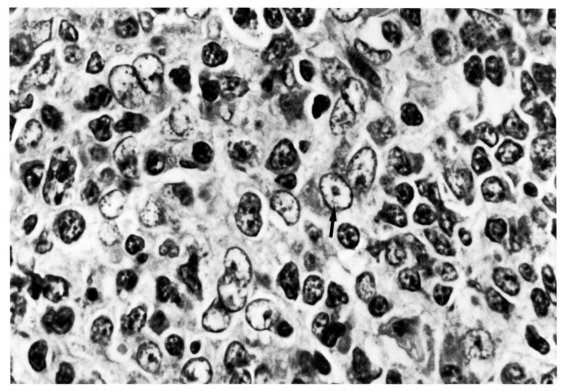

Fig. 482. Infectious mononucleosis of the tonsil: Mononucleosis cells (immunoblasts – arrow) (19-year-old female, ×800).

Tumors of the hypopharynx
(postcricoid area, piriform sinus, posterior pharyngeal wall)

T – primary tumor

Tis = preinvasive carcinoma (carcinoma in situ)

T 0 = no evidence of primary tumor

T 1 = tumor confined to one site

T 2 = tumor with extension to an adjacent site or region without fixation of the hemi-larynx

T 3 = tumor with extension to an adjacent site or region with fixation of the hemi-larynx

T 4 = tumor with extension to bone, cartilage, or soft tissue

T x = the minimal requirements to assess the primary tumor cannot be met (clinical examination, endoscopy, and radiography)

N – regional lymph nodes
(cervical nodes)

N 0 = no evidence of lymph node involvement

N 1 = evidence of involvement of the movable homolateral regional lymph nodes

N 2 = evidence of involvement of the movable contralateral or bilateral regional lymph nodes

N 3 = evidence of involvement of the fixed regional lymph nodes

N x = the minimal requirements to assess the regional lymph nodes cannot be met (clinical examination)

M – distant metastases

M 0 = no evidence of distant metastases

M 1 = evidence of distant metastases

M x = the minimal requirements to assess the presence of distant metastases cannot be met (clinical examination and radiography)

pTNM – postsurgical histopathological classification
the pTNM categories correspond to the TNM categories

Stage grouping

Stage I	T 1	N 0	M 0
Stage II	T 2	N 0	M 0
Stage III	T 3	N 0	M 0
	T 1, T 2, T 3	N 1	M 0
Stage IV	T 4	N 0, N 1	M 0
	any T	N 2, N 3	M 0
	any T	any N	M 1

M-8070/3
T 148.9

1. Squamous cell carcinoma (WHO)

General Remarks

Incidence: Carcinomas of the hypopharynx are rare. The majority (about 80%) of these tumors are squamous cell carcinomas.
Age: The peak age is the 5th to 7th decades.
Sex: Females are considerably more frequently affected than males.
Site: Squamous cell carcinomas can occur at one of the above-mentioned sites; of special interest is the

M-8070/3
T 148.0
General Remarks

Postcricoid squamous cell carcinoma

Incidence: Postcricoid carcinomas develop mostly in elderly or middle-aged women. Postcricoid carcinoma is occasionally associated with squamous cell carcinoma of the tongue and the buccal mucosa and carcinoma of the lip.

Macroscopy

The tumor develops in the postcricoid area of the hypopharynx without infiltrating the larynx.

Histology

The tumor is composed of malignant squamous cells, which are well differentiated.

Spread

1. Local infiltration into the larynx is very rare; the cartilage of the thyroid is more often involved.
2. Infiltration into the lymphatics with regional lymph node metastases.

Clinical Findings

a) Signs of stenosis at the pharynx.
b) Postcricoid carcinomas are often associated with iron and vitamin deficiency and atrophic epithelium on the lips, oropharynx, and esophagus with dysphagia, achlorhydria, and hypochromic anemia.

Treatment

Surgery:
Radical surgery [109].
Radiation therapy:
Up to 70 Gy in 5 to 7 weeks.
Postoperative radiotherapy seems to give a better 5-year survival rate than preoperative irradiation [118, 119].

Prognosis

Carcinoma of the hypopharynx:
5-year survival, 31%
5-year survival after low-dose preoperative radiation and partial laryngopharyngectomy, 59%.
5-year survival after total laryngectomy, partial pharyngectomy, and irradiation, 21%.
5-year survival with palliative radiation, surgery, or chemotherapy, 4% [70].

---

[70] Marks et al. 1978.
[109] Shepperd 1977.
[118] Taylor 1977.
[119] Vandenbrouck et al. 1977.

**Further
Information**

a) Exceedingly rare are **adenocarcinomas** (WHO) in the postcricoid area.
b) The histology of the lymph nodes in the draining area of carcinomas of the head and neck could perhaps be related to a certain degree to the prognosis:
Lymph nodes with a depleted lymphocytic pattern seem to indicate a poorer prognosis than lymph nodes with an increased number of germinal centers [10, 22].

**M-8070/3
T 146.8**

2. Squamous cell carcinoma originating in a branchial cleft

On very rare occasions a squamous cell carcinoma, infiltrating or in situ, can develop in the epithelium of a branchiogenic cleft. The wall of the cleft should be identified to determine that the squamous cell carcinoma originates in the wall (containing lymphoid tissue) (Figs. 483 and 484) [96].

[10] Berlinger et al. 1976.
[22] Cottier et al. 1972.
[96] Rossberg and Rosemann 1964.

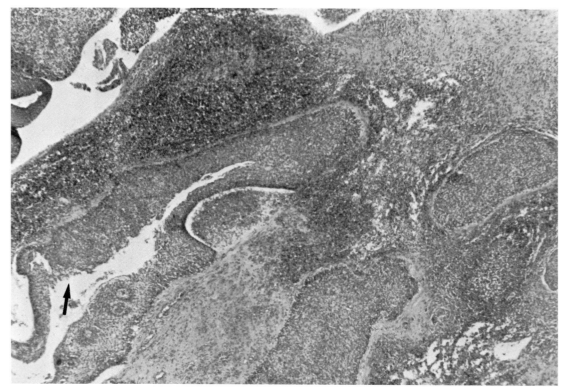

Fig. 483. Branchiogenic carcinoma originating from the wall of the cyst (arrow) (44-year-old male, × 40).

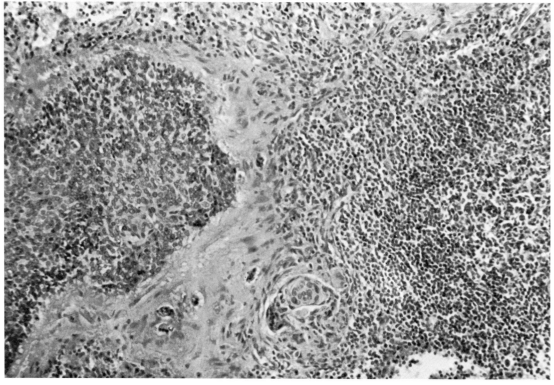

Fig. 484. Branchiogenic carcinoma, infiltrating area (see Fig. 483) (× 125).

3. Tumor-like lesions (WHO)

M-2650/0
T 193.9

a) Thyroglossal duct cyst

Thyroglossal duct cysts are localized in the midline of the neck.
The cysts are lined by squamous cell epithelium or respiratory epithelium. Both cell types can be present in one cyst. The wall does not contain lymphoid tissue (Fig. 485).
It has been reported that very rarely a carcinoma can develop from the epithelium of a thyroglossal duct cyst [61].

(M-2270/7)
M-9172/0
T 171.0

b) Hygroma cysticum colli congenitum

This lesion is composed of a multilocular lymphangioma growing at the base of the neck. The tumor occurs in childhood.

M-9351/0

c) Hamartoma

Hamartomas are very rarely found in the neck or in the tongue.

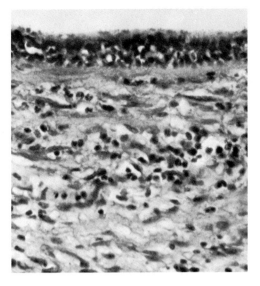

Fig. 485. Thyroglossal duct cyst lined by respiratory epithelium (64-year-old female, × 200).

[61] Joseph and Komorowski 1975.

T 160.0
T 160.9

Tumors of the nose and paranasal sinuses

1. Nasal and paranasal papilloma

M-8121/0, 1

(Schneiderian papilloma)

(Ewing's papilloma)

M-8053/0 (transitional cell papilloma, inverted type – WHO)

M-8052/0 (squamous cell papilloma – WHO)

**General
Remarks**

Incidence: Compared with the nasal (inflammatory) polyps, the papillomatous neoplasms are relatively rare lesions [112].

Age: The neoplasm can occur at any age; however, the older age group is more frequently affected.

Sex: These tumors are more frequently observed in men than in women.

Site: These papillomas can occur in one or both nasal cavities, in the nasal sinuses, or in both.

Macroscopy

Papillomas can be solitary or multiple polypoid neoplasms. They have a grayish-whitish cut surface. Their consistency is firmer than the nasal mucosa in cases of polyps.

Easy bleeding might occur if the papillomas are touched.

The majority of papillomas have a space-occupying, exophytic growth pattern. Occasionally, however, the tumor can grow into the mucosa and only a small polypoid tumor is detected (inverted papilloma).

Histology

The origin of the papilloma is the respiratory epithelium. Papillomas are therefore covered by columnar cells; among them mucin-producing cells can occasionally be detected (Figs. 486 and 487).

Other papillomas are covered by squamous cell layers. In these cases keratin layers can be found.

The epithelial cell layers in papillomas do not infiltrate the submucosa. However, occasionally the epithelium might contain foci of atypical cells (dysplasias) (Fig. 488) or foci of carcinoma in situ.

In about 10% of the cases, infiltrating carcinomatous growth develops.

These foci of infiltrating carcinoma might be hidden in the large papillomatous masses; multiple sections and a careful search for those foci are therefore required.

**Differential
Diagnosis**

1. Nasal (and paranasal) papilloma **with inflammatory polyp:**

   Inflammatory polyps are covered by regular respiratory epithelium, which is supported by a loose connective tissue containing plasma cells, lymphocytes, and eosinophilic granulocytes (Fig. 489). Inflammatory polyps are often bilateral.

2. Inverted papilloma **with infiltrating squamous cell carcinoma:**

   The basal layer in inverted papillomas is intact and separates the epithelium from the underlying connective tissue. However, cellular atypias and mitoses can be observed in inverted papillomas (Figs. 490 to 497).

   Inverted papillomas are usually localized in the lateral wall of the nasal cavity.

---

[112] Snyder and Perzin 1972.

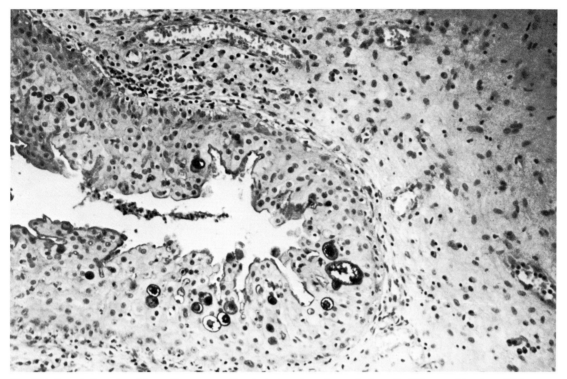

Fig. 486. Inverted nasal papilloma: Squamous cell metaplasia and mucin-producing cells (68-year-old male, × 125).

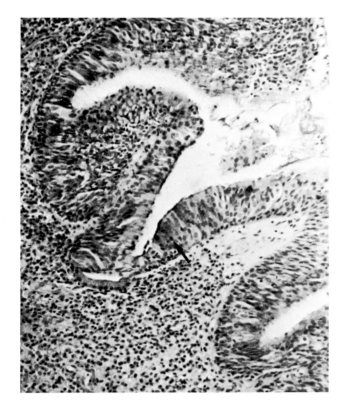

Fig. 487. Nasal polyp with small foci of squamous cell metaplasia (arrow) (78-year-old female, × 125).

488

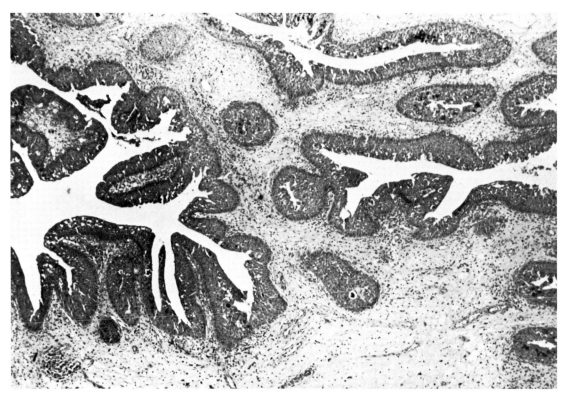

Fig. 488. Inverted nasal papilloma: Squamous cell metaplasia and dysplasia (68-year-old male, × 40).

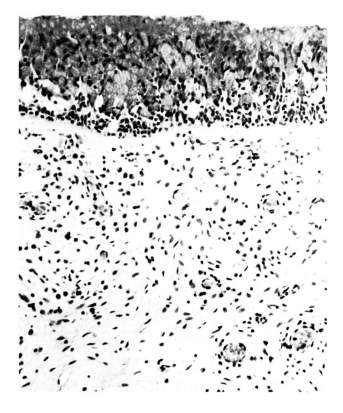

Fig. 489. Inflammatory polyp of the nose: Respiratory epithelium (21-year-old female, × 50).

489

Nasal papilloma

Clinical Findings   Signs of nasal obstruction.

Treatment   **Surgical removal** of the tumor.

In cases of malignant tumor (carcinoma), a combined treatment with surgery and **radiation therapy** including **chemotherapy** should be attempted according to the individual situation [34].

Prognosis

1. Nasal and paranasal papillomas are usually benign tumors.
2. About 70% of the cases recur.
   The recurrence cannot be predicted by histological findings.
3. The danger of recurrence is particularly high when the extent of the disease is great and elderly patients are affected.
4. About 3% of the cases develop a carcinoma after several recurrences [92].
   However, very rarely the transition of an initial papilloma into a carcinoma can be demonstrated [66].
5. A squamous cell carcinoma developing in a papilloma was most probably malignant from the beginning.

---

[34] Frommhold et al. 1978.
[66] Lasser et al. 1976.
[92] Ridolfi et al. 1977.

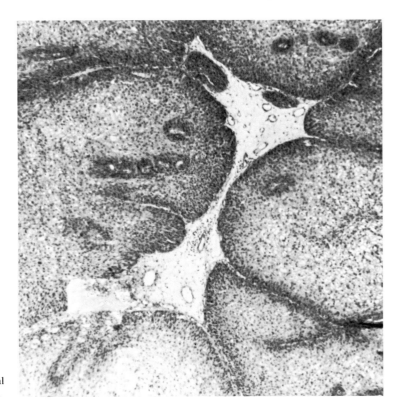

Fig. 490. Inverted keratotic nasal papilloma (64-year-old male, ×40).

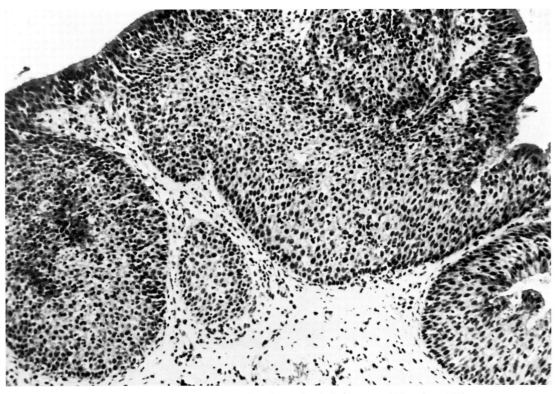

Fig. 491. Inverted nasal papilloma: Inflammation and moderate dysplasia (64-year-old female, ×125).

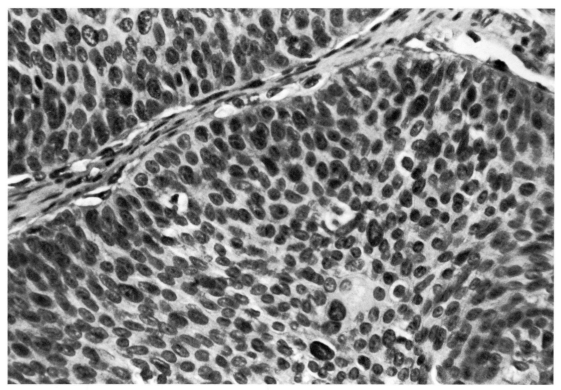

Fig. 492. Inverted nasal papilloma: Foci of atypical nuclei, no infiltration (64-year-old male, × 200).

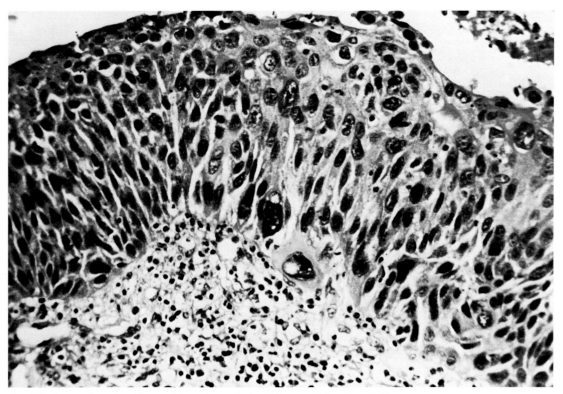

Fig. 493. Inverted nasal papilloma with carcinoma in situ (64-year-old female, × 200).

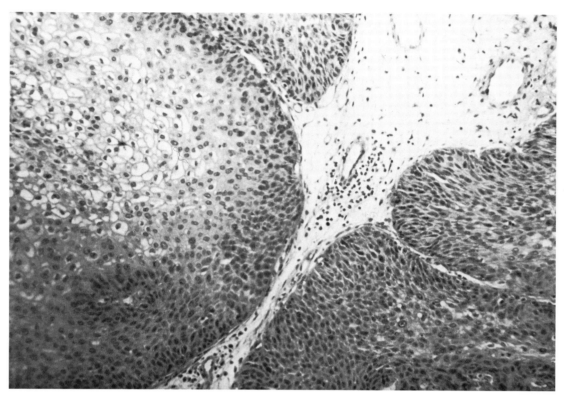

Fig. 494. Inverted keratotic nasal papilloma: Foci of dysplasia, no infiltration (64-year-old male, × 125).

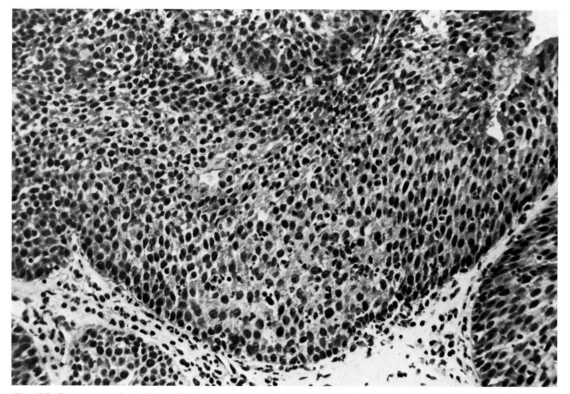

Fig. 495. Inverted nasal papilloma: Slight dysplasia and inflammation, no infiltration (64-year-old female, × 200).

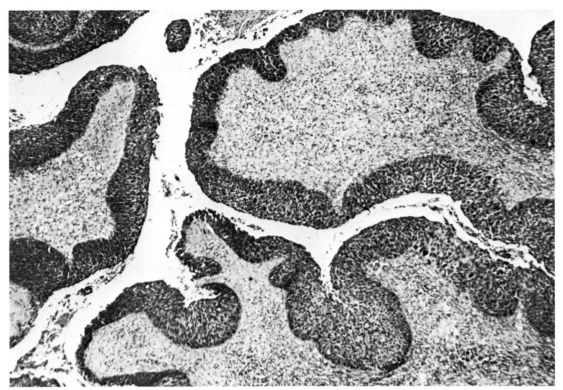

Fig. 496. Inverted nasal papilloma with extensive carcinoma in situ (64-year-old female, × 40).

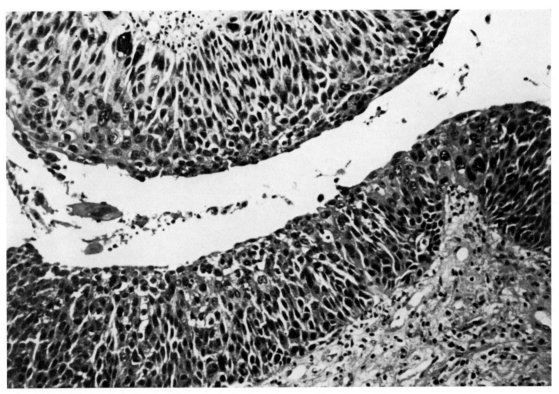

Fig. 497. Inverted nasal papilloma with carcinoma in situ (64-year-old female, × 125).

494

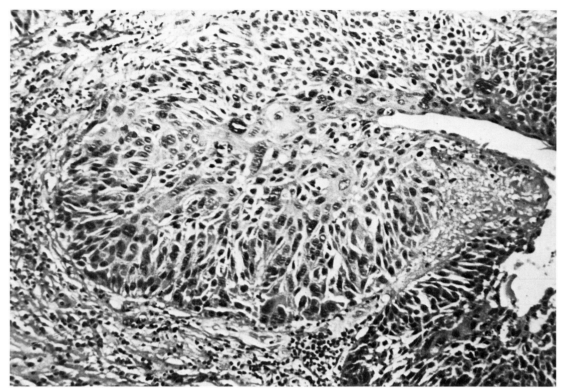

Fig. 498. Exophytic and inverted nasal papilloma: Area of carcinoma (64-year-old female, × 200).

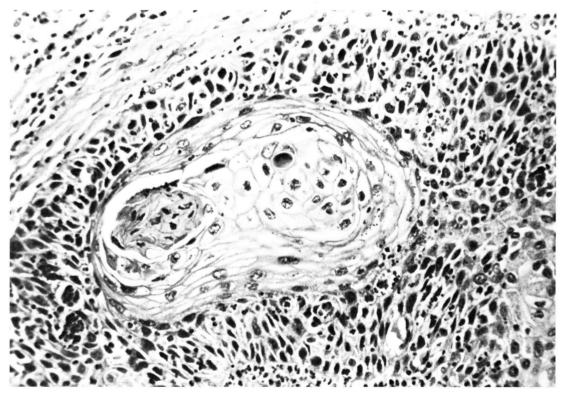

Fig. 499. Papillomatous carcinoma of the nose with squamous cell metaplasia (64-year-old female, × 200).

M-8070/3
T 160.0, 9

2. Squamous cell carcinoma (WHO)

General Remarks

Incidence: Squamous cell carcinomas at this location are rare tumors; however, they are the most common malignant tumors in this region.
Age: Patients of the older age group are most commonly affected.
Sex: Men are more frequently affected than women.

Macroscopy

Squamous cell carcinoma presents mostly as a verrucous-papillomatous tumor.

Histology
M-8052/3

The tumor is composed of malignant squamous cells, which grow in a **papillary pattern.** The degree of differentiation in this tumor is different from area to area (Figs. 498 to 501).

M-8122/3

– Admixture of spindle cells and squamous cells: **Spindle cell carcinoma** (WHO).

M-8121/3

– Tumor composed of transitional epithelium-like cells: **"Transitional" carcinoma** (WHO).

M-8051/3

– Very rarely the tumor cells grow in the **verrucous type of squamous cell carcinoma.**

Differential Diagnosis

Squamous cell carcinoma **with benign papilloma** (Figs. 488 to 497):
The differential diagnosis might be difficult, especially in cases of highly differentiated squamous cell carcinomas versus papillomas with numerous atypias.
The decision is made on evidence of malignant infiltration into the underlying tissue (occasionally multiple sections are required to ascertain this finding).

Spread

1. The tumor infiltrates locally.
2. Lymphatic spread into the regional lymph nodes: About 10% of the patients already have lymph node metastases at the time of admission to the hospital.
3. Hematogenous metastases are relatively rare and occur late.

Treatment

Extensive tumors are treated by combined **surgery** and **chemotherapy** (bleomycin) [2].
Localized, early carcinomas might be treated by surgery of alternatively by **radiation therapy** (up 80 Gy in 7 to 8 weeks) [76].

Prognosis

The overall 5-year survival rate is about 30 to 40%.
The 5-year survival rate for very small carcinomas without lymph node metastases is about 90% [14].

---

[2] Alth and Kollabek 1976.
[14] Bosch et al. 1976.
[76] Müller et al. 1979.

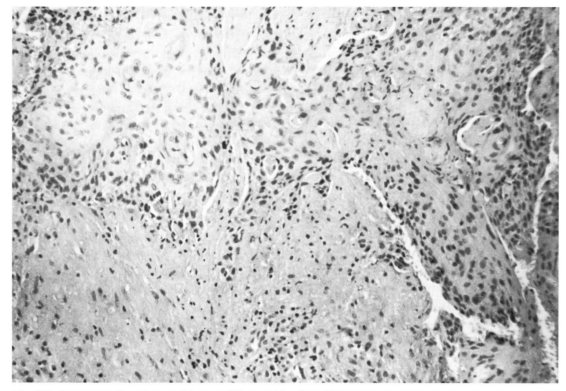

Fig. 500. Squamous cell carcinoma of the nose (67-year-old male, × 125).

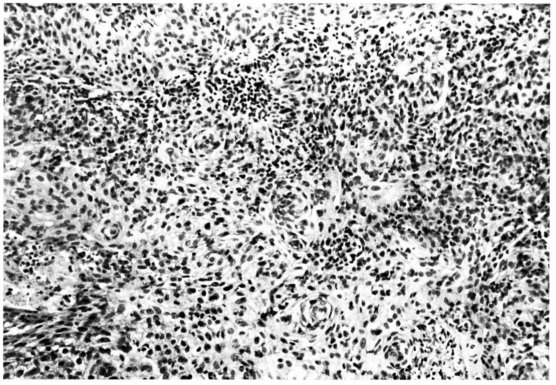

Fig. 501. Squamous cell carcinoma of the nose (Grade II) (67-year-old male, × 125).

M-8140/3
T 160.0, 9

3. Adenocarcinoma (WHO)

**General
Remarks**

Incidence: Adenocarcinomas at this location are very rare.
Of all carcinomas at this site about 5% are adenocarcinomas.
Age: The tumor is mostly observed in patients in the 5th decade.
Sex: Men are considerably more frequently affected than women.

Macroscopy

Exophytic mucinous tumor, soft, with a grayish-whitish cut surface.

Histology

M-8481/3

The adenocarcinoma at this location is a mucin-producing tumor. The tumor cells are columnar (Fig. 502). The glands that are formed by these tumor cells might be filled with mucin. The tumor has a resemblance to adenocarcinoma of the colon [98].
Occasionally adenocarcinomas at this location grow in a fashion similar to a signet ring cell carcinoma [43].

Spread

1. Local invasion.
2. Lymphatic spread into lymph nodes.
3. Hematogenous metastases occur rarely and late in the course of the disease.

Treatment

Surgery, eventually combined with **chemotherapy.**

Prognosis

Adenocarcinomas recur frequently.
They are locally aggressive.
The overall 5-year survival rate is about 50%.

[43] Gamez-Araujo et al. 1975.
[98] Sanchez-Casis et al. 1971.

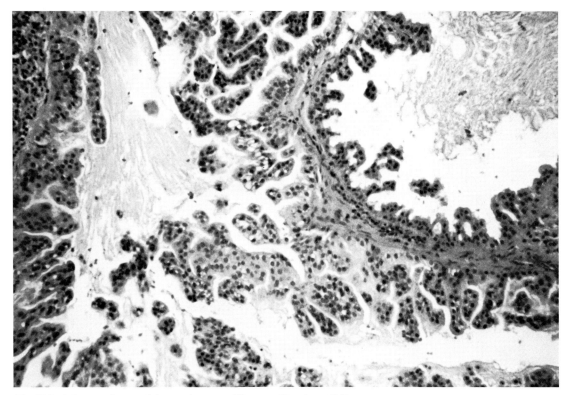

Fig. 502. Adenocarcinoma of the nasal mucosa (59-year-old male, × 125).

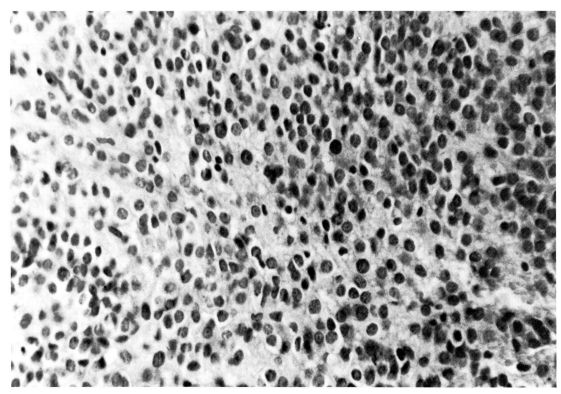

Fig. 503. Olfactory neuroblastoma: Rather cellular tumor, small cells, rather regular (26-year-old male, × 310).

M-9522/3
T 160.0

4. Olfactory neuroblastoma [9, 58]
(esthesioneuroblastoma; esthesioneuroma; olfactory neurogenic tumor – WHO)

General
Remarks
T 160.0
T 160.3
T 160.2

Incidence: Olfactory neuroblastomas are very rare tumors.
Site: Nasal cavity, often above the middle turbinate or at the site of the ethmoid sinus, at the cribriform plate, or even in the maxillary sinus [5].
Further notes: Most probably the tumor arises from the neuroectodermal olfactory membrane [52, 83].

Macroscopy

Polypoid tumor with a pink to whitish-grayish cut surface. The tumor contains hemorrhages and necroses.

Histology

Neuroblastomas are cellular tumors. The cells are small (similar to middle-sized lymphocytes) (Fig. 503). The chromatin is coarse or granular.
The cells look relatively uniform and grow in clusters. Occasionally rosette formation is observed.
The cytoplasm of these cells is scanty, and occasionally the impression prevails that naked nuclei compose the tumor. Between the tumor cells are fibrils (neurites), forming a network (Figs. 504 and 505). These neurofibrils are diagnostic for the tumor.

Electron
Microscopy

The ultrastructure of the tumor cell shows different degrees of neurosecretory granules in the cytoplasm [94, 117, 122].
The tumor cells contain microtubules, filaments, and secretory granules (Figs. 506 and 507) [83, 117].

Differential
Diagnosis

1. Olfactory neuroblastoma **with undifferentiated carcinoma.**
2. Olfactory neuroblastoma **with malignant lymphoma.**
3. Olfactory neuroblastoma **with amelanotic melanoma** (Figs. 508 to 510):
   The differential diagnosis might be difficult, especially between olfactory neuroblastoma and undifferentiated (small cell) carcinoma.
   Evidence of neurofibrils is an important finding for the diagnosis of olfactory neuroblastoma.
   When it is impossible to separate the different tumors by light microscopy, electron microscopy showing neurosecretory granules in the tumor cells might give the diagnosis (Figs. 506 and 507) [75].

Spread

1. Aggressive infiltration into the surrounding tissue (nasopharynx, orbit, base of the skull, brain).
2. Lymphatic spread into lymph nodes.
3. Hematogenous spread.
   About 30% of the cases develop metastases [81].

[5] Ash et al. 1964.
[9] Berger and Coutard 1926.
[52] Herrold 1964.
[58] Hutter et al. 1963.
[75] Micheau 1977.
[81] Obert et al. 1960.
[83] Osamura and Fine 1976.
[94] Romansky et al. 1978.
[117] Taxy and Hidvegi 1977.
[122] Wilander et al. 1977.

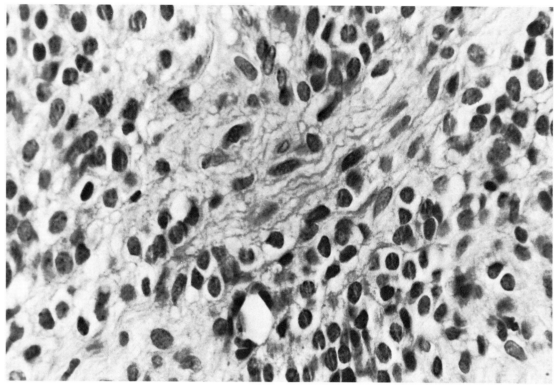

Fig. 504. Olfactory neuroblastoma: Numerous neurofibrils, oval nuclei, scanty cytoplasm (26-year-old male, × 500).

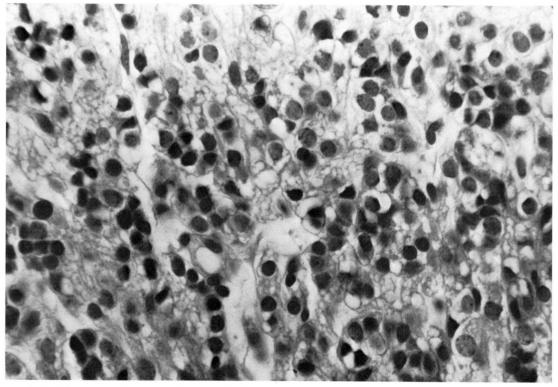

Fig. 505. Olfactory neuroblastoma: Note neurofibrils (26-year-old male, × 310).

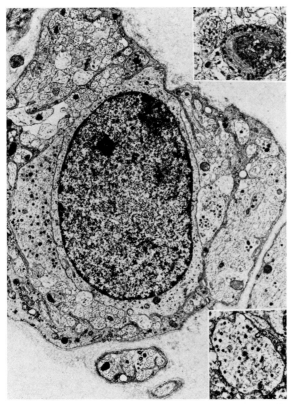

Fig. 506. Olfactory neuroblastoma (esthesioneuroblastoma): Tumor cells with microtubules and neurosecretory granules (×8200) (Taxy and Hidevegy, Cancer *39* (1977) 131-138).

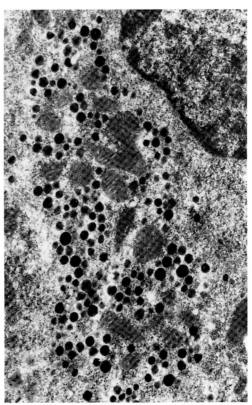

Fig. 507. Olfactory neuroblastoma (esthesioneuroblastoma): Neurosecretory granules (×14,800) (Wilander et al., Virchows Arch. A. Path. Anat. and Histol. *375* (1977) 125-128).

Clinical Findings	Recurrent epistaxis, anosmia, or nasal obstruction (unilateral).
Treatment	The tumor is radiosensitive: **Surgery** combined with **radiation therapy** has been recommended (30 to 40 Gy in 3 to 4 weeks).
	Chemotherapy:
	Several effective drugs are known: Cyclophosphamide, vincristine, adriamycin, prednisone, or the combination cyclophosphamide and vincristine.
Prognosis	Olfactory neuroblastomas are slow-growing tumors. The prognosis is more favorable than for neuroblastomas at other sites.
	However, the course of the disease is unpredictable [80].

[80] Oberman and Rice 1976.

M-8720/3
T 160.0, 9

5. Malignant melanoma (WHO)

Malignant melanomas at this site are rare. However, they are more frequently observed than benign nevi (Figs. 508 to 511) [54].

6. Soft tissue tumors (WHO)

T 160.0, 9

Soft tissue tumors in the nasal and paranasal sinuses are very rare (page 7).
A variety of different soft tissue tumors, however, have been observed:

M-8890/3

a) leiomyosarcoma [35],

M-8910/3

b) embryonal rhabdomyosarcoma [36], **rhabdomyoma** [36],

M-8850/0, 3

c) lipoma and liposarcoma [39, 99],

M-9540/0

d) neurofibroma,

M-8840/0

e) myxoma [38],

M-8810/0, 3
M-7610/0

f) fibroma, fibromatosis, and fibrosarcoma [37].

7. Tumors of the salivary glands

All types of salivary gland tumors can occur in the nose and paranasal sinuses (see page 561).

[35] Fu and Perzin 1975.
[36] Fu and Perzin 1976.
[37] Fu and Perzin 1976.
[38] Fu and Perzin 1977.
[39] Fu and Perzin 1977.
[54] Holdcraft and Gallagher 1969.
[99] Saunders et al. 1979.

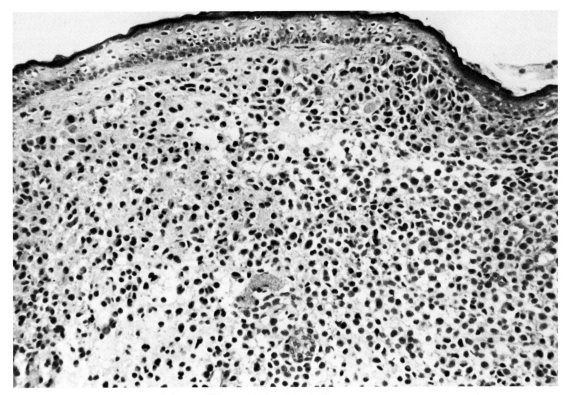

Fig. 508. Malignant melanoma of the nose (67-year-old female, ×125).

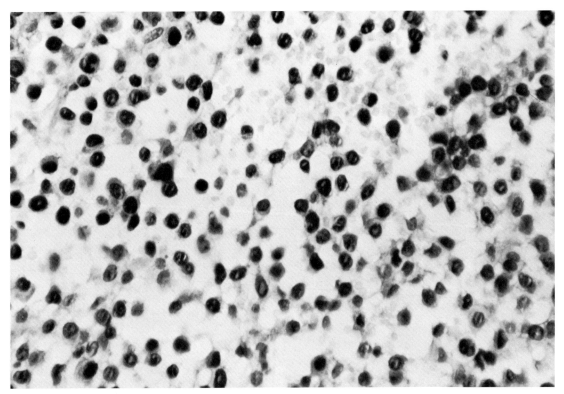

Fig. 509. Malignant melanoma of the nose: Small cell type (67-year-old female, ×310).

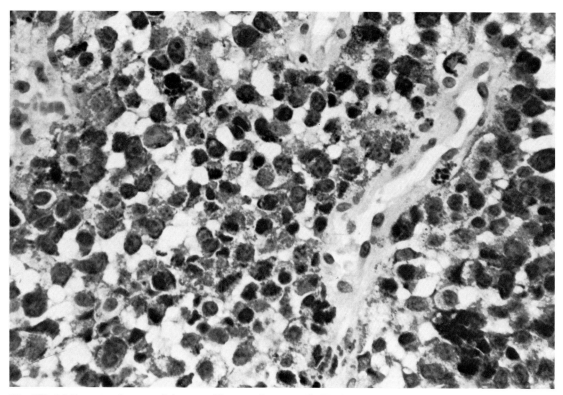

Fig. 510. Malignant melanoma of the nose: Pigmented tumor cells. Unpigmented area has been confused with olfactory neuroblastoma (55-year-old male, × 310).

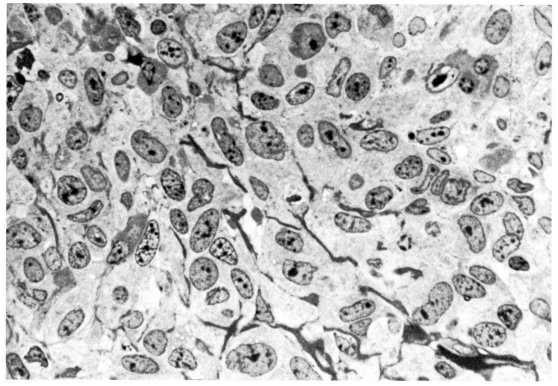

Fig. 511. Malignant melanoma of the nose: Tumor cells with atypical nuclei (55-year-old male, × 400).

M-9590/3
M-9730/3
T 160.0, 9

8. Malignant lymphoma and plasmacytoma [40] (WHO)

Both tumors can occur as primary tumors in the nose and paranasal sinuses; this is, however, rare [41] (see page 1247).

M-9080/0, 3
T 160.0, 9

9. Teratomas in infants and children (WHO) [13]

The benign and malignant teratomas can also (however, very rarely) develop at this location (see Testicular tumors, Tumors of the retroperitoneum, and Soft tissue tumors, pages 130, 154 and 1484).

M-9084/0
T 160.0

10. Dermoid cyst
(teratoma – WHO)

T 145.5

This variety of benign teratoma is usually located in the midline. The lesion may also be observed in the sella turcica and in the palate.

M-2616/0
T 160.0

11. Nasal glioma (WHO)

Nasal gliomas are composed of astrocytes that are multinucleated. Nasal gliomas contain glial fibers.
Nasal gliomas are due to a herniation from cerebral vesicles through the skull.
This malformation can be found in an intranasal position or in a subcutaneous localization.
Nasal gliomas are found in newborns or infants.

---

[13] Boies Jr. and Harris 1965.
[40] Fu and Perzin 1978.
[41] Fu and Perzin 1979.

12. Tumor-like lesions (WHO)

a) Lethal midline granuloma (WHO)
(granuloma gangraenescens nasi; Kraus-Chatelier's disease)

Lethal midline granuloma is a malignant inflammation that destroys the septum nasi and the palate and can reach the trachea [62].

The clinical findings indicate malignant tumor.

Histologically, the inflammatory tissue reaction contains capillaries, loose connective tissue, and numerous plasma cells, lymphocytes, and monocytes. Occasionally the blood vessels show thickening of the wall with proliferation of endothelial cells.

The lethal midline granuloma is occasionally associated with Wegener's granulomatosis.

M-3320/0
T 160.3
T 160.2

b) Mucocele of the ethmoidal sinuses and maxillary sinuses (WHO)

The mucocele in this region contains cysts with mucin in the lumen and mucin-producing epithelium. The epithelium is columnar and might show metaplasia.

If the mucocele is not removed, the surrounding bone might be destroyed due to the expansive pressure of the cystic lesion.

---

[62] Kassel et al. 1969.

Tumors of the ear

Tumors of the ear are rare.
The origin of the tumor can be the skin, the ceruminous glands, or the soft tissues including the bone:

M-8070/3
T 160.1

1. Squamous cell carcinoma (WHO)
(Figs. 512 and 513)

M-8090/3

2. Basal cell carcinoma (WHO)
(Figs. 1118 to 1125)

3. Tumors of the skin appendages
(see Tumors of the skin, page 1129) (Fig. 514)

4. Soft tissue tumors (WHO)
(see page 7)

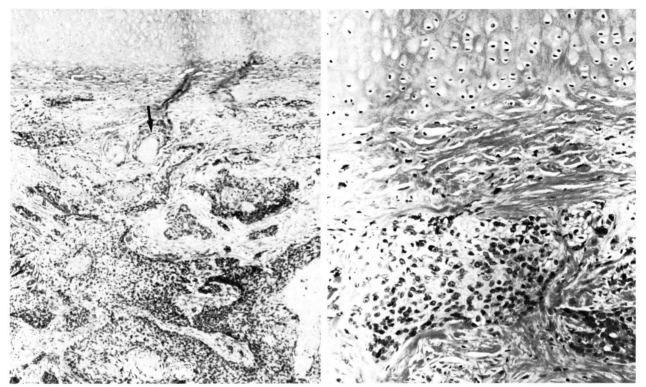

Fig. 512. Squamous cell carcinoma of the ear growing toward the cartilage (arrow) (68-year-old male, × 50).

Fig. 513. Squamous cell carcinoma of the ear: Tumor cells reaching the cartilage (68-year-old male, × 125).

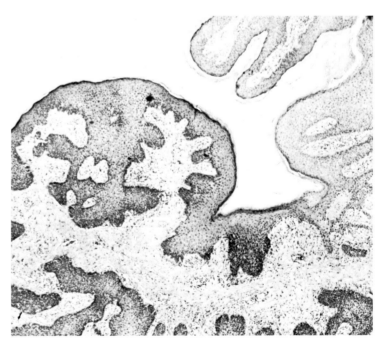

Fig. 514. Papillomatous keratosis with inflammation in the auditory duct (28-year-old female, × 40).

509

M-8420/3
T 173.2

5. Ceruminous adenocarcinoma (WHO)

Tumors originating from the ceruminous glands are very unusual [74].
This adenocarcinoma can rarely cause an extramammary Paget's disease in the overlying epithelium [33].

M-8420/0
T 173.2

6. Ceruminous adenoma (WHO)

Adenomas originating from the ceruminous glands can also occur (Figs. 515 and 516). This again is rare.

7. Tumor-like lesions

a) Chondrodermatitis nodularis chronica helicis (WHO)

This chronic inflammation appears at the external ear.
The inflammation involves both the epidermis and the cartilage.
In the cartilage the inflammation grows in a granulomatous pattern.
Since the ulceration of the epidermis can induce hyperplasia, differential diagnosis with a squamous cell carcinoma of the epidermis is occasionally necessary (Fig. 517).

M-7290/0
T 160.1

b) Cholesteatoma (WHO)

Cholesteatomas usually develop in the middle ear.
The lesion is composed of squamous cells that are surrounded by granulation tissue. This granulation tissue contains keratin and histiocytes, which often are loaded with iron pigment (Figs. 518 and 519).

---

[33] Fligiel and Kaneko 1975.
[74] Michel et al. 1978.

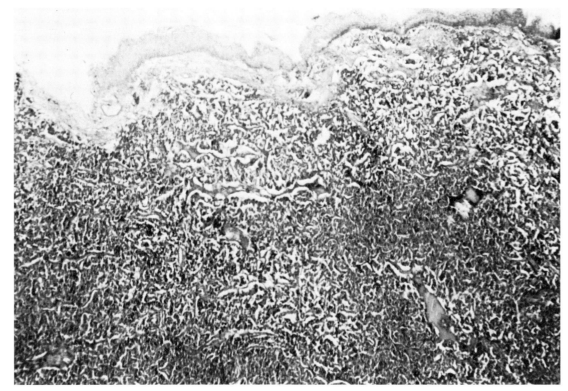

Fig. 515. Adenoma of the ceruminous glands (× 40).

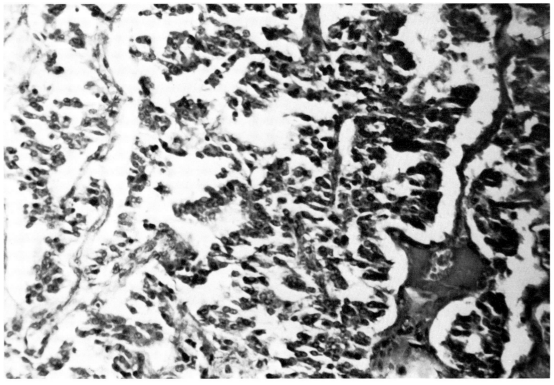

Fig. 516. Adenoma of the ceruminous glands (× 200).

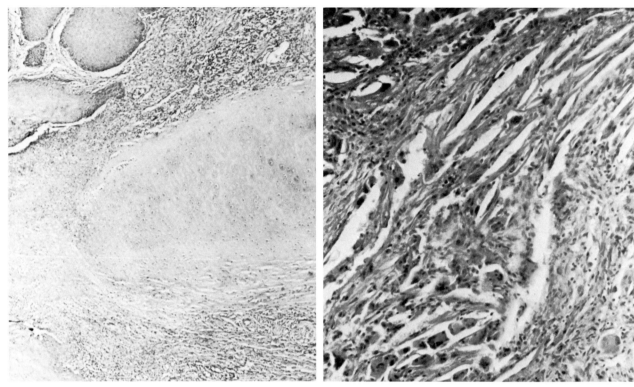

Fig. 517. Chondrodermatitis nodularis chronica helicis: Pseudocarcinomatous proliferation of the epithelium close to cartilage (72-year-old male, × 40).

Fig. 518. Cholesteatoma: Area of foreign body reaction and cholesterol crystals (66-year-old female, × 125).

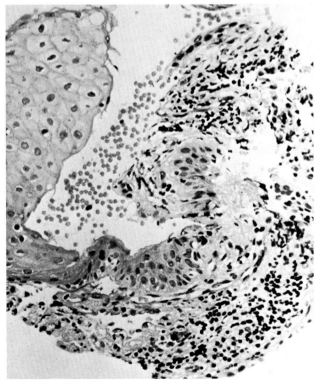

Fig. 519. Cholesteatoma: Chronic inflammation and islet of squamous epithelium (30-year-old female, × 200).

Tumors of the larynx

a) Supraglottis T – primary tumor

Tis = preinvasive carcinoma (carcinoma in situ)

T 0 = no evidence of primary tumor

T 1 = tumor confined to the region with normal mobility

> T 1 a = tumor confined to the laryngeal surface of the epiglottis, an aryepiglottic fold, a ventricular cavity, or to a ventricular band
>
> T 1 b = tumor involving the epiglottis and extending to the ventricular cavities or bands

T 2 = tumor confined to the larynx with extension to an adjacent site or sites or to the glottis without fixation

T 3 = tumor confined to the larynx with fixation and/or other evidence of deep infiltration

T 4 = tumor with direct extension beyond the larynx

T x = the minimal requirements to assess the primary tumor cannot be met (clinical examination, laryngoscopy, and radiography)

b) Glottis T – primary tumor

Tis = preinvasive carcinoma (carcinoma in situ)

T 0 = no evidence of primary tumor

T 1 = tumor confined to the region with normal mobility

> T 1 a = tumor confined to one cord
>
> T 1 b = tumor involving both cords

T 2 = tumor confined to the larynx with extension to either the supraglottic or the subglottic region with normal or impaired mobility

T 3 = tumor confined to the larynx with fixation of one or both cords

T 4 = tumor with direct extension beyond the larynx

T x = the minimal requirements to assess the primary tumor cannot be met (clinical examination, laryngoscopy, and radiography)

c) Subglottis T – primary tumor

Tis = preinvasive carcinoma (carcinoma in situ)

T 0 = no evidence of primary tumor

T 1 = tumor confined to the region

> T 1 a = tumor confined to one side of the region
>
> T 1 b = tumor involving both cords

T 2 = tumor confined to the larynx with extension to one or both cords with normal or impaired mobility

T 3 = tumor confined to the larynx with fixation of one or both cords

T 4 = tumor with destruction of cartilage and/or with direct extension beyond the larynx

T x = the minimal requirements to assess the primary tumor cannot be met (clinical examination, laryngoscopy, and radiography)

N – regional lymph nodes

(cervical nodes)

N 0 = no evidence of regional lymph node involvement

N 1 = evidence of involvement of the movable homolateral regional lymph nodes

N 2 = evidence of involvement of the movable contralateral or bilateral regional lymph nodes

N 3 = evidence of involvement of the fixed regional lymph nodes

N x = the minimal requirements to assess the regional lymph nodes cannot be met (clinical examination)

M – distant metastases

M 0 = no evidence of distant metastases

M 1 = evidence of distant metastases

M x = the minimal requirements to assess the presence of distant metastases cannot be met (clinical examination and radiography)

pTNM – postsurgical histopathological classification

the pTNM categories correspond to the TNM categories

Stage grouping

Stage I	T 1	N 0	M 0
Stage II	T 2	N 0	M 0
Stage III	T 3	N 0	M 0
	T 1, T 2, T 3	N 0	M 0
Stage IV	T 4	N 0, N 1	M 0
	any T	N 2, N 3	M 0
	any T	any N	M 1

M-8070/3
T 161.9

1. Squamous cell carcinoma (WHO)

General Remarks

Incidence: About 1% of all malignant tumors are squamous cell carcinomas of the larynx.

99% of all neoplasms of the larynx are squamous cell carcinomas.

Age: The peak age is the 5th to 7th decades, average age 60 years.

Sex: Men are considerably more frequently affected than women (10:1).

Site: Squamous cell carcinomas can be unilateral tumors or of multifocal origin.

T 161.0 About 60% of the tumors grow in the vocal cord (intrinsic carcinomas).

T 161.1 The remaining carcinomas develop beyond the vocal cords (extrinsic carcinomas).

Macroscopy

Carcinomas are ulcerated lesions with hardening of the underlying connective tissue. The tumor is friable.

Very rarely carcinomas can be of the verrucous type (Fig. 520).

Histology
M-8071/3

The tumor can be composed of **keratinizing** malignant squamous cells (Figs. 521 to 524).

M-8073/3 In a certain number of cases the tumor is of the **nonkeratinized** type (Figs. 525 to 527).

Electron Microscopy

The squamous cell carcinoma shows microfilaments and tonofibril attachment in the cytoplasm of tumor cells [100] and desmosomal attachment (Figs. 528 and 529).

Spread

1. Local aggressiveness into the surrounding tissue.
2. Lymphatic spread into the regional lymph nodes [72].
   The frequency of lymph node metastases depends on the site of the carcinoma:

T 161.0

a) Glottic carcinoma

In cases of carcinoma of the vocal cords, lymph node metastases of the homolateral side are rare and occur only in T 2 carcinomas.

T 161.1

b) Supraglottic carcinoma

In cases of carcinoma of the false cord and the epiglottis, 30% have lymph node metastases at the time of diagnosis.

Undetected metastases are rare.

T 161.2

c) Infraglottic carcinoma (subglottic carcinoma)

In cases of carcinoma of the true vocal cord with subglottic extension, lymph node metastases are almost always clinically undetected, but exist in about 20% of the cases.

T 161.9

d) Transglottic carcinoma

When the carcinoma has crossed the laryngeal ventricle, more than 50% of the cases have developed lymph node metastases.

3. The tumor extends also through the glands of the larynx [15].

---

[15] Bridger and Nassar 1972.
[72] McGavran et al. 1961.
[100] Schenk 1977.

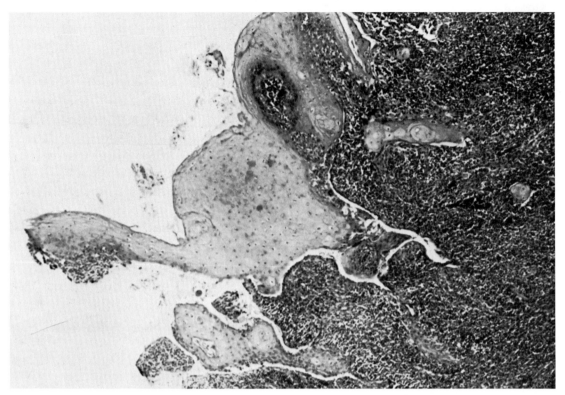

Fig. 520. Squamous cell carcinoma of the larynx, dominantly verrucous type (49-year-old male, × 50).

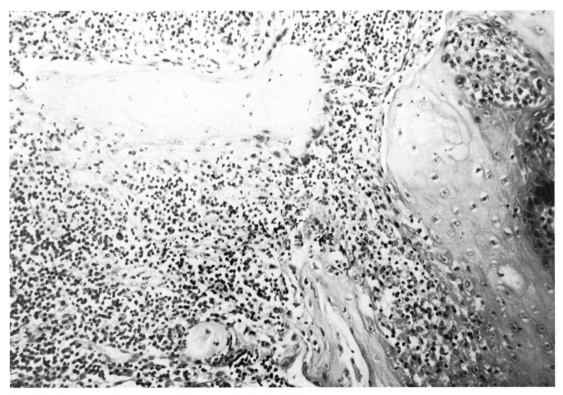

Fig. 521. Squamous cell carcinoma of the larynx, Grade I (× 125).

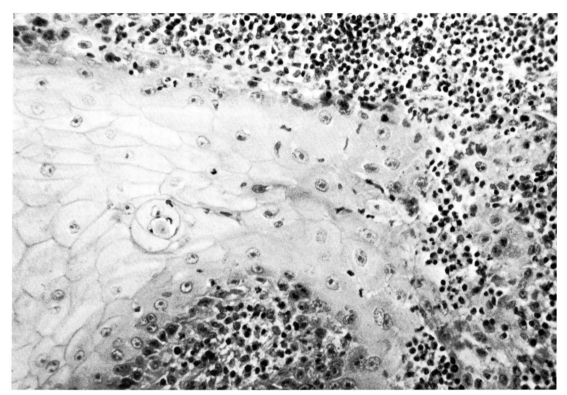

Fig. 522. Squamous cell carcinoma of the larynx, well-differentiated (Grade I) (× 200).

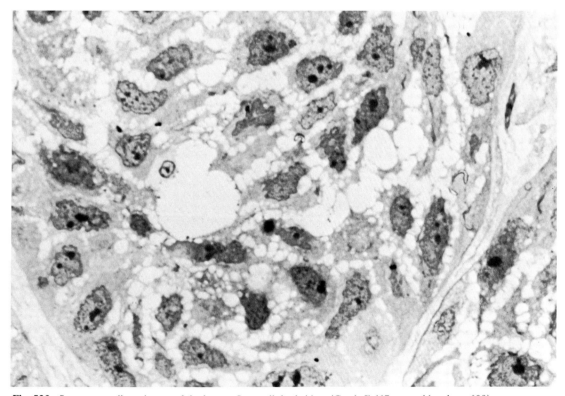

Fig. 523. Squamous cell carcinoma of the larynx: Intercellular bridges (Grade I) (67-year-old male, × 600).

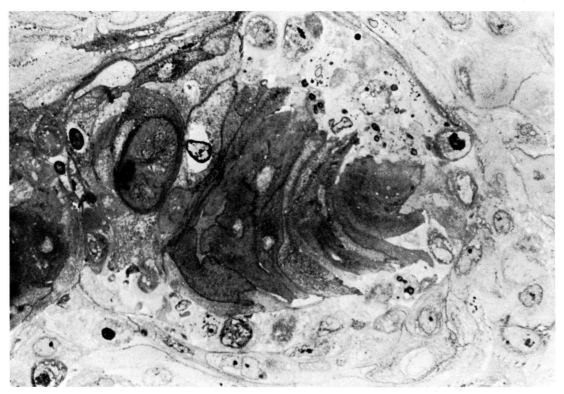

Fig. 524. Pearl formation in a squamous cell carcinoma of the larynx: Lamellated keratin in tumor cells (78-year-old male, ×400).

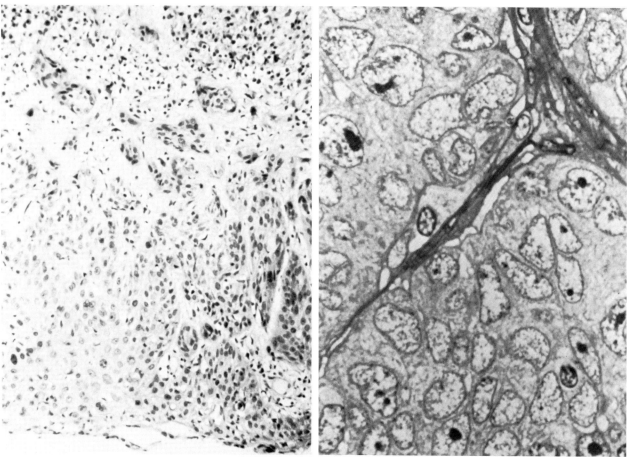

Fig. 525. Nonkeratinized squamous cell carcinoma of the larynx (Grade II) (67-year-old male, × 125).

Fig. 526. Squamous cell carcinoma, nonkeratinized, of the larynx: Pleomorphic large nucleoli, no intercellular bridges (69-year-old male, × 800).

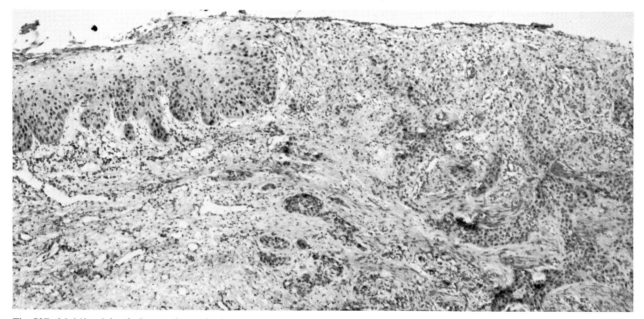

Fig. 527. Multifocal dysplasias, carcinoma in situ, and infiltrating carcinoma of the true vocal cord (67-year-old male, × 50).

Squamous cell carcinoma

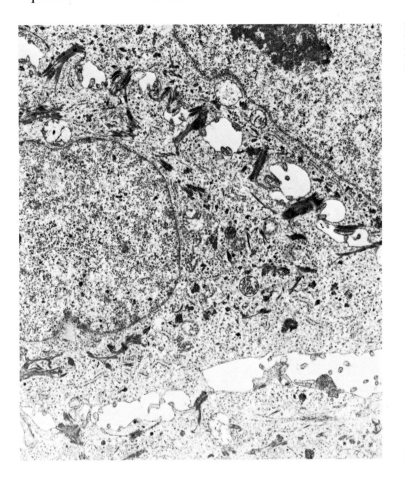

Figs. 528 and 529. Squamous cell carcinoma of the larynx: Tumor cells with numerous desmosomes. Bundles of filaments attached to the desmosomes (Fig. 528, × 10,000; Fig. 529, × 22,300).

Fig. 528.

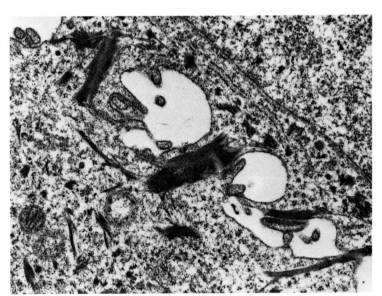

Fig. 529.

520

Clinical Findings

Hoarseness, cough, and occasionally pain.
Hoarseness is an early symptom in intrinsic (glottic) carcinoma, while in extrinsic (supraglottic and subglottic) carcinoma hoarseness is a late sign of the tumor (especially when the true vocal cord is not involved).

Treatment

Surgery.
Radiation therapy.
The possibilities for a cure are rather good [63, 79, 118].
Chemotherapy:
In cases of disseminated disease, chemotherapy with bleomycin, methotrexate, and 5-fluorouracil is recommended [123].
Radiation therapy as an alternative to surgery is sometimes applied in cases of small, localized carcinomas of the middle third of the vocal cord.

The therapeutic methods vary according to the site of the tumor:

a) Carcinoma of the subglottic area with or without involvement of the true vocal cord:
In most instances, total resection of the larynx.
Elective lymph node dissection.
Postoperative irradiation (60 to 70 Gy in 5 to 7 weeks) [78], particularly if
– the tumor could not be resected entirely,
– lymph node metastases are suspected,
– the tumor is close to the resection border.

b) Transglottic carcinoma (tumor arising in the anterior commissure with involvement of both true vocal cords):
Laryngectomy and lymph node dissection.
Postoperative irradiation (60 to 70 Gy in 6 to 7 weeks).

c) Supraglottic carcinoma:
Partial supraglottic laryngectomy followed by radiation therapy (60 to 70 Gy in 6 to 7 weeks).
Lymph node dissection.

d) Glottic carcinoma (T 1, N 0; T 2)
– Cordectomy or
– radiation therapy alone (up to 70 Gy in 6 weeks).
T 3:
– Surgery is preferred to radiation therapy:
  Hemilaryngectomy or total laryngectomy, according to the extension of the tumor.

e) Very small superficially growing (verrucous) carcinomas can be treated by endoscopic biopsy alone.

---

[63] Kirchner and Owen 1977.
[78] Niederer et al. 1977.
[79] Nordman and Kytta 1978.
[118] Taylor 1977.
[123] Wittes et al. 1977.

Squamous cell carcinoma

Prognosis

1. The overall 5-year survival rate is 40 to 50%.
2. In individual cases the prognosis is determined by the extension of the tumor.
3. Cancer of the larynx (T 1): 5-year survival, about 90%.
4. Failure of treatment in cases of localized Carcinoma is due to new disease because of the multifocal origin of the tumor (see also Carcinoma in situ) [86].
5. The success of treatment should be evaluated 5-years after the initiation of treatment and by the duration of the first remission [19, 20].
6. It has been debated whether late "recurrence" might be induced by the previous radiation therapy [44].

[19] Cachin 1975.
[20] Cachin 1978.
[44] Glanz and Kleinsasser 1976.
[86] Pêne and Fletcher 1976.

M-8051/3
T 161.0

2. Verrucous carcinoma (WHO) (Fig. 520)

Verrucous carcinomas of the larynx are rare.
The tumor is well differentiated and contains extensive keratinization.
The malignancy is low, and lymph node metastases are very rare [64].

M-8980/3
T 161.9

3. Carcinosarcoma

Carcinosarcomas in the larynx are rare.
The tumor is composed of malignant epithelial and mesenchymal cell populations (Figs. 1361 to 1364).
The tumor usually grows in a polypoid fashion.
The prognosis is claimed to be better than for other laryngeal cancers [4].

M-8042/3
T 161.9

4. Oat cell carcinoma

Oat cell carcinomas of the larynx are exceedingly rare [31, 77].

M-8200/3
T 161.1

5. Adenoid cystic carcinoma (WHO) (Figs. 588 to 592)

Adenoid cystic carcinomas originate from the mucous glands of the larynx. The tumor is extremely rare and grows in almost all instances in the supraglottic area [82].

[4] Appelman and Oberman 1965.
[31] Eusebi et al. 1978.
[64] Kraus and Perez-Mesa 1966.
[77] Mullins et al. 1979.
[82] Olofsson and van Nostrand 1977.

M-8070/2
T 161.9

6. Carcinoma in situ (WHO)

**General
Remarks**

Incidence: Infiltrating carcinomas are in 75% of the cases associated with foci of carcinoma in situ [8].

Site: Carcinomas in situ can be observed at a single site; often, however, they are of a multifocal origin.

Macroscopy

Carcinoma in situ is distinguished by a discrete thickening of the vocal cord.

Histology

Carcinoma in situ is composed of atypical cells, which occupy the epithelial layer. The underlying tissue is not infiltrated.

The atypical cells contain numerous hyperchromatic nuclei, mitotic figures, and intracytoplasmic keratinization (Figs. 527, 530, and 531).

**Differential
Diagnosis**

1. Carcinoma in situ **with infiltrating squamous cell carcinoma:**
   Occasionally foci of early infiltration might develop out of a carcinoma in situ (Fig. 532). In case of doubt new biopsies or multiple sections of the obtained tissue should be performed.

M-7400/6
M-7400/7
M-7400/8

2. Carcinoma in situ **with dysplasia with keratosis of a mild, moderate, or severe degree:**
   Foci of dysplasia contain atypical cells. The basal cell layer of the epithelium is intact. The degree of extension of atypical cells in the epithelium, the degree of hyperchromatism, and the number of atypical cells determine the degree of dysplasia (Figs. 531 and 533 to 535).
   Dysplasias rarely develop into a squamous cell carcinoma.

**Clinical
Findings**

Carcinoma in situ: Hoarseness.

Treatment

Surgical removal or biopsy.
Eventually **radiation therapy.**
Failures of treatment are due to the multifocal origin of these lesions and not to true recurrences [86].

Prognosis

Untreated carcinoma in situ might develop into an infiltrating carcinoma.

**Further
Information**

1. Dysplasias and carcinoma in situ are often observed in singers and smokers.
2. Dysplasias and carcinoma in situ lesions are related to polyploidy [6].

[6] Avtandilov and Kazantseva 1973.
[8] Bauer and McGavran 1972.
[86] Pêne and Fletcher 1976.

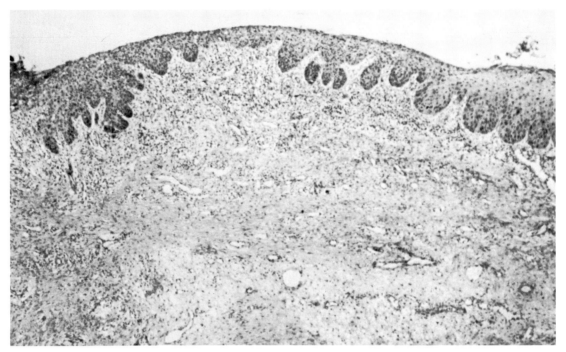

Fig. 530. Numerous foci of dysplasia and carcinoma in situ of the true vocal cord (× 30).

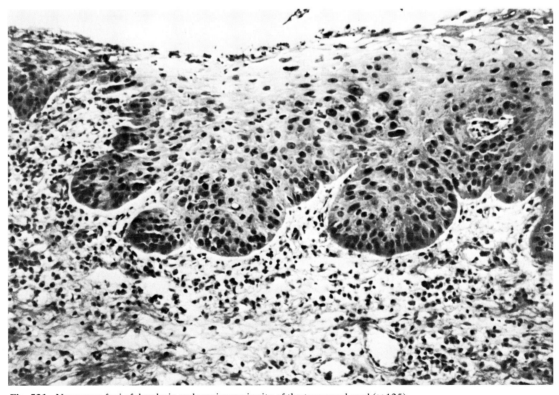

Fig. 531. Numerous foci of dysplasia and carcinoma in situ of the true vocal cord (× 125).

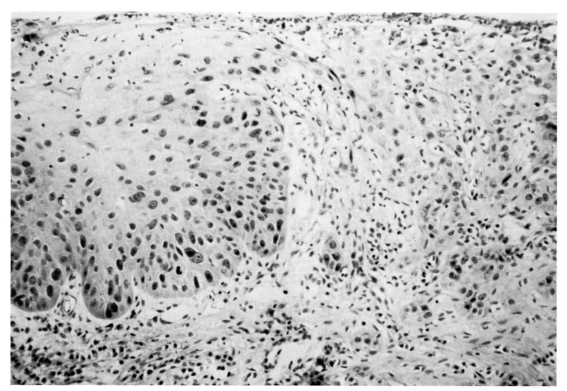

Fig. 532. Carcinoma in situ plus infiltrating carcinoma of the true vocal cord (× 125).

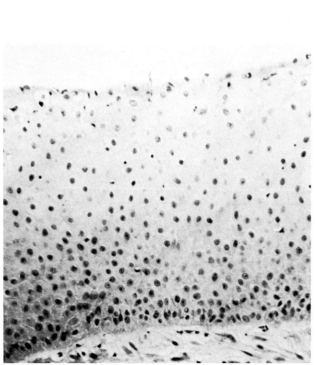

Fig. 533. Squamous cell hyperplasia of the true vocal cord (67-year-old male, × 125).

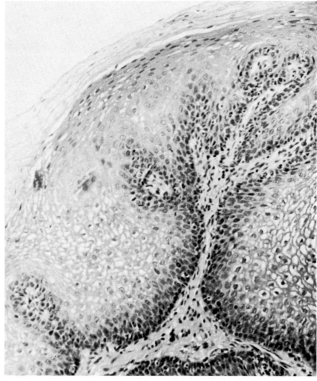

Fig. 534. Marked keratosis with discrete inflammation of the true vocal cord (71-year-old male, × 125).

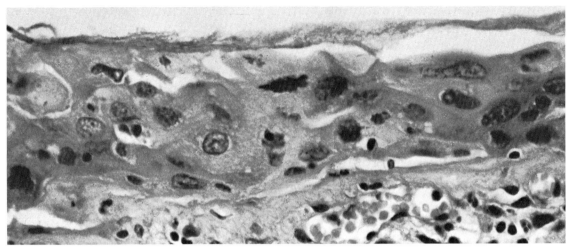

Fig. 535. Cellular atypias at the larynx following irradiation of a carcinoma (62-year-old male, × 310).

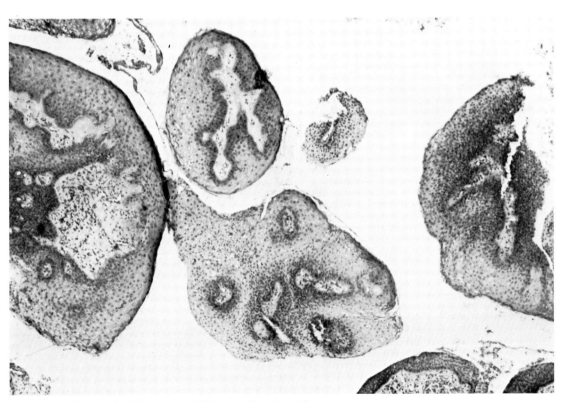

Fig. 536. Papillomatosis of the false cord (57-year-old male, × 50).

M-8050/0
(M-8060/0)
T 161.9

7. Squamous cell papilloma of the larynx
(papillomatosis) (WHO)

General
Remarks

Incidence: Papillomatosis of the larynx is relatively rare.
Age: This lesion can be observed at any age; usually, however, adults are affected.
Site: Papillomatosis can develop on the true vocal cords; less frequently it is observed on the false cords and the epiglottis.
Occasionally in children a generalized papillomatosis can develop with involvement of the trachea and the bronchi.

Macroscopy

Papillomas of the larynx can be solitary or multiple. Some of the papillomas are sessile; some are pedunculated.

Histology

The tumor is composed of squamous cells, which have regular nuclei (Figs. 536 to 538). The squamous cells are supported by connective tissue with blood vessels.

Electron
Microscopy

The surface of the papillomatous cells in papilloma of the larynx shows short, thick microvilli. Occasionally virus-like particles are found [59].

Clinical
Findings

Hoarseness.
In cases of multiple papillomas, embarrassment of the respiration can occur.

Treatment

Removal of the papilloma.

Prognosis

Papillomas of the larynx are most probably of a viral origin:
The papillomas have a strong tendency to recur.
Recurrences can also be observed after complete removal of the tumor.
Whereas papillomas in children are never malignant, those developing in adults occasionally can become malignant after a number of recurrences.

---

[59] Incze et al. 1977.

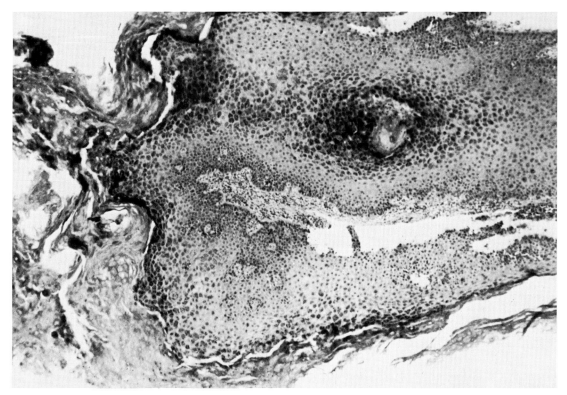

Fig. 537. Papilloma of the vocal cord (49-year-old male, × 30).

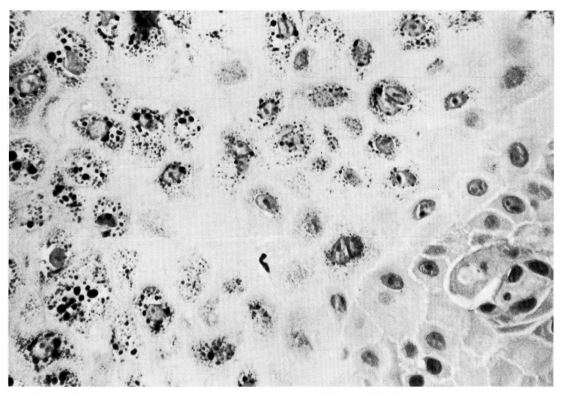

Fig. 538. Papilloma of the vocal cord with basophilic inclusion bodies (viral origin) (49-year-old male, × 310).

T 161.9

8. Soft tissue tumors (WHO) (see page 7)

Soft tissue tumors in the larynx are very rare.

M-9180/3 **a) osteosarcoma** [24]

M-8900/0 **b) rhabdomyoma** [12]

M-8830/3 **c) malignant fibrous histiocytoma** [32]

M-9040/3 **d) synovial sarcoma** (tumor in the neck) [102]

M-9160/0 **e) angiofibroma** (Fig. 539)

M-8900/3 **f) rhabdomyosarcoma**

M-9560/0 **g) neurilemoma**

M-8810/3 **h) fibrosarcoma**

M-9220/3 **i) chondrosarcoma**

M-9580/0 **k) granular cell tumor** [27]:
Granular cell tumors grow in the vocal cords.

M-9120/0 **l) hemangioma** (Fig. 540):
Hemangiomas are usually observed in infants and are often associated with hemangiomas at other locations (for instance, hemangiomas in the skin).
The majority of hemangiomas develop in the glottic area.
Hemangiomas can be treated by low dose radiation therapy.

[12] Bianchi and Muratti 1975.
[24] Dahm et al. 1978.
[27] Domansky and Schoen 1977.
[32] Ferlito 1978.
[102] Schöndorf and Seeliger 1977.

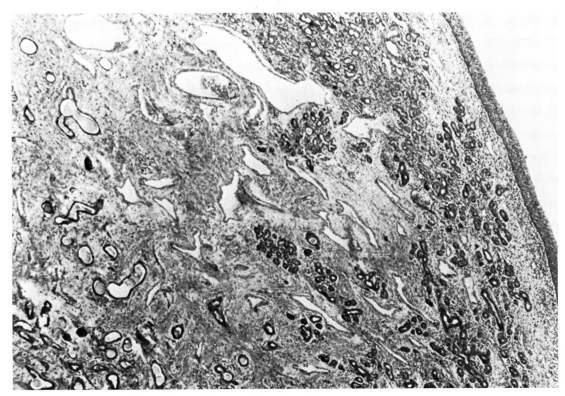

Fig. 539. Angiofibroma of the epiglottis (69-year-old female, × 40).

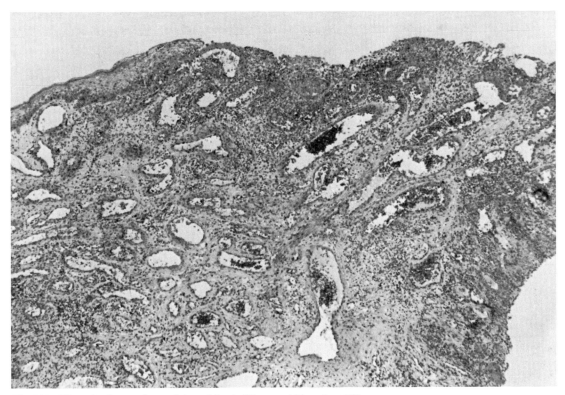

Fig. 540. Ulcerating hemangioma of the epiglottis (38-year-old female, × 50).

M-8693/1
T 161.9

9. Chemodectoma (WHO) [53] (Fig. 743)

Chemodectomas in the larynx are very rare.

M-8240/1
T 161.9

10. Carcinoid tumor (WHO)

Very rarely primary carcinoid tumors of the larynx can occur.

M-9590/3
T 161.9

11. Malignant lymphoma (WHO)

M-7229/0

All types of malignant lymphoma can grow in the larynx, including plasmacytoma. Occasionally the differential diagnosis with **pseudolymphoma** must be solved.

M-8000/6
T 161.9

12. Metastatic tumors in the larynx

Metastases into the larynx are rare. They can in most instances originate from a primary thyroid carcinoma (Fig. 541).

---

[53] Hohbach and Mootz 1978.

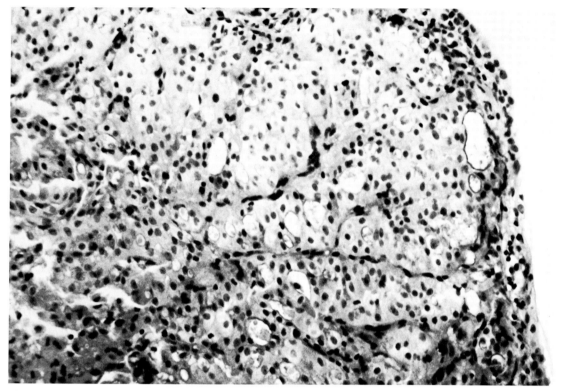

Fig. 541. Micrometastasis from follicular thyroid carcinoma in the false cord (62-year-old female, × 200).

M-7682/0
T 161.0

13. Laryngeal nodule
(vocal cord polyp – WHO)

This is a tumor-like lesion in which the connective tissue contains numerous blood vessels, foci of fibrinoid degeneration, and hyalinization (Figs. 542 to 544).
The overlying epithelium is thickened, without signs of atypias.

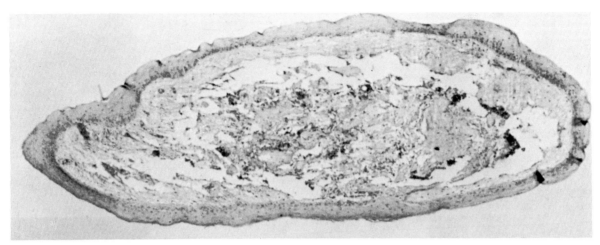

Fig. 542. Laryngeal polyp (30-year-old male, × 50).

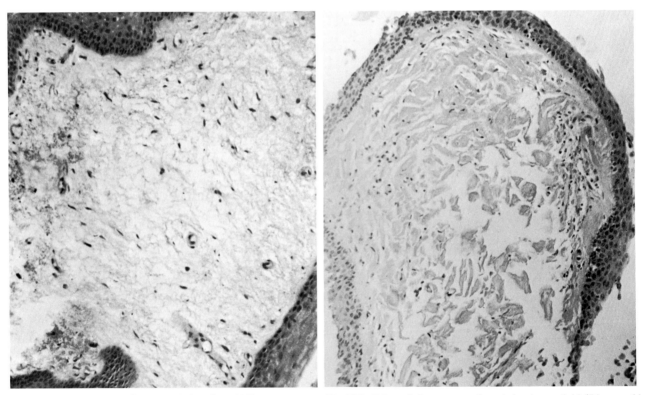

Fig. 543. Laryngeal polyp (65-year-old female, × 125).

Fig. 544. Polyp of the true vocal cord due to amyloid (74-year-old male, × 125).

Recommendations for differential diagnosis
in tumors of the head and neck

(oropharynx, nasopharynx, hypopharynx, nose, paranasal sinuses, larynx)

squamous cell carcinoma	with	– pseudocarcinomatous (pseudo-epitheliomatous) hyperplasia
ulcerating squamous cell carcinoma	with	– verrucous squamous cell carcinoma
squamous cell carcinoma		– grading according to the malignancy
poorly differentiated squamous cell carcinoma (especially in the tonsils)	with	– malignant lymphoma (electron microscopy) – poorly differentiated sarcoma
lymphoepithelial carcinoma	with	– undifferentiated carcinoma – malignant lymphoma (eventually electron microscopy)
leukoplakia	with	– definition of the underlying epithelial lesion – detection of infiltrating carcinoma
olfactory neuroblastoma	with	– undifferentiated carcinoma – malignant lymphoma – chronic inflammation – embryonal rhabdomyosarcoma – malignant melanoma
benign papilloma (paranasal and nasal)	with	– papillary carcinoma – squamous cell carcinoma – inflammatory polyp
well-differentiated squamous cell carcinoma (paranasal and nasal)	with	– inverted squamous cell papilloma
mucoepidermoid carcinoma	with	– squamous cell carcinoma – adenocarcinoma

Tumors of the trachea

Tumors localized in the trachea are very rare [57].

M-8070/3
T 162.0

1. Squamous cell carcinoma (WHO)

Squamous cell carcinomas in the trachea are very rare.
The tumor develops in the lower third of the trachea.
The prognosis is very poor.

M-8200/3
T 162.0

2. Adenoid cystic carcinoma (WHO)

The adenoid cystic carcinoma in the trachea is very rare and corresponds to the tumor observed in the salivary glands (Figs. 588 to 592).
Adenoid cystic carcinoma grows slowly and infiltrates the lymphatics.
Adenoid cystic carcinomas develop mainly in the upper third of the trachea [50].

M-8050/0
T 162.0

3. Squamous cell papilloma and papillomatosis (WHO)

Papillomas and papillomatosis originating from the epithelium of the trachea are very rare (Figs. 537 and 538).
These papillomas (papillomatosis) correspond to those observed in the larynx.

M-8240/0
T 162.0

4. Carcinoid tumor

Very rarely observations have been made of carcinoid tumors originating in the trachea [16].

---

[16] Briselli et al. 1978.
[50] Hajdu et al. 1970.
[57] Houston et al. 1969.

Odontogenic tumors (WHO)

The interaction between oral epithelium and mesenchymal cells determines the development of teeth. Odontogenic tumors are most probably due to a defective interplay between these two components.

According to the amount of epithelial or mesenchymal components in the individual odontogenic tumor, the cellular and structural aspect of these neoplasms varies considerably.

Therefore, numerous types of odontogenic tumors have been identified [89].

Tumors of the jaws (mandible and maxilla)

M-9310/0, 3

1. Ameloblastoma (WHO)

(adamantinoma)

**General
Remarks**

Incidence: Ameloblastomas are very rare tumors: About 1% of all neoplasms of the jaw, including cysts, are ameloblastomas.

Age: The tumor can be observed in any age group including children. The majority of patients are in the 3rd to 6th decades.

Sex: Men are affected slightly more often than women.

Site: The majority of ameloblastomas develop in the mandible (about 80%).

Further notes: The tumor is particulary frequent in East Africa.

Macroscopy

Ameloblastomas are solid tumors with cyst formations. The cysts might dominate the macroscopic picture. The cysts contain fluid, which can be mucinous. The cyst walls are smooth; occasionally papillary formations are observed.

Ameloblastomas can become very large.

Histology

Ameloblastomas are composed of epithelial cells. The cells have regular nuclei. The cytoplasm is often clear.

The growth pattern of these cells is variable:

The tumor can form large cords, which form anastomoses (Fig. 545).

In other instances the tumor cells form larger cell nests, which might be surrounded by palisading cells, giving to the tumor a basaloid appearance (Fig. 546).

The tumor cells can undergo squamous cell metaplasia. Occasionally the cells form small follicles (Figs. 547 and 548).

The surrounding tissue might be infiltrated by these cells.

Other areas in ameloblastomas can be similar to mesenchymal tumors with spindle-shaped cells.

---

[89] Pindborg and Kramer 1971.

Ameloblastoma

Histology

The epithelial cell nest might undergo cystic degeneration. The cysts are lined by columnar cells. Pseudomucinous material can be found in the lumina of the cysts (Fig. 549).
The connective tissue in ameloblastomas contains foci of lymphocytic infiltration. The amount of connective tissue is different [65].

Spread

Very rarely ameloblastomas develop distant metastases.

Clinical Findings

Ameloblastomas show a painless enlargement in the area of the slow-growing tumor.
On radiography the bone is destroyed, and unilocular or multilocular neoplasms can be seen.

Treatment

Ameloblastomas are excised radically with a large safe margin. However, it is controversial whether the ameloblastoma should be treated aggressively or by a more conservative approach [23].

Prognosis

a) Amelobastomas are locally infiltrating tumors (Figs. 550 and 551). About 30% of the treated patients suffer recurrences.
b) Life is threatened by local extension of the tumor to the base of the skull.
Unicystic ameloblastomas are less aggressive than multicystic or solid ameloblastomas [93].

Further Information

There is one reported case in which an ameloblastoma was associated with renal calculi and hypercalcemia [105].

[23] Crawley and Levin 1978.
[65] Krempien et al. 1979.
[93] Robinson and Martinez 1977.
[105] Seward et al. 1975.

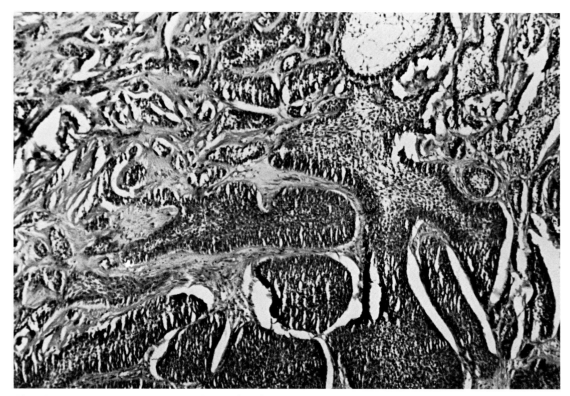

Fig. 545. Ameloblastoma: Solid and cystic areas (× 60).

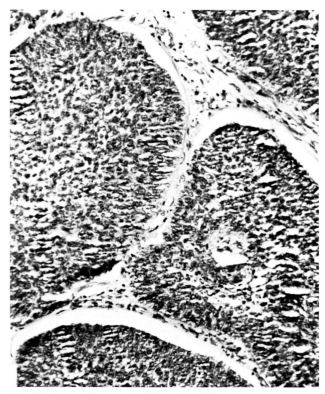

Fig. 546. Ameloblastoma: Solid area (× 200).

Ameloblastoma

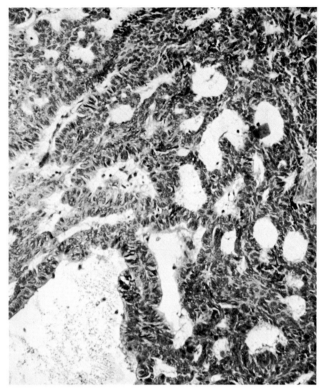

Fig. 547. Ameloblastoma, plexiform type (× 125).

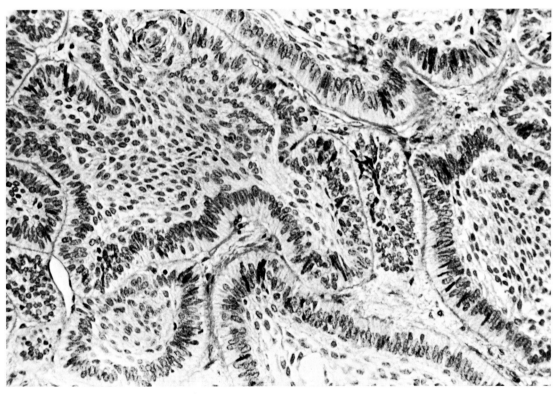

Fig. 548. Ameloblastoma, follicular type (× 200).

540

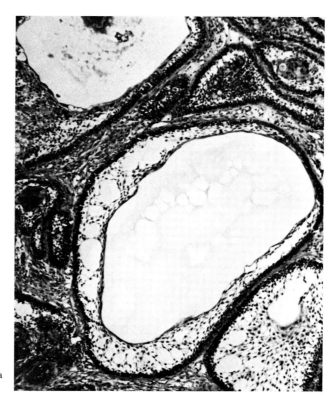

Fig. 549. Ameloblastoma with cysts and squamous cell metaplasia (× 125).

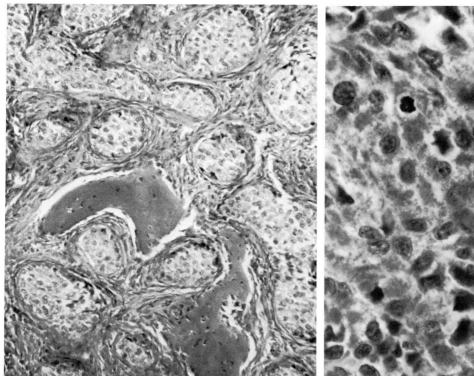

Fig. 550. Malignant ameloblastoma infiltrating the bone (× 125).

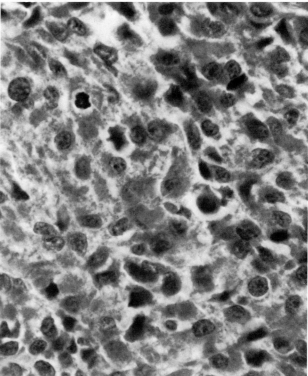

Fig. 551. Malignant ameloblastoma with hyperchromatic nuclei and mitotic figures (× 400).

M-9340/0

2. Calcifying epithelial odontogenic tumor (WHO)

General Remarks

Incidence: This is a very rare tumor.

Age: The age distribution corresponds to that of ameloblastoma; the majority of the patients are in the 4th to 5th decade.

Sex: Males and females are equally affected.

Site: The majority (about two-thirds) of the cases develop in the premolar and molar region of the mandible.

Histology

The tumor is composed of eosinophilic epithelial cells, which are very large. The nulei are slightly pleomorphic and are large (Figs. 552 and 553). Between the cells there are intercellular bridges.

The tumor cells grow in a connective tissue that contains both calcifications, which occasionally resemble psammoma bodies, and amyloid substance.

Clinical-Findings

This is a very slowly growing tumor of discrete aggressiveness.

Treatment

Resection of the tumor.

Prognosis

Recurrences are observed in about 20% of the cases.

There are no reported metastases.

Further Information

The amyloid-like material is most probably produced by the tumor cells [84, 90].

---

[84] Page et al. 1975.

[90] Ranløv and Pindborg 1966.

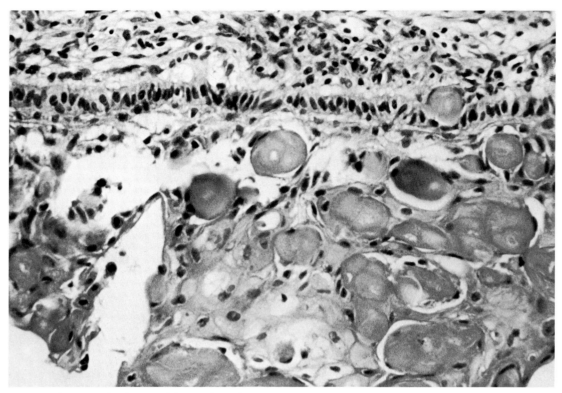

Fig. 554. Odontogenic adenomatoid tumor (×200).

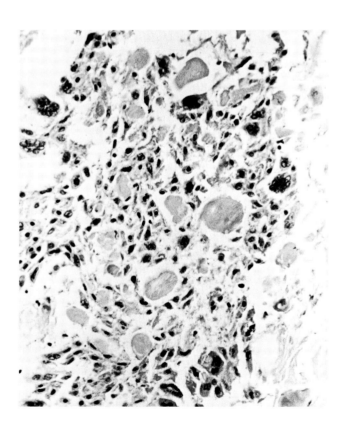

Fig. 555. Odontogenic adenomatoid tumor with giant cells (×200).

M-9330/0

4. Ameloblastic fibroma (WHO)

**General
Remarks**

Incidence: This is a rare variety of ameloblastoma.

Age: This ameloblastic fibroma usually develops in patients of younger ages: adolescents and children (peak age, 2nd decade).

Sex: Males and females are equally affected.

T 170.1

Site: The majority of these ameloblastic fibromas develop in the premolar-molar region of the mandible.

Histology

The odontogenic benign epithelial cells grow in strands or form small cell nests. These cells grow in a loose connective tissue, which contains spindle cells (Fig. 556). The connective tissue might show zones of hyalinization. Occasionally dysplastic dentin can be detected.

Compared with other ameloblastomas, this tumor is partly dominated by the connective tissue.

Treatment

The tumor is removed by curettage.

Prognosis

Excellent; recurrences are almost never observed.

Very rarely the mesenchymal component of this tumor can show a malignant sarcomatous behavior:

**M-9330/3
T 170.1**

Ameloblastic sarcoma

The transition of an amelobastic fibroma into an ameloblastic fibrosarcoma (WHO) has rarely been observed [47].

---

[47] Goldstein et al. 1976.

M-9290/0
T 170.0

5. Ameloblastic fibro-odontoma (WHO)

(fibroameloblastic odontoma)

General Remarks

Incidence: This variety of ameloblastoma is very rare.
Age: The tumor affects the younger age groups (2nd decade).
Sex: Males and females are equally affected.

Macroscopy

Ameloblastic fibro-odontomas can become very large and destroy the bone.

Histology

The tumor composition is similar to that of ameloblastic fibroma, with small strands of epithelial cells embedded in connective tissue. Besides these structures, the tumor contains foci of dentin and enamel (Fig. 557).

Treatment

The tumor is removed by curettage.

Prognosis

This is a benign lesion without recurrences.

M-9320/0
T 170.0

6. Odontogenic myxoma (WHO)

(myxofibroma)

Histology

This tumor is dominated by a myxomatous ground substance, which shows a positive mucin stain.
In this ground substance, cells grow that exhibit signs of nuclear atypias.
The tumor is not encapsulated and infiltrates into the surrounding tissue.
Rarely, foci of collagen fibers or odontogenic cells might be detected.

Treatment

The tumor must be removed surgically.
Complete removal might be difficult (see Myxoma, page 54).

Prognosis

After removal, recurrences must be expected.

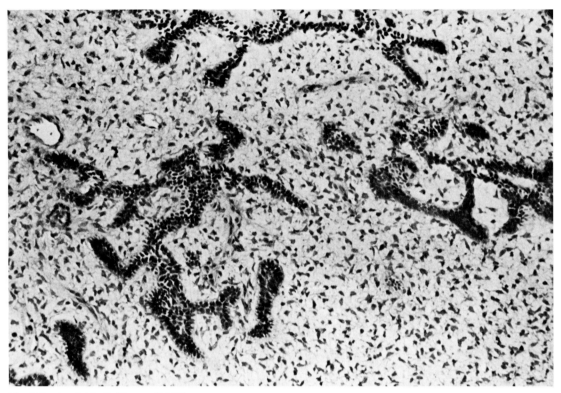

Fig. 556. Ameloblastic fibroma (× 125).

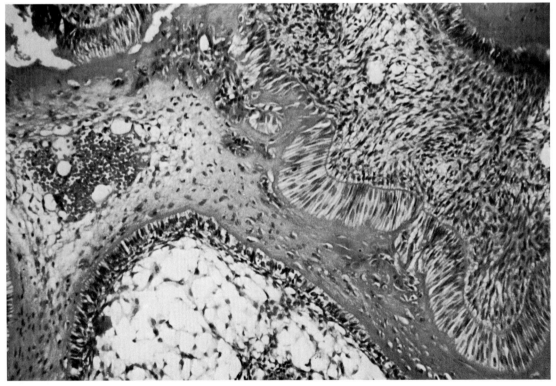

Fig. 557. Ameloblastic fibro-odontoma (× 125).

548

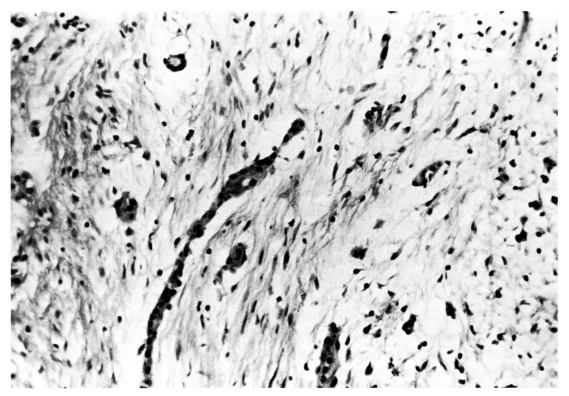

Fig. 558. Odontogenic fibroma (× 200).

M-9321/0
T 170.0

7. Odontogenic fibroma (WHO)
(central odontogenic epithelial hamartoma)

Histology

This tumor is composed of collagen fibers, which can form interlacing bundles. The mesenchymal component can dominate the picture. The nuclei are regular and spindle-shaped.

Between these collagen fibers, nests of odontogenic epithelial cells are observed. They can form small nests, small strands, or larger complexes, which can anastomose with each other. The connective tissue may furthermore show foci of osteoid material (Fig. 558).

M-9272/0

8. Cementoma (WHO)

General Remarks

Site: Cementomas usually develop in the lower jaw around the root of the molar or premolar tooth.

Histology

The tumor is composed of basophilic material. This material shows areas of mineralized and unmineralized zones with basophilic lines between (Fig. 559). This gives the tumor an irregular aspect similar to that observed in Paget's disease of bone.

This material is deposited in a connective tissue. The material might be surrounded by osteoclasts and osteoblasts.

Treatment

Removal of the tumor by extraction of the affected tooth.

Prognosis

Cementomas are benign lesions.
There are no recurrences.

Further Information

Cementoma areas can also be found in other odontogenic tumors.

M-9274/0

Cementoma in fibroma:
Cementifying fibroma (WHO).

M-9275/0

Gigantiform cementoma (WHO) (familial multiple cementomas):
In this disease cementomas develop symmetrically on both sides in the jaws.

M-9272/0

Periapical cemental dysplasia (WHO) (periapical fibrous dysplasia):
This lesion develops mainly in the mandible and affects middle-aged females.
The cementum-like material is deposited in a loose connective tissue.

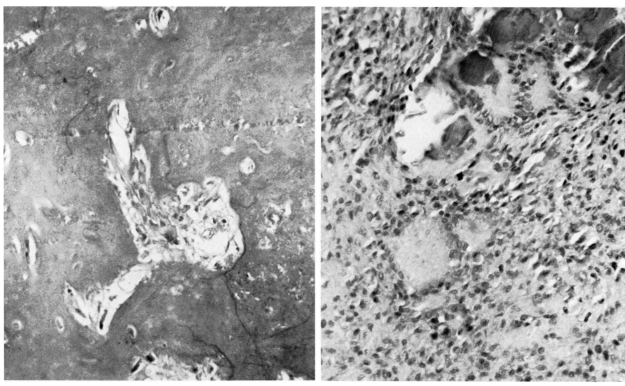

Fig. 559. Cementoma (cementoblastoma): Basophilic lines (× 200).

Fig. 560. Dentinoma: Calcified and noncalcified dentin and odontogenic epithelial cells (× 200).

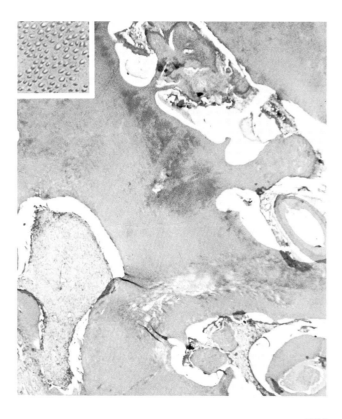

Fig. 561. Odontoma: Tooth-like structures (× 40; inset, × 200).

M-9271/0
T 170.0

9. Dentinoma (WHO)

General
Remarks

Incidence: Dentinomas are very rare tumors.
Site: The tumor is observed mostly within the bone.

Histology

The tumor contains connective tissue in which odontogenic epithelial cells grow.
The connective tissue shows foci of dentin, which is dysplastic and poorly mineralized.
These islets of dentin are surrounded by connective fibers and by odontogenic epithelium
(Fig. 560).

M-9311/0
T 170.0

10. Odontoameloblastoma (WHO)

This very rare neoplasm contains dentin combined with odontogenic epithelial cells and
an enamel matrix.
The epithelial cells can occasionally form a pattern similar to an ameloblastoma.

M-9282/0
T 170.0

11. Complex odontoma (WHO)

General
Remarks

Incidence: This is a rare tumor-like malformation [49].
Age: The tumor is usually observed in young patients.
Sex: Complex odontomas are more frequently observed in females than in males.
Site: Complex odontomas affect mainly the premolar or molar region.

Histology

The tumor has similarities with ameloblastic fibromas or fibro-odontomas. There are also a number of toothlike formations (Fig. 561).
If the toothlike formations dominate the picture, the malformation is called

M-9281/0
T 170.0

12. Compound odontoma (WHO)

Treatment

Removal of the lesion.

Prognosis

Complex odontoma and compound odontoma: Excellent.

M-9270/3
T 170.0

13. Odontogenic carcinoma (WHO)

(primary intraosseous squamous cell carcinoma; intraalveolar carcinoma)

Very rarely squamous cell carcinoma can develop from remnants of the odontogenic epithelium.
The tumor infiltrates the lymphatics and causes regional lymph node metastases.

Differential
Diagnosis

1. Odontogenic carcinoma **with extension of carcinomas from the tongue, mouth, or gingiva.**
2. Odontogenic carcinoma **with tumors of the salivary glands** (possibly displaced salivary glands).
3. Odontogenic carcinoma **with metastatic lesions to the jaws:**
   Metastases have been observed from tumors of the kidney, thyroid, breast, and bronchus and (in children) from neuroblastomas.

[49] Häupl and Riedel 1966.

T 170.0
T 170.1

14. Bone tumors in the jaws

The jaws can be the site of malignant bone tumors such as

M-9180/3   — **osteosarcoma,**

M-9220/3   — **chondrosarcoma,**

M-8810/3   — **fibrosarcoma.**

Tumor-like lesions such as

M-3364/0   — **aneurysmal bone cyst** (WHO),
M-3340/4   — **simple bone cyst** (WHO),
M-4411/0   — **giant cell reparative granuloma** (WHO) can also be observed (see Bone tumors, page 1107).

M-7491/0

15. Fibrous dysplasia of the jaws (WHO)

This tumor-like condition due to developmental failure of the skeletal system is observed in young patients and often is located in the jaws (see Bone tumors, page 1106).

16. Cherubism (WHO)

Cherubism is a tumor-like lesion, in which solitary or multiple cysts develop in the jaws.
This familial disease is observed in young patients.
The cysts are surrounded by connective tissue, which contains multiple giant cells and histiocytes.
With the continuation of the cysts, the connective tissue shows bone formation and the number of cells diminishes.

M-9750/3
T 170.0
T 170.1

17. Malignant lymphoma in the jaws

All types of non-Hodgkin's lymphomas might develop in the jaws.
Burkitt's lymphoma has a very strong predilection for this location (see Malignant lymphomas, page 1296).

M-9363/0
T 170.0

18. Melanotic neuroectodermal tumor of infancy (WHO)

(melanoameloblastoma; melanotic progonoma)

General Remarks

Incidence: This is a rare tumor, which is benign and develops from the neural crest (see Tumors of the peripheral nerves, page 174).
Age: This lesion is observed in infants, usually under the age of 1 year.
Site: The majority of melanotic neuroectodermal tumors develop in the maxilla, and this lesion is rarely observed in the mandible.

Macroscopy

The tumor resembles epulis. The cut surface is black.

Histology

Melanotic neuroectodermal tumor is composed of cells that form tubular structures or nests. The cytoplasm of these cells contains melanin pigment.
The tumor cells resemble those observed in a fetal pineal gland [28].

Further Information

A case has been reported in which melanotic neuroectodermal tumor was associated with brain heterotopia in the oropharynx [67].

---

[28] Dooling et al. 1977.
[67] Lee et al. 1976.

References

[1] Akanuma, A.: High-dose rate intracavitary radiation therapy for advanced head and neck tumors. Cancer *40* (1977) 1071-1076.

[2] Alth, G., und H. Kollabek: Malignome der Nasennebenhöhlen. Wien. Klin. Wschr. *88* (1976) 660-664.

[3] Ammon, J., R. Löffler, H. Stockberg und H. Zeumer: Systematisierte, am TNM-System orientierte Strahlentherapie von Tumoren im Kopf-Hals-Bereich. Strahlentherapie *154* (1978) 511-519.

[4] Appelman, H.D., and H.A. Oberman: Squamous cell carcinoma of the larynx with sarcoma-like stroma; a clinicopathologic assessment of spindle cell carcinoma and "pseudosarcoma". American J. Clin. Pathol. *44* (1965) 135-145.

[5] Ash, J.E., M.R. Beck, and J.D. Wilkes: Tumors of the upper respiratory tract and ear. Atlas of tumor pathology. A.F.I.P. Washington, D.C. 1964.

[6] Avtandilov, G.G., and I.A. Kazantseva: Comparative microspectrophotometric study of the DNA content in the diagnosis of pre-tumorous processes and cancer. Virchows Arch. A Path. Anat. and Histol. *359* (1973) 289-297.

[7] Barton, R.T., and A. Ucmakli: Treatment of squamous cell carcinoma of the floor of the mouth. Surg. Gynecol. Obstet. *145* (1977) 21-27.

[8] Bauer, W.C., and M.H. McGavran: Carcinoma in situ and evaluation of epithelial changes in laryngopharyngeal biopsies. JAMA *221* (1972) 72-75.

[9] Berger, L., et H. Coutard: L'esthésioneurocytome olfactif. Bull de l'Assoc. franç. p. l'étude du cancer *15* (1926) 404-414.

[10] Berlinger, N.T., V. Tsakraklides, K. Pollak, G.L. Adams, M. Yang, and R.A. Good: Immunologic assessment of regional lymph node histology in relation to survival in head and neck carcinoma. Cancer *37* (1976) 697-705.

[11] Berthelsen, A., H.S. Hansen, and J. Rygard: Radiation therapy of squamous carcinoma of the floor of mouth and the lower alveolar ridge. J. Laryngol. Otol. *91* (1977) 489-499.

[12] Bianchi, C., and G. Muratti: Rhabdomyoma (adult type) of the larynx. (Fallbericht eines Rhabdomyosarkoms vom adulten Typ im Kehlkopf). Beitr. Path. *156* (1975) 75-79.

[13] Boies, L.R. Jr., and D. Harris: Nasopharyngeal dermoid of the newborn. Laryngoscope *75* (1965) 763-767.

[14] Bosch, A., L. Vallecillo, and Z. Frias: Cancer of the nasal cavity. Cancer *37* (1976) 1458-1463.

[15] Bridger, G.P., and V.H. Nassar: Cancer spread in the larynx. Arch. Otolaryng. *95* (1972) 497-505.

[16] Briselli, M., G.J. Mark, and H.C. Grillo: Tracheal carcinoids. Cancer *42* (1978) 2870-2879.

[17] Burkhardt, A., W.-J. Höltje, and J.-O. Gebbers: Vascular lesions following perfusion with bleomycin. Electron-microscopic observations. Virchows Arch. A Path. Anat. and Histol. *372* (1976) 227-236.

[18] Burkhardt, A., und G. Seifert: Morphologische Klassifikation der oralen Leukoplakie. Dtsch. Med. Wschr. *102* (1977) 223-229.

[19] Cachin, Y.: Cancers of the head and neck: Prognostic factors and criteria of response to treatment. In: Cancer therapy: Prognostic factors and criteria of response, edited by M.J. Staquet, Raven Press, New York 1975.

[20] Cachin, Y.: Cancer of the head and neck. In: Randomized trials in cancer: A critical review by sites, edited by M.J. Staquet, Raven Press, New York 1978.

[21] Coates, H.L., G.R. Pearson, H.B. Neel III, L.H. Weiland, and K.D. Devine: An immunologic basis for detection of occult primary malignancies of the head and neck. Cancer *41* (1978) 912-918.

[22] Cottier, H., J. Turk, and L. Sobin: A proposal for a standardized system of reporting human lymph node morphology in relation to immunological function. Bull. WHO *47* (1972) 375-417.

[23] Crawley, W.A., and L.S. Levin: Treatment of the ameloblastoma. A controversy. Cancer *42* (1978) 357-363.

[24] Dahm, L.J., St.D. Schaefer, H.M. Carder, and F. Vellios: Osteosarcoma of the soft tissue of the larynx. Report of a case with light and electron microscopic studies. Cancer *42* (1978) 2343-2351.

[25] Deutsch, M., R. Mercado Jr., and J.A. Parsons: Cancer of the nasopharynx in children. Cancer *41* (1978) 1128-1133.

[26] Dold, U.W., und H. Sack: Praktische Tumortherapie. Thieme, Stuttgart 1975.

[27] Domanski, R., und U. Schoen: Das sogenannte Myoblastenmyom des Kehlkopfes. HNO *25* (1977) 172-174.

[28] Dooling, E.C., J.G. Chi, and F.H. Gilles: Melanotic neuroectodermal tumor of infancy. Its histological similarities to fetal pineal gland. Cancer *39* (1977) 1535-1541.

[29] Einhorn, J., and J. Wersäll: Incidence of oral carcinoma in patients with leukoplakia of the oral mucosa. Cancer *20* (1967) 2189-2193.

[30] Eneroth, C.-M.: Incidence and prognosis of salivary-gland tumours at different sites; a study of parotid, submandibular and palatal tumours in 2632 patients. Acta Otolaryngol. (Stockholm) *263* (1970) 174-178.

[31] Eusebi, V., C.M. Betts, and F. Giangaspero: Primary oat-cell carcinoma of the larynx. Virchows Arch. A Path. Anat. and Histol. *380* (1978) 349-354.

[32] Ferlito, A.: Histiocytic tumors of the larynx. A clinicopathological study with review of the literature. Cancer *42* (1978) 611-622.

[33] Fligiel, Z., and M. Kaneko: Extramammary Paget's disease of the external ear canal in association with ceruminous gland carcinoma. A case report. Cancer 36 (1975) 1072-1076.

[34] Frommhold, H., R. Janson und K. Scherholz: Zur Strahlenbehandlung von Tumoren der Nase und der Nasennebenhöhlen. I. Mitteilung. Strahlentherapie 154 (1978) 813-819.

[35] Fu, Y.-S., and K.H. Perzin: Nonepithelial tumors of the nasal cavity, paranasal sinuses, and nasopharynx: A clinicopathologic study. IV. Smooth muscle tumors (leiomyoma, leiomyosarcoma). Cancer 35 (1975) 1300-1308.

[36] Fu, Y.-S., and K.H. Perzin: Nonepithelial tumors of the nasal cavity, paranasal sinuses, and nasopharynx. A clinicopathologic study. V. Skeletal muscle tumors (rhabdomyoma and rhabdomyosarcoma). Cancer 37 (1976) 364-376.

[37] Fu, Y.-S., and K.H. Perzin: Nonepithelial tumors of the nasal cavity, paranasal sinuses, and nasopharynx. A clinicopathologic study. VI. Fibrous tissue tumors (fibroma, fibromatosis, fibrosarcoma). Cancer 37 (1976) 2912-2928.

[38] Fu, Y.-S., and K.H. Perzin: Nonepithelial tumors of the nasal cavity, paranasal sinuses, and nasopharynx: A clinicopathologic study. VII. Myxomas. Cancer 39 (1977) 195-203.

[39] Fu, Y.-S., and K.H. Perzin: Nonepithelial tumors of the nasal cavity, paranasal sinuses, and nasopharynx. A clinicopathologic study. VIII. Adipose tissue tumors (lipoma and liposarcoma). Cancer 40 (1977) 1314-1317.

[40] Fu, Y.-S., and K.H. Perzin: Nonepithelial tumors of the nasal cavity, paranasal sinuses, and nasopharynx. A clinicopathologic study. IX. Plasmocytomas. Cancer 42 (1978) 2399-2406.

[41] Fu, Y.-S., and K.H. Perzin: Nonepithelial tumors of the nasal cavity, paranasal sinuses, and nasopharynx. A clinicopathologic study. X. Malignant lymphomas. Cancer 43 (1979) 611-621.

[42] Gamel, J.W., I.W. McLean, W.D. Foster, and L.E. Zimmerman: Uveal melanomas. Correlation of cytologic features with prognosis. Cancer 41 (1978) 1897-1901.

[43] Gamez-Araujo, J.J., A.G. Ayala, and O. Guillamondegui: Mucinous adenocarcinomas of nose and paranasal sinuses. Cancer 36 (1975) 1100-1105.

[44] Glanz, H., und O. Kleinsasser: Radiogene Zweitcarcinome des Larynx. HNO 24 (1976) 48-59.

[45] Glanzmann, Ch.: Strahlentherapie in der Behandlung von Karzinomen der anterioren zwei Drittel der Zunge und des Mundbodens. Erfahrungen bei 266 Patienten aus dem Zeitraum 1950 bis 1975. Strahlentherapie 154 (1978) 368-379.

[46] Goldhaber, P.: Oral manifestations of disease. In: Harrison's Principles of internal medicine. Eighth edition, McGraw-Hill Book Company, New York–Düsseldorf etc. 1977.

[47] Goldstein, G., F.P. Parker, and G.S.F. Hugh: Ameloblastic sarcoma. Pathogenesis and treatment with chemotherapy. Cancer 37 (1976) 1673-1678.

[48] Griffin, T.W., G.E. Laramore, R.G. Parker, A.J. Gerdes, D.W. Hebard, J.C. Blasko, and M. Groudine: An evaluation of fast neutron beam teletherapy of metastatic cervical adenopathy from squamous cell carcinomas of the head and neck region. Cancer 42 (1978) 2517-2520.

[49] Häupl, K., und H. Riedel: Zähne und Zahnhalteapparat. In: Spezielle pathologische Anatomie. Band I, Hrsg. W. Doerr, E. Uehlinger. Springer, Berlin–Heidelberg–New York 1966.

[50] Hajdu, S.I., A.G. Huvos, J.T. Goodner, F.W. Foote Jr., and E.J. Beattie Jr.: Carcinoma of the trachea; clinicopathologic study of 41 cases. Cancer 25 (1970) 1448-1456.

[51] Hendricks, J.L., B.C. Mendelson, and J.E. Woods: Invasive carcinoma of the lower lip. Surg. Clin. North. Am. 57 (1977) 837-844.

[52] Herrold, K.M.: Induction of olfactory neuroepithelial tumors in Syrian hamsters by diethylnitrosamine. Cancer 17 (1964) 114-121.

[53] Hohbach, C., and W. Mootz: Chemodectoma of the larynx. A clinico-pathological study. Virchows Arch. A Path. Anat. and Histol. 378 (1978) 161-172.

[54] Holdcraft, J., and J.C. Gallagher: Malignant melanomas of the nasal and paranasal sinus mucosa. Ann. Otol. Rhinol. Laryngol. 78 (1969) 5-20.

[55] Hoppe, R.T., D.R. Goffinet, and M.A. Bagshaw: Carcinoma of the nasopharynx. Eighteen years' experience with megavoltage radiation therapy. Cancer 37 (1976) 2605-2612.

[56] Hornback, N.B., and H. Shidnia: Carcinoma of the lower lip. Treatment results at Indiana University Hospitals. Cancer 41 (1978) 352-357.

[57] Houston, H.E., W.S. Payne, E.G. Harrison Jr., and A.M. Olsen: Primary cancers of the trachea. Arch. Surg. 99 (1969) 132-140.

[58] Hutter, R.V.P., J.S. Lewis, F.W. Foote, and H.R. Tollefsen: Esthesioneuroblastoma. A clinical and pathologic study. Am. J. Surg. 106 (1963) 748-753.

[59] Incze, J.S., P.S. Lui, M.S. Strong, C.W. Vaughan, and M.P. Clemente: The morphology of human papillomas of the upper respiratory tract. Cancer 39 (1977) 1634-1646

[60] Johnston, W.D., and R.M. Byers: Squamous cell carcinoma of the tonsil in young adults. Cancer 39 (1977) 632-636.

[61] Joseph, T.J., and R.A. Komorowski: Thyroglossal duct carcinoma. Hum. Pathol. 6 (1975) 717-729.

[62] Kassel, S.H., R.A. Echevarria, and F.P. Guzzo: Midline malignant reticulosis (so-called lethal midline granuloma). Cancer 23 (1969) 920-935.

[63] Kirchner, J.A., and J.R. Owen: Five hundred cancers of the larynx and pyriform sinus. Results of treatment by radiation and surgery. Laryngoscope 87 (1977) 1288-1303.

[64] Kraus, F.T., and C. Perez-Mesa: Verrucous

557

carcinoma; clinical and pathologic study of 105 cases involving oral cavity, larynx, and genitalia. Cancer *19* (1966) 26-38.

[65] Krempien, B., W. E. Brandeis und R. Singer: Metastasierendes Ameloblastom im Kindesalter. Licht- und elektronenmikroskopische Befunde. Virchows Arch. A Path. Anat. and Histol. *381* (1979) 211-222.

[66] Lasser, A., P. R. Rothfeld, and R. S. Shapiro: Epithelial papilloma and squamous cell carcinoma of the nasal cavity and paranasal sinuses. A clinicopathological study. Cancer *38* (1976) 2503-2510.

[67] Lee, S. C., M. M. Henry, and F. Gonzalez-Crussi: Simultaneous occurrence of melanotic neuroectodermal tumor and brain heterotopia in the oropharynx. Cancer *38* (1976) 249-253.

[68] Lee, Y. W., and S. D. Gisser: Squamous cell carcinoma of the tongue in a nine year renal transplant survivor. A case report with a discussion of the risk of development of epithelial carcinomas in renal transplant survivors. Cancer *41* (1978) 1-6.

[69] Mantravadi, R. V. P., E. J. Liebner, and J. V. Ginde: An analysis of factors in the successful management of cancer of tonsillar region. Cancer *41* (1978) 1054-1058.

[70] Marks, J. E., B. Curnik, W. E. Powers, and J. H. Ogura: Carcinoma of the pyriform sinus. An analysis of treatment results and patterns of failure. Cancer *41* (1978) 1008-1015.

[71] Mashberg, A., and H. Meyers: Anatomical site and size of 222 early asymptomatic oral squamous cell carcinomas. A continuing prospective study of oral cancer. II. Cancer *37* (1976) 2149-2157.

[72] McGavran, M. H., W. C. Bauer, and J. H. Ogura: The incidence of cervical lymph node metastases from epidermoid carcinoma of the larynx and their relationship to certain characteristics of the primary tumor; a study based on the clinical and pathological findings for 96 patients treated by primary en bloc laryngectomy and radical neck dissection. Cancer *14* (1961) 55-66.

[73] McGavran, M. H., D. G. Sessions, R. F. Dorfman, D. O. Davis, and J. H. Ogura: Nasopharyngeal angiofibroma. Arch. Otolaryng. *90* (1969) 68-78.

[74] Michel, R. G., B. H. Woodward, J. D. Shelburne, and E. H. Bossen: Ceruminous gland adenocarcinoma. A light and electron microscopic study. Cancer *41* (1978) 545-553.

[75] Micheau, C.: A new histochemical and biochemical approach to olfactory esthesioneuroma. A nasal tumor of neural crest origin. Cancer *40* (1977) 314-318.

[76] Müller, R.-P., W. Castrup, S. Baumeister und G. Burkhardtsmaier: Zur Therapie der Malignome der Nasenhaupt- und -nebenhöhlen. Strahlentherapie *155* (1979) 149-153.

[77] Mullins, J. D., R. K. Newman, and C. A. Coltman Jr.: Primary oat cell carcinoma of the larynx. A case report and review of the literature. Cancer *43* (1979) 711-717.

[78] Niederer, J., N. V. Hawkins, W. D. Rider, and J. E. Till: Failure analysis of radical radiation therapy of supraglottic laryngeal carcinoma. Int. J. Radiat. Oncol. Biol. Phys. *2* (1977) 621-629.

[79] Nordman, E. M., and J. T. Kytta: Five year survival of patients with larynx carcinoma treated with irradiation. Strahlentherapie *154* (1978) 245-248.

[80] Oberman, H. A., and D. H. Rice: Olfactory neuroblastomas. A clinicopathologic study. Cancer *38* (1976) 2494-2502.

[81] Obert, G. J., K. D. Devine, and J. R. MacDonald Jr.: Olfactory neuroblastomas. Cancer *13* (1960) 205-214.

[82] Olofsson, J., and A. W. P. van Nostrand: Adenoid cystic carcinoma of the larynx. A report of four cases and a review of the literature. Cancer *40* (1977) 1307-1313.

[83] Osamura, R. Y., and G. Fine: Ultrastructure of the esthesioneuroblastoma. Cancer *38* (1976) 173-179.

[84] Page, D. L., S. W. Weiss, and J. C. Eggleston: Ultrastructural study of amyloid material in the calcifying epithelial odontogenic tumor. Cancer *36* (1975) 1426-1435.

[85] Patel, D. D., and R. I. Dave: Carcinoma of the anterior tongue in adolescence. Cancer *37* (1976) 917-921.

[86] Pène, F., and G. H. Fletcher: Results in irradiation of the in situ carcinomas of the vocal cords. Cancer *37* (1976) 2586-2590.

[87] Pigneux, J., P. M. Richaud, and C. Lagarde: The place of interstitial therapy using ^{192}iridium in the management of carcinoma of the lip. Cancer *43* (1979) 1073-1077.

[88] Pindborg, J. J., O. Jølst, G. Renstrup, and B. Roed-Petersen: Studies in oral leukoplakia: A preliminary report on the period prevalence of malignant transformation in leukoplakia based on a follow-up study of 248 patients. J. Am. Dent. Assoc. *76* (1968) 767-771.

[89] Pindborg, J. J., and I. R. H. Kramer: Histological typing of odontogenic tumours, jaw cysts and allied lesions. WHO, Geneva 1971.

[90] Ranløv, P., and J. J. Pindborg: The amyloid nature of the homogeneous substance in the calcifying epithelial odontogenic tumour. Acta Pathol. Microbiol. Scand. *68* (1966) 169-174.

[91] Rapidis, A. D., J. D. Langdon, M. F. Patel, and P. W. Harvey: STNMP. A new system for the clinico-pathological classification and identification of intraoral carcinomata. Cancer *39* (1977) 204-209.

[92] Ridolfi, R. L., P. H. Lieberman, R. A. Erlandson, and O. S. Moore: Schneiderian papillomas: A clinicopathologic study of 30 cases. Am. J. Surg. Path. *1* (1977) 43-53.

[93] Robinson, L., and M. G. Martinez: Unicystic ameloblastoma. A prognostically distinct entity. Cancer *40* (1977) 2278-2285.

[94] Romansky, S., D. W. Crocker, and K. N. F. Shaw: Ultrastructural studies on neuroblastoma. Evaluation of cytodifferentiation and correlation of morphology and biochemical and survival data. Cancer *42* (1978) 2392-2398.

[95] Rominger, C. J., and F. J. Santore: Juvenile na-

sopharyngeal fibroma in a female adult: Report of a case. Arch. Otolaryng. *88* (1968) 177-179.

[96] Rossberg, G., und G. Rosemann: Über das „branchiogene Karzinom". Zeitschrift f. Laryngologie-Rhinologie-Otologie *43* (1964) 141-147.

[97] Roth, J.A., F.M. Enzinger, and M. Tannenbaum: Synovial sarcoma of the neck: A follow-up study of 24 cases. Cancer *35* (1975) 1243-1253.

[98] Sanchez-Casis, G., K.D. Devine, and L.H. Weiland: Nasal adenocarcinomas that closely simulate colonic carcinomas. Cancer *28* (1971) 714-720.

[99] Saunders, J.R., D.A. Jaques, P.F. Casterline, B. Percarpio, and S. Goodloe: Liposarcomas of the head and neck. A review of the literature and addition of four cases. Cancer *43* (1979) 162-168.

[100] Schenk, P.: Cytoplasmatische Mikrofilamente in malignen Keratinocyten des Larynxcarcinoms. HNO *25* (1977) 413-418.

[101] Schmauz, R., W. Hoppe und H. zur Hausen: Okkultes Nasopharynxkarzinom. Deutsche Medizinische Wochenschrift *100* (1975) 2527-2529.

[102] Schöndorf, J., und H. Seeliger: Maligne Synovialome im Halsbereich. HNO *25* (1977) 99-101.

[103] Schulz, U., M. Bamberg und E. Scherer: Lokalrezidive bei verhornenden Plattenepithelkarzinomen der Mundhöhle. Auftreten, Ursachen und Therapie nach kurativer Primärbehandlung. Strahlentherapie *155* (1979) 154-159.

[104] Seifert, G.: Mundhöhle, Mundspeicheldrüsen, Tonsillen und Rachen. In: Spezielle pathologische Anatomie. Band I, Hrsg. W. Doerr und E. Uehlinger. Springer, Berlin–Heidelberg–New York 1966.

[105] Seward, G.R., S.J. Beales, N.W. Johnson, and E.G.S. Lumsden: A metastasising ameloblastoma associated with renal calculi and hypercalcaemia. Cancer *36* (1975) 2277-2285.

[106] Shafer, W.G., and C.A. Waldron: Erythroplakia of the oral cavity. Cancer *36* (1975) 1021-1028.

[107] Shaw, H.J., and M. Hardingham: Cancer of the floor of the mouth: Surgical management. J. Laryngol. Otol. *91* (1977) 467-488.

[108] Shear, M., D.M. Hawkins, and H.W. Farr: The prediction of lymph node metastases from oral squamous carcinoma. Cancer *37* (1976) 1901-1907.

[109] Shepperd, H.W.: Surgery for the post-cricoid carcinoma: Report on 23 cases in which replacement by stomach was attempted. J. Otolaryngol. *6* (1977) 271-276.

[110] Silverman, S. Jr., K. Bhargava, N.J. Mani, L.W. Smith, and A.M. Malaowalla: Malignant transformation and natural history of oral leukoplakia in 57,518 industrial workers of Gujarat, India. Cancer *38* (1976) 1790-1795.

[111] Snow, G.B., R.P. Boom, J.F. Delemarre, and J.A. Bangert: Squamous carcinoma of the oropharynx. Clin. Otolaryngol. *2* (1977) 93-103.

[112] Snyder, R.N., and K.H. Perzin: Papillomatosis of nasal cavity and paranasal sinuses (inverted papilloma, squamous papilloma). A clinicopathologic study. Cancer *30* (1972) 668-677.

[113] Spanos, W.J. Jr., L.J. Shukovsky, and G.H. Fletcher: Time, dose, and tumor volume relationships in irradiation of squamous cell carcinomas of the base of the tongue. Cancer *37* (1976) 2591-2599.

[114] Szpak, C.A., M.J. Stone, and E.P. Frenkel: Some observations concerning the demo-graphic and geographic incidence of carcinoma of the lip and buccal cavity. Cancer *40* (1977) 343-348.

[115] Takagi, M., Y. Sakota, S. Takayama, and G. Ishikawa: Adenoid squamous cell carcinoma of the oral mucosa. Report of two autopsy cases. Cancer *40* (1977) 2250-2255.

[116] Taxy, J.B.: Juvenile nasopharyngeal angiofibroma. An ultrastructural study. Cancer *39* (1977) 1044-1054.

[117] Taxy, J.B., and D.F. Hidvegi: Olfactory neuroblastoma. An ultrastructural study. Cancer *39* (1977) 131-138.

[118] Taylor, R.F.: Late recurrence of cancer in the larynx and hypopharynx after irradiation. ORL *39* (1977) 251-256.

[119] Vandenbrouck, C., H. Sancho, R.L. Fur, J.M. Richard, and Y. Cachin: Results of a randomized clinical trial of preoperative irradiation versus postoperative in treatment of tumors of the hypopharynx. Cancer *39* (1977) 1445-1449.

[120] Wahi, P.N.: Histological typing of oral and oropharyngeal tumours. WHO, Geneva 1971.

[121] Waldron, C.A., and W.G. Shafer: Leukoplakia revisited. A clinicopathologic study of 3256 oral leukoplakias. Cancer *36* (1975) 1386-1392.

[122] Wilander, E., H. Nordlinder, L. Grimelius, L.-I. Larsson, and C. Angelborg: Esthesioneuroblastoma. Histological, histochemical and electron microscopic studies of a case. Virchows Arch. A Path. Anat. and Histol. *375* (1977) 123-128.

[123] Wittes, R.E., R.H. Spiro, J. Shah, F.P. Gerold, B. Koven, and E.W. Strong: Chemotherapy of head and neck cancer: Combination treatment with cyclophosphamide, adriamycin, methotrexate, and bleomycin. Med. Pediatr. Oncol. *3* (1977) 301-309.

14 Tumors of the salivary glands

Salivary glands

1. Tumors of the salivary glands arise mainly from epithelial cells, which form the acini or line the ducts.
2. The dual epithelial origin of salivary gland tumors is responsible for the variability of growth patterns observed in these neoplasms.
   The architecture of even one tumor can be so pleomorphic that a large group of these neoplasms of the salivary glands have been called "mixed tumors."
3. There are two subgroups of salivary glands: The major salivary glands – parotid, submandibular, and sublingual glands – and minor (smaller) salivary glands distributed in the oral cavity, bronchi, nasopharynx, trachea, and lacrimal glands.
4. The structure of the different salivary glands is identical; the incidence of the tumors arising from these various glands is different.
5. The majority of salivary gland tumors develop in the parotid gland. The majority of pleomorphic adenomas, mucoepidermoid carcinomas, and Whartin tumors are observed in the parotid glands.
6. Due to the pleomorphic appearance of salivary gland tumors, a number of differential diagnoses occasionally must be solved.
   Important in the differential diagnosis is the recognition of malignant lymphomas versus salivary gland inflammation, the recognition of adenoid cystic carcinoma, and the diagnosis of a carcinoma arising in a pleomorphic adenoma.
7. The percentage of malignant tumors in relation to the overall tumor growth is higher in the submandibular gland than in the parotid gland:
   17% of the tumors in the parotid gland are malignant, 38% in the submandibular glands, and 44% in salivary glands of the palate are malignant [6].

----

[6] Eneroth 1970.

M-8561/0
T 142.0

1. Adenolymphoma (WHO)

(Whartin tumor, papillary cystadenoma lymphomatosum)

General Remarks	**Incidence:** About 6% of the epithelial salivary gland tumors are adenolymphomas. About 70% of the bilateral salivary gland tumors are adenolymphomas [38]. **Age:** All ages can be affected. The majority of patients are around 40 years old. **Sex:** Almost all adenolymphomas are observed in males (80 to 90%).
T 142.0	**Site:** Adenolymphomas are almost always tumors of the parotid gland. The tumor can develop in the parotid gland or in the immediate neighborhood. Adenolymphomas can be solitary or multiple tumors: About 15% are bilateral. Rarely, foci of adenolymphomas can be observed in lymph nodes.
Macroscopy	Adenolymphomas are cystic tumors, which are encapsulated. The tumor is smooth, and it is lobulated or round. The size is about 2 to 5 cm, rarely 8 cm across. Adenolymphomas are adherent to the skin.
Histology	The tumor is composed of lymphatic tissue with germinal centers and epithelial cells (Fig. 562). The epithelial cells line the tubular and cystic structures in the tumor. These cells are acidophilic and are similar to oncocytes. The cysts are lined by a second cell row underneath the epithelial cell layer. These cells are smaller and indistinct. The cells lining the cysts can follow a papillary growth pattern, which projects into the lumen of the cysts (Figs. 563 and 564). The connective tissue between the cysts is the site of the lymphatic tissue.
Electron Microscopy	The lining epithelial cells are packed with mitochondria similar to the oxyphilic cells in oncocytomas (Fig. 565).
Clinical Findings	Adenolymphomas are slow-growing tumors almost always affecting the parotid gland. A rather considerable percentage of the tumors are bilateral.
Treatment	Resection of the tumor.
Prognosis	Adenolymphomas are benign tumors with an excellent prognosis.
Further Information	1. Adenolymphomas are of a multifocal origin. The recurrences after surgery are partly due to the outgrowth of new adenolymphomas. The recurring tumor remains benign. 2. The histogenesis of adenolymphomas might be the growth of heterotopic salivary gland tissue within lymph nodes. Occasionally lymph nodes contain remnants of this adenolymphoma. These adenolymphoma islets in lymph nodes should not be mistaken for metastatic lesions.

---

[38] Turnbull and Frazell 1969.

563

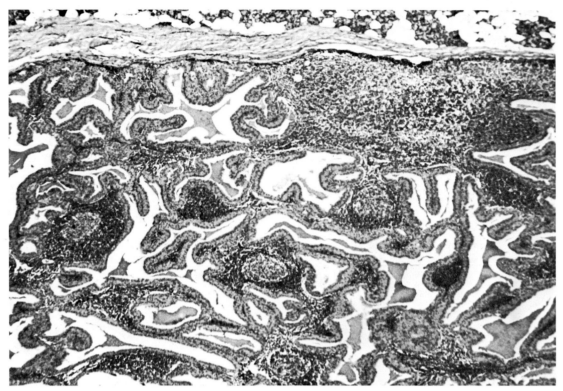

Fig. 562. Adenolymphoma (76-year-old female, × 125).

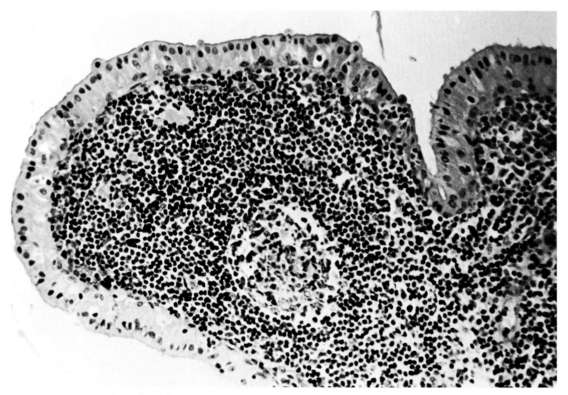

Fig. 563. Adenolymphoma (× 200).

564

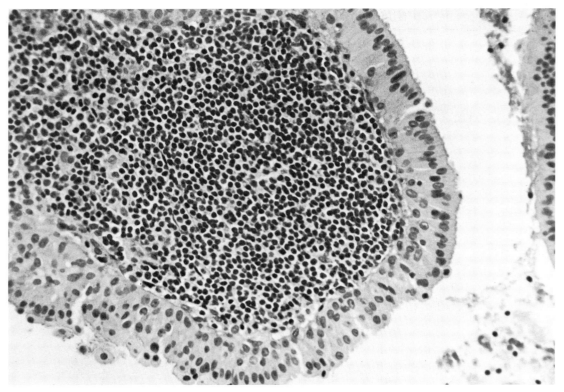

Fig. 564. Adenolymphoma (53-year-old male, × 200).

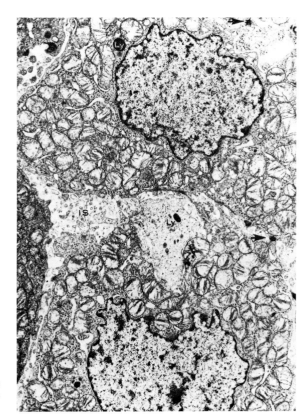

Fig. 565. Oncocytoma: Numerous mitochondria (× 14,000) (Lee and Roth, Cancer *37* [1976] 1607-1614).

M-8290/0
T 142.9

2. Oxyphilic adenoma (WHO)

(oncocytoma) [12]

**General
Remarks**

Incidence: Oxyphilic adenomas are very rare.

Macroscopy

Oxyphilic adenomas are encapsulated and soft.
The tumor is small and does not exceed 5 cm in diameter.
The cut surface is pink; cyst formations are rare.

Histology

The tumor is composed of acidophilic large cells [12]. These cells have vesicular, regular, or pycnotic nuclei. The nuclei contain a nucleolus. Mitoses are very rare (Figs. 566 and 567).
Between the tumor cells there is only a discrete connective tissue, which organizes the tumor in lobes and lobules [35].

**Clinical
Findings**

This is a slow-growing, unilateral tumor.

Treatment

The benign oxyphilic adenoma is treated by simple excision.

Prognosis

Excellent, no recurrences.

**Further
Information
M-8290/3
T 142.9**

Malignant oncocytomas have been reported very rarely [2, 12, 21].

[2] Bazaz-Malik and Gupta 1968.
[12] Hamperl 1962.
[21] Lee and Roth 1976.
[35] Tandler et al. 1970.

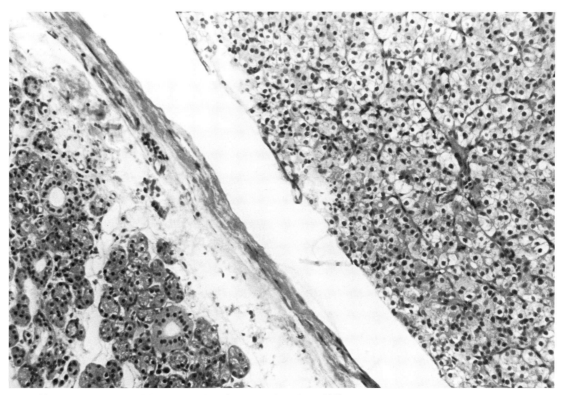

Fig. 566 Oxyphil adenoma of the parotid gland (76-year-old male, ×125).

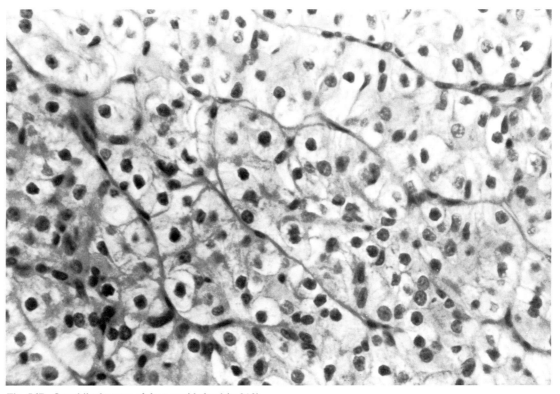

Fig. 567. Oxyphil adenoma of the parotid gland (×310).

M-8146/0
T 142.0

3. Adenoma (monomorphic) of the salivary glands (WHO)

General
Remarks

Incidence: Monomorphic adenomas are rare.
Site: The majority of these adenomas grow in the parotid gland.
The adenomas originate from ductal cells.

Macroscopy

Monomorphic adenomas are encapsulated tumors. The cut surface contains cysts in most instances.

Histology

Monomorphic adenomas are composed of epithelial cells that have regular round or spindle-shaped nuclei.
These cells can show a fascicular growth pattern, solid complexes, or tubular structures.
According to the growth pattern and the type of cells, the monomorphic adenomas are subclassified as

M-8310/0

a) Adenoma of clear cell type (WHO)
This adenoma is composed of clear cells (similar to those in renal cell carcinoma). The tumor cells form large complexes that are surrounded by very discrete connective tissue.

M-8190/0

b) Trabecular adenoma (WHO)
The tumor cells in this adenoma form a trabecular growth pattern and are embedded in a very loose connective tissue with few cells (Fig. 568).

M-8211/0

c) Tubular adenoma (WHO)
In this adenoma the entire tumor is composed of epithelial cells that are arranged in a tubular growth pattern (Figs. 569 and 570).

M-8147/0

d) Basal cell type adenoma (WHO)
In this adenoma the tumor cells form large complexes that are surrounded by cells in a palisade position (Fig. 571) (resembling the structure of basal cell tumors in the skin) [1, 5].

Electron
Microscopy

Some cells of the basal cell type of adenoma contain tonofilaments with prominent desmosomes, mitochondria, and a small Golgi apparatus with many small secretory vesicles [14].

[1] Batsakis 1972.
[5] Crumpler et al. 1976.
[14] Headington et al. 1977.

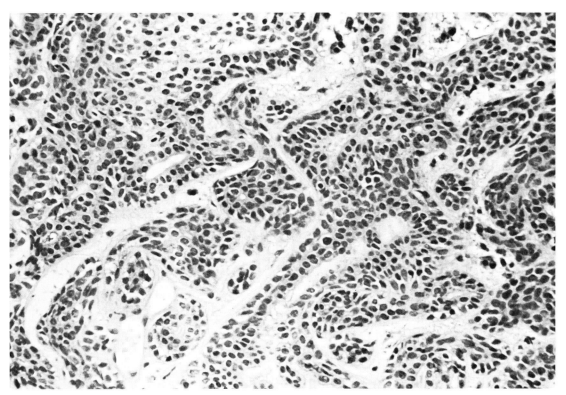

Fig. 568. Monomorphic adenoma, trabecular type (× 200).

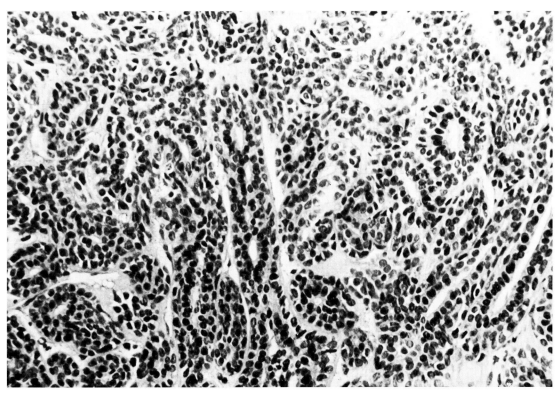

Fig. 569. Monomorphic adenoma, tubular type (55-year-old male, × 200).

Monomorphic adenoma

Differential Diagnosis

1. Monomorphic adenoma **with pleomorphic adenoma** (Figs. 572 to 576):
   The pleomorphic adenoma contains an epithelial component and an important mesenchymal component, which is lacking in monomorphic adenomas [24].
2. Monomorphic adenoma **with adenoid cystic carcinoma** (Figs. 588 to 592):
   Occasionally the monomorphic adenoma can form cystic spaces.
   The adenoid cystic carcinoma shows atypical nuclei and there is almost always an invasion of tumor cells into the lymphatics.

Further Information

1. Monomorphic adenomas are also oxyphilic adenomas and adenolymphomas [3a].
2. Occasionally there is an association between multiple dermal cylindromas (turban tumor) and multiple cylindromas of the dermal type in both parotid glands [27].

[3a] Cameron and Stenram 1979.
[24] Nelson and Jacoway 1973.
[27] Reingold et al. 1977.

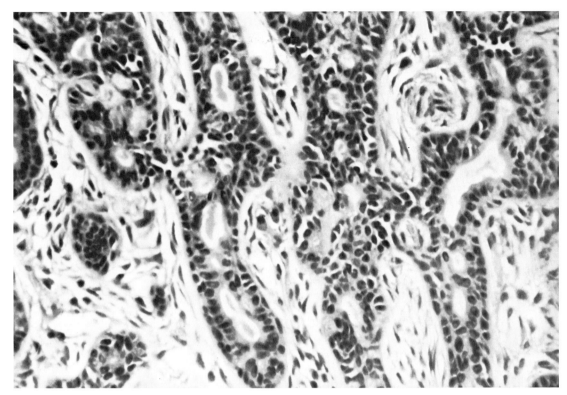

Fig. 570. Monomorphic adenoma, tubular type (× 310).

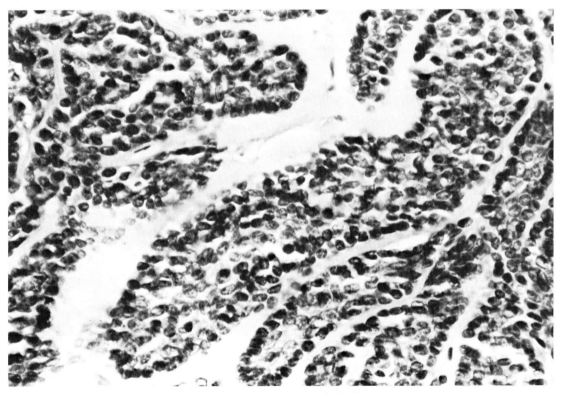

Fig. 571. Monomorphic adenoma, basaloid type, of the parotid gland (× 310).

M-8940/0
T 142.9

4. Pleomorphic adenoma (WHO)

(mixed tumor)

**General
Remarks**

Incidence: This is the most common tumor in the salivary glands.

Age: The peak age is the 5th decade. Elderly persons can be equally affected as often as children [19].

Sex: Females are more frequently affected than males.

T 142.0
T 142.1

Site: Pleomorphic adenomas occur mainly in the parotid gland (about 85%), whereas the other salivary glands are less frequently affected (10% in the submandibular gland and 5% in other salivary glands).

In the parotid gland 50% of the tumors are in the tail, 25% are in the anterior portion.

Macroscopy

Pleomorphic adenomas are surrounded by a thin capsule. The tumor is usually about 5 cm across; occasionally it is larger.

The tumor may be firm or soft. On the cut surface there are signs of lobulation, occasionally cysts, and the appearance and consistency of cartilage. Occasionally the cut surface is mucinous.

The tumor grows in the salivary gland. Occasionally it can also be observed outside the salivary gland (parotid gland).

Histology

Pleomorphic adenomas are composed of an epithelial and a mesenchymal component. Since both components can have different appearances in their cytological aspect and their growth pattern, a great variability is characteristic for this tumor (Fig. 572).

The mesenchymal component contains mucoid substances. Occasionally the stroma has a myxomatous appearance with a PAS-positive staining. Furthermore, there are areas of cartilage (Fig. 573).

The epithelial component can form solid nests, sheets, or tubular or adenoid structures. Occasionally there are areas of keratinization (Fig. 574).

Sometimes the tumor tissue is very rich in epithelial cells. Sometimes they are very sparse (Fig. 575).

The epithelial cells occasionally exhibit signs of mucin production.

In pleomorphic adenoma the histological picture can be dominated by the mesenchymal component, including cartilage, or by the epithelial cells.

The majority of pleomorphic adenomas are very rich in connective tissue (about 50% of the cases), while in 15% the cellular epithelial component dominates.

In about 10% the mesenchymal component contains foci of mucoid-chondroid or mucoid stroma (20%) [29] (Fig. 576).

These differences in the composition of pleomorphic adenoma are also reflected in tumor cell culture [33].

**Electron
Microscopy**

Evidence of clear and dark cells (Fig. 577).

---

[19] Krolls et al. 1972.
[29] Seifert et al. 1977.
[33] Takeuchi et al. 1975.

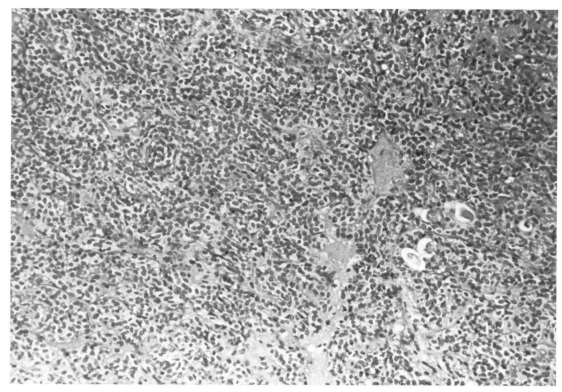

Fig. 572. Pleomorphic adenoma of the parotid gland: Epithelial component with solid cell nests and some ductal structures (×125).

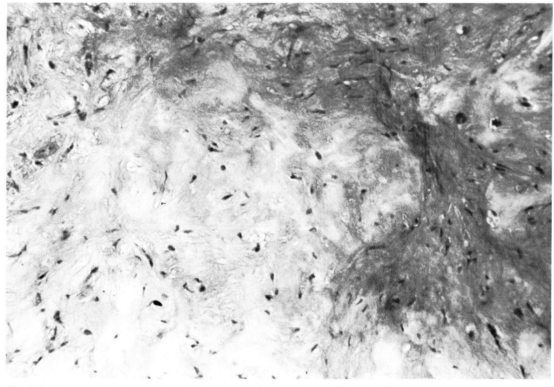

Fig. 573. Pleomorphic adenoma: Mucoid and chondroid area (73-year-old male, ×125).

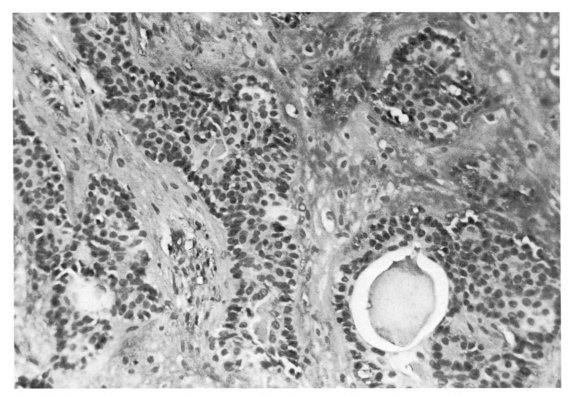

Fig. 574. Pleomorphic adenoma: Epithelial strands and ductal structures (41-year-old female, × 200).

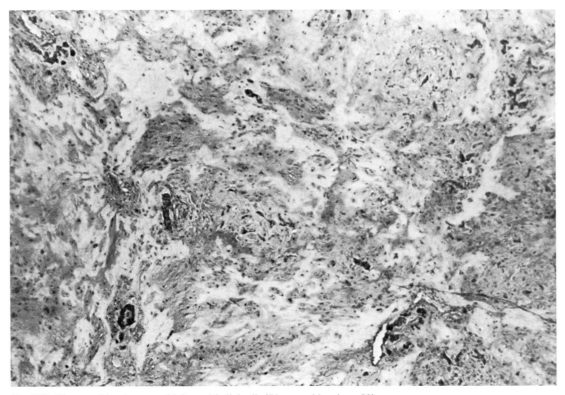

Fig. 575. Pleomorphic adenoma with few epithelial cells (73-year-old male, × 50).

574

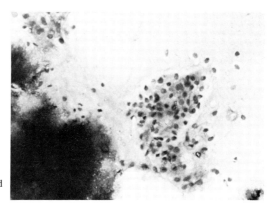

Fig. 576. Pleomorphic adenoma of the parotid gland: Area of epithelial cells and mesenchymal ground substance (dark) (May-Grünwald-Giemsa stain, × 400).

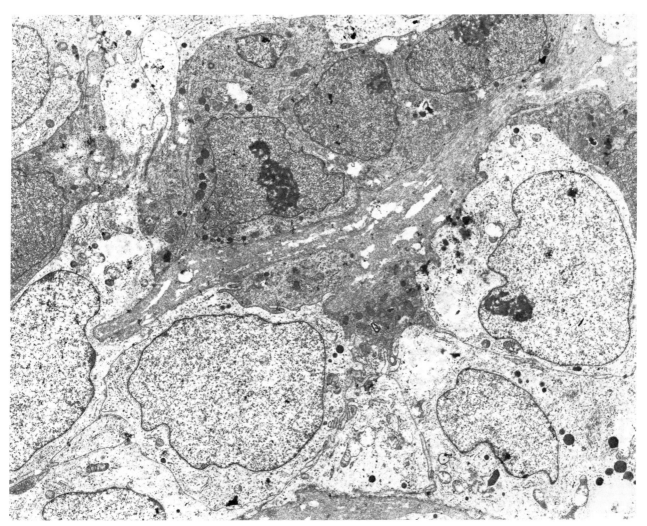

Fig. 577. Pleomorphic adenoma, parotid gland: Demonstration of a clear and dark cell type due to different densities of the cytoplasm and the nucleus (× 10,500).

575

Pleomorphic adenoma

Differential Diagnosis

Pleomorphic adenoma **with carcinoma in pleomorphic adenoma:**
The benign adenoma contains foci of high cellularity, hyperchromatic nuclei, and occasionally mitotic figures. Benign pleomorphic adenoma can mimic infiltration into the capsule and the surrounding tissue and even lymph node metastases (heterotopic tissue) (Figs. 578 and 579).
Proof of malignancy is the invasion of perineural spaces. In case of doubt the differential diagnosis is supported by the following facts:
- Carcinomas develop more frequently in pleomorphic adenomas, which are dominated by epithelial cells [29].
- Carcinomas in pleomorphic adenomas are in more than 50% of the undifferentiated type or adenocarcinomas (see page 578).

Clinical Findings

At the site of the parotid gland just beneath the lobule of the ear, there is a movable tumor.
The tumor causes pain.
Pleomorphic adenomas are slow-growing.

Treatment

The complete removal of the pleomorphic adenoma is important (high recurrence rate).

Prognosis

The complete removal of the adenoma practically always means cure for the patient [18].
Multiple recurrences are common. Complete resection of recurrent tumors is more difficult than that of primary tumors.
Recurrences might be due to a multifocal origin of the tumor.
The frequency of recurrences in the parotid gland is about 15% and in the submandibular gland it is about 15%, while the pleomorphic adenoma at other sites rarely recurs.
The majority of recurrences occur 1 to 2 years after operation; they can, however, appear many years following the surgical intervention.
Numerous recurrences are not equivalent with malignant tumors; however, with the second and subsequent recurrences the incidence of malignancy becomes higher, about 25% [8]. It can be postulated that these malignant pleomorphic adenomas were carcinomas from the onset.
There is one report of metastases of a pleomorphic adenoma into the lung and other organs [11].

[8] Frazell 1954.
[11] Gerughty et al. 1969.
[18] Kirklin et al. 1951.
[29] Seifert et al. 1977.

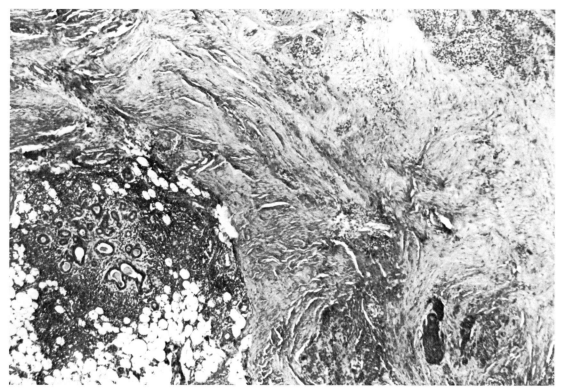

Fig. 578. Pleomorphic adenoma: Ectopic tumor tissue mimicking malignant infiltration (53-year-old female, × 40).

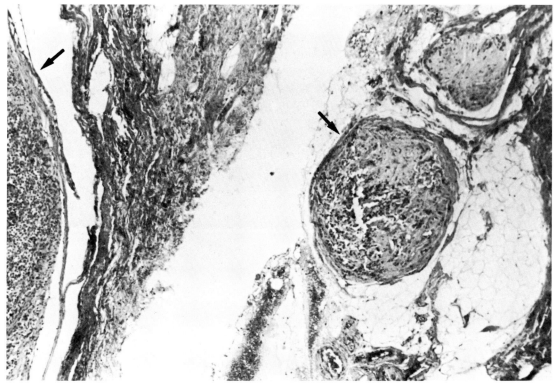

Fig. 579. Pleomorphic adenoma (arrow): Ectopic tumor tissue, no malignancy (double arrow) (28-year-old male, × 40).

577

M-8940/3
T 142.9

5. Carcinoma in pleomorphic adenoma (WHO)

(malignant mixed tumor)

General
Remarks

T 142.0

T 142.1

T 145.9

Incidence: Carcinomas develop in 4.5% of pleomorphic adenomas [6, 23].

The incidence of carcinoma is different in the different glands:

– About 5% of the pleomorphic adenomas in the parotid gland contain carcinomas.
– The submandibular gland is very rarely affected.
– At other locations about 10% of the adenomas become carcinomatous (minor salivary glands in the oral cavity, hard palate, soft palate, tonsilar region, tongue, gingiva, buccal mucosa).

Age: The peak age for carcinomas is the 7th and 8th decades [29].

Further notes: Probably carcinomas develop in long-persisting pleomorphic adenomas [6, 23].

Macroscopy

Pleomorphic adenomas with carcinomatous components are similar to benign pleomorphic adenoma.

Some differences can, however, occasionally be observed:

– Carcinomas in pleomorphic adenomas are larger than the benign tumor.
– There are adhesions with the surrounding structures, including the skin. The skin can be ulcerated.
– The malignant pleomorphic adenoma is more bosselated than the benign tumor.
– Carcinomas are not encapsulated.
– The consistency is less firm and the tumor is friable.
– The cut surface contains necroses and hemorrhages with multiple cysts.

Histology

In pleomorphic adenoma there can be all types of carcinomas, which also grow as primary tumors in the salivary glands.

In pleomorphic adenomas the following tumors are observed:

a) Undifferentiated carcinoma in about 35% of the cases,

b) adenocarcinoma in about 27% of the cases,

c) adenoid cystic carcinoma in about 10% of the cases (Figs. 588 to 592),

d) mucoepidermoid carcinoma in about 15% of the cases (Fig. 580),

e) squamous cell carcinoma in about 10% of the cases (Fig. 581),

f) acinic cell tumor (Figs. 593 and 594) [29].

The carcinomatous component in pleomorphic adenoma is announced by the appearance of very atypical cells, atypical nuclei and nulceoli, and an increase in mitotic figures.

The infiltration into the surrounding structures can be detected (however, this can also be found in benign adenomas).

Perineural invasion of the tumor cells definitively indicates malignant tumor in pleomorphic adenoma.

[6] Eneroth 1970.
[23] Moberger and Eneroth 1968.
[29] Seifert et al. 1977.

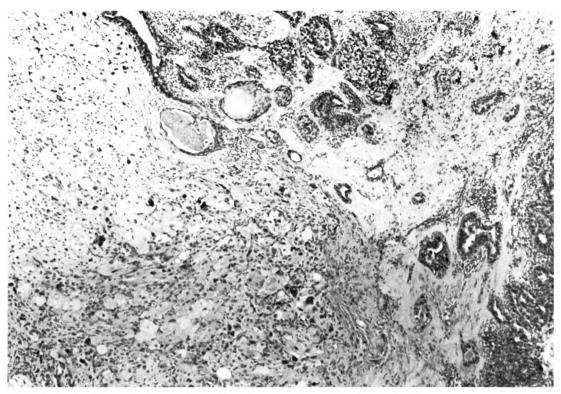

Fig. 580. Poorly differentiated mucoepidermoid carcinoma in pleomorphic adenoma (× 50).

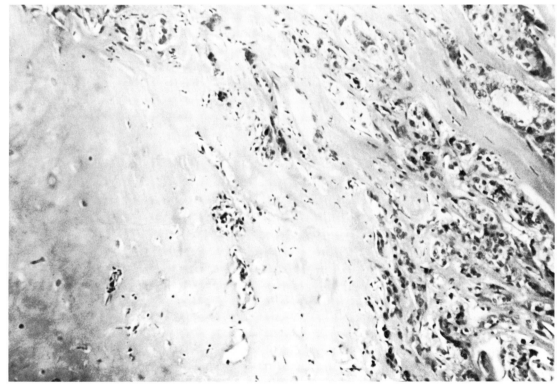

Fig. 581. Carcinoma in pleomorphic adenoma (× 125).

Carcinoma in pleomorphic adenoma

Differential Diagnosis

Carcinoma in pleomorphic adenoma **with benign pleomorphic adenoma:**
The most important feature is the invasion of the perineural spaces.

Spread

1. The degree of spread, including the local infiltration, depends on the type of carcinoma:
   High grade malignant tumors are more aggressive than low grade tumors (for instance, the well-differentiated mucoepidermoid carcinoma).
2. The tumor infiltrates the lymphatics and causes regional lymph node metastases.
3. Hematogenous spread into bone, lung, and other organs.

Clinical Findings

The symptoms are due to the onset of infiltration and rapid growth of the carcinoma in a pleomorphic adenoma:
Appearance of pain, facial paralysis, adherence to the skin with ulceration, infiltration of the surrounding structures (facial paralysis), and rapid increase of the tumor size.
Important is the appearance of facial paralysis, which is observed in about one-third of the cases of tumor of the parotid gland.

Treatment

Surgery:
Radical resection of the salivary gland in which the tumor grows, including the surrounding tissue with possibly a wide safe margin.
The surgery can be combined with neck dissection.
Radiation therapy:
The tumor cells in carcinoma in a pleomorphic adenoma have low radiosensitivity.
Postoperative irradiation should, however, be tried so as to reduce the number of recurrences [10, 26, 31].
Adjuvant postoperative chemotherapy should be tried in order to avoid recurrences as much as possible [28].

Prognosis

The 5-year survival rate is determined by the type of the carcinoma, the extension of the tumor, and the site of the tumor:
a) Carcinomas in pleomorphic adenomas in salivary glands of the palate have a better prognosis than carcinomas arising in the major salivary glands [22].
b) Carcinomas arising in the submandibular gland have a worse prognosis than those growing in other salivary glands.
c) The 5-year survival rate for mucoepidermoid carcinoma in pleomorphic adenoma is 60 to 80%.
   for squamous cell carcinoma: about 20%
   for adenocarcinoma and undifferentiated carcinoma: about 20%.
d) Recurrences of carcinomas in the salivary glands indicate a poor prognosis, regardless of treatment [17].

[10] Fu et al. 1977.
[17] Kagan et al. 1976.
[22] LiVolsi and Perzin 1977.
[26] Rafla 1977.
[28] Rentschler et al. 1977.
[31] Soni et al. 1977.

M-8430/3
T 142.0

6. Mucoepidermoid carcinoma (WHO)

General Remarks

Incidence: About 5 to 10% of tumors of the major salivary glands are mucoepidermoid carcinomas.

About 20% of the tumors of the minor salivary glands are mucoepidermoid carcinomas.

In the parotid gland mucoepidermoid carcinoma is the most frequently observed malignant tumor.

Age: The peak ages are the 4th and 5th decades.

Sex: Females are clearly more frequently affected than males.

T 145.9

Site: In the minor salivary glands, the mucoepidermoid carcinoma is usually observed in the palate.

T 142.0

90% of mucoepidermoid carcinomas grow in the parotid gland.

Macroscopy

Mucoepidermoid carcinomas are of different sizes, measuring from millimeters to 5 cm across and more.

Mucoepidermoid carcinomas are well circumscribed, but usually do not have a capsule.

The grayish-whitish-pinkish cut surface shows cysts.

Tumors larger than 5 cm are considered to be more malignant than smaller ones. Signs of infiltration into the surrounding tissue can be observed.

Histology

The tumor is composed of epithelial squamous cells (Fig. 582). These cells can form solid complexes or line cysts. (Fig. 583). The lining cells and the cells in the solid formations might produce mucin (Fig. 584). Occasionally there are foci of keratinization in the solid complexes (Fig. 585).

The number of cysts and the number of mucin-producing cells varies from tumor to tumor (Figs. 586 and 587).

The tumor infiltrates the lymphatics and grows into the surrounding structures.

Differential Diagnosis

1. Mucoepidermoid carcinoma **with squamous cell carcinoma** (Fig. 581):

   Occasionally the mucoepidermoid carcinoma can contain numerous foci of keratinization and few mucin-producing epithelial cells. Mucicarmine-positive staining in the epithelial cells indicates mucoepidermoid carcinoma; however, sometimes multiple sections are required to find these foci.

2. Mucoepidermoid carcinoma **with adenocarcinoma:**

   In some mucoepidermoid carcinomas the cysts with mucin-producing cells dominate the picture.

   Foci of squamous cell complexes lining the cysts indicate mucoepidermoid carcinoma.

Grading

Mucoepidermoid carcinomas of **low grade malignancy:**

The tumor contains multiple cysts with mucin in the lumen.

The mucin-producing cells dominate the picture; squamous cells are rare (Fig. 583).

Mucoepidermoid carcinoma of **high grade malignancy:**

There are considerably more squamous cells with nuclear atypias than mucin-producing cells (which occasionally can be found only with difficulty) (Fig. 587).

There are few cysts.

This tumor shows clear infiltration into the neighboring structures.

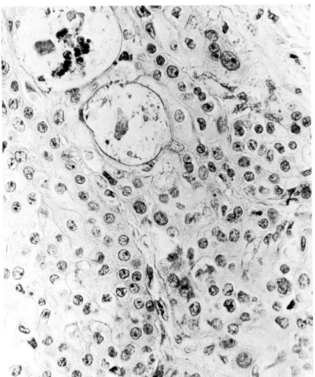

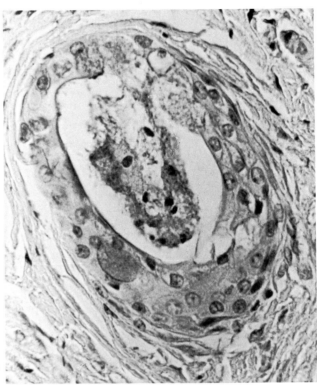

Fig. 582. Mucoepidermoid carcinoma: Gland formation (75-year-old female, × 200).

Fig. 583. Mucoepidermoid carcinoma: Epithelial duct (gland) formation (× 200).

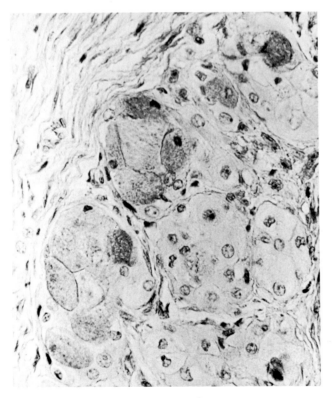

Fig. 584. Mucoepidermoid carcinoma: Mucin production in individual tumor cells, solid cell nests (× 200).

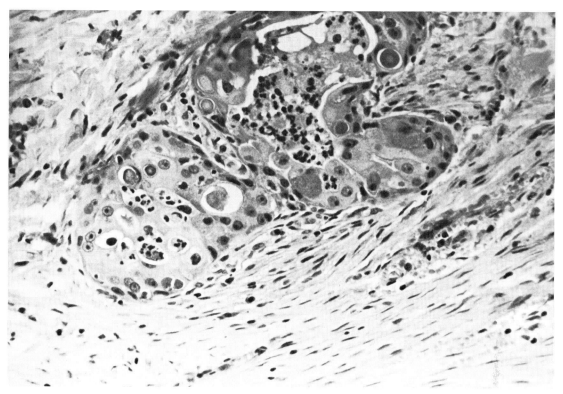

Fig. 585. Gland formation in mucoepidermoid carcinoma (69-year-old female, × 200).

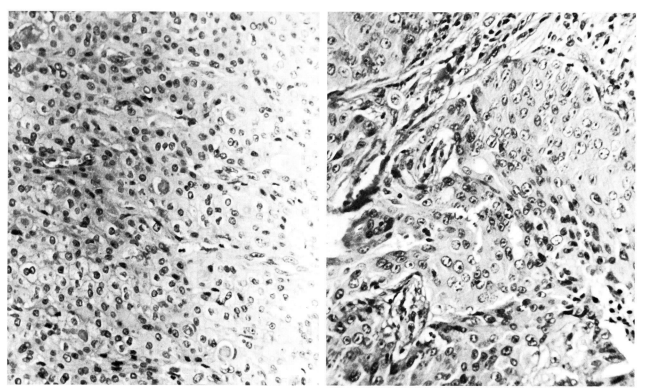

Fig. 586. Mucoepidermoid carcinoma: Solid cell growth and few glandular structures (× 125).

Fig. 587. Mucoepidermoid carcinoma, poorly differentiated (58-year-old male, × 200).

Spread

Mucoepidermoid carcinomas can metastasize by lymphatic and hematogenous spread. The low grade tumors metastasize less frequently than the high grade malignant mucoepidermoid carcinomas.

The overall rate of metastases in mucoepidermoid carcinomas is, however, low.

Clinical Findings

Slow-growing tumor without pain and without facial paralysis in almost all instances.

Treatment

Removal of the tumor.

Prognosis

a) 5-year survival rate for low grade mucoepidermoid carcinoma, about 100%.
b) 5-year survival rate for high grade malignancy, about 60% [15, 16].
c) Recurrence rate, about 15%.
d) Mucoepidermoid carcinoma in the submandibular gland has a worse prognosis than that arising in other salivary glands.

M-8070/3
T 142.9

7. Squamous cell carcinoma
(epidermoid carcinoma – WHO)

General Remarks

Incidence: Squamous cell carcinomas of the salivary glands are rare.

Macroscopy

The tumor is hard and infiltrates the surrounding tissue.
The tumor is adherent to the skin, which is sometimes ulcerated.

Histology

The tumor is composed of cells of a malignant squamous cell carcinoma with keratinizations.
There are no foci of mucin production by the tumor cells (mucin stain).

Spread

Squamous cell carcinomas are malignant tumors with early metastases into the regional lymph nodes.

Treatment

Radical **surgery** followed by **radiation therapy.**

Prognosis

Squamous cell carcinomas have a very poor prognosis due to rapid growth into the surrounding tissue and early metastases.

---

[15] Healey et al. 1970.
[16] Jakobsson et al. 1968.

584

M-8200/3
T 142.9

8. Adenoid cystic carcinoma (WHO)

("cylindroma")

**General
Remarks**

Incidence: About 7% of the salivary gland tumors are malignant adenoid cystic carcinomas.

About 20% of the tumors in the submandibular glands are adenoid cystic carcinoma; this malignant neoplasm is found in about 5% of the tumors of the parotid gland.

Age: The peak age is the 5th and 6th decades.

Site: Adenoid cystic carcinomas can occur in any salivary gland:

– Adenoid cystic carcinoma is the most frequent malignant neoplasm in the palatal salivary glands and in the submandibular gland. It is almost always a unilateral tumor.

Further notes: Adenoid cystic carcinomas can also occur in other parts of the organism: breast, bronchus, vagina.

Macroscopy

The tumor may be of various size, mostly measuring 2 to 6 cm across. The grayish-whitish cut surface is homogeneous and contains cysts only rarely.

There are signs of infiltration into the neighboring tissue.

Histology

Adenoid carcinomas have a cribriform appearance (Fig. 588).

The tumor cells show signs of discrete nuclear atypias; mitotic figures are rare.

The tumor cells are rich in glycosaminoglycan [34] and can produce PAS-positive material or mucin.

The tumor cells can form small, solid trabecular structures without an organoid imitation; in most instances, however, they imitate glandular structures (adenoid growth pattern) and ductlike tubular formations (Figs. 589 to 591).

These spaces are often lined by two cell rows: the inner epithelial lining and the outer myoepithelial cells.

The PAS-positive material that is produced by the tumor cells can be found in the lumen of the spaces or surrounding the myoepithelial cells [36].

The tumor cells in adenoid cystic carcinoma have a strong tendency to infiltrate the lymphatics and the perineural spaces (Fig. 592).

**Differential
Diagnosis**

1. Adenoid cystic carcinoma **with metastases from breast carcinoma.**
2. Adenoid cystic carcinoma **with benign adenoma:**
   The tumor cells in adenoid cystic carcinoma have only discrete signs of malignancy. However, the tumor is always malignant and should be treated accordingly [30].
   Evidence of invasion of the lymphatics ascertains the diagnosis of malignant tumor (Fig. 592).
3. Adenoid cystic carcinoma **with mucoepidermoid carcinoma** (Figs 582 to 587):
   Extensive invasion of the lymphatics indicates adenoid cystic carcinoma.

---

[30] Smith et al. 1965.
[34] Takeuchi et al. 1976.
[36] Thackray 1972.

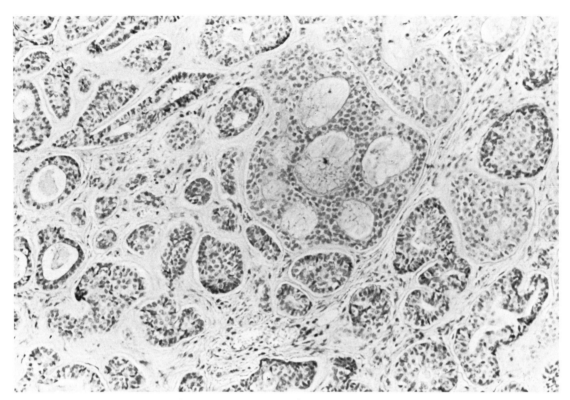

Fig. 588. Adenoid cystic carcinoma (37-year-old female, × 125).

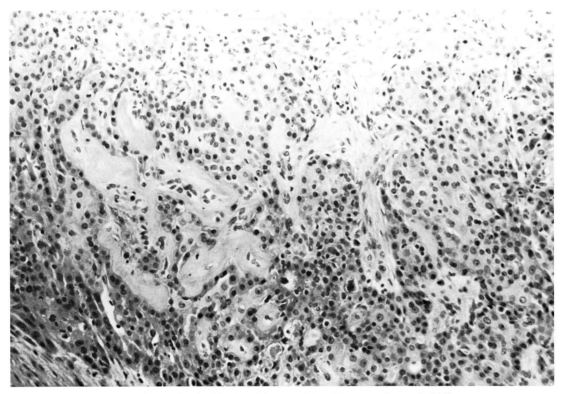

Fig. 589. Adenoid cystic carcinoma: Bands of PAS-positive material, solid tumor cell nests (× 200).

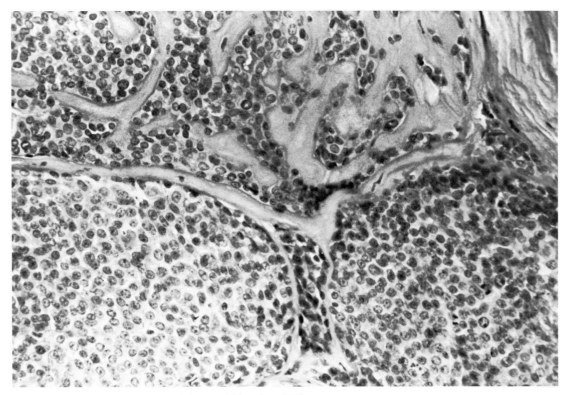

Fig. 590. Adenoid cystic carcinoma (38-year-old female, × 310).

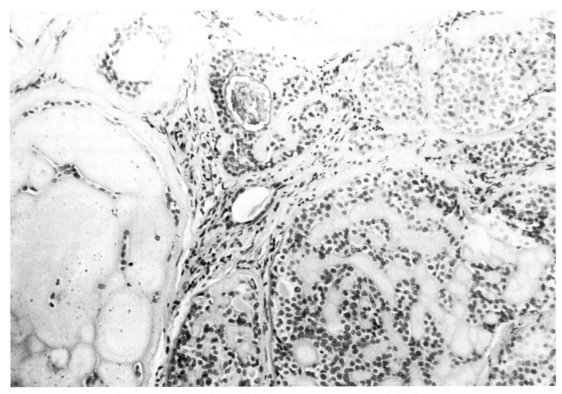

Fig. 591. Adenoid cystic carcinoma: Extensive hyalinization, solid tumor cell nests (× 200).

587

Adenoid cystic carcinoma

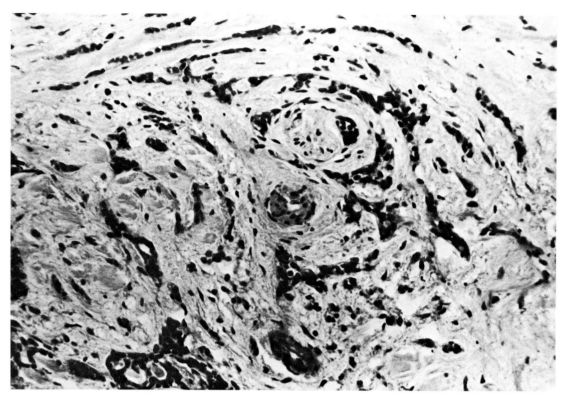

Fig. 592. Adenoid cystic carcinoma: Lymphatic invasion (62-year-old female, × 125).

Spread

1. The lymphatics are rapidly involved with regional lymph node metastases in about 30% of the cases at the time of diagnosis.
2. Early infiltration into the surrounding tissue.
3. Hematogenous metastases into the lung, bone, brain, and skin develop in about 50% of all treated patients [37].

Clinical Findings

Adenoid cystic carcinomas are unilateral tumors in the submandibular or parotid gland. The adenoid cystic carcinoma is a slow-growing tumor. The time lapse between the first symptoms caused by the tumor and hospital admission is about 5 years.

Treatment

Surgery:
Radical surgery.
Radiation therapy:
Postoperative radiation therapy or irradiation for large, unresectable tumors or recurrences: 60 Gy in 5 to 6 weeks.

---

[37] Thackray and Lucas 1974.

588

Prognosis

In the individual case the prognosis is determined by the site of the tumor and the extent of tumor infiltration at the time of diagnosis:
- 5-year survival rate for adenoid cystic carcinoma that can be treated radically, 25%.
- Adenoid cystic carcinoma of the submandibular gland has a worse prognosis than that arising in the parotid gland and the small salivary glands of the palate, which have the best prognosis.

Frequent recurrences end in metastases.

Untreated adenoid cystic carcinoma (or insufficiently resected tumors) will finally be lethal due to hematogenous distant metastases [22a].

M-8140/3
T 142.9

9. Adenocarcinoma (WHO)

General Remarks

Incidence: Adenocarcinomas in the salivary glands are very rare.

Histology

The adenocarcinomas show a glandular growth pattern. The tumor cells often develop papillary formations into the spaces.

Mucin production can be found; other areas are composed of undifferentiated tumor cells.

Differential Diagnosis

1. Adenocarcinoma **with mucoepidermoid carcinoma** [3]:
   Evidence for foci of squamous cell complexes in the glands decide for mucoepidermoid carcinoma.
2. Adenocarcinoma **with metastases from other primary tumors.**

Treatment

Resection of the tumor; eventually postoperative **irradiation.**

Prognosis

Adenocarcinomas in the submandibular gland have a worse prognosis than those growing in other salivary glands.

---

[3] Blanck et al. 1971.
[22a] Marsh and Allen 1979.

M-8550/3
T 142.9

10. Acinic cell adenocarcinoma (WHO)

General Remarks

Incidence: Acinic cell adenocarcinomas are very rare.
Site: Acinic cell adenocarcinomas are unilateral tumors.

Macroscopy

Acinic cell adenocarcinomas are similar to adenomas: They are encapsulated and have a whitish-grayish cut surface.
They are about 2 to 4 cm in diameter.
The cut surface contains numerous cysts.
From the gross inspection the malignant tumor is often not expected [13].

Histology

Acinic cell adenocarcinomas are composed of clear cells, which are similar in aspect to those observed in renal cell carcinomas: The cytoplasm is granular and occasionally shows a basophilic staining (Fig. 593) [7].
The nuclei are regular, small, often pyknotic, and located in the periphery of the cell (Fig. 594).
These tumor cells form solid sheets or trabecular structures.
Occasionally they are arranged in small tubular structures in which the lining cells are flat.
The trabecular structures are surrounded by a very discrete connective tissue.
Between the basophilic and clear cells, there are foci of eosinophilic cells resembling oncocytes.
Very rarely, signs of malignant infiltration or invasion of the lymphatics can be detected.

Electron Microscopy

The tumor cells of acinic adenocarcinoma form small acinar lumina. The cytoplasm contains secretory granules, which are also observed in the acinar lumina. There are many mitochondria, frequently a Golgi zone, and some tonofilaments [4].

Differential Diagnosis

1. Acinic cell adenocarcinoma **with metastatic renal cell carcinoma.**
2. Acinic cell adenocarcinoma **with benign adenoma:**
   These differential diagnoses are often very difficult to solve.
   The decision is occasionally only possible when metastases occur.

Spread

Acinic cell adenocarcinomas can invade the lymphatics and cause regional lymph node metastases in about 20% of the cases.

Clinical Findings

Clinically the unilateral tumor mimics a pleomorphic adenoma.

Treatment

Radical **surgery.**
Subtotal parotidectomy is effective when the tumor is small.

---

[4] Chen et al. 1978.
[7] Eneroth and Jakobsson 1966.
[13] Hanson 1975.

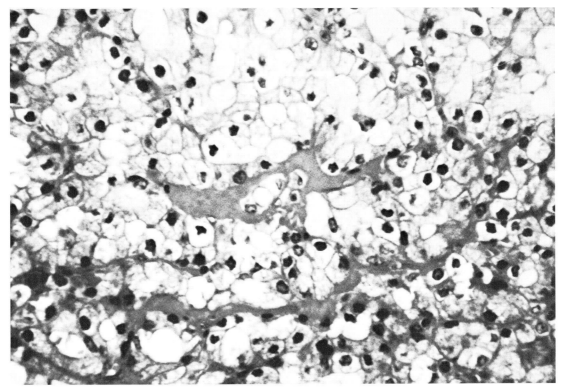

Fig. 593. Acinic cell adenocarcinoma: Mucin production (× 310).

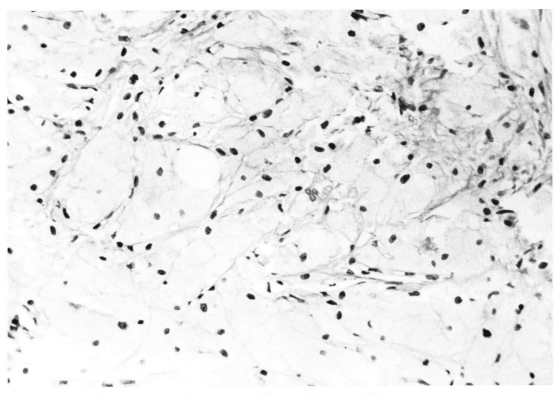

Fig. 594. Acinic cell adenocarcinoma: Pyknotic nuclei (77-year-old female, × 200).

Prognosis

a) Overall 5-year survival rate, about 76 to 90%.
   10-year survival, 63%; 15-year survival, 55% [32].
b) Overall 20-year survival, about 55% [7].
c) Local recurrences, about 25%.
d) In the individual case the extension of the tumor determines the outcome of the disease:
   Extensive acinic cell carcinomas have a high recurrence rate and finally become lethal regardless of the extent of surgery [32].

Further Information

Sialosis (WHO)
This lesion is composed of acinar cells that are swollen and increased in size. The nuclei are regular and located at the base (periphery) of the cells (Fig. 595).
This is a benign, tumor-like lesion.
Usually the parotid gland is affected; however, rarely the submandibular glands can show this sialosis.

**M-8020/3
T 142.9**

11. Undifferentiated carcinoma (WHO)

Undifferentiated carcinomas are growths of malignant epithelial cells that do not form organoid structures and do not permit a classification into one of the above-mentioned tumors (Figs. 596 to 598).
Occasionally these undifferentiated carcinomas can exhibit a sarcomatous-like growth and the appearance of malignant cells (Fig. 599).

---

[7] Eneroth and Jakobsson 1966.
[32] Spiro et al. 1978.

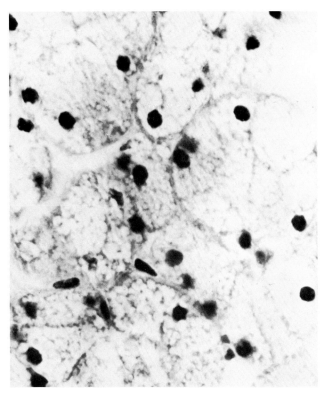

Fig. 595. Sialosis of the parotid gland (33-year-old female, × 600).

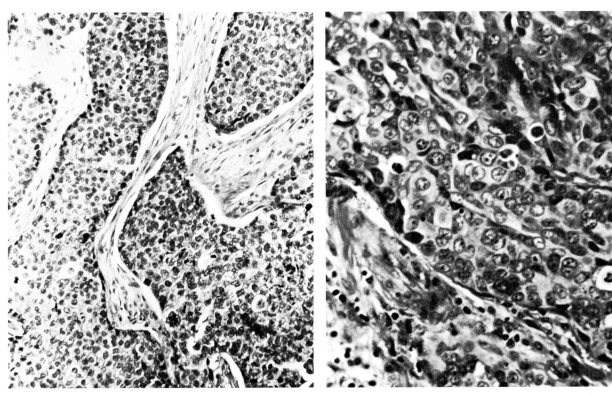

Fig. 596. Undifferentiated carcinoma of the parotid gland (77-year-old female, × 200).

Fig. 597. Undifferentiated carcinoma of the parotid gland (× 200).

Undifferentiated carcinoma

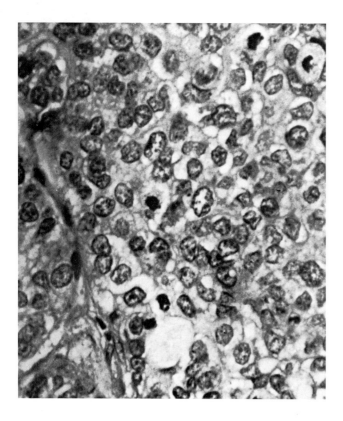

Fig. 598. Undifferentiated carcinoma of the parotid gland (77-year-old female, ×310).

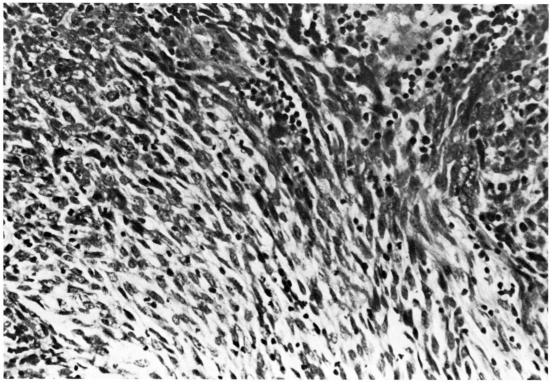

Fig. 599. Undifferentiated carcinoma of the parotid gland, sarcoma-like component (55-year-old female, ×200).

M-9590/3
T 142.9

12. Malignant lymphoma
(non-Hodgkin's lymphoma)

General Remarks

Incidence: Malignant lymphomas of the salivary glands are rare.
Site: Primary malignant lymphomas are almost always unilateral. Salivary glands can also be affected by disseminated malignant lymphoma.
The parotid gland is affected more frequently by primary malignant lymphoma than the submandibular gland.
Further notes: Hodgkin's disease probably does not involve the salivary glands.

Macroscopy

Malignant lymphomas are unilateral soft tumors with a pinkish-whitish cut surface.

Histology

The salivary gland is infiltrated by cells of a malignant non-Hodgkin's lymphoma.
Any type of malignant lymphoma can be encountered (Figs. 600 to 602); however, the well-differentiated lymphocytic malignant lymphoma of a nodular or diffuse growth pattern is usually observed [9].

Differential Diagnosis

Malignant lymphoma **with benign lymphoepithelial lesion** (WHO) (benign lymphoid hyperplasia):
A number of inflammatory diseases of the salivary glands are characterized by dense lymphocytic infiltrations. The glandular structures are atrophic (which might give the impression of an infiltrating tumor).
In a number of cases the myoepithelial cells of the ducts proliferate (Figs. 603 and 604).
According to the clinical symptoms and the histological picture, these lymphocytic inflammations with atrophy of the glands are observed in Sjögren's syndrome and Mikulicz's syndrome.
The differential diagnosis of lymphocytic inflammation with malignant lymphoma in the salivary glands might be very difficult. The appearance of germinal centers in the lymphocytic infiltrates are helpful in recognizing benign lesion.
Clinical signs of Sjögren's syndrome are another indication for the benign lesion.
However, in Sjögren's syndrome and Mikulicz's syndrome malignant lymphomas can develop [20, 39].

Treatment

Primary malignant lymphoma is treated by radical **surgery** and **radiation therapy** (up to 50 Gy in 5 weeks).

Prognosis

Primary malignant lymphoma of the salivary glands seems to have a better prognosis than the usual lymphoma with dissemination [25].

Further Information

Sjögren's syndrome is a benign lymphocytic inflammation of the salivary glands accompanied by keratoconjunctivitis, xerostomia, rheumatoid arthritis, and hypergammaglobulinemia.
Mikulicz's syndrome is an enlargement of the salivary and lacrimal glands, occasionally due to lymphocytic inflammation but also due to sarcoidosis (Heerfordt's syndrome), tuberculosis, sarcoma, and malignant lymphoma.

[9] Friedmann 1971.
[20] Lapes et al. 1976.
[25] Nime et al. 1976.
[39] Zulman et al. 1978.

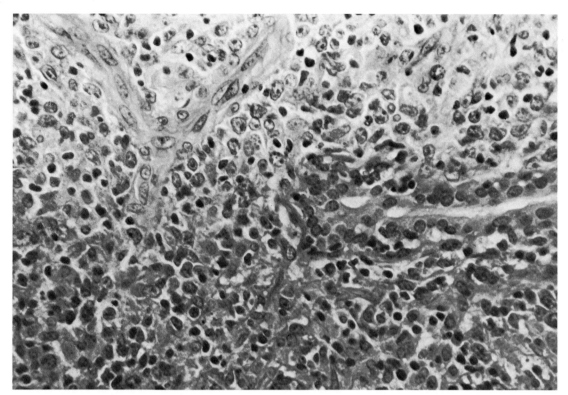

Fig. 600. Malignant lymphoma of the parotid gland (69-year-old female, × 200).

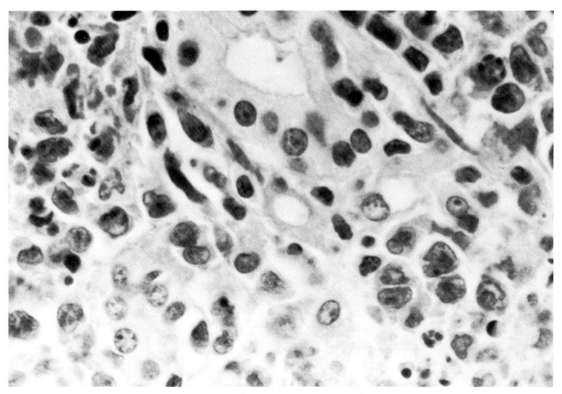

Fig. 601. Malignant lymphoma in the parotid gland (69-year-old female, × 600).

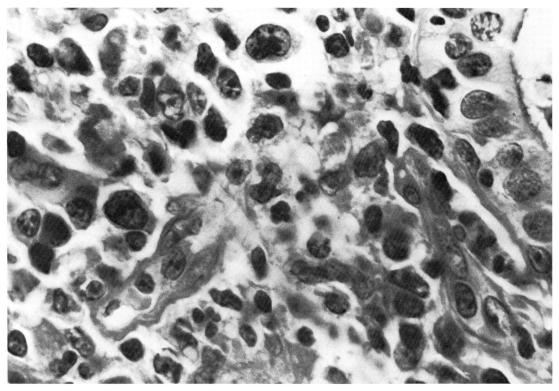

Fig. 602. Malignant lymphoma in the parotid gland (58-year-old female, × 800).

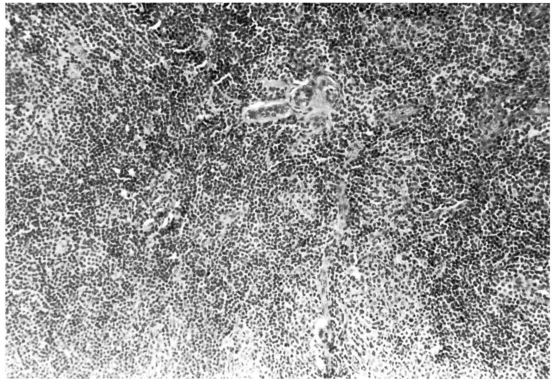

Fig. 603. Myoepithelial sialadenitis (54-year-old female, × 50).

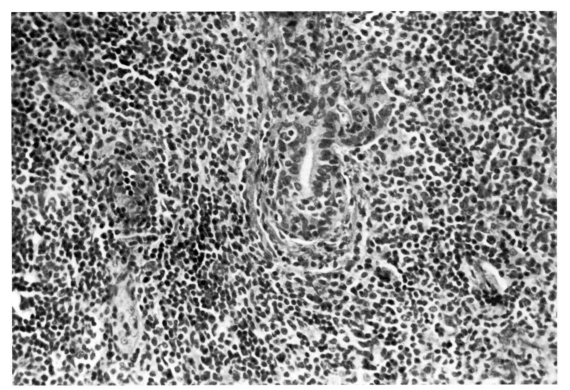

Fig. 604. Myoepithelial sialadenitis: Proliferation of ductal epithelial cells (54-year-old female, × 125).

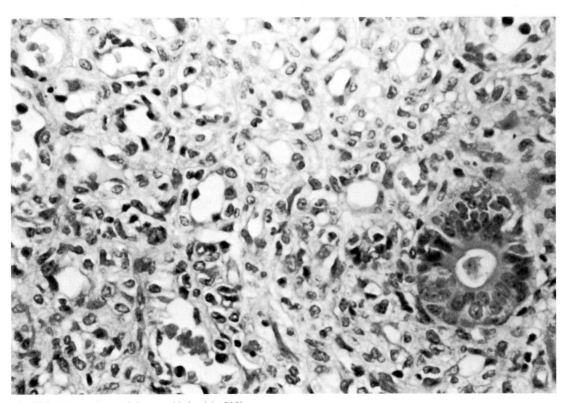

Fig. 605. Hemangioma of the parotid gland (× 310).

13. Soft tissue tumors of the salivary glands

M-9120/0
T 142.0

a) Hemangioma (WHO)
This is the most frequently observed benign soft tissue tumor in the salivary glands, particularly in the parotid gland (Fig. 605).

M-9560/0
T 142.0

b) Neurilemoma
This tumor usually originates from the sheath of the facial nerve.

M-7410/0
T 142.9

c) Lipomatosis
Occasionally the salivary glands are occupied by mature adipose tissue that grows between the acini.

M-8000/3
T 142.9

14. Unclassified tumors

Recommendations for differential diagnosis in tumors of the salivary glands

monomorphic adenoma	with	– pleomorphic adenoma – adenoid cystic carcinoma
pleomorphic adenoma	with	– carcinoma (of different types) in pleomorphic adenoma – adenoid cystic carcinoma
mucoepidermoid carcinoma	with	– squamous cell carcinoma – adenocarcinoma – adenoid cystic carcinoma – squamous cell metaplasia
adenoid cystic carcinoma	with	– pleomorphic adenoma – carcinoma in pleomorphic adenoma – benign adenoma – mucoepidermoid carcinoma – metastases from other primary tumors (for instance, breast)
acinic cell adenocarcinoma	with	– metastatic renal cell carcinoma – benign adenoma – sialosis – alveolar soft part sarcoma
malignant lymphoma (non-Hodgkin's)	with	– benign lymphoepithelial lesion (chronic lymphocytic sialadenitis with glandular atrophy) – Sjögren's syndrome – Mikulicz's syndrome – undifferentiated carcinoma

References

[1] Batsakis, J.G.: Basal cell adenoma of the parotid gland. Cancer 29 (1972) 226-230.

[2] Bazaz-Malik, G., and D.N. Gupta: Metastasizing (malignant) oncocytoma of the parotid gland. Z. Krebsforsch. 70 (1968) 193-197.

[3] Blanck, C., C.-M. Eneroth, and P.Å. Jakobsson: Mucus-producing adenopapillary (non-epidermoid) carcinoma of the parotid gland. Cancer 28 (1971) 676-685.

[3a] Cameron, W.R., and U. Stenram: Adenoma of parotid gland with sebaceous and oncocytic features. Cancer 43 (1979) 1429-1433.

[4] Chen, S.-Y., R.B. Brannon, A.S. Miller, D.K. White, and S.P. Hooker: Acinic cell adenocarcinoma of minor salivary glands. Cancer 42 (1978) 678-685.

[5] Crumpler, C., J.C. Scharfenberg, and R.J. Reed: Monomorphic adenomas of salivary glands. Trabecular-tubular, canalicular, and basaloid variants. Cancer 38 (1976) 193-200.

[6] Eneroth, C.-M.: Incidence and prognosis of salivary-gland tumours at different sites; a study of parotid, submandibular, and palatal tumours in 2632 patients. Acta Otolaryngol. (Stockholm) Suppl. 263 (1970) 174-178.

[7] Eneroth, C.-M., and P.A. Jakobsson: Acinic cell carcinoma of the parotid gland. Cancer 19 (1966) 1761-1772.

[8] Frazell, E.L.: Clinical aspects of tumors of the major salivary glands. Cancer 7 (1954) 637-659.

[9] Friedmann, I.: Electron microscopy in head and neck oncology. Acta Otolaryngol. (Stockholm) 71 (1971) 115-122.

[10] Fu, K.K., S.A. Leibel, M.L. Levine, L.M. Friedlander, R. Boles, and T.L. Phillips: Carcinoma of the major and minor salivary glands. Analysis of treatment results and sites and causes of failures. Cancer 40 (1977) 2882-2890.

[11] Gerughty, R.M., H.H. Scofield, F.M. Brown, and G.R. Hennigar: Malignant mixed tumors of salivary gland origin. Cancer 24 (1969) 471-486.

[12] Hamperl, H.: Benign and malignant oncocytoma. Cancer 15 (1962) 1019-1027.

[13] Hanson, T.A.S.: Acinic cell carcinoma of the parotid salivary gland presenting as a cyst. Report of two cases. Cancer 36 (1975) 570-575.

[14] Headington, J.T., J.G. Batsakis, T.F. Beals, T.E. Campbell, J.L. Simmons, and W.D. Stone: Membranous basal cell adenoma of parotid gland, dermal cylindromas, and trichoepitheliomas. Comparative histochemistry and ultrastructure. Cancer 39 (1977) 2460-2469.

[15] Healey, W.V., K.H. Perzin, and L. Smith: Mucoepidermoid carcinoma of salivary gland origin; classification, clinical-pathologic correlation, and results of treatment. Cancer 26 (1970) 368-388.

[16] Jakobsson, P.Å., C. Blanck, and C.-M. Eneroth: Mucoepidermoid carcinoma of the parotid gland. Cancer 22 (1968) 111-124.

[17] Kagan, A.R., H. Nussbaum, S. Handler, R. Shapiro, H.A. Gilbert, M. Jacobs, J.W. Miles, P.Y.M. Chan, and P.T. Calcaterra: Recurrences of malignant parotid salivary gland tumors. Cancer 37 (1976) 2600-2604.

[18] Kirklin, J.W., J.R. McDonald, S.W. Haarington, and G.B. New: Parotid tumors; histopathology, clinical behavior, and end results. Surg. Gynecol. Obstet. 92 (1951) 721-733.

[19] Krolls, S.O., J.N. Trodahl, and R.C. Boyers: Salivary gland lesions in children; a survey of 34 cases. Cancer 30 (1972) 145-155.

[20] Lapes, M., K. Antoniades, W. Gartner Jr., and R. Vivacqua: Conversion of a benign lymphoepithelial salivary gland lesion to lymphocytic lymphoma during dilantin therapy. Correlation with dilatin-induced lymphocyte transformation in vitro. Cancer 38 (1976) 1318-1322.

[21] Lee, S.C., and L.M. Roth: Malignant oncocytoma of the parotid gland. Cancer 37 (1976) 1607-1614.

[22] LiVolsi, V.A., and K.H. Perzin: Malignant mixed tumors arising in salivary glands. I. Carcinomas arising in benign mixed tumors: A clinicopathologic study. Cancer 39 (1977) 2209-2230.

[22a] Marsh, W.L., and M.S. Allen: Adenoid cystic carcinoma. Biologic behavior in 38 patients. Cancer 43 (1979) 1463-1473.

[23] Moberger, J.G., and C.-M. Eneroth: Malignant mixed tumors of the major salivary glands; special reference to the histologic structure in metastases. Cancer 21 (1968) 1198-1211.

[24] Nelson, J.F., and J.R. Jacoway: Monomorphic adenoma (canalicular type). Report of 29 cases. Cancer 31 (1973) 1511-1520.

[25] Nime, F.A., H.S. Cooper, and J.C. Eggleston: Primary malignant lymphomas of the salivary glands. Cancer 37 (1976) 906-912.

[26] Rafla, S.: Malignant parotid tumors: Natural history and treatment. Cancer 40 (1977) 136-144.

[27] Reingold, I.M., L.E. Keasbey, and J.H. Graham: Multicentric dermal-type cylindromas of the parotid glands in a patient with florid turban tumor. Cancer 40 (1977) 1702-1710.

[28] Rentschler, R., M.A. Burgess, and R. Byers: Chemotherapy of malignant major salivary gland neoplasms. A 25-year review of M.D. Anderson Hospital experience. Cancer 40 (1977) 619-624.

[29] Seifert, G., J. Schulz und K. Donath: Pathomorphologische Subklassifikation der Carcinome in pleomorphen Speicheldrüsenadenomen. HNO 25 (1977) 337-348.

[30] Smith, L.C., N. Lane, and R.M. Rankow: Cylindroma (adenoid cystic carcinoma). A report of fifty-eight cases. Am. J. Surg. 110 (1965) 519-526.

[31] Soni, S.C., F.R. Khan, J.M. Paul, and J. Ovadia: Electron beam treatment of malignant tumors of salivary glands. J. Radiol. Electrol. Med. Nucl. 58 (1977) 677-679.

[32] Spiro, R.H., A.G. Huvos, and E.W. Strong: Acinic cell carcinoma of salivary origin. A clinicopathologic study of 67 cases. Cancer *41* (1978) 924-935.

[33] Takeuchi, J., M. Sobue, M. Yoshida, T. Esaki, and Y. Katoh: Pleomorphic adenoma of the salivary gland. With special reference to histochemical and electron microscopic studies, and biochemical analysis of glycosaminoglycans in vivo and in vitro. Cancer *36* (1975) 1771-1789.

[34] Takeuchi, J., M. Sobue, Y. Katoh, T. Esaki, M. Yoshida, and K. Miura: Morphologic and biologic characteristics of adenoid cystic carcinoma cells of the salivary gland. Cancer *38* (1976) 2349-2356.

[35] Tandler, B., R.V.P. Hutter, and R.A. Erlandson: Ultrastructure of oncocytoma of the parotid gland. Lab. Invest. *23* (1970) 567-580.

[36] Thackray, A.C.: Histological typing of salivary gland tumours. WHO, Geneva 1972.

[37] Thackray, A.C., and R.B. Lucas: Tumors of the major salivary glands. Atlas of tumor pathology, A.F.I.P. – Washington, D.C. 1974.

[38] Turnbull, A.D., and E.L. Frazell: Multiple tumors of the major salivary glands. Am. J. Surg. *118* (1969) 787-789.

[39] Zulman, J., R. Jaffe, and N. Talal: Evidence that the malignant lymphoma of Sjögren's syndrome is a monoclonal B-cell neoplasm. N. Engl. J. Med. *299* (1978) 1215-1220.

15 Tumors of the thyroid and parathyroid gland

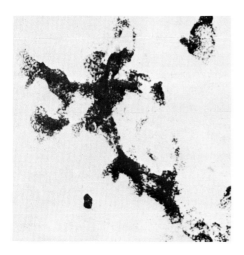

Fig. 606. Cytological preparation in a case of papillary carcinoma of the thyroid: Papillary arrangement of the material in low power view (Papanicolaou, × 4).

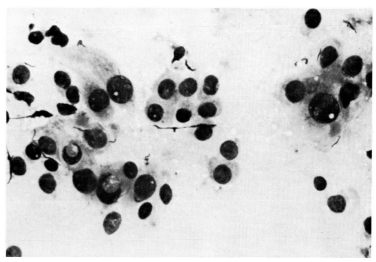

Fig. 607. Cytology of papillary carcinoma of the thyroid: Nuclei of different sizes, no pleomorphic nuclei. Cytoplasm with clear cell borders. Intranuclear inclusions of cytoplasm in several cells (May-Grünwald-Giemsa stain, × 40).

Tumors of the thyroid gland

1. One to 2% of all malignant tumors are carcinomas of the thyroid.
2. Malignant mesenchymal tumors in the thyroid are exceedingly rare.
3. Thyroid carcinomas can occur at all ages. The peak ages are the 3rd, 4th, and 6th decades.

   The majority of undifferentiated carcinomas are observed in elderly patients.
4. With the exception of medullary carcinoma, carcinomas of the thyroid are strongly predominant in females. This is true also for children and young adults.
5. Medullary carcinomas are usually spontaneously occurring tumors. However, about 20% are of a familial occurrence with a probably autosomal-dominant heredity.
6. Solitary nodules in the thyroid are carcinomatous in 5 to 20% of the cases [26].
7. Nodular goiter is not a precancerous lesion [4].
8. The classification of thyroid tumors respects the degree of differentiation reflected by the organoid growth pattern [23].

   65% of all thyroid tumors are follicular or papillary carcinomas [24].
9. The prognosis is determined by the degree of differentiation: Well-differentiated thyroid carcinomas infiltrate and metastasize slowly, while undifferentiated carcinomas are malignant due to early spread.

   The stage of the tumor at the time of diagnosis determines the outcome of the disease.

[4] Ashley 1978.
[23] Hedinger 1974.
[24] Heitz et al. 1976.
[26] Ingbar and Woeber 1977.

10. A considerable number of thyroid carcinomas are detected only by lymph node metastases.

11. Thyroid carcinomas can be indicated clinically by rapid recent growth and diminished or absent function on scintiscan.

12. Irradiation of the thymus with 6 to 12 Gy in early childhood can cause thyroid carcinoma [10, 14, 17, 39].

    These carcinomas are of the papillary type.

13. Thyroid cancer is rather often associated with thyroiditis.

    This inflammation is probably a reaction to the cancer and not a precursor of the tumor.

    However, lymphocytic thyroiditis might be a precursor of malignant lymphoma in the thyroid.

    Cytological studies might be helpful to detect malignant tumors [30] (Figs. 606 and 607).

T – primary tumor

Tis = preinvasive carcinoma (carcinoma in situ)

T 0 = no evidence of primary tumor

T 1 = single nodule in one lobe with or without deformity of the gland and with no limitation of mobility

T 2 = multiple nodules in one lobe with or without deformity of the gland and with no limitation of mobility

T 3 = bilateral tumor with or without deformity of the gland and with no limitation of mobility or a single nodule of the isthmus

T 4 = tumor with extension beyond the gland capsule

T x = the minimal requirements to assess the primary tumor cannot be met (clinical examination, radiography, endoscopy, and isotope scanning)

N – regional lymph nodes

(jugular nodes, bilateral tracheoesophageal nodes, upper anterior mediastinal nodes, nodes on the thyroid cartilage, and retropharyngeal nodes)

N 0 = no evidence of regional lymph node involvement

N 1 = evidence of involvement of the movable homolateral regional lymph nodes

N 2 = evidence of involvement of the movable contralateral or bilateral regional lymph nodes

N 3 = evidence of involvement of the fixed regional lymph nodes

N x = the minimal requirements to assess regional lymph nodes cannot be met (clinical examination and radiography)

[10] Cady et al. 1979.
[14] Curtin et al. 1977.
[17] Favus et al. 1976.
[30] Lang et al. 1978.
[39] Refetoff et al. 1975.

M – distant metastases

M 0 = no evidence of distant metastases

M 1 = evidence of distant metastases

M x = the minimal requirements to assess the presence of distant metastases cannot be met (clinical examination, radiography, and isotope scanning)

pTNM – postsurgical histopathological classification

pT – primary tumor

pTis = preinvasive carcinoma (carcinoma in situ)

pT 0 = no tumor found on examination of the specimen

pT 1 = single nodule 1 cm or less in diameter not invading beyond the thyroid capsule

pT 2 = single nodule more than 1 cm in diameter not invading beyond the thyroid capsule

pT 3 = multiple nodules (uni- or bilateral) and/or isthmus nodule not invading beyond the thyroid capsule

pT 4 = tumor with invasion beyond the thyroid capsule

pT x = the extent of invasion cannot be assessed

pN – regional lymph nodes

the pN categories correspond to the N categories

pM – distant metastases

the pM categories correspond to the M categories

Stage grouping

no stage grouping is at present recommended.

M-8334/0
T 193.9

1. Adenoma (WHO)

General Remarks

Site: Adenomas in the thyroid might be found at any site of this gland.
In most instances adenomas are solitary lesions.

Macroscopy

Adenomas are usually small tumors that are encapsulated. The cut surface may be fleshy or brownish. The adenomas are soft.
The cut surface may contain signs of regressive changes:
Calcifications, cysts, zones of edema, hemorrhages, and fibrosis.

Histology

The thyroid adenoma is composed of cells that imitate the regular pattern of the thyroid gland.
These cells form colloid-containing follicles that can be rather large (Fig. 608).

M-8330/0

Besides the **follicular adenoma** (WHO) other subclassifications for the adenomas have been established according to the arrangement of the epithelial cells:

M-8191/0

Embryonal adenoma (WHO), in which the epithelial cells form a small trabecular pattern,

M-8211/0

tubular adenoma (WHO), with a tubular arrangement of the epithelial cells,

M-8334/0

normomacrofollicular adenoma (WHO), according to the size of the follicles,

M-8333/0

microfollicular adenoma (fetal adenoma) (WHO) when the follicles have only discrete colloid in the small lumen.

Occasionally oxyphilic cells or clear cells may be observed in adenomas. There are adenomas that are dominated by these cells:

M-8290/0

Oxyphil adenoma (Hürthle cell adenoma) (Figs. 609 and 610).

The adenomas may contain hyalinizations, calcifications, bone formation, areas of edema, and hemorrhages with iron pigment deposits in histiocytes.
The capsule that surrounds the adenoma is not infiltrated by the cells.
The thyroid tissue surrounding the adenoma is compressed (Fig. 611).

Differential Diagnosis

1. Adenoma **with carcinoma:**
   Adenomas do not show invasion of the capsule; there is no invasion of blood vessels.
2. Adenoma **with changes in colloid goiter:**
   It might be difficult to separate adenomas from lesions in an adenomatous goiter.
   This is especially true for the **papillary adenomas,** which often can be observed in adenomatous goiters.
   Helpful for the separation of both are these facts:
   – Adenomas are encapsulated,
   – in most instances adenomas are solitary lesions,
   – adenomas compress the surrounding thyroid tissue,
   – adenomas have a rather uniform growth pattern and cellular type.

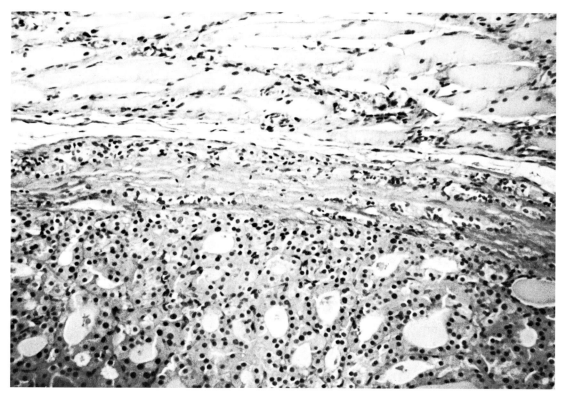

Fig. 608. Follicular adenoma of thyroid: Regular cells, no signs of invasion, colloid-containing follicles (×125).

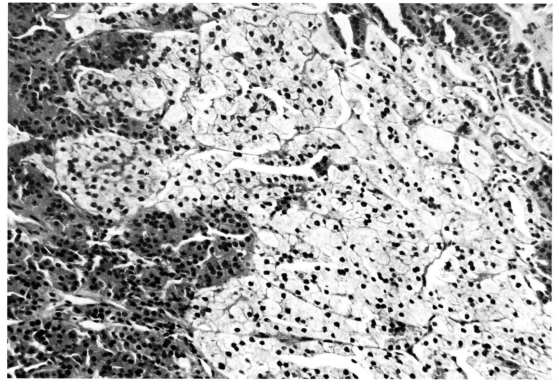

Fig. 609. Adenoma of thyroid: Clear cells and oxyphilic cells (×125).

609

Adenoma

**Clinical
Findings**

a) Solitary adenomas (in most instances follicular adenomas) grow slowly over many years.

b) Adenomas are autonomous tissue, independent of TSH stimulation.
  - In their early development, they can accumulate 131 J: **Warm nodule.**
  - During their later development they might concentrate 131 J only in the region of the adenoma: **Hot adenoma, toxic adenoma.**
  - In cases of regressive changes, there is no 131 J storage: **Cold adenoma.**

c) Regressive changes with bleeding and edematous areas in the tumor might mimic rapid growth and suggest malignant tumor (especially in cold adenomas).

Treatment

Removal of the adenoma.

Prognosis

Excellent.

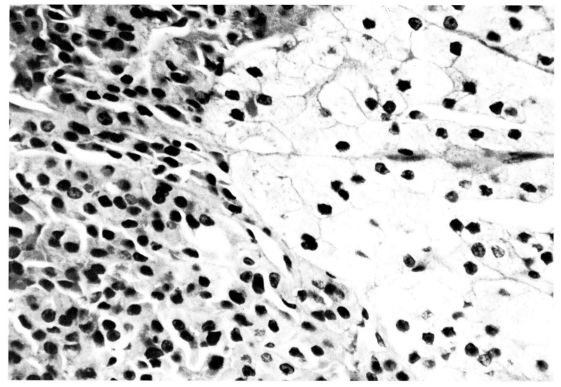

Fig. 610. Follicular adenoma: Clear cells and oxyphilic cells. No malignant infiltration (× 310).

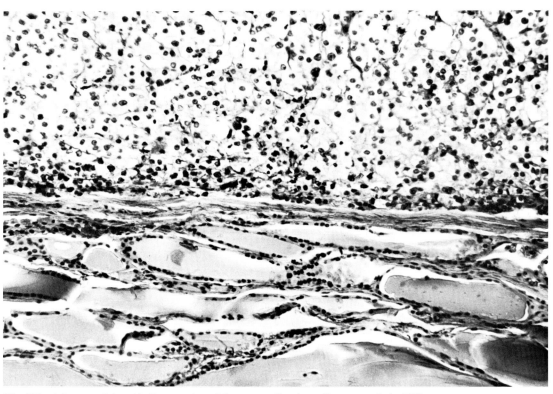

Fig. 611. Adenoma of thyroid: Compression of the surrounding tissue. Intact capsule (× 125).

2. Papillary carcinoma (WHO)

M-8260/3
T 193.9

General Remarks

Incidence: The most frequently observed carcinoma of the thyroid is the papillary carcinoma.

Age: Papillary carcinomas occur at all ages, including children and young adults. The peak ages are in the 2nd and 3rd decades and in later life.

Sex: Females are considerably more frequently affected than males.

Site: Papillary carcinomas are of a multifocal origin.

Macroscopy

Papillary carcinomas can be very small or rather large.

Occasionally the papillary carcinoma resembles a scar.

Papillary carcinomas infiltrate the surrounding thyroid tissue.

The cut surface is grayish-whitish.

Histology

The tumor cells in papillary carcinomas grow in a papillary pattern: These papillary formations are supported by connective tissue containing capillaries.

The covering tumor cells usually grow in multilayers over the surface of the connective tissue. The nuclei are of different sizes and shapes. Often they are indented. The interior contains finely dispersed chromatin in an otherwise empty nucleus (so-called ground glass appearance) (Figs. 612 and 613).

Papillary carcinomas contain psammoma bodies (Fig. 614).

M-8340/3
T 193.9

Besides the papillary growth of the tumor there are almost always follicular areas:
Papillary and follicular carcinoma (Fig. 615).

Occasionally papillary carcinomas can develop in a very small area. In these instances the tumor is embedded in a scarlike tissue with dense collagen fibers. This area also shows the atypical cellular arrangements and psammoma bodies:

M-8350/3
T 193.9

Sclerosing (occult) nonencapsulated carcinoma (WHO) (Fig. 616).

In all instances the cells of a papillary carcinoma invade the lymphatics; occasionally the blood vessels may also be invaded.

Electron Microscopy

The cells of papillary carcinoma of the thyroid are similar to those observed in follicular carcinoma.

The nuclei are lobulated and irregularly shaped [27, 51].

Differential Diagnosis

1. Papillary carcinoma **with papillary adenoma:**

   It is advisable to consider any papillary lesion in the thyroid (except a goiter) as possibly carcinomatous.

   Papillary adenomas are exceedingly rare [23]. It is even possible that all papillary tumors in the thyroid are malignant [1].

   Evidence for malignant growth is
   - invasion of the lymphatics, and
   - psammoma bodies.

---

[1] Ackerman and Rosai 1974.
[23] Hedinger 1974.
[27] Johannessen et al. 1978.
[51] Valenta and Michel-Béchet 1977.

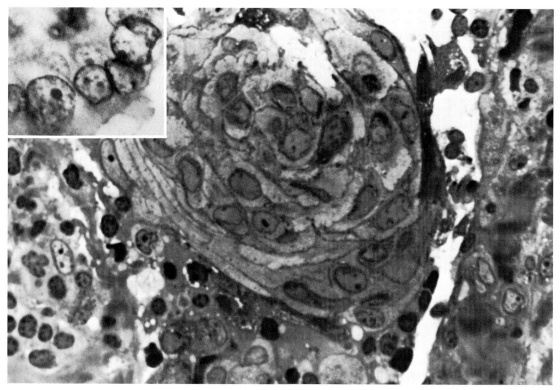

Fig. 612. Papillary carcinoma of the thyroid: Vesicular nuclei (× 600; Inset, × 600).

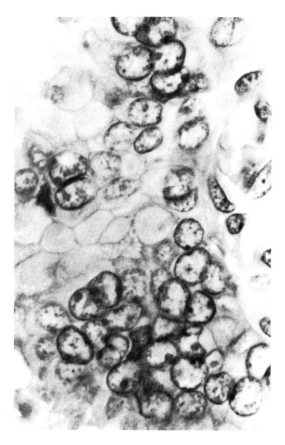

Fig. 613. Papillary carcinoma of the thyroid: Vesicular nuclei (× 600).

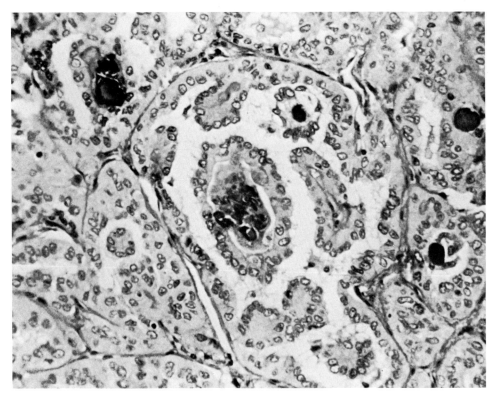

Fig. 614. Papillary carcinoma of the thyroid: Vesicular tumor nuclei, psammoma bodies (52-year-old female, × 200).

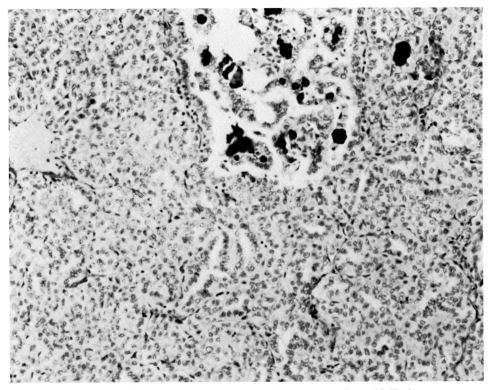

Fig. 615. Papillary and follicular carcinoma of the thyroid: Psammoma bodies and follicular arrangement of tumor cells (× 125).

614

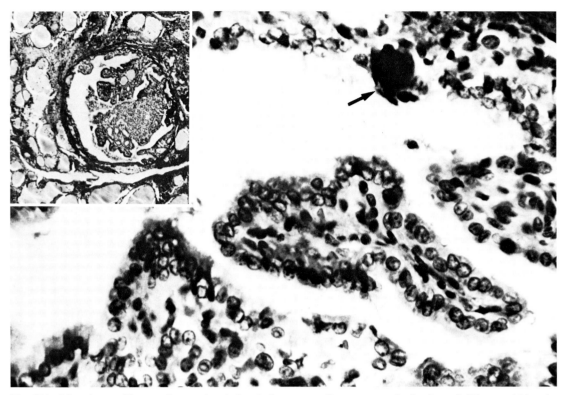

Fig. 616. Sclerosing papillary carcinoma: Atypical vesicular tumor cells, psammoma bodies (arrow) (51-year-old female, ×310; inset, ×50).

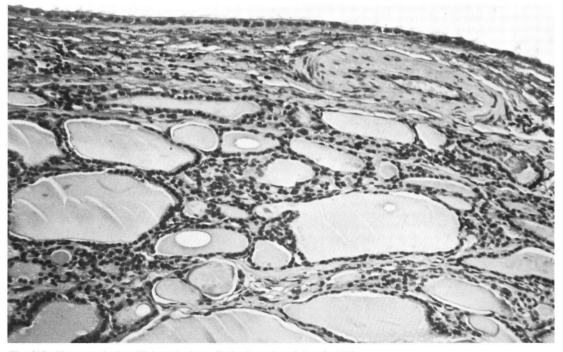

Fig. 617. Heterotopic thyroid tissue in the wall of a thyroglossal duct (×125).

Papillary carcinoma

Differential Diagnosis M-7160/0

2. Papillary carcinoma **with papillary growth in goiters:**
   In these instances the papillary formations are without psammoma bodies and there is no invasion of the lymphatics.
3. Papillary carcinoma metastatic in lymph nodes **with ectopic thyroid tissue in lymph nodes:**
   Metastatic growth of papillary carcinomas in lymph nodes can replace the entire lymphatic structure. The impression of ectopic thyroid tissue may exist.
   However, ectopic thyroid tissue in the lymph nodes is very rare and is never arranged in a papillary growth pattern (Fig. 617).

Spread

1. Dissemination by lymphatic spread occurs frequently.
   The metastases develop mainly in cervical lymph nodes, which for a long time might be the only site of a metastatic lesion.
   In about 25% of the cases lymph node metastases are present at the time of diagnosis. Often these lymph node metastases are the first sign of the (occult) papillary carcinoma.
2. Hematogenous metastases are relatively rare and usually involve lung, bone, and brain.

Clinical Findings

Papillary carcinomas are slow-growing tumors of a multifocal origin.
Rather often the primary tumor is not detected unless cervical lymph node metastases reveal the origin of the assumed malignant tumor.
Papillary carcinoma does not accumulate 131 J (since the tumor often contains follicular components, there might be uptake of 131 J in follicular-papillary carcinomas).

Treatment

Surgery:
Total thyroidectomy (papillary carcinomas are of a multifocal origin).
Radical neck dissection (frequently there are early cervical lymph node metastases) [52].
Radiation therapy:
Postoperative irradiation can be useful, especially in cases of incomplete tumor removal (about 50 Gy in 5 weeks).
The usefulness of radioiodine is debatable [52].
Treatment with **thyroid hormone** can be added to surgery and radiation therapy.
Chemotherapy [7].

Prognosis

1. Small (occult) papillary carcinoma has an excellent prognosis [42].
2. Papillary carcinoma with metastases:
   – 10-year survival, about 80%.
3. Papillary carcinoma with extrathyroidal extension:
   – 10-year survival, about 50%.
4. The majority of patients die from the consequences of extrathyroidal extension.
5. In the individual case, the prognosis depends on the stage of the tumor at the time of diagnosis [28].

[7] Benker et al. 1977.
[28] Keminger et al. 1975.
[42] Russell et al. 1975.
[52] Wahl et al. 1977.

**Further
Information**

1. 25% of thyroid carcinomas in children are papillary carcinomas.
2. A papillary carcinoma originates as a malignant tumor. There is no proven relationship between papillary carcinomas and adenomatous goiter, remnants of the thyroglossal duct, or chronic thyroiditis.
3. A relationship between Grave's disease and papillary carcinoma has been reported [32].
4. Papillary carcinomas can be mixed with follicular carcinomas.
   The designation of the tumor should be made according to the predominant growth pattern.
5. In cases of metastatic papillary-follicular carcinoma, the follicular component is responsible for the uptake of 131 J.

---

[32] Meissner and Warren 1969.

M-8330/3
T 193.9

3. Follicular carcinoma (WHO)

General Remarks

Incidence: Follicular carcinomas are observed less frequently than papillary carcinomas: About 10% of the tumors of the thyroid are follicular carcinomas.

Age: The tumor can be observed in children and in adults; the incidence increases with age.

Sex: Females are considerably more frequently affected than males.

Site: Any site of the thyroid can be affected.

In most instances follicular carcinomas are solitary tumors.

Macroscopy

Follicular carcinomas are small or large tumors. The tumor seems to be well delineated, but has no capsule.

The fleshy cut surface shows signs of degeneration with calcifications, fibrosis, scar formation, and recurrent hemorrhages.

Occasionally the surrounding tissue is involved; very rarely tumor infiltration into blood vessels can be seen on gross inspection.

In other instances follicular carcinomas are very similar to adenomas.

Histology

Follicular carcinomas are composed of malignant follicular cells that imitate the follicular growth pattern of the normal thyroid. The tumor produces colloid.

The epithelial cells might show discrete or moderate signs of nuclear atypias (Figs. 618 and 619).

Some of the tumors contain areas of poorly differentiated carcinoma or papillary carcinoma.

Follicular carcinomas infiltrate mainly the blood vessels (Fig. 620), rarely the lymphatics.

Electron Microscopy

The cytoplasm of the tumor cells in follicular carcinoma of the thyroid contains multiple vesicles of rough endoplasmic reticulum, relatively few mitochondria, and numerous dense bodies (they are almost indistinguishable from the secretory granules described in medullary thyroid carcinoma) [27, 51].

Differential Diagnosis

1. Follicular carcinoma **with follicular adenoma** (Fig. 608):
   Besides cellular atypias, which might be very discrete, the carcinomatous growth is indicated by invasion of the blood vessels.
2. Follicular carcinoma **with Hashimoto's thyroiditis:**
   In Hashimoto's thyroiditis there are numerous lymphocytes between the follicular cells. There is no blood vessel invasion (Figs. 621 to 623).

[27] Johannessen et al. 1978.
[51] Valenta and Michel-Béchet 1977.

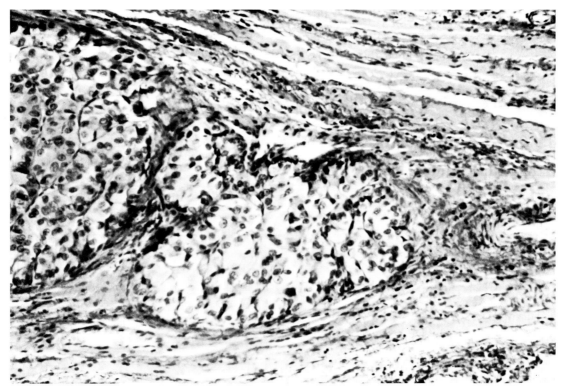

Fig. 618. Follicular carcinoma, moderately differentiated: Clear nuclear atypias, no colloid (× 200).

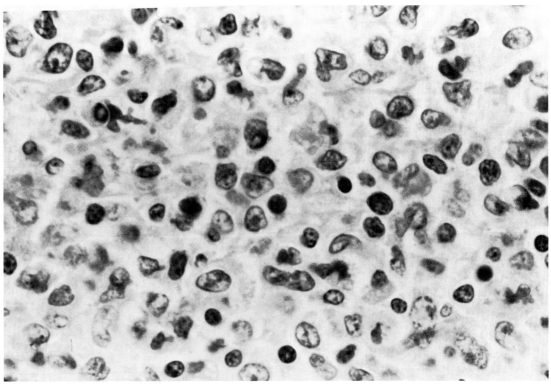

Fig. 619. Poorly differentiated follicular thyroid carcinoma (78-year-old male, × 800).

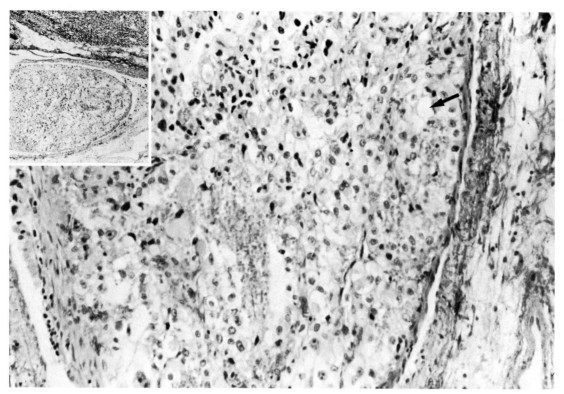

Fig. 620. Follicular carcinoma of thyroid: Invasion of blood vessels (arrow) (23-year-old female, × 125; inset, × 40).

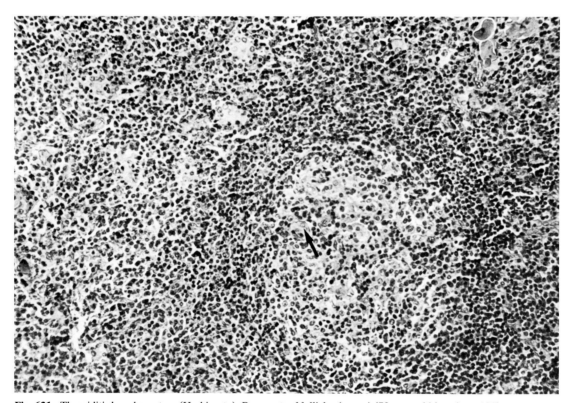

Fig. 621. Thyroiditis lymphomatosa (Hashimoto): Remnants of follicles (arrow) (72-year-old female, × 125).

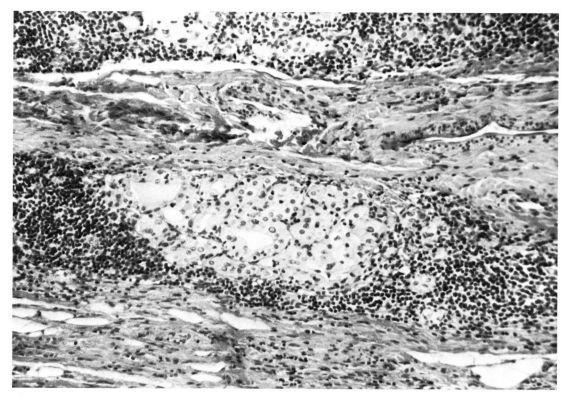

Fig. 622. Thyroiditis lymphomatosa (Hashimoto): Remnants of follicular structures mimicking infiltrating carcinoma (36-year-old female, ×200).

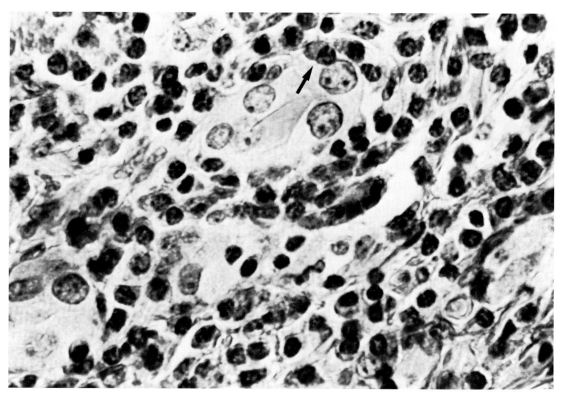

Fig. 623. Thyroiditis lymphomatosa (Hashimoto): Lymphocytes between the follicular cells (arrow) (×400).

Follicular carcinoma

Grading

Well-differentiated and moderately differentiated follicular carcinoma (WHO) ("malignant adenoma," "metastasizing goiter," "wuchernde Struma Langhans," "encapsulated angioinvasive type of follicular carcinoma," "low grade carcinoma," "carcinoma arising in adenoma"):

All of these designations describe a follicular carcinoma that shows a follicular or trabecular growth pattern.

These tumors may be extremely similar to adenomas.

Only evidence for invasion of the blood vessels proves the carcinomatous nature of this lesion (multiple sections with a special stain for elastic fibers in the wall of the blood vessels are often required).

Spread

1. In follicular carcinoma, hematogenous dissemination is frequently observed but lymphatic dissemination is rare (the opposite is true in papillary carcinoma).
   Hematogenous metastases can develop in bone, lung, or other organs (for instance, kidney) [15].
2. Lymphatic spread into the regional lymph nodes is relatively rare (Fig. 624).

Clinical Findings

Frequently a pre-existing goiter has been present for many years when the slow growth of the carcinoma leads to enlargement of the thyroid.

Follicular carcinomas (primary tumor and metastatic lesions) take up 131 J (whole body scan).

Treatment

Surgery:
– Lobectomy, when the other lobe is free of tumor.
– Total thyroidectomy, when both lobes are involved.
– Radical neck dissection has been recommended to remove lymph node metastases [52].
– The usefulness of radical neck dissection is still debated.
Radiation therapy in cases of lymph node metastases (up to 60 Gy in 6 weeks).
Suppressive doses of **thyroid hormone.**
Application of **131 J.**
Most probably, tumor tissue is not destroyed by radioactive iodine.

Prognosis

1. Follicular carcinomas are more malignant than papillary carcinomas.
2. The overall 5-year survival rate is about 65 to 85% [18].
3. In the individual case the prognosis is determined by the stage of the tumor at the time of diagnosis.
   – Minimal invasion of the blood vessels: excellent prognosis.
   – Local invasion of the tumor with development of hematogenous metastases: 5-year survival rate is less than 50%.

---

[15] Davis and Corson 1979.
[18] Gerard-Marchant and Bok 1975.
[52] Wahl et al. 1977.

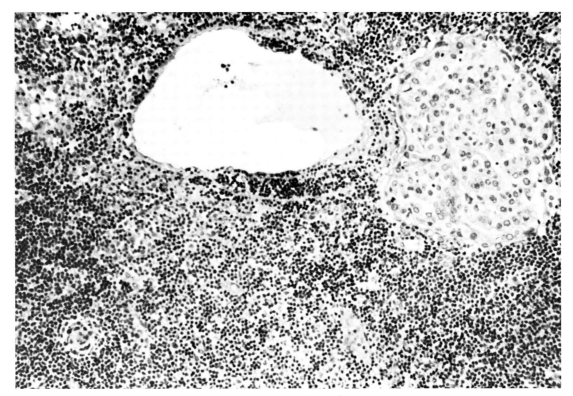

Fig. 624. Lymph node metastasis of follicular thyroid carcinoma (× 125).

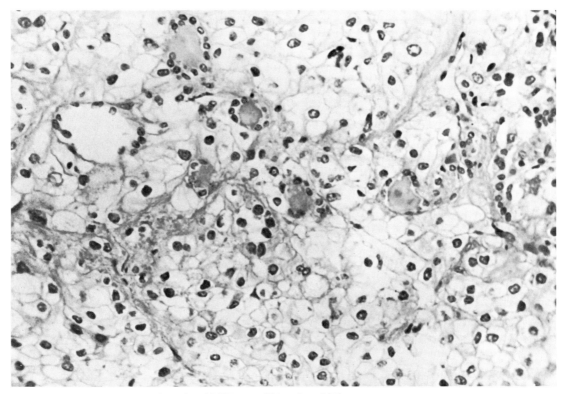

Fig. 625. Clear cell carcinoma of the thyroid (57-year-old female, × 200).

Follicular carcinoma

Further Information

M-8310/3

M-8290/3

1. Two variations of follicular carcinomas have been described:

   a) Clear cell carcinoma (WHO)
   In this case the tumor is composed of clear cells, resembling the cells of a renal cell carcinoma (Fig. 625).

   b) Hürthle cell carcinoma (oxyphil carcinoma) (WHO)
   This is a follicular carcinoma in which the tumor cells have an acidophilic, abundant cytoplasm due to numerous mitochondria (see Figs. 565, 609, and 610).
   Both tumors show signs of malignancy by invasion of tumor cells into the blood vessels.

2. Follicular carcinomas are more malignant than papillary carcinomas, which is shown by local invasion and the rapid development of distant metastases.
   In mixed tumors, therefore, the component of follicular carcinoma determines the prognosis, especially when this type dominates the picture.

3. Metastatic thyroid tumors may entirely replace the lymphatic tissue in lymph nodes.
   Therefore the question of whether the finding corresponds to a metastatic carcinoma of the thyroid or to ectopic thyroid tissue might arise although the great majority of thyroid tissue in lymph nodes represents metastases.
   Ectopic thyroid tissue is observed in the course of the thyroglossal tract, in the mediastinum between muscle bundles, and very rarely in a subthyroid, intratracheal, intralaryngeal, or intraesophageal location.
   Ectopic thyroid tissue always has follicles and never has papillary structures.
   Ectopic thyroid tissue does not show signs of malignancy.

4. Lymph node metastases from an occult carcinoma has also been called
   "lateral aberant thyroid" (WHO).

<table>
<tr><td>

M-8511/3
T 193.9
M-8510/3
</td><td>

4. Medullary carcinoma (WHO) [22]
(medullary carcinoma with amyloid stroma; parafollicular cell carcinoma;
C-cell carcinoma)
</td></tr>
</table>

General Remarks

Incidence: About 5% of the thyroid carcinomas are medullary carcinomas.

Age: The majority of the patients are over 40 years old; the tumor has also been observed in children.

Sex: Medullary carcinomas are more frequent in males than in females.

Site: Medullary carcinomas can grow in every part of the thyroid. The tumor is of a multifocal origin.

Further notes: About 20% of medullary carcinomas are familial. This form of medullary carcinoma is probably of a dominant-autosomal heredity. (See further details in Clinical findings and Further information).

Macroscopy

Medullary carcinomas are firm-to-hard tumors. They are well demarcated from the surrounding tissue; however, capsules are rare.

The size of these tumors varies, and the diameter ranges from 2 to 8 cm.

The cut surface is whitish.

Occasionally the invasion of the tumor into blood vessels can be seen on gross inspection.

Histology

Medullary carcinomas are composed of cells that are polygonal, oval, or spindle-shaped. The cytoplasm is abundant and acidophilic. The cell membrane is sometimes distinct and sometimes indistinct (Fig. 626).

The tumor cells can grow in different patterns: Sometimes they form alveolar structures, sometimes they grow in solid sheets and cords (Fig. 627); papillary formations with psammoma bodies (Fig. 628) or follicular structures are equally observed.

In some instances the tumor cells resemble plasma cells (Fig. 629). These tumor cells, which have a great variability in growth pattern and aspect, grow in a connective tissue that contains amyloid (Figs. 630 and 631). The amount of amyloid differs from tumor to tumor; sometimes it might be difficult to detect this protein.

Electron Microscopy

The tumor arises from C cells: The cells contain secretory granules, which are surrounded by a single membrane.

Histochemistry

Fluorescamine induces fluorescence in the cells of human thyroid medullary carcinoma but not in non-neoplastic C cells [48].

Immunohisto-chemistry

Occasionally calcitonin can be observed in the amyloid stroma and in the tumor cells [3].

[3] Arnal-Monreal et al. 1977.
[22] Hazard et al. 1959.
[48] Sundler et al. 1974.

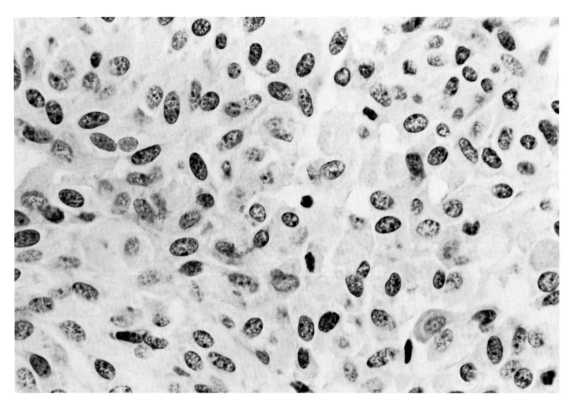

Fig. 626. Medullary carcinoma of the thyroid: Ill-defined cytoplasm, irregular malignant nuclei (48-year-old female, ×400).

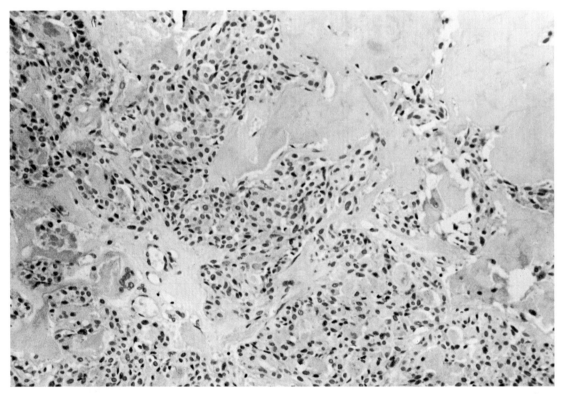

Fig. 627. Medullary carcinoma of the thyroid: Solid complexes of tumor cells and amyloid (48-year-old female, ×125).

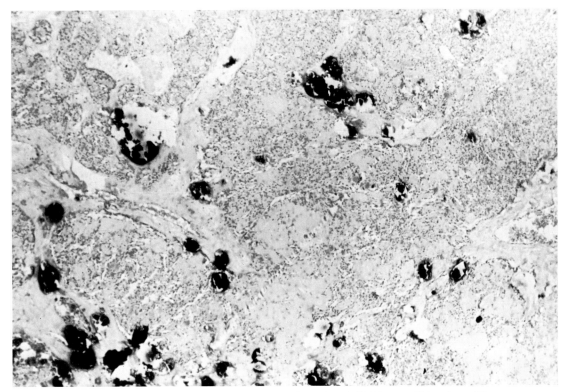

Fig. 628. Medullary carcinoma of the thyroid: Psammoma bodies and amyloid (48-year-old female, × 40).

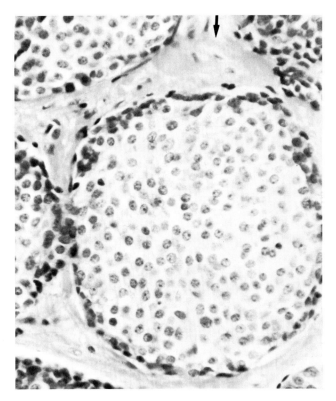

Fig. 629. Medullary carcinoma of the thyroid: Cell nests resembling small cell carcinoma or plasma cells, amyloid deposits (arrow) (30-year-old female, ×310).

627

Medullary carcinoma

Differential Diagnosis

Due to the great variability of the growth pattern of medullar carcinomas, different tumors should be taken into consideration.
1. Medullary carcinoma **with other thyroid carcinomas.**
2. Medullary carcinoma **with metastatic lesions** from
   - undifferentiated carcinoma,
   - paraganglioma (Fig. 1741),
   - carcinoid (Fig. 322).

The diagnosis of medullary carcinoma is supported by the evidence of amyloid (which occasionally cannot be seen on light microscopy, but is detectable on electron microscopy).

Spread

1. Lymphatic dissemination into the cervical and supraclavicular lymph nodes.
2. Hematogenous metastases into the lung, liver, bone, adrenal glands, and other organs.

Clinical Findings

1. A common symptom is diarrhea.
2. Medullary carcinomas do not take up 131 J.
3. Occasionally Cushing's syndrome develops in patients with medullary carcinoma.
4. In the familial medullary carcinoma, there is a high incidence of hyperparathyroidism due to parathyroid hyperplasia and the simultaneous occurrence of parathyroid adenoma.
5. Other tumors associated with the familial type of medullary carcinomas are pheochromocytoma (often bilateral) and neurofibromatosis von Recklinghausen [35, 40].
6. The C cells produce thyrocalcitonin with induction of hypocalcemia.
   It has been recommended that a calcium infusion test be given to families with medullary carcinoma: Abnormally high serum calcitonin after this test indicates a tumor before metastatic dissemination [8, 20, 47].

Treatment

The only efficient treatment is **surgical removal** (total thyroidectomy and radical neck dissection) [37].

Prognosis

Medullary carcinomas grow slowly; however, most of the patients have metastases at the time of diagnosis.

Early detection in familial medullary carcinoma is therefore important.

The 5-year survival rate is better for medullary carcinoma than for undifferentiated thyroid carcinomas but worse than for papillary and follicular carcinoma:

The 5- to 10-year overall survival rate is less than 50 to 80% [18].

Further Information

1. Medullary carcinomas can occur sporadically or familially. Sporadic carcinoma occurs in middle or late life and is usually unilateral.
   Familial medullary carcinoma occurs in younger age groups (the first 3 decades) and is multifocal.

---

[8] Block et al. 1978.
[18] Gerard-Marchant and Bok 1975.
[20] Graze et al. 1978.
[35] Obara et al. 1977.
[37] Potts Jr. 1977.
[40] Rocklin et al. 1977.
[47] Stepanas et al. 1979.

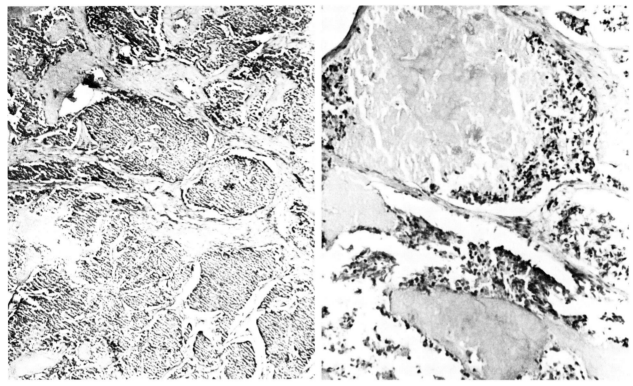

Fig. 630. Medullary carcinoma of the thyroid: Tumor cell groups surrounded by amyloid deposits (× 40).

Fig. 631. Medullary carcinoma of the thyroid: Abundant amyloid deposits (× 125).

Further Information

2. There is a report of medullary carcinoma of the thyroid being observed in 3 generations [50].

3. The tumor cells in medullary carcinoma can secrete thyrocalcitonin [33], 5-hydroxy-tryptamine, prostaglandins [53], histaminase [6, 49], somatostatin, and ACTH.

4. Occasionally, medullary thyroid carcinoma is composed of C cells and other endocrine-active cells, causing the multiple endocrine cell type of carcinoma [11].

5. Occasionally, thyroid carcinomas other than the medullary type are associated with parathyroid adenoma, causing hyperparathyroidism [31].

[6] Baylin et al. 1972.
[11] Capella et al. 1978.
[31] LiVolsi and Feind 1976.
[33] Meyer and Abdel-Bari 1968.
[49] Szijj et al. 1969.
[50] Toyoda et al. 1977.
[53] Williams et al. 1968.

M-8020/3
T 193.9

5. Undifferentiated (anaplastic) carcinoma (WHO)

**General
Remarks**

Incidence: 15% of the thyroid carcinomas are undifferentiated carcinomas.
Age: Undifferentiated carcinomas occur mostly in elderly patients.
Sex: Females are considerably more frequently affected than males.
Site: Undifferentiated carcinomas grow in large parts of the thyroid gland.

Macroscopy

Undifferentiated carcinomas have a fleshy cut surface. They are large and grow in both lobes. The tumor infiltrates the surrounding thyroid tissue and the adjacent structures: Muscle, esophagus, trachea.

Histology

Undifferentiated carcinomas are composed of malignant cells with marked nuclear atypias: Hyperchromasia and atypical mitotic figures. It is very rare to find an organoid growth pattern like follicular or papillary areas in undifferentiated carcinomas.
The tumor shows infiltration into the surrounding tissue and invasion of the lymphatics and blood vessels.
The tumor cells can be quite variable in appearance and occasionally imitate sarcomatous growth.
According to the size of the tumor cells, a subclassification has been established:

M-8041/3
T 193.9

a) Small cell carcinoma (WHO)

In this case the tumor cells are very small and the nuclear pleomorphism is rather discrete. The tumor cells form large nests that are surrounded by connective tissue (compact type) (Figs. 632 and 633).
This tumor might resemble the medullary carcinoma; however, there is no detectable amyloid.

M-8031/3
T 193.9

b) Giant cell carcinoma (WHO)

Giant cell carcinomas are observed more frequently than small cell carcinomas. They occur mostly in patients over 60 years old.
The tumor cells can be very large and multinucleated giant cells may be detected. The nuclear pleomorphism is extensive; there are numerous mitotic figures (Figs. 634 and 635).
Especially in this type of tumor sarcoma-like structures may be encountered (Figs. 636 and 637).

**Electron
Microscopy**

The nuclei of small cell carcinoma are irregular, dense bodies randomly distributed throughout the cytoplasm; the atypical nuclei contain hypertrophic nucleoli. The mitochondria are abnormal and may entirely lack the cristae [51].

---

[51] Valenta and Michel-Béchet 1977.

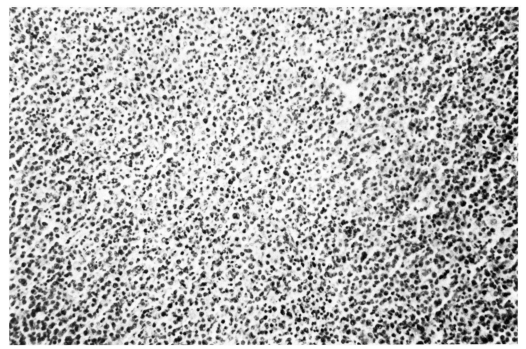

Fig. 632. Undifferentiated carcinoma of the thyroid, small cell type: Diffuse growth pattern (78-year-old male, ×125).

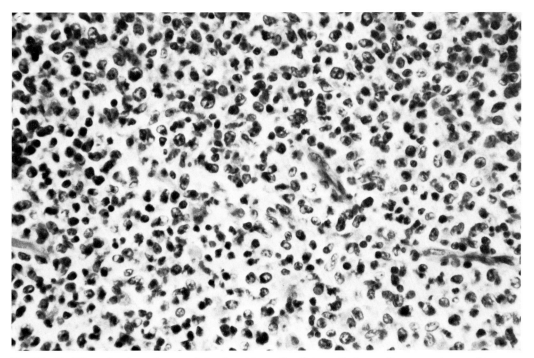

Fig. 633. Undifferentiated carcinoma of the thyroid, small cell type: Rather uniform aspect, resemblance to malignant lymphoma (78-year-old male, ×310).

631

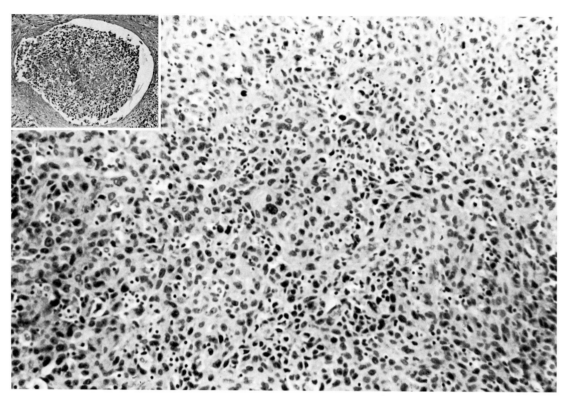

Fig. 634. Undifferentiated carcinoma of the thyroid, giant cell type: Blood vessel invasion (inset) (78-year-old male, ×125; inset, ×125).

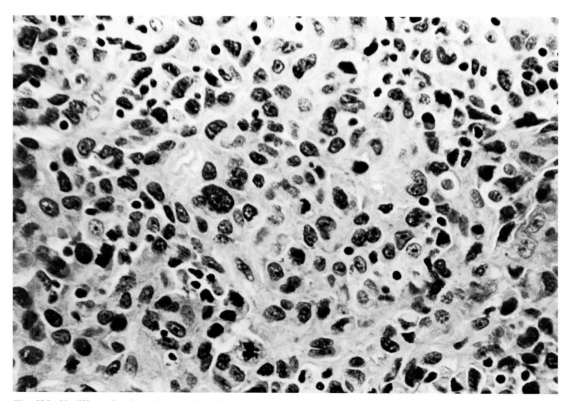

Fig. 635. Undifferentiated carcinoma of the thyroid, giant cell type: Occasional spindle-shaped cells (78-year-old male, ×310).

632

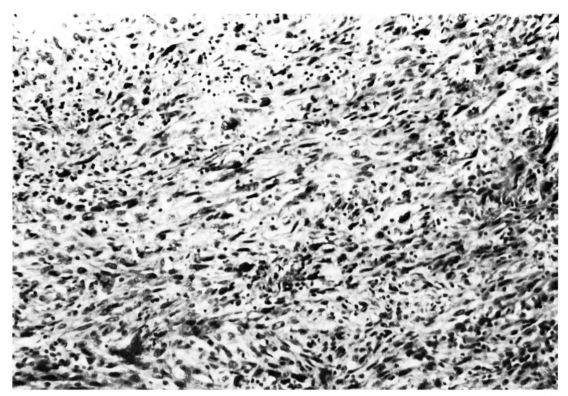

Fig. 636. Undifferentiated carcinoma of the thyroid, giant cell type: Sarcoma-like growth pattern (57-year-old female, ×125).

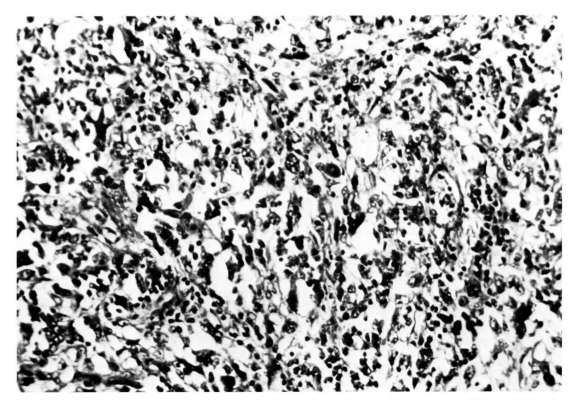

Fig. 637. Undifferentiated carcinoma of the thyroid, giant cell type: Sarcoma-like appearance (74-year-old female, ×200).

Undifferentiated carcinoma

Differential Diagnosis

1. Undifferentiated carcinoma, small cell type **with malignant lymphoma:**
   The tumor might be very difficult to separate from malignant lymphoma; however, on several sections one might find remnants of follicular structures.

2. Undifferentiated carcinoma, small cell type **with medullary carcinoma** (Figs. 626 to 631):
   Medullary carcinomas contain amyloid in the stroma.

3. Undifferentiated carcinoma, giant cell type, **with sarcoma:**
   Sarcomas of the thyroid are very rare tumors.
   In case of doubt an intensive search should be made for the epithelial growth pattern of the tumor (reticulin stain).

M-8000/6
T 193.9

4. Undifferentiated carcinoma **with metastatic carcinoma into the thyroid:**
   Metastatic lesions in the thyroid are rather frequent: About 10% of the carcinomas disseminate into the thyroid gland [46].
   In the individual case it might be very difficult to separate metastatic lesions from undifferentiated primary carcinoma.

5. Undifferentiated carcinoma **with invasive chronic fibrosing thyroiditis** (Riedl's thyroiditis):
   The differential diagnosis is indicated by
   a) The localized development of this inflammation in the thyroid (mimicking a tumor).
   b) The hardness of the lesion because of abundant fibrous tissue.
   c) Extension of the lesion into the surrounding structures (muscle), imitating malignant infiltration (Fig. 638).
   d) Histologically the connective scar tissue leaves only remnants of the normal thyroid tissue (mimicking malignant epithelial cells).
   Indicating Riedl's thyroiditis are the facts that connective tissue dominates with large areas of hyalinization, and that infiltration occurs by collagen fibers and not by epithelial cells. There are few inflammatory cells in this lesion.
   Riedl's thyroiditis occurs more frequently in women than in men. The disease usually affects patients in the 4th to 7th decades [55].

6. Undifferentiated carcinoma **with subacute thyroiditis de Quervain** (granulomatous thyroiditis):
   Differential diagnosis might be required, especially in frozen sections.
   Subacute granulomatous thyroiditis occasionally involves local areas in the thyroid; usually the entire gland is involved.
   The gland is enlarged and the affected areas are firm.
   The de Quervain thyroiditis does not infiltrate the surrounding structures; there is no adherence between thyroid gland, muscle, and connective tissue.
   On histological analysis the de Quervain thyroiditis is composed of numerous granulocytes and foreign body giant cells, which are arranged around colloid (Fig. 639).

Spread

Undifferentiated carcinomas metastasize early by hematogenous and lymphatic dissemination.

[46] Shimaoka et al. 1962.
[55] Woolner et al. 1975.

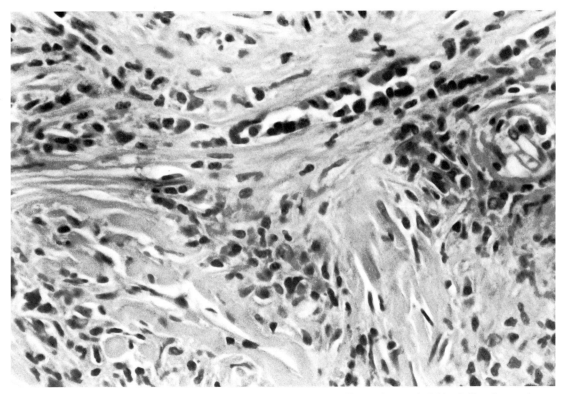

Fig. 638. Riedl's thyroiditis: Nests of inflammatory cells between dense fibrous tissue, mimicking infiltrating carcinoma (57-year-old female, × 310).

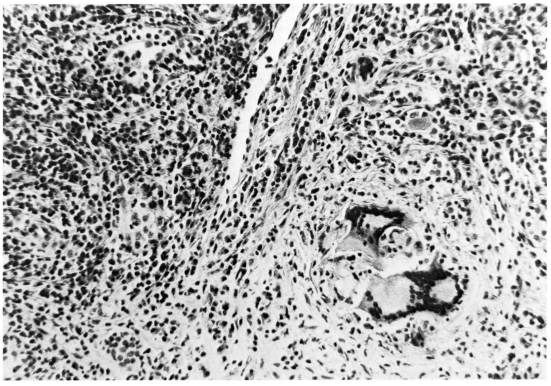

Fig. 639. Subacute thyroiditis de Quervain: Inflammatory cells and foreign body giant cells with colloid (× 125).

635

Clinical Findings

Undifferentiated carcinomas present as rapidly growing tumors, usually without a previous history of goiter.

Elderly patients, mainly women, are affected.

Treatment

If possible radical **surgery** should be tried; however, in most instances the tumor has infiltrated the surrounding tissue.

Postoperative high voltage **irradiation** could be tried as an adjunctive measure.

Chemotherapy and **endocrine therapy** with thyroxine or adriamycin can be tried; the response rate is about 75%. There has been no demonstrated improvement in survival.

Prognosis

1. Undifferentiated carcinomas have a very poor prognosis:

   5-year survival for small cell carcinoma, about 20% [44]

   5-year survival for giant cell carcinoma, about 5% [18]

   Average survival from the time of diagnosis for giant cell carcinoma, around 5 months [32].

2. In the individual case the prognosis is always determined by the stage of the tumor at the time of diagnosis.

3. Since the poorly differentiated carcinoma correlates with early dissemination, the prognosis of these thyroid carcinomas is always also determined by the degree of differentiation [28].

M-8070/3
T 193.9

6. Squamous cell carcinoma (WHO)

Primary squamous cell carcinomas in the thyroid are exceedingly rare.

Both sexes are equally affected.

The peak age is the 5th and 6th decades.

The tumor occasionally contains keratin and shows intercellular bridges.

The great majority of squamous cell carcinomas found in the thyroid are metastatic tumors.

[18] Gerard-Marchant and Bok 1975.
[28] Keminger et al. 1975.
[32] Meissner and Warren 1969.
[44] Schoumacher et al. 1977.

M-9590/3
T 193.9

7. Malignant lymphoma (WHO)

<table>
<tr><td>

**General
Remarks**

</td><td>

Incidence: Primary malignant lymphomas in the thyroid are rare.
Age: Elderly patients are affected.
Sex: Primary malignant lymphoma usually develops in females.
Site: The malignant lymphoma involves the entire thyroid gland.
Further notes: Malignant lymphoma can be associated with Hashimoto's thyroiditis [38].

</td></tr>
</table>

Macroscopy

The enlarged thyroid shows a whitish-grayish, sometimes pinkish cut surface.
Occasionally adhesions to the surrounding tissue might be observed.

**Differential
Diagnosis**

1. Malignant lymphoma **with undifferentiated carcinoma, small cell type** (Figs. 632 and 633):
   The differential diagnosis might be very difficult. Occasionally only the evidence for malignant lymphoma involving the adjacent lymph nodes decides the diagnosis.
2. Malignant lymphoma **with Hashimoto's disease:**
   In cases of highly differentiated lymphocytic malignant lymphoma the differential diagnosis might be difficult (Figs. 621 and 640).

M-9650/3
T 193.9

3. Malignant lymphoma **with Hodgkin's disease:**
   Hodgkin's disease is very rare in the thyroid. Reed-Sternberg cells will reveal the nature of the lesion.

M-9731/1
T 193.9

4. Malignant lymphoma **with plasmacytoma:**
   Plasmacytomas are exceedingly rare in the thyroid; however, they can be found in localized areas in the thyroid tissue.

**Clinical
Findings**

Enlargement of the thyroid.

Treatment

Surgery:
Total thyroidectomy should be applied in cases of malignant lymphoma limited to the thyroid gland.
Radiation therapy:
Postoperative radiation therapy with an average tumor dose of 40 Gy [9].
In cases of malignant lymphoma extending beyond the thyroid gland, radiation therapy and **chemotherapy** should be applied.
Malignant lymphomas in the thyroid as part of the systemic disease are more frequently observed than primary malignant lymphoma. The treatment is accordingly that for disseminated lymphoma (see page 1252).
Plasmacytomas can be treated by subtotal thyroidectomy with subsequent irradiation of the thyroid [1, 45].

[1] Ackerman and Rosai 1974.
[9] Burke et al. 1977.
[38] Ranström 1957.
[45] Shaw and Smith 1940.

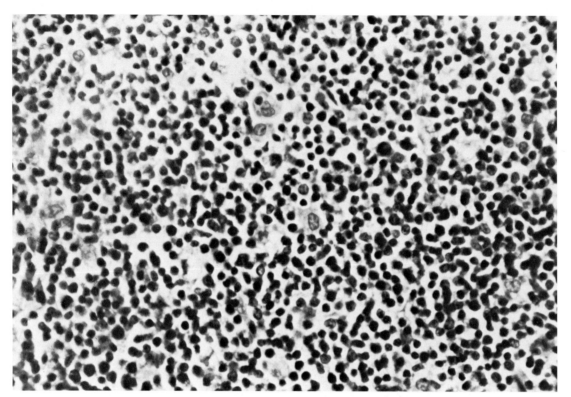

Fig. 640. Malignant lymphocytic lymphoma in the thyroid (56-year-old male, × 310).

Prognosis

1. Malignant lymphoma confined to the thyroid: 5-year survival, around 75%.
2. The mortality rate increases after the tumor has infiltrated the capsule and reached the surrounding tissue [56].

The overall 5-year survival rate for primary malignant lymphoma of the thyroid is about 50% [9].

Further Information

Occasionally remnants of a chronic lymphocytic thyroiditis can be discovered in cases of residual thyroid tissue in malignant lymphomas.

This might indicate a relation between chronic lymphocytic thyroiditis and primary malignant lymphoma in the thyroid [9].

[9] Burke et al. 1977.
[56] Woolner et al. 1966.

M-8800/3
T 193.9

8. Sarcomas of the thyroid (WHO)

Malignant mesenchymal tumors in the thyroid are very rare.

Due to the great variability of undifferentiated carcinoma with sarcoma-like structures of the tumor cells, the sarcoma most probably is more often diagnosed than it exists in reality.

There are reports on

M-9120/3

angiosarcoma (WHO) (however, the existence of angiosarcomas as tumor in the thyroid gland is still debated) [1].

M-8810/3

fibrosarcoma (WHO),

M-9180/3

osteogenic sarcoma,

M-9150/3

malignant hemangiopericytoma.

There is a report in which a sarcoma of the thyroid was associated with a carcinoma of the colon [19].

Sarcomas of the thyroid gland have a very poor prognosis.

Benign soft tissue tumors also occur in the thyroid (page 7).

M-8980/3
T 193.9

9. Carcinosarcoma (WHO)

Carcinosarcomas of the thyroid are exceedingly rare.

After studying the growth pattern of undifferentiated carcinoma, one might question whether this tumor exists at all.

---

[1] Ackerman and Rosai 1974.
[19] Giersch and Noltenius 1978.

M-9080/0, 3
T 193.9

10. Teratoma (WHO)

Teratomas of the thyroid are very rare; they may occur in children and sometimes are observed in newborns.
A primary malignant teratoma has been reported in the thyroid. These tumors are very rare [5, 29, 34].

M-8000/6
T 193.9

11. Metastatic tumors (WHO)

Metastases may simulate primary neoplasms. Metastases from renal cell carcinoma occasionally may resemble thyroid carcinoma.

M-8000/3
T 193.9

12. Unclassified tumors (WHO)

---

[5] Bale 1950.
[29] Kimler and Muth 1978.
[34] Newstedt and Shirkey 1964.

Recommendations for differential diagnosis in tumors of the thyroid

papillary carcinoma	with	– papillary adenoma – papillary growth in goiters
follicular carcinoma	with	– follicular adenoma – Hashimoto's disease – subacute thyroiditis – nodular goiter
undifferentiated carcinoma small cell type	with	– malignant lymphoma – chronic sclerosing (Riedl's) thyroiditis – Hashimoto's disease – metastatic lesions of the thyroid

undifferentiated carcinoma
giant cell type
	with	– metastatic lesions of the thyroid
		– metaplastic giant cell reaction in
		  follicular carcinoma
		– subacute granulomatous thyroiditis
		  de Quervain
		– sarcoma

medullary carcinoma	with	– other thyroid carcinomas – adenomas – nodular goiter – metastatic lesions of the thyroid – plasmacytoma – thyroiditis – carcinoid – paraganglioma

squamous cell carcinoma	with	– squamous cell metaplasia in follicular
		  epithelial cells (for instance, associated
		  with thyroiditis or papillary carcinoma)

malignant lymphoma	with	– thyroiditis – small cell carcinoma – Hodgkin's disease – plasmacytoma
plasmacytoma	with	– medullary carcinoma – thyroiditis
ectopic thyroid tissue	with	– metastatic thyroid carcinoma
thyroiditis (sclerosing chronic (Riedl's) thyroiditis; subacute granulomatous thyroiditis de Quervain; Hashimoto's disease)	with	– undifferentiated carcinoma – follicular carcinoma

Differential diagnosis of thyroid tumors in frozen sections

Usually the undifferentiated type of carcinoma is not difficult to diagnose.
The well-differentiated carcinomas might be difficult to separate from benign adenomas or thyroiditis.
Helpful for the frozen sections are
– evidence of psammoma bodies (papillary carcinoma),
– evidence of germinal centers in lymphoid tissue (Hashimoto's disease),
– invasion of tumor cells into the blood vessels,
– the extremely hard consistency of Riedl's thyroiditis tissue.

Tumors of the parathyroid gland

M-8321/0
T 194.1

1. Parathyroid adenoma

**General
Remarks**

Incidence: Parathyroid adenomas are rare [41].

Age: The peak age is the 4th decade; however, any age can be affected, including children.

Sex: Women are more frequently affected than men (3 : 1).

Site: The inferior parathyroid bodies are more frequently affected than the superior glands [4].

The majority of tumors develop as a solitary neoplasm; however, two or four parathyroid glands may be affected [54].

Occasionally parathyroid adenomas can be found in the anterior or posterior mediastinum.

Macroscopy

Parathyroid adenomas are encapsulated tumors of a lobular architecture and brownish color (similar to lymph nodes).

Adenomas of the parathyroid are small: Mean weight about 7 g, size around 1 to 3 cm, weight from 0.4 to 120 g [1].

The gross recognition of adenomas might be so difficult that the surgeon needs the help of frozen sections.

Histology

Adenomas of the parathyroid contain the cells that normally occur in this gland: Water-clear cells, chief cells, and oxyphilic cells (Figs. 641 and 642).

The tumor cells can have very pleomorphic nuclei with hyperchromasia (Fig. 643).

The adenoma may be dominated by one of the cytological subgroups.

The tumor cells can form alveolar structures or tubular formations or may grow in solid complexes (Figs. 644 and 645).

The cells can form cysts containing colloid-like material in their lumina. This structure gives a thyroid-like aspect to the adenoma (Fig. 646).

Mitotic figures are very rare [12].

**Electron
Microscopy**

The tumor cells contain secretory granules of different size.

**Differential
Diagnosis**

Parathyroid adenoma **with hyperplasia of the parathyroid gland:**

The hyperplasia involves all glands in the majority of cases, while adenomas in the majority of cases develop only in one gland [13, 16].

Hyperplasia involves the entire gland, while remnants of the unaffected parathyroid gland can be found at the periphery of adenomas.

[1] Ackerman and Rosai 1974.
[4] Ashley 1978.
[12] Castleman 1952.
[13] Castleman et al. 1976.
[16] Dorado et al. 1976.
[41] Russ et al. 1979.
[54] Woolner et al. 1952.

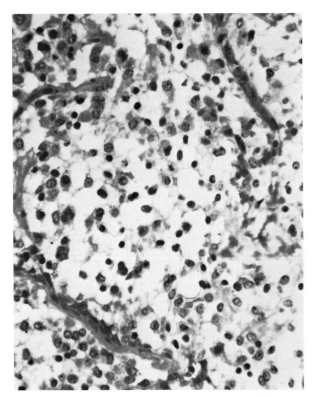

Fig. 641. Parathyroid adenoma: Water clear cells (× 310).

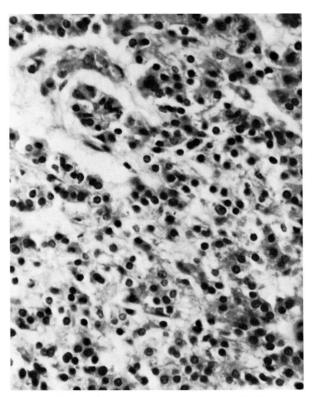

Fig. 642. Parathyroid adenoma, dominated by chief cell type (× 310).

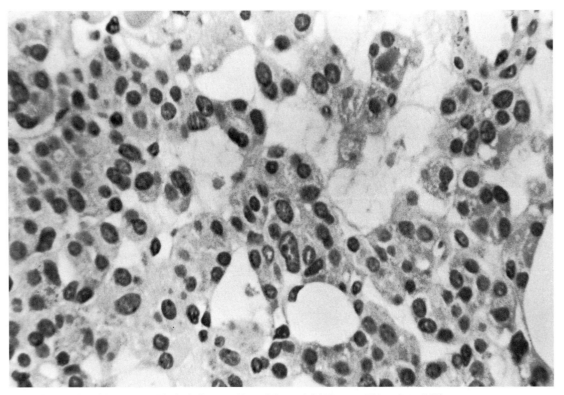

Fig. 643. Parathyroid adenoma: Marked pleomorphism of the nuclei (65-year-old female, × 360).

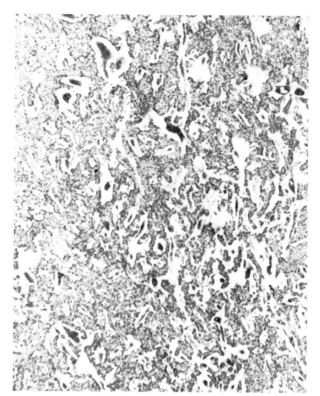

Fig. 644. Parathyroid adenoma: Alveolar growth pattern (×40).

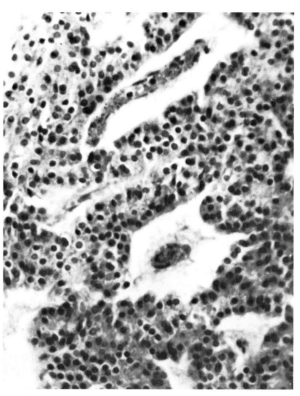

Fig. 645. Parathyroid adenoma mainly composed of chief cells: Occasional alveolar and tubular formations (×200).

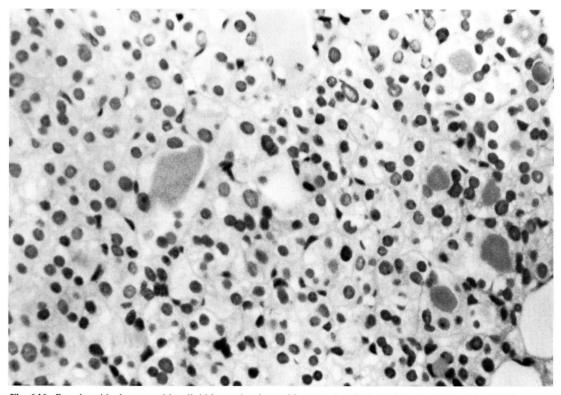

Fig. 646. Parathyroid adenoma with colloid formation (resemblance to thyroid tissue (65-year-old female, ×310).

M-8321/3
T 194.1

2. Parathyroid carcinoma

Parathyroid carcinomas are exceedingly rare.

The adenoma might contain numerous atypical nuclei, which are therefore not evidence for carcinoma.

However, the increased number of mitotic figures indicates malignancy [2, 43].

Evidence for parathyroid carcinoma is invasive growth into the surrounding tissue at the time of the first surgical intervention!

Spread

Parathyroid carcinoma metastasizes into the cervical lymph nodes in 32% of the cases and into the lung in 26% of the cases [25].

Clinical Findings

Adenoma and carcinoma:

Adenomas or carcinomas may or may not cause primary hyperparathyroidism.

Primary hyperparathyroidism can also be caused by chief cell hyperplasia [21, 36].

The hyperparathyroidism can cause osteitis fibrosa cystica, nephrolithiasis, discrete symptoms of gastrointestinal tract or duodenal ulcer, and psychic and neurological disturbances.

The cell type of the tumor does not completely correlate with the clinical symptoms; however, oxyphil adenomas are usually silent.

The size of the tumor does not correlate with the clinical symptoms.

Treatment

Surgery:

The parathyroid adenoma should be removed.

The remaining glands should be checked to rule out hyperplasia.

The surgical intervention should be accompanied by frozen sections to check the removed tissue.

Surgical intervention in cases of carcinoma should also include resection of the thyroid lobe on the side of tumor growth, the regional lymph nodes, and the surrounding tissue [25].

Prognosis

Parathyroid adenomas have an excellent prognosis.

Parathyroid carcinomas: 5-year survival rate, about 40% [25, 43].

Further Information

1. Hyperparathyroidism with hypercalcemia can also be observed in multiple endocrine neoplasia (MEN I or MEN II).

   In MEN II there is an association of bilateral pheochromocytomas, parathyroid hyperplasia, and medullary carcinoma.

2. Hypercalcemia due to hyperparathyroidism can be part of a paraneoplastic syndrome.

3. There is an increased incidence of nonmedullary thyroid carcinoma in cases of hyperparathyroidism [31].

[2] Altenähr and Saeger 1973.   [31] LiVolsi and Feind 1976.
[21] Haff et al. 1970.   [36] Potts Jr. 1977.
[25] Holmes et al. 1969.   [43] Schantz and Castleman 1973.

References

[1] Ackerman, C.V., and J. Rosai: Surgical pathology. Fifth ed., C.V. Mosby Company 1974.

[2] Altenähr, E., and W. Saeger: Light and electron microscopy of parathyroid carcinoma. Report of three cases. Virchows Arch. A Path. Anat. and Histol. *360* (1973) 107-122.

[3] Arnal-Monreal, F.M., D. Goltzman, J. Knaack, N. Wang, and S. Huang: Immunohistologic study of thyroidal medullary carcinoma and pancreatic insulinoma. Cancer *40* (1977) 1060-1070.

[4] Ashley, D.J.B.: In: Evan's histological appearances of tumours. Churchill Livingstone, Edinburgh–London–New York 1978.

[5] Bale, G.F.: Teratoma of the neck in the region of the thyroid gland; a review of the literature and report of four cases. Am. J. Path. *26* (1950) 565-579.

[6] Baylin, S.B., M.A. Beaven, L.M. Buja, and H.R. Keiser: Histaminase activity: A biochemical marker for medullary carcinoma of thyroid. Am. J. Med. *53* (1972) 723-733.

[7] Benker, G., K. Hackenberg, H.G. Hoff, S. Seeber, J. Ebke, R. Windeck und D. Reinwein: Zytostatische Kombinationsbehandlung metastasierender Schilddrüsenkarzinome mit Doxorubicin und Bleomycin. Ergebnisse bei 21 Patienten. Dtsch. Med. Wschr. *102* (1977) 1908-1913.

[8] Block, M.A., C.E. Jackson, and A.H. Tashjian: Management of occult medullary thyroid carcinoma. Evidenced only by serum calcitonin level elevations after apparently adequate neck operations. Arch. Surg. *113* (1978) 368-372.

[9] Burke, J.S., J.J. Butler, and L.M. Fuller: Malignant lymphomas of the thyroid. A clinical pathologic study of 35 patients including ultrastructural observations. Cancer *39* (1977) 1587-1602.

[10] Cady, B., C.E. Sedgwick, W.A. Meissner, M.S. Wool, F.A. Salzman, and J. Werber: Risk factor analysis in differentiated thyroid cancer. Cancer *43* (1979) 810-820.

[11] Capella, C., C. Bordi, G. Monga, R. Buffa, P. Fontana, S. Bonfanti, G. Bussolati, and E. Solcia: Multiple endocrine cell types in thyroid medullary carcinoma. Evidence for calcitonin, somatostatin, ACTH, 5 HT, and small granule cells. Virchows Arch. A Path. Anat. and Histol. *377* (1978) 111-128.

[12] Castleman, B.: Tumors of the parathyroid glands. Atlas of tumor pathology. A.F.I.P., Washington, D.C. 1952.

[13] Castleman, B., A. Schantz, and S.I. Roth: Parathyroid hyperplasia in primary hyperparathyroidism. A review of 85 cases. Cancer *38* (1976) 1668-1675.

[14] Curtin, C.T., B. McHeffy, and A.J. Kolarsick: Thyroid and breast cancer following childhood radiation. Cancer *40* (1977) 2911-2913.

[15] Davis, R.I., and J.M. Corson: Renal metastases from well differentiated follicular thyroid carcinoma. A case report with light and electron microscopic findings. Cancer *43* (1979) 265-268.

[16] Dorado, A.E., G. Hensley, and B. Castleman: Water clear cell hyperplasia of parathyroid. Autopsy report of a case with supernumerary glands. Cancer *38* (1976) 1676-1683.

[17] Favus, M.J., A.B. Schneider, M.E. Stachura, J.E. Arnold, U.Y. Ryo, S.M. Pinsky, M. Colman, M.J. Arnold, and L.A. Frohman: Thyroid cancer occurring as a late consequence of head and neck irradiation. Evaluation of 1056 patients. N. Engl. J. Med. *294* (1976) 1019-1025.

[18] Gerard-Marchant, R., and B. Bok: Cancer of the thyroid: Prognostic factors and criteria of response. In: Cancer therapy: Prognostic factors and criteria of response, edited by M.J. Staquet, Raven Press, New York 1975.

[19] Giersch, H., und H. Noltenius: Maligner Schilddrüsentumor mit epithelialen und mesenchymalen Anteilen bei gleichzeitigem Auftreten eines Kolonkarzinoms. Zbl. Allg. Path. *122* (1978) 70-74.

[20] Graze, K., I.J. Spiler, A.H. Tashjian, K.E.W. Melvin, S. Cervi-Skinner, R.F. Gagel, H.H. Miller, H.J. Wolfe, R.A. DeLellis, L. Leape, Z.T. Feldman, and S. Reichlin: Natural history of familial medullary thyroid carcinoma. Effect of a program for early diagnosis. N. Engl. J. Med. *299* (1978) 980-985.

[21] Haff, R.C., W.C. Black, and W.F. Ballinger: Primary hyperparathyroidism: Changing clinical, surgical and pathological aspects. Ann. Surg. *171* (1970) 85-92.

[22] Hazard, J.B., W.A. Hawk, and G. Crile Jr.: Medullary (solid) carcinoma of the thyroid – a clinicopathologic entity. J. Clin. Endocrinol. Metab. *19* (1959) 152-161.

[23] Hedinger, C.: Histological typing of thyroid tumours. WHO (Geneva) 1974.

[24] Heitz, P., H. Moser, and J.J. Staub: Thyroid cancer. A study of 573 thyroid tumors and 161 autopsy cases observed over a thirty-year period. Cancer *37* (1976) 2329-2337.

[25] Holmes, E.C., D.L. Morton, and A.S. Ketcham: Parathyroid carcinoma: A collective review. Ann. Surg. *169* (1969) 631-640.

[26] Ingbar, S.H., and K.A. Woeber: Diseases of the thyroid. In: Harrison's Principles of internal medicine. Eighth edition. McGraw-Hill Book Company, New York–Düsseldorf etc. 1977.

[27] Johannessen, J.V., V.E. Gould, and W. Jao: The fine structure of human thyroid cancer. Hum. Pathol. *9* (1978) 385-400.

[28] Keminger, K., K. Dinstl und D. Depisch: Struma maligna. In: Krebsbehandlung als interdisziplinäre Aufgabe. Hrsg. von K.H. Kärcher. Springer, Berlin–Heidelberg–New York 1975.

[29] Kimler, S.C., and W.F. Muth: Primary malignant teratoma of the thyroid. Case report and literature review of cervical teratomas in adults. Cancer *42* (1978) 311-317.

[30] Lang, W., Z. Atay und A. Georgii: Die cytologische Unterscheidung follikulärer Tumoren in der Schilddrüse. Virchows Arch. A Path. Anat. and Histol. *378* (1978) 199-211.

[31] LiVolsi, V.A., and C.R. Feind: Parathyroid adenoma and nonmedullary thyroid carcinoma. Cancer *38* (1976) 1391-1393.

[32] Meissner, W.A., and S. Warren: Tumors of the thyroid gland. Atlas of tumor pathology. A.F.I.P., Washington, D.C. 1969.

[33] Meyer, J.S., and W. Abdel-Bari: Granules and thyrocalcitonin-like activity in medullary carcinoma of the thyroid gland. N. Engl. J. Med. *278* (1968) 523-529.

[34] Newstedt, J.R., and H.C. Shirkey: Teratoma of the thyroid region. Report of a case with seven-year follow-up. Am. J. Dis. Child. *107* (1964) 88-95.

[35] Obara, T., Y. Fujimoto, A. Oka, M. Fukumitsu, K. Abe, K. Yamaguchi, and T. Wada: Medullary thyroid carcinoma and pheochromocytoma accompanied with nodular hyperplasia in multiple endocrine neoplasia type 2. Jpn. J. Surg. *7* (1977) 235-245.

[36] Potts, J.T.Jr.: Disorders of parathyroid glands. In: Harrison's Principles of internal medicine. Eighth edition. McGraw-Hill Book Company, New York–Düsseldorf etc. 1977.

[37] Potts, J.T.Jr.: Medullary carcinoma of the thyroid and calcitonin. In: Harrison's Principles of internal medicine. Eighth edition. McGraw-Hill Book Company, New York–Düsseldorf etc. 1977.

[38] Ranström, S.: Malignant lymphoma of the thyroid and its relation to Hashimoto's and Brill-Symmers' disease. Acta Chir. Scand. *113* (1957) 185-193.

[39] Refetoff, S., J. Harrison, B.T. Karanfilski, E.L. Kaplan, L.J. De Groot, and C. Dekerman: Continuing occurrence of thyroid carcinoma after irradiation to the neck in infancy and childhood. N. Engl. J. Med. *292* (1975) 171-175.

[40] Rocklin R.E., R. Gagel, Z. Feldman, and A.H. Tashjian Jr.: Cellular immune responses in familial medullary thyroid carcinoma. N. Engl. J. Med. *296* (1977) 835-838.

[41] Russ, J.E., E.F. Scanlon, and F. Sener: Parathyroid adenomas following irradiation. Cancer *43* (1979) 1078-1083.

[42] Russell, M.A., E.F. Gilbert, and W.F. Jaeschke: Prognostic features of thyroid cancer. A long-term followup of 68 cases. Cancer *36* (1975) 553-559.

[43] Schantz, A., and B. Castleman: Parathyroid carcinoma. A study of 70 cases. Cancer *31* (1973) 600-605.

[44] Schoumacher, P., R. Metz, P. Bey, and A.M. Chesneau: Anaplastic carcinoma of the thyroid gland. Eur. J. Cancer *13* (1977) 381-383.

[45] Shaw, R.C., and F.B. Smith: Plasmocytoma of the thyroid gland. Report of a case. Arch. Surg. *40* (1940) 646-657.

[46] Shimaoka, K., J.E. Sokal, and J.W. Pickren: Metastatic neoplasms in the thyroid gland; pathological and clinical findings. Cancer *15* (1962) 557-565.

[47] Stepanas, A.V., N.A. Samaan, C. Hill Jr., and R.C. Hickey: Medullary thyroid carcinoma. Importance of serial serum calcitonin measurement. Cancer *43* (1979) 825-837.

[48] Sundler, F., L.-I. Larsson, R. Håkanson, and O. Ljungberg: Fluorescamine-induced fluorescence in C cell tumours of the thyroid. Virchows Arch. A Path. Anat. and Histol. *363* (1974) 17-20.

[49] Szijj, I., Z. Csapó, F.A. Lászkó, and K. Kovács: Medullary cancer of the thyroid gland associated with hypercorticism. Cancer *24* (1969) 167-173.

[50] Toyoda, H., Y. Kawaguchi, K. Shirasawa, and A. Muramatsu: Familial medullary carcinoma of the thyroid through 3 generations. Acta Path. Jap. *27* (1977) 111-121.

[51] Valenta, L.J., and M. Michel-Béchet: Ultrastructure and biochemistry of thyroid carcinoma. Cancer *40* (1977) 284-300.

[52] Wahl, R., J. Nievergelt, H.D. Röher und B. Oellers: Radikale Thyreoidektomie wegen maligner Schilddrüsentumoren. Dtsch. Med. Wschr. *102* (1977) 13-20.

[53] Williams, E.D., S.M.M. Karim, and M. Sandler: Prostaglandin secretion by medullary carcinoma of the thyroid; a possible cause of the associated diarrhoea. Lancet *1* (1968) 22-23.

[54] Woolner, L.B., F.R. Keating Jr., and B.M. Black: Tumors and hyperplasia of the parathyroid glands; a review of the pathological findings in 140 cases of primary hyperparathyroidism. Cancer *5* (1952) 1069-1088.

[55] Woolner, L.B., W.M. McConahey, and O.H. Beahrs: Granulomatous thyroiditis (De Quervain's thyroiditis). J. Clin. Endocrinol. Metab. *17* (1975) 1202-1221.

[56] Woolner, L.B., W.M. McConahey, O.H. Beahrs, and B.M. Black: Primary malignant lymphoma of the thyroid; review of forty-six cases. Am. J. Surg. *111* (1966) 502-523.

648

16 Tumors of the mediastinum

The mediastinum can be involved by primary tumors or metastatic neoplasms.

The mediastinal tumors can originate from the heart, the thymus, the soft tissues, the lymphatic tissue, the thyroid, the parathyroid, and the sympathetic ganglia and paraganglionic structures. Furthermore, tumors can develop from embryonal tissue.

These neoplasms and tumor-like lesions (cysts) have preferred sites in the mediastinum [1].

mediastinum			
superior	**middle**	**anterior**	**posterior**
– thymoma	– malignant	– malignant	– neurofibroma
– malignant	lymphomas	lymphomas	– neurilemoma
lymphoma	– pericardial	– fibroma	– malignant
– thyroid tumors	cysts	– teratoma	schwannoma
– parathyroid	– branchiogenic	– thyroid tumors	– ganglioneuroma
tumors	cysts	– parathyroid	– ganglioneuro-
		adenoma	blastoma
		– hemangioma	– neuroblastoma
		– lipoma	– paraganglioma
		– paraganglioma	– gastroenteric cysts

---

[1] Ackerman and Rosai 1974.

Tumors of the heart

1. Myxoma

M-8840/0
T 164.1

General Remarks

Incidence: Myxomas of the heart are very rare.
About half of the tumors of the heart are myxomas.
Site: Myxomas are usually observed in the left atrium in association with the fossa ovalis. Multiple myxomas in the heart have also been reported [30].

Macroscopy

Myxomas are soft tumors that are well circumscribed. Calcifications may be found.

Histology

The tumor is composed of a ground substance that stains positive with PAS.
In this substance there are a few stellate cells with long fibrillary processes (Figs. 49 and 50).

Clinical Findings

According to the site of the tumor.
According to the main site at the left atrium, the symptoms are due to mitral valve disease (insufficiency of stenosis).

Treatment

Resection of the tumor [13].

Further Information

It is still debated whether cardiac myxomas are true tumors or are organized thrombi. Most probably, the majority of myxomas are true tumors; this is supported by electron microscopic studies [12, 27].

[12] Feldman et al. 1977.
[13] Frede et al. 1975.
[27] Mikuz et al. 1978.
[30] Nichols and Hennigar 1959.

M-8810/0
T 164.1

2. Fibroma
(intramural fibroma)

Fibromas of the heart are very rare.
The tumor is considered a (fibroelastic) hamartoma.
This tumor is usually observed in infants and children.

Macroscopy   Grossly the tumor resembles a leiomyoma.

Histology   The tumor is composed of collagen fibers.

Treatment   Intramural fibroma is removed by surgery [11].

M-8900/0
T 164.1

3. Rhabdomyoma

Rhabdomyomas in the heart are most often observed in young children.
The main site is the left ventricle.
Rhabdomyomas of the heart are often associated with tuberous sclerosis.

Histology   Rhabdomyomas are composed of striated muscle cells. These cells are of different sizes.
The cytoplasm is vacuolated.

Electron
Microscopy   The myofibrils in rhabdomyomas show different degrees of differentiation [46].
The extracardiac rhabdomyoma has filaments arranged in a more disorderly fashion than
the cardiac rhabdomyoma (Fig. 647) [45, 46].

Clinical
Findings   Rhabdomyomas of the heart are stationary without symptoms of a growing tumor.

[11] Feldman and Meyer 1976.
[45] Silverman et al. 1978.
[46] Silverman et al. 1976.

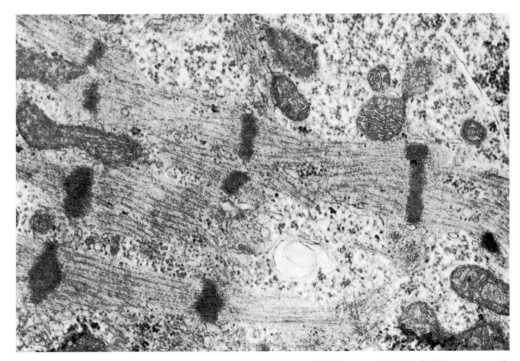

Fig. 647. Rhabdomyoma of heart with thick Z bands and myosin filaments (×12,000) (Silverman et al., Cancer *42* (1978) 189-193).

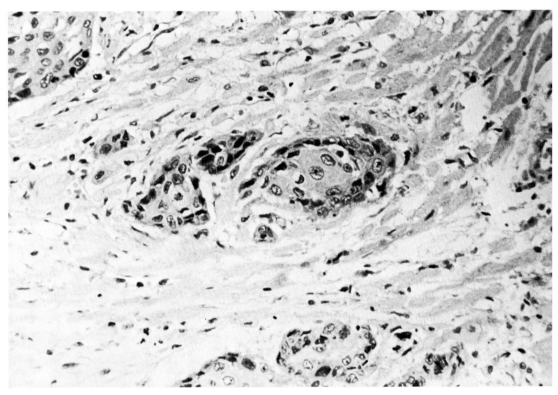

Fig. 648. Metastasis into the heart: Squamous cell carcinoma (60-year-old male, × 200).

653

M-9140/3
T 164.1

4. Kaposi's sarcoma (Figs. 84 to 86)

Kaposi's sarcoma in the heart is extremely rare.
There is a case reported to be a primary Kaposi's sarcoma of the heart [22].

M-8895/3
T 164.1

5. Myosarcoma

Myosarcomas in the heart are exceedingly rare [3].

M-9120/3
T 164.1

6. Angiosarcoma

Primary angiosarcomas of the heart are exceedingly rare [14, 38, 40].

M-8711/0
T 164.1

7. Cardiac glomus tumor

There is one report of a cardiac glomus tumor [39].

[3] Ashley 1978.
[14] Gröntoft and Hellquist 1977.
[22] Levison and Semple 1976.
[38] Poole-Wilson et al. 1976.
[39] Riesner and Böcker 1975.
[40] Rossi et al. 1976.

M-8830/3
T 164.1

8. Malignant fibrous histiocytoma

This malignant soft tissue tumor is extremely rare in the heart. One tumor has been reported, presenting as an atrial myxoma [44].

M-8000/6
T 164.1

9. Metastatic lesions in the heart

The heart can be involved by metastatic lesions including leukemias, myelomas, and malignant lymphomas.
Among the most frequently encountered tumors growing in the heart are the malignant melanoma and thyroid carcinoma (Fig. 48).

M-9120/0

10. Hemangioma

M-8850/0
T 164.1

11. Lipoma

Hemangiomas and lipomas are of great rarity. Lipomas can cause cardiac dysrhythmia [20].

---

[20] Klein and Schaefer 1973.
[44] Shah et al. 1978.

M-9084/0
M-9080/0
T 164.1

12. Benign cystic teratoma
(dermoid cyst)

These benign lesions in the heart are rare and have been reported only occasionally. They can develop in the pericardial cavity [19].

M-8880/0
T 164.1

13. Multiple hibernomas (Fig. 56)

There is one report describing the observation of multiple hibernomas in the heart [18].

[18] Kindblom and Svensson 1977.
[19] Klammer 1976.

Tumors of the thymus

M-8580/0, 1, 3
T 164.0

14. Thymoma

General Remarks

Incidence: 10 to 15% of tumors of the mediastinum are thymomas. Thymomas are rare.
Age: Most of the patients are adults; the tumor is very rare in patients under 20 years old.
Sex: There is a slight preference for females.
Site: Thymomas grow in the anterior or superior mediastinum; the entire mediastinum may be occupied, however.

Macroscopy

Thymomas are firm, encapsulated tumors with a yellowish cut surface.
Occasionally hemorrhages and cyst formations are observed. The majority of thymomas are well separated from the surrounding tissue; in about 20% of the cases, however, signs of infiltration into the surrounding structures can be observed.
The thymomas are small or rather large (up to 15 cm across).

Histology

Thymomas are in most instances composed of epithelial and lymphocytic cells [26] (Figs. 649 and 650).
The epithelial cells are of different sizes and shapes. Some of the thymomas are composed of spindle-shaped epithelial cells; in other areas they are round or oval. The cells grow in a whorl-like pattern (Figs. 651 to 657).
Adjacent to the epithelial structures or admixed with these cells are lymphocytes.
Occasionally the lymphocytic structures dominate the entire tumor; in other instances the epithelial cells constitute the main element of the thymoma.
Hassall's corpuscles are rarely found.
The tumor cells show a low number of mitotic figures.
In some of the thymomas infiltration into the surrounding tissue can be seen [5].

Electron Microscopy

The lymphocytes in thymoma might have the appearance of partly transformed lymphoid cells with large nuclei, discrete heterochromatin, and numerous ribosomes.
The surface of these cells is smooth (scanning electron microscopy).
The epithelial cells show tonofilaments and desmosomes [8, 21, 37].

Differential Diagnosis

1. Thymoma **with malignant lymphoma:**
   This differential diagnosis comes to mind when the lymphocytic component dominates the picture of a thymoma.
   The evidence of epithelial cells indicates the diagnosis of thymoma.
2. Thymoma **with Hodgkin's disease:**
   Infiltration by Hodgkin's disease (often the nodular sclerosis type) (Figs. 1223 to 1225) might occupy the region of the thymus.
   The evidence of Reed-Sternberg cells proves the nature of the tumor.

---

[5] Castleman 1955.
[8] Cossman et al. 1978.
[21] Levine and Bensch 1972.
[26] Masaoka et al. 1977.
[37] Pascoe and Miner 1976.

657

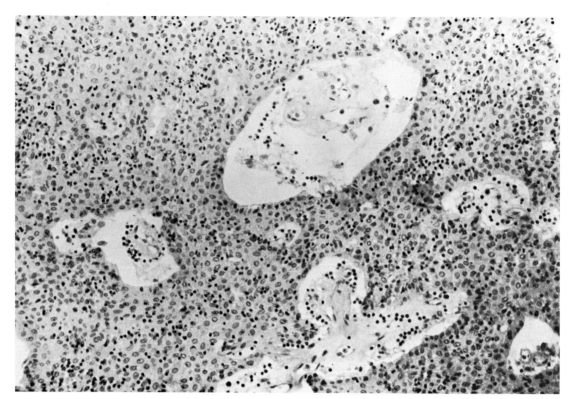

Fig. 649. Epithelioid thymoma (74-year-old male, no myasthenia gravis, ×125).

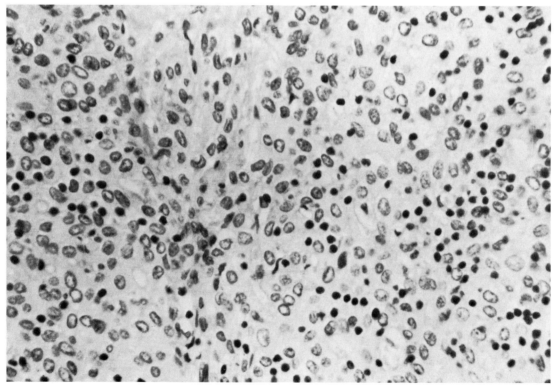

Fig. 650. Epithelioid thymoma (74-year-old male, ×310).

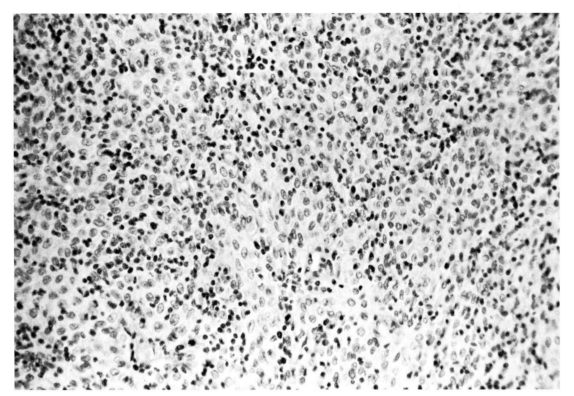

Fig. 651. Thymoma: Lymphoepithelial cell proliferation (myasthenia gravis, 42-year-old male, × 200).

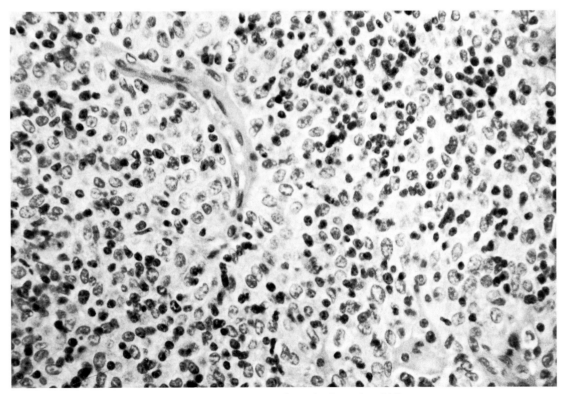

Fig. 652. Thymoma: Slight predominance of epithelial cells (myasthenia gravis, × 310).

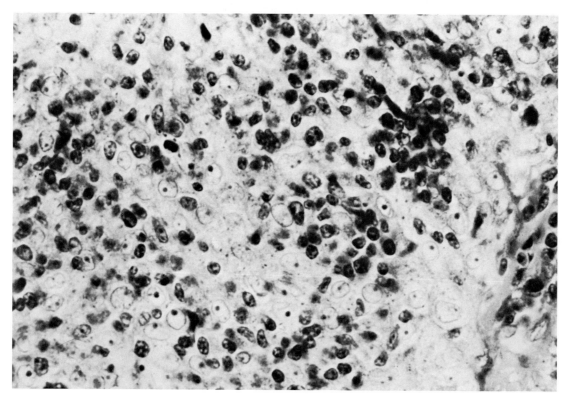

Fig. 653. Thymoma with myasthenia gravis: Area of large epithelial cells with vesicular nuclei (× 500).

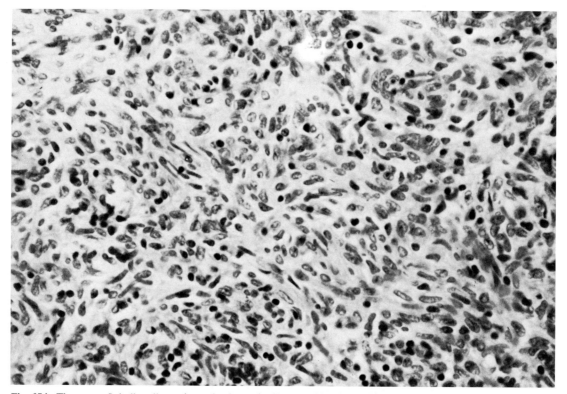

Fig. 654. Thymoma: Spindle cell type (myasthenia gravis, 68-year-old male, × 310).

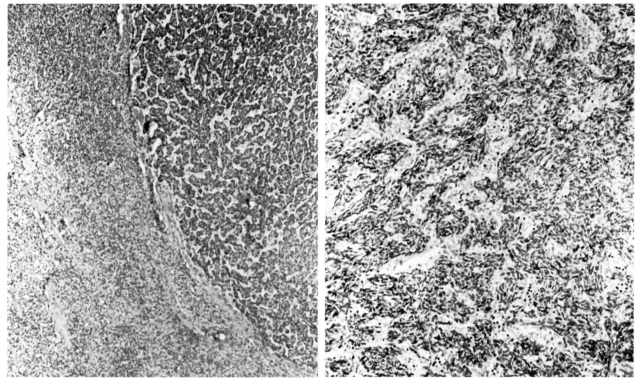

Fig. 655. Lobulated growth pattern of thymoma (64-year-old female, no myasthenia gravis, × 40).

Fig. 656. Spindle cell type of thymoma (64-year-old female, × 125).

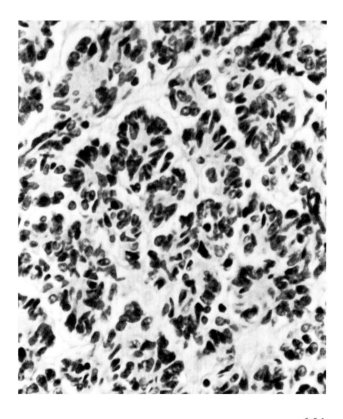

Fig. 657. Papillary type of thymoma (65-year-old female, × 310).

Thymoma

Differential Diagnosis

3. Thymoma **with metastatic carcinoma:**
   In thymomas the epithelial component dominates the picture.
   The great variability of epithelial elements in thymomas adds to the occasional difficulties in recognizing and separating metastatic tumor from a thymoma.

4. Thymoma **with hemangiopericytoma:**
   In cases of very vascular tumors and spindle-shaped epithelial elements, the structure of thymoma might mimic hemangiopericytomas. The reticulin fiber stain will help to clarify the situation: In hemangiopericytoma the pericytes are individually surrounded by reticulin fibers (Fig. 93).

M-7229/0
T 164.0

5. Thymoma **with thymic hyperplasia:**
   In thymic hyperplasia the lymphatic tissue contains germinal centers in the thymic medulla (Figs. 658 to 660).

Spread

In cases of malignant thymoma the tumor infiltrates the surrounding tissue.
Distant metastases from thymoma are rare [24].

Clinical Findings

About 20% of patients with thymoma suffer from myasthenia gravis [16].
Occasionally there is an association between thymic hyperplasia and myasthenia gravis.
- Thymomas can be associated with autoimmune disease.
- Occasionally thymomas show signs of Cushing's syndrome (ACTH production) [15],
- are associated with aplastic anemia, or
- produce ADH.

Treatment

Surgery:
Thymectomy.
Radiation therapy:
Thymomas (especially malignant thymomas) are sensitive to radiation therapy: Up to 60 Gy in 6 weeks [25].
Chemotherapy:
Chemotherapy in cases of dissemination of thymomas should be according to the treatment of non-Hodgkin's lymphoma (see page 1268).

Prognosis

1. The prognosis is determined by the associated syndrome (myasthenia gravis) and whether the tumor infiltrates the surrounding tissue at the time of operation [41].
   The histological type of the thymoma does not correlate with the prognosis.
2. About 30% of the thymomas are malignant.
   About 20% (up to 30%) of thymomas are associated with myasthenia gravis.
3. 10-year survival:
- Benign thymoma with myasthenia gravis, 32%,
- thymoma without myasthenia gravis, 67%,
- encapsulated thymoma without myasthenia gravis, about 100%,
- malignant thymoma with myasthenia gravis, 0% [49].

Further Information

It seems that myasthenia gravis is associated with the histological picture of epithelial cells with a plump shape [1].

---

[1] Ackerman and Rosai 1974.
[15] Imura et al. 1975.
[16] Jochem and Greschuchna 1974.
[24] McDonald et al. 1978.
[25] Marks et al. 1978.
[41] Salyer and Eggleston 1976.
[49] Wilkins Jr. et al. 1966.

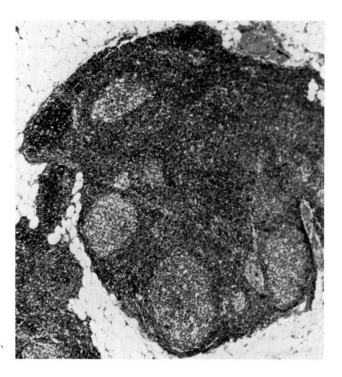

Fig. 658. Thymic hyperplasia (56-year-old male, myasthenia gravis, ×40).

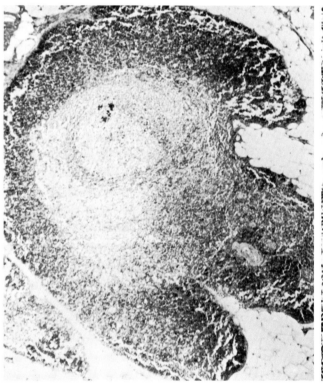

Fig. 659. Thymic hyperplasia (42-year-old male, myasthenia gravis, ×40).

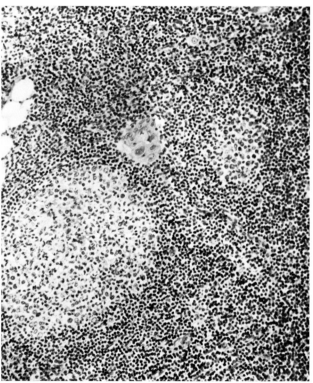

Fig. 660. Thymic hyperplasia with follicles (56-year-old male, ×125).

M-8070/3
T 164.0

15. Squamous cell carcinoma of the thymus

Squamous cell carcinomas of the thymus are rare.
The tumor is radiosensitive and should be treated by radical surgical excision and irradiation (Figs. 661 and 662)

M-8240/1
T 164.0

16. Carcinoid tumor of the thymus

Carcinoid tumors of the thymus are rare [7, 33].
This carcinoid is not related to myasthenia gravis. The tumor is more aggressive than thymoma [42].

M-8850/0
T 164.0

17. Thymolipoma

Thymolipomas can be very large. They are encapsulated. The cut surface is yellowish and histologically they are composed of adipose tissue intermingled with thymic tissue.

[7] Chalk and Donald 1977.
[33] Otto and Hüsselmann 1976.
[42] Salyer et al. 1976.

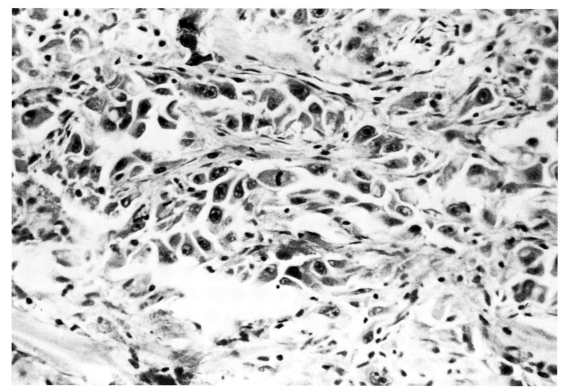

Fig. 661. Poorly differentiated squamous cell carcinoma of the thymus (× 200).

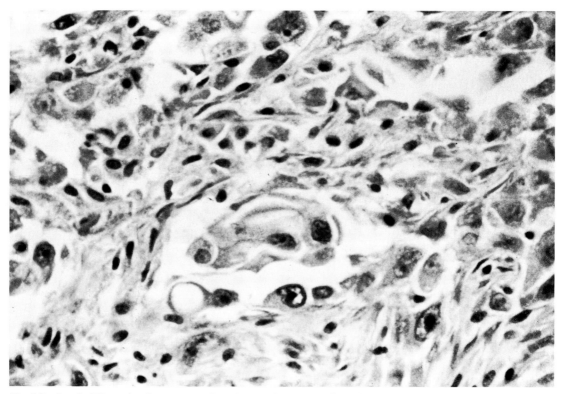

Fig. 662. Poorly differentiated squamous cell carcinoma of the thymus (× 310).

M-9080/0
T 164.0

18. Teratoma in the thymus

Benign and malignant (seminoma) teratomas can arise in the thymic gland [1, 5] (Figs. 663 to 669).

M-9650/3
T 164.0

19. Hodgkin's disease of the thymus

The thymic gland can be infiltrated by Hodgkin's disease, usually the nodular sclerosis type (Figs. 1223 to 1225).

The nodular sclerosing type of Hodgkin's disease in the thymus has also been interpreted as granulomatous thymoma [10, 17, 23].

M-9590/0
T 164.0

20. Castleman tumor [6]
(localized mediastinal lymph node hyperplasia (Figs. 736 and 737)

Castleman tumors are benign lymphomatous tumors growing in the mediastinum adjacent to the thymic gland.

Histology

The tumor contains lymphoid tissue with follicles. These follicles show an onion-like arrangement of the cells and hyalinizations in their center. This picture mimics Hassall's bodies.

Castleman tumors are rich in blood vessels, which extend into the follicles [2].

Differential Diagnosis

1. Castleman tumor **with thymoma** (Fig. 651).
2. Castleman tumor **with malignant lymphoma.**

Prognosis

Castleman tumors are benign lesions. After surgical excision there are no recurrences even if remnants of the tumor were left behind.

[1] Ackerman and Rosai 1974.
[2] Albrich et al. 1973.
[5] Castleman 1955.
[6] Castleman et al. 1956.
[10] Fechner 1969.
[17] Katz and Lattes 1969.
[23] Lowenhaupt and Brown 1951.

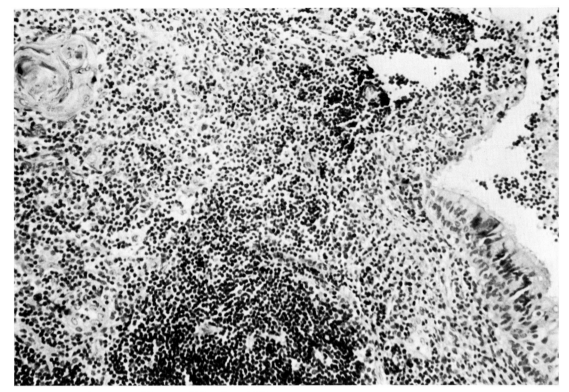

Fig. 663. Thymic teratoma (44-year-old female, × 125).

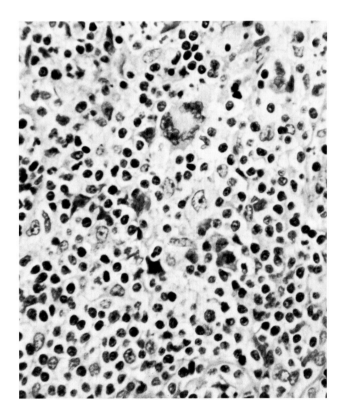

Fig. 664. Thymic teratoma: Areas of giant cells induced by epidermoid cyst (× 400).

667

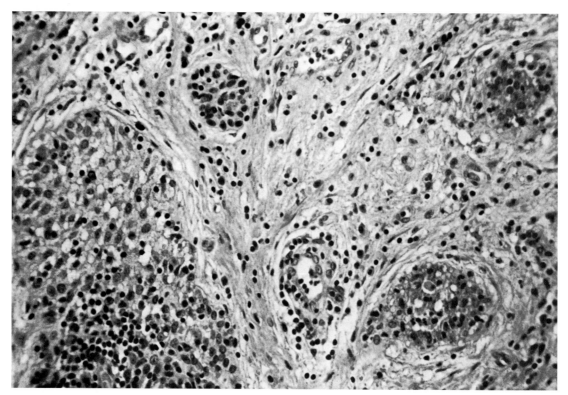

Fig. 665. Thymic teratoma: Islets of epithelial cell nests (× 200).

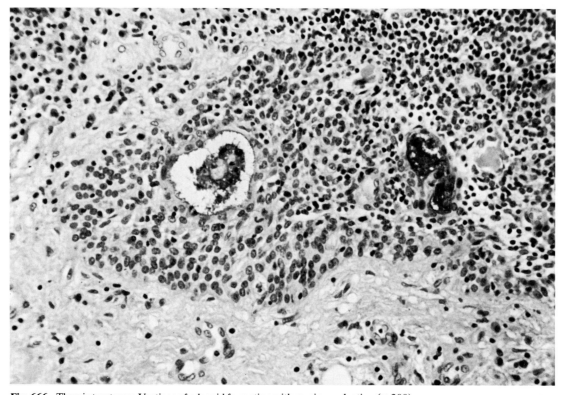

Fig. 666. Thymic teratoma: Vestiges of adenoid formation with mucin production (× 200).

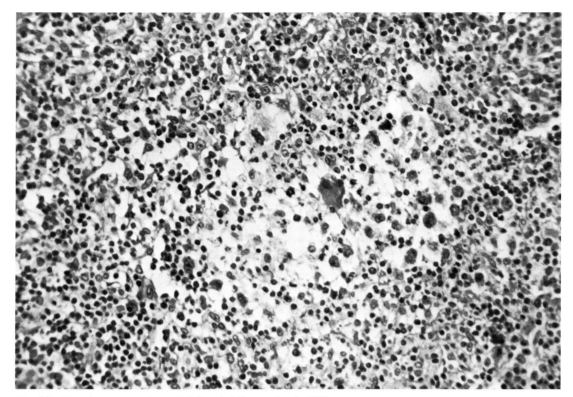

Fig. 667. Thymic teratoma: Area of histiocytic inflammation (× 200).

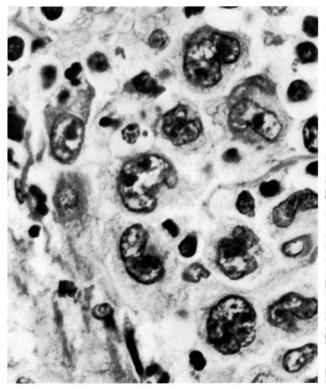

Fig. 668. Thymic teratoma: Giant cells similar to Reed-Sternberg cells (same case as Fig. 667) (× 800).

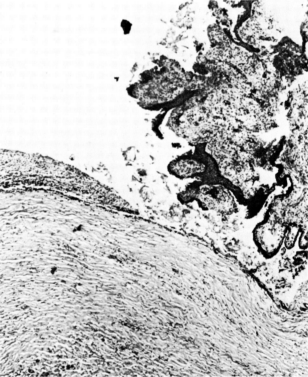

Fig. 669. Epidermoid cyst in the mediastinum (59-year-old female, × 40).

Recommendations for differential diagnosis in tumors of the thymus

thymic hyperplasia	with	– thymoma – Castleman tumor
benign thymoma	with	– malignant thymoma – malignant lymphoma – Hodgkin's disease – metastatic carcinoma – hemangiopericytoma
primary carcinoid tumor of the thymus	with	– metastatic carcinoid tumor – malignant thymoma
malignant teratoma in the thymus	with	– metastases of a malignant teratoma
primary squamous cell carcinoma	with	– metastatic squamous cell carcinoma

Other tumors of the mediastinum

T 164.9

21. Soft tissue tumors of the mediastinum

Benign and malignant soft tissue tumors can occur in the mediastinum, including
- **hemangiopericytomas,**
- **leiomyomas,**
- **benign mesenchymomas** (Fig. 670) [34-36, 43],
- **rhabdomyomas** [28],
- **liposarcomas,**
- **fibrosarcomas,** and
- **embryonal rhabdomyosarcoma** [1] (see page 7).

M-9560/0, 3
M-9540/0
T 164.3

22. Tumors of nerve sheath origin

Neurilemomas, malignant schwannomas, and neurofibromas are usually observed in the posterior mediastinum (Fig. 671).
Gross inspection shows large encapsulated tumors with regressive changes.
The benign varieties of these tumors have an excellent prognosis when treated surgically. (For further information see page 163).

M-9590/3
T 164.9

23. Malignant lymphoma

Malignant lymphomas of the mediastinum grow mostly in the middle part of the mediastinum.
The posterior mediastinum is almost never affected.
The majority of malignant lymphomas are of Hodgkin's type.
The nodular sclerosis is the most frequently observed subtype of Hodgkin's disease in the mediastinum (see page 1253).

---

[1] Ackerman and Rosai 1974.
[28] Miller et al. 1978.
[34] Pachter and Lattes 1963.
[35] Pachter and Lattes 1963.
[36] Pachter and Lattes 1963.
[43] Schlumberger 1951.

24. Tumors of the sympathetic ganglia
(see page 1792)

M-9490/0
T 164.9

a) Ganglioneuroma (Fig. 1735)
This is the most frequently encountered neoplasm of this group, occurring in elderly patients.
The tumor is encapsulated and soft, with cysts in a yellowish cut surface.

M-9490/1
T 164.9

b) Ganglioneuroblastoma
This tumor is rare and is composed of an admixture of the cells of a neuroblastoma and ganglion cells.
The tumor is encapsulated and lobulated and shows areas of calcification.

M-9490/3
M-9500/3
T 164.9

c) Neuroblastoma (Figs. 1730 to 1732)
This tumor is rare in the mediastinum and is observed in children.
This malignant tumor is not encapsulated and infiltrates the surrounding tissue.

M-8680/1, 3
T 164.9

25. Tumors of the paraganglionic structures
(paragangliomas of the mediastinum)
(see page 1801)

Paragangliomas in the mediastinum can have an aggressive behavior [9] (Fig. 1746).
Very occasionally mediastinal pheochromocytomas are observed. They are always benign [32] (see Fig. 1736).
The great majority of paragangliomas grow in the anterior-superior mediastinum associated with the aortic chemoreceptor bodies.

---

[9] Edmunds Jr. 1966.
[32] Olson and Salyer 1978.

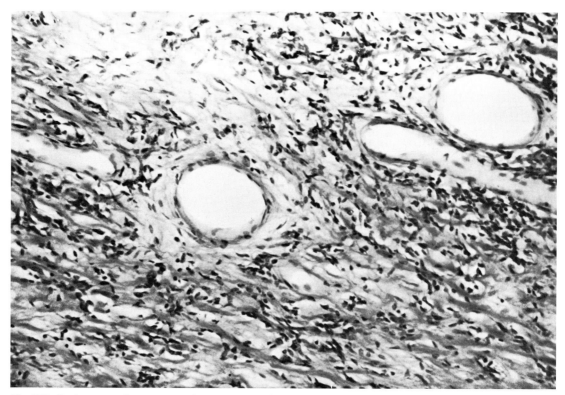

Fig. 670. Benign mesenchymoma, anterior mediastinum (61-year-old female, × 125).

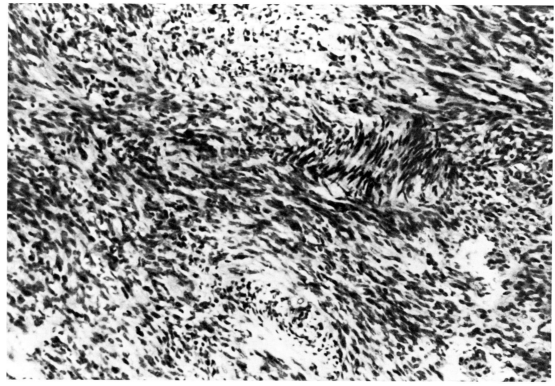

Fig. 671. Neurilemoma in the mediastinum (50-year-old female, × 125).

26. Teratomas

Benign and malignant teratomas can occur in the mediastinum; they usually grow in the anterior mediastinum.

These tumors are large, cystic, and encapsulated; they might contain sebaceous material and hairs in the cysts.

Benign-looking teratomas might occasionally disseminate [4].

About 5% of all mediastinal teratomas are malignant (Figs. 672 to 679):

– **seminoma** [31],

– **choriocarcinoma** [48],

– **embryonal carcinoma** [47],

– **yolk sac tumor** [29, 47] (see page 1469).

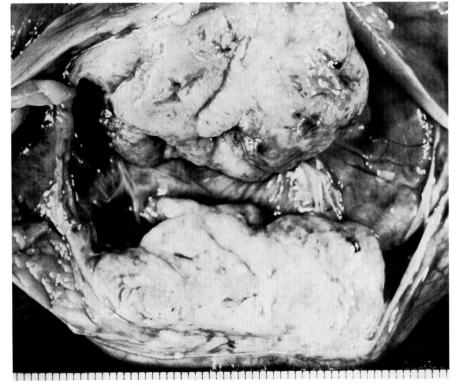

Fig. 672. Malignant cystic teratoma of the anterior mediastinum (same case as Figs. 673 to 679) (31-year-old male, ×2).

[4] Canty and Siemens 1978.
[29] Mukai and Adams 1979.
[31] Oberman and Libcke 1964.
[47] Teilmann et al. 1967.
[48] Wenger et al. 1968.

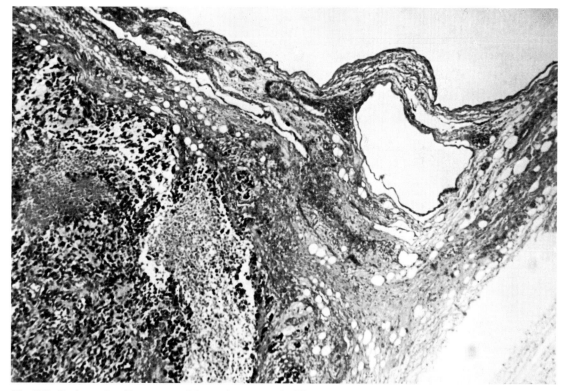

Fig. 673. Benign and malignant area of the cystic teratoma (×40).

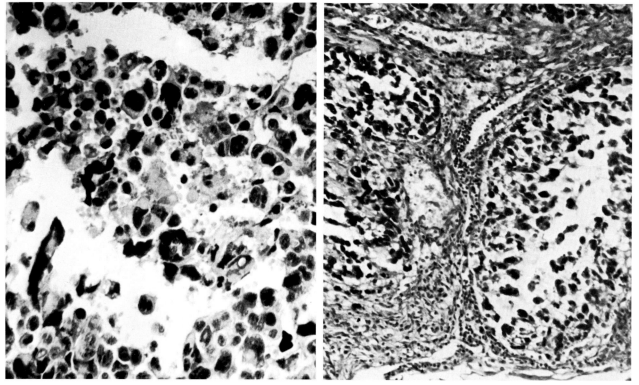

Fig. 674. Unclassifiable malignant part of the mediastinal teratoma (×125).

Fig. 675. Retroperitoneal metastasis of the mediastinal teratoma: Choriocarcinoma (×200).

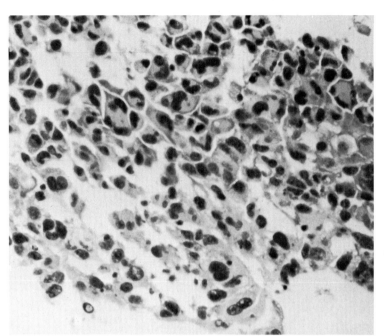

Fig. 676. Metastasis in the parotid gland of the mediastinal teratoma: Rhabdomyosarcoma (×200).

Fig. 677.

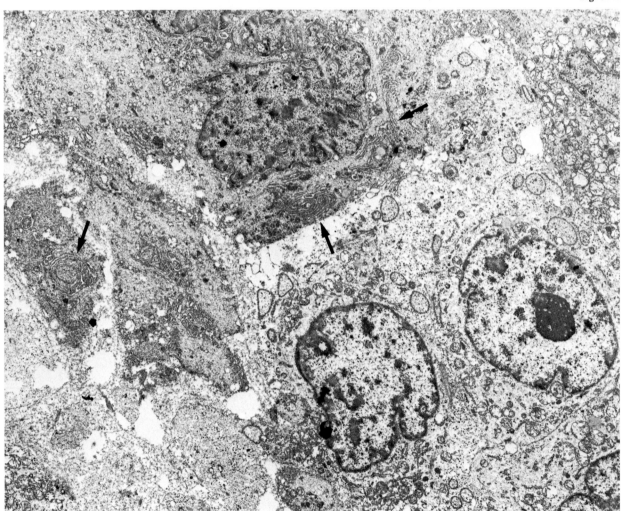

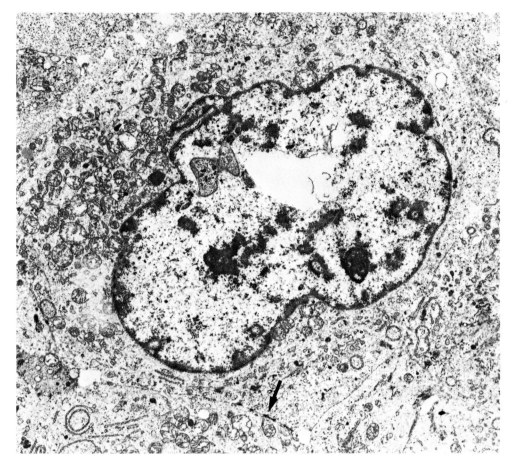

Fig. 678.

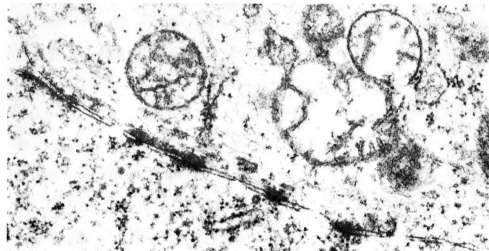

Fig. 679.

Figs. 678 and 679. Malignant teratoma of the mediastinum: Tumor cell with mitochondria, some of them rather closely packed, and occasionally cisterns of rough endoplasmic reticulum. Some circumscribed desmosome-like contacts with the adjacent tumor cell (arrow and Fig. 679) (Fig. 678, × 6800; Fig. 679, × 35,000).

◁ **Fig. 677.** Malignant teratoma of the mediastinum: Several dark and clear cells. The dark cells contain cisterns of the rough endoplasmic reticulum, partly in a concentric arrangement. The clear cells with some dilated cisterns of the rough endoplasmic reticulum contain material of moderate density (× 5200).

677

27. Mediastinal cysts

Cysts in the mediastinum can clinically and pathologically mimic tumors.
These tumor-like lesions are congenital malformations.
These cysts occur in the thymus, the esophagus, the tracheobronchial tree, the pericardium, and the gastrointestinal tract.

a) Esophageal cyst

The cysts are observed in adults in the lower half of the esophagus.
Esophageal cysts are lined by squamous epithelium or by pseudostratified, ciliated epithelium, or by both.

M-2666/0
T 164.3

b) Gastric and enterogenic cyst

These cysts are found in the posterior mediastinum. They are attached to the esophagus or develop in the wall of the esophagus (in the muscular layer).
These cysts are lined by intestinal epithelium or gastric epithelium.
Cysts lined by gastric epithelium can be complicated clinically by the development of a peptic ulcer with bleeding and perforation of the cystic wall.

c) Bronchial cyst

These cysts are found in the mediastinum immediately above the diaphragma and posterior to the carina.
These cysts do not communicate with the lumen of the trachea or bronchus.
Grossly, these are small cysts that contain fluid or mucinous material.
The cysts are lined by ciliated columnar epithelium. The wall contains hyalin cartilage, smooth muscle fibers, and occasionally nerve fibers.
The clinical symptoms are determined by the size and the site of the cyst: cough, dysphagia, or respiratory distress.

d) Pericardial cyst

These cysts are lined by mesothelium.
The cysts very rarely communicate with the pericardial cavity, are adherent to the pericardium, and are found in the right cardiophrenic angle.

e) Thymic cyst

These cysts are found in the neck or in the mediastinum.
The cysts are lined by squamous or columnar epithelium.
The wall contains thymic tissue.
In the wall of these cysts cholesterol granulomas can be found.

References

[1] Ackerman, L. V., and J. Rosai: Surgical pathology. Fifth edition. C. V. Mosby Company 1974.

[2] Albrich, W., K. O. Schmid, G. Friehs, W. Köle und H. L. Seewann: Das Castleman-Lymphom. Virchows Arch. A Path. Anat. and Histol. *358* (1973) 163-171.

[3] Ashley, D. J. B.: In: Evans' histological appearances of tumours. Third edition, Churchill Livingstone, Edinburgh–London–New York 1978.

[4] Canty, T. G., and R. Siemens: Malignant mediastinal teratoma in a 15-year-old girl. Cancer *41* (1978) 1623-1626.

[5] Castleman, B.: Tumors of the thymus gland. Atlas of tumor pathology. A. F. I. P. Washington, D.C. 1955.

[6] Castleman, B., L. Iverson, and V. P. Menendez: Localized mediastinal lymph-node hyperplasia resembling thymoma. Cancer *9* (1956) 822-830.

[7] Chalk, S., and K. J. Donald: Carcinoid tumour of the thymus. A case report including discussion of the morphological diagnosis and the cell of origin. Virchows Arch. A. Path. Anat. and Histol. *377* (1977) 91-96.

[8] Cossman, J., M. J. Deegan, and B. Schnitzer: Thymoma: An immunologic and electron microscopic study. Cancer *41* (1978) 2183-2191.

[9] Edmunds, L. H. Jr.: Mediastinal pheochromocytoma. Ann. Thorac. Surg. *2* (1966) 742-751.

[10] Fechner, R. E.: Hodgkin's disease of the thymus. Cancer *23* (1969) 16-23.

[11] Feldman, P. S., and M. W. Meyer: Fibroelastic hamartoma (fibroma) of the heart. Cancer *38* (1976) 314-323.

[12] Feldman, P. S., E. Horvath, and K. Kovacs: An ultrastructural study of seven cardiac myxomas. Cancer *40* (1977) 2216-2232.

[13] Frede, K. E., F. Follath, J. Hasse, G. Wolff und E. Grädel: Herzmyxome. Klinische Erscheinungsformen, Diagnosen und chirurgische Therapie. Dtsch. Med. Wschr. *100* (1975) 2270-2275.

[14] Gröntoft, O., and H. Hellquist: Cardiac haemangio-endotheliosarcoma. Review of the literature and report of a case. Acta. Pathol. Microbiol. Scand. Sect. A *85* (1977) 33-41.

[15] Imura, H., S. Matsukura, H. Yamamoto, Y. Hirata, Y. Nakai, J. Endo, A. Tanaka, and M. Nakamura: Studies on ectopic ACTH-producing tumors. II. Clinical and biochemical features of 30 cases. Cancer *35* (1975) 1430-1437.

[16] Jochem, B., und D. Greschuchna: Diagnostik von Mediastinaltumoren. Med. Klin. *69* (1974) 735-744.

[17] Katz, A., and R. Lattes: Granulomatous thymoma or Hodgkin's disease of thymus? A clinical and histologic study and a re-evaluation. Cancer *23* (1969) 1-15.

[18] Kindblom, L. G., and U. Svensson: Multiple hibernomas of the heart. A case report. Acta Pathol. Microbiol. Scand. Sect. A *85* (1977) 122-126.

[19] Klammer, A.: Primäres Teratoma coetaneum des Herzens und der Lunge in Kombination mit einer hypertrophischen Pylorusstenose. Z. Kinderchir. *19* (1976) 365-376.

[20] Klein, P. J., und H. E. Schaefer: Das interatriale Lipom des Herzens. Z. Krebsforsch. *79* (1973) 11-18.

[21] Levine, G. D., and K. G. Bensch: Epithelial nature of spindle-cell thymoma; an ultrastructural study. Cancer *30* (1972) 500-511.

[22] Levison, D. A., and P. d'A. Semple: Primary cardiac Kaposi's sarcoma. Thorax (Lond.) *31* (1976) 595-600.

[23] Lowenhaupt, E., and R. Brown: Carcinoma of the thymus of granulomatous type. Clinical and pathological study. Cancer *4* (1951) 1193-1209.

[24] McDonald, J., J. C. Parker, S. Brown, L. K. Page, and D. E. Wolfe: Cerebral metastasis from a malignant thymoma. Surg. Neurol. *9* (1978) 58-60.

[25] Marks, R. D., K. M. Wallace, and H. S. Pettit: Radiation therapy control of nine patients with malignant thymoma. Cancer *41* (1978) 117-119.

[26] Masaoka, A., Y. Nagaoka, M. Maeda, Y. Monden, and Y. Seike: Study on the ratio of lymphocytes to epithelial cells in thymoma. Cancer *40* (1977) 1222-1228.

[27] Mikuz, G., F. Hofstädter, H. Hausen und J. Hager: Das sog. Endokardmyxom. Histologische, elektronenmikroskopische, immunfluoreszenz- und biochemische Untersuchungen an drei Fällen. Virchows Arch. A Path. Anat. and Histol. *380* (1978) 221-236.

[28] Miller, R., S. M. Kurtz, and J. M. Powers: Mediastinal rhabdomyoma. Cancer *42* (1978) 1983-1988.

[29] Mukai, K., and W. R. Adams: Yolk sac tumor of the anterior mediastinum. Case report with light- and electron microscopic examination and immunohistochemical study of alpha-fetoprotein. Am. J. Surg. Path. *3* (1979) 77-83.

[30] Nichols, J., and G. Hennigar: A case of bilateral multicentric cardiac myxoma. Am. Med. Ass. Arch. Pathol. *67* (1959) 24-29.

[31] Oberman, H. A., and J. H. Libcke: Malignant germinal neoplasms of the mediastinum. Cancer *17* (1964) 498-507.

[32] Olson, J. L., and M. W. R. Salyer: Mediastinal paragangliomas (aortic body tumor). A report of four cases and a review of the literature. Cancer *41* (1978) 2405-2412.

[33] Otto, H. F., und H. Hüsselmann: Thymus-Carcinoid. Fallbericht und Literaturübersicht. Z. Krebsforsch. *88* (1976) 55-67.

[34] Pachter, M. R., and R. Lattes: Mesenchymal tumors of the mediastinum. I: Tumors of fibrous tissue, adipose tissue, smooth muscle, and striated muscle. Cancer *16* (1963) 74-94.

[35] Pachter, M. R., and R. Lattes: Mesenchymal

tumors of the mediastinum. II: Tumors of blood vascular origin. Cancer *16* (1963) 95-107.

[36] Pachter, M.R., and R. Lattes: Mesenchymal tumors of the mediastinum. III: Tumors of lymph vascular origin. Cancer *16* (1963) 108-117.

[37] Pascoe, H.R., and M.S. Miner: An ultrastructural study of nine thymomas. Cancer *37* (1976) 317-326.

[38] Poole-Wilson, P.A., A. Farnsworth, M.V. Braimbridge, and H. Pambakian: Angiosarcoma of pericardium. Problems in diagnosis and management. Br. Heart J. *38* (1976) 240-243.

[39] Riesner, K., und W. Böcker: Cardialer Glomustumor. Licht- und elektronenoptische Befunde. Z. Krebsforsch. *84* (1975) 59-66.

[40] Rossi, N.P., J.M. Kioschos, C.A. Aschenbrener, and J.L. Ehrenhaft: Primary angiosarcoma of the heart. Cancer *37* (1976) 891-894.

[41] Salyer, W.R., and J.C. Eggleston: Thymoma. A clinical and pathological study of 65 cases. Cancer *37* (1976) 229-249.

[42] Salyer, W.R., G.C. Salyer, and J.C. Eggleston: Carcinoid tumors of thymus. Cancer *37* (1976) 958-973.

[43] Schlumberger, H.G.: Tumors of the mediastinum. Atlas of tumor pathology. A.F.I.P., Washington, D.C. 1951.

[44] Shah, A.A., A. Churg, J.A. Sbarbaro, J.M. Sheppard, and J. Lamberti: Malignant fibrous histiocytoma of the heart presenting as an atrial myxoma. Cancer *42* (1978) 2466-2471.

[45] Silverman, J.F., S. Kay, and C.H. Chang: Ultrastructural comparison between skeletal muscle and cardiac rhabdomyomas. Cancer *42* (1978) 189-193.

[46] Silverman, J.F., S. Kay, C.M. McCue, R.R. Lower, A.J. Brough, and C.H. Chang: Rhabdomyoma of the heart. Ultrastructural study of three cases. Lab. Invest. *35* (1976) 596-606.

[47] Teilmann, I., H. Kassis, and G. Pietra: Primary germ cell tumor of the anterior mediastinum with features of endodermal sinus tumor (mesoblastoma vitellinum). Acta Pathol. Microbiol. Scand. *70* (1967) 267-278.

[48] Wenger, M.E., D.E. Dines, D.L. Ahmann, and C.A. Good: Primary mediastinal choriocarcinoma. Mayo Clin. Proc. *43* (1968) 570-575.

[49] Wilkins, E.W. Jr., L.H. Edmunds Jr., and B. Castleman: Cases of thymoma at the Massachusetts General Hospital. J. Thoracic Surg. *52* (1966) 322-330.

17 Tumors of the lung and pleura

681

1. Carcinomas of the lung are the most common malignant tumor in males.
2. 25% of deaths by malignant tumors are caused by carcinomas of the lung.
3. In the most common types of carcinoma of the lung, there is a strong relationship between cancer and heavy cigarette smoking.
4. According to the different cells and growth patterns, cancer of the lung has been subdivided into different histological types (WHO) [116].

   Rather often, mixtures of these different tumor types can be observed in one tumor. However, other tumors are distinctly composed of uniform cell types.

   This separation seems justified, especially for the separation of squamous cell carcinoma (epidermoid carcinoma) and small cell carcinoma.
5. **Paraneoplastic syndromes** are rather often associated with cancer of the lung:

Cushing's syndrome	small cell carcinoma carcinoid tumor [35, 139]
carcinoid syndrome	small cell carcinoma carcinoid tumor
hyperparathyroidism	squamous cell carcinoma
gonadotropin secretion (gynecomastia)	all tumor types
cortical-cerebellar degeneration	all tumor types
hyponatremia due to inappropriate secretion of ADH	small cell carcinoma squamous cell carcinoma
MSH production (hyperpigmentation)	squamous cell carcinoma
psychosis	small cell carcinoma
encephalomyelitis, sensorineuropathy, and myopathic myasthenic syndrome	small cell carcinoma

6. The primary approach for treatment of lung cancer is surgery.

   Radiation therapy is indicated for palliation purposes.

   Chemotherapy can be tried for advanced tumor diseases.

   Polychemotherapy with different combinations has been tried (adriamycin + vincristine + cyclophosphamide;

   cyclophosphamide + methotrexate + CCNU;

   BCNU + cyclophosphamide + vincristine + procarbacine).

   Small cell carcinomas respond particulary well to radiotherapy, chemotherapy, or a combination of both.

[35] Cohen et al. 1960
[116] Sobin 1979.
[139] Yalow 1979.

7. The prognosis depends to a certain degree on the histological type:
The best prognosis seems to be for the squamous cell carcinomas, followed by adeno-carcinoma, large cell carcinoma, and small cell carcinoma.
   a) The overall 5-year survival rate of all bronchogenic carcinomas, about 5%.
   b) The 5-year survival of bronchogenic carcinoma following radical surgery: about 20%.
   c) Inoperable tumors, the overall survival time is 5 to 14 months. The 1-year survival after diagnosis: about 10%.
   d) Median survival from the first treatment in patients with limited, but inoperable tumor disease: 36 weeks [80], with extensive disease: 14 weeks.
8. In the individual case factors determining the prognosis are (besides the histological type) the degree of weight loss, the existence or nonexistence of supraclavicular metastases [95, 127], the age of the patient, and probably the CEA level in the serum. Marked elevation of CEA seems to be linked with very poor prognosis [38].

T – primary tumor

Tis = preinvasive carcinoma (carcinoma in situ)

T0 = no evidence of primary tumor

T1 = tumor 3 cm or less in its greatest dimension, surrounded by lung or visceral pleura and with no evidence of invasion proximal to lobar bronchus on bronchoscopy

T2 = tumor more than 3 cm in its greatest dimension or tumor of any size which, with its associated atelectasis or obstructive pneumonitis, extends to the hilar region. On bronchoscopy the proximal extent of demonstrable tumor must be at least 2 cm distal to the carina. Any associated atelectasis or obstructive pneumonitis must involve less than an entire lung and there must be no pleural effusion.

T3 = tumor of any size with direct extension to adjacent structures such as the chest wall, diaphragma, or mediastinum and its contents; tumor on bronchoscopy less than 2 cm distal to the carina; or tumor associated with atelectasis or obstructive pneumonitis of an entire lung or pleural effusion

Tx = any tumor that cannot be assessed or proven by the presence of malignant cells in pulmonary secretions but not visualized by radiography or bronchoscopy (clinical examination, radiography, and endoscopy)

N – regional lymph nodes
(intrathoracic nodes)

N0 = no evidence of regional lymph node involvement

N1 = evidence of involvement of the peribronchial and/or homolateral hilar lymph nodes, including direct extension of the primary tumor

N2 = evidence of involvement of the mediastinal lymph nodes

Nx = the minimal requirements to assess the regional lymph nodes cannot be met (clinical examination, radiography, and endoscopy)

[38] Dent et al. 1978.
[80] Lanzotti et al. 1977.
[95] Mountain and Hermes 1979.
[127] Underwood Jr. et al. 1979.

M – distant metastases

M 0 = no evidence of distant metastases

M 1 = evidence of distant metastases

M x = the minimal requirements to assess the presence of distant metastases cannot be met (clinical examination and radiography)

pTNM – postsurgical histopathological classification
pT – primary tumor

the pT categories correspond to the T categories

G – histopathological grading

G 1 = high degree of differentiation

G 2 = medium degree of differentiation

G 3 = low degree of differentiation or undifferentiated

pN – regional lymph nodes

the pN categories correspond to the N categories

pM – distant metastases

the pM categories correspond to the M categories

Stage grouping

Occult cancer	T x	N 0	M 0
Stage I a	T 1	N 0	M 0
	T 2	N 0	M 0
Stage I b	T 0, T 1	N 1	M 0
Stage II	T 2	N 1	M 0
Stage III	T 3	N 0, N 1	M 0
	any T	N 2	M 0
Stage IV	any T	any N	M 1

M-8070/3
T 162.9

1. Squamous cell carcinoma
(epidermoid carcinoma – WHO) [76]

General Remarks

Incidence: About 25% of all malignant tumors are cancer of the lung. Cancer of the lung is the most important cause of death from cancer. About 60% of cancers of the lung are squamous cell carcinomas.

Age: The peak age is the 6th decade; in women, this tumor occurs some years earlier. A large number of patients are affected by this tumor in the 5th or 7th decade.

Sex: The great majority of squamous cell carcinoma occurs in males.

Site: The main site for squamous cell carcinoma is the major bronchi.

The right lung is more often affected than the left lung.

The tumor often originates peripheral to the first bifurcation of the bronchi.

Further notes: The great majority of patients are heavy smokers.

Macroscopy

Squamous cell carcinomas originate from the mucosa of the bronchus and present as grayish tumors with sudden ulceration and destruction of the bronchial epithelium.

Squamous cell carcinomas are of different sizes; they can be very small. Large tumors show areas of necrosis on the cut surface.

The tumor infiltrates the surrounding peribronchial tissue and occasionally can resemble pneumonia.

Often the tumor grows into the lumen of the bronchus, causing obstruction.

Histology

The tumor cells have a large cytoplasm, which sometimes is eosinophilic. There are nuclear atypias and mitotic figures.

Often the tumor cells are polygonal.

The tumor forms large complexes.

The tumor cells often invade the lymphatics.

Besides foci of infiltrating squamous cell carcinoma, areas of carcinoma in situ might be found in the neighborhood of the tumor. The infiltrating carcinoma might originate from those foci of carcinoma in situ [91].

Squamous cell carcinomas have different degrees of keratinization. The grading is done on the degree of keratinization including dyskeratosis and on the degree of nuclear atypias.

The degrees of differentiation are expressed by:

M-8071/3

– **highly differentiated** (WHO)
(well-differentiated, keratinized squamous cell carcinoma) (Figs. 680 and 681),

– **moderately differentiated** (WHO) (Figs. 682 to 685),

M-8072/3

– **poorly differentiated** (WHO)
(nonkeratinized squamous cell carcinoma) (Figs. 686 and 687).

Occasionally the tumor cells are without signs of organoid structure and cannot be differentiated any further.

---

[76] Kreyberg et al. 1967.
[91] Melamed et al. 1977.

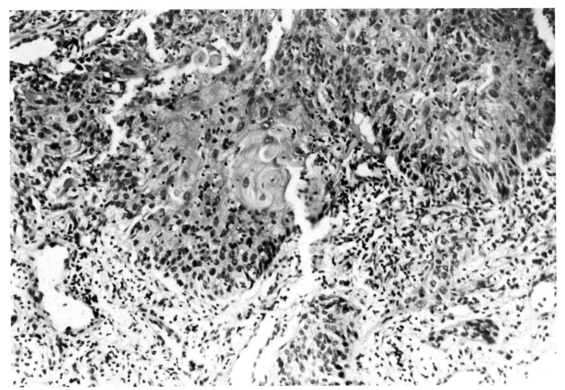

Fig. 680. Highly differentiated keratinized squamous cell carcinoma of the bronchus (60-year-old male, × 200).

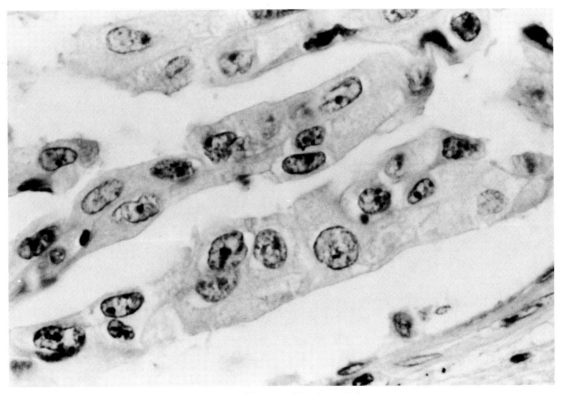

Fig. 681. Squamous cell carcinoma of the bronchus (61-year-old male, × 600).

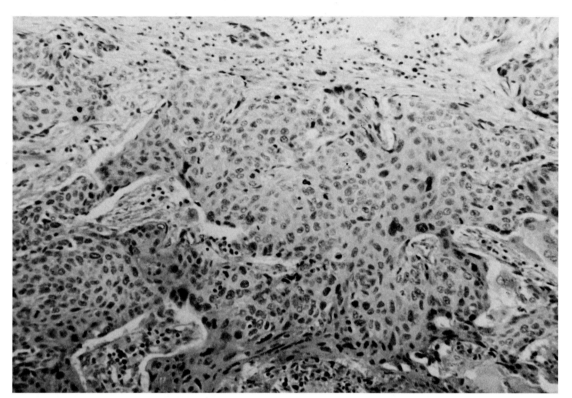

Fig. 682. Moderately differentiated bronchogenic squamous cell carcinoma (60-year-old male, × 200).

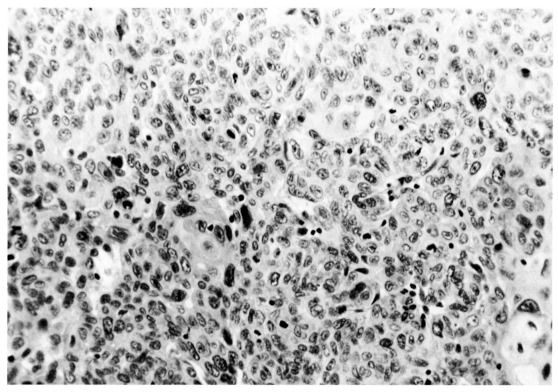

Fig. 683. Moderately differentiated bronchogenic squamous cell carcinoma: Remnants of keratinization, marked nuclear atypia (49-year-old male, × 200).

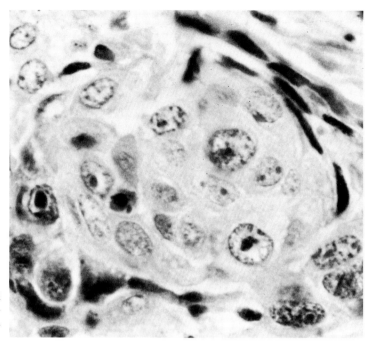

Fig. 684. Moderately differentiated poorly keratinizing squamous cell carcinoma of the bronchus (60-year-old male, ×600).

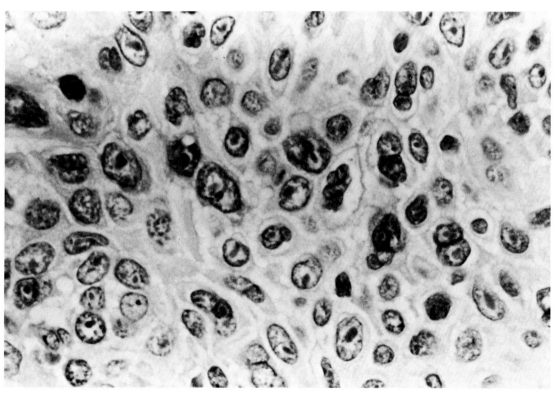

Fig. 685. Poorly differentiated, nonkeratinizing squamous cell carcinoma of the bronchus (60-year-old male, ×600).

Squamous cell carcinoma

Differential Diagnosis

Squamous cell carcinoma **with other bronchogenic carcinomas:**
Indicating squamous cell carcinoma are
— presence of keratin formation,
— intercellular bridges in nonkeratinized squamous cell carcinoma,
— foci of carcinoma in situ, or foci of squamous cell metaplasia in the mucosa of the bronchus surrounding the tumor [10],
— whorl formation (in cases of nonkeratinization).

Spread

1. Squamous cell carcinomas often directly invade the surrounding lung parenchyma.
2. Invasion of the lymphatics with regional lymph node metastases.
3. Hematogenous metastases into liver, adrenal, brain, bone, and other organs.

Clinical Findings

a) Early symptom: Cough.
b) Symptoms due to bronchial obstruction:
   Fever, hemoptysis, localized bronchopneumonia, atelectasis.
c) Loss of weight, hoarseness.
d) Squamous cell carcinoma can show an increased level of carcinoembryonic antigen (CEA) in the serum.
e) **Pancoast tumor:**
   Horner's syndrome.
   Intractable pain.
   Pancoast tumors are almost always squamous cell carcinomas.
   In this case the surrounding structures are involved early:
   Pleura, chest wall, cervical sympathetic plexus, tracheal plexus, bone.
f) In **preclinical stages** malignant cells may be shed into the sputum, including those cells that derive from foci of carcinoma in situ.
   Cytology might be an important tool for the early detection of cancer of the bronchus (Figs. 688 and 689).

Treatment

Surgery:
— Radical surgery with pneumectomy or lobectomy according to the extent of the tumor [101, 130].
  Removal of the regional lymph nodes.
— About 15 to 25% of the patients are eligible for curative surgical therapy when they first ask for medical care.
— **Contraindication** for pneumectomy or lobectomy:
  — intra- or extrathoracic spread of the tumor,
  — lymph node metastases,
  — superior vena caval obstruction,
  — recurrent laryngeal or phrenic nerve paralysis.
Radiation therapy:
— Radiation therapy alone is seldom curative.
— The main purpose of radiation therapy is palliation.
— Occasionally, preoperative external irradiation has been recommended, yielding a higher 5-year survival [72].

[10] Auerbach et al. 1957.
[72] Kent and Schwade 1979.
[101] Rilke et al. 1979.
[130] Viereck et al. 1974.

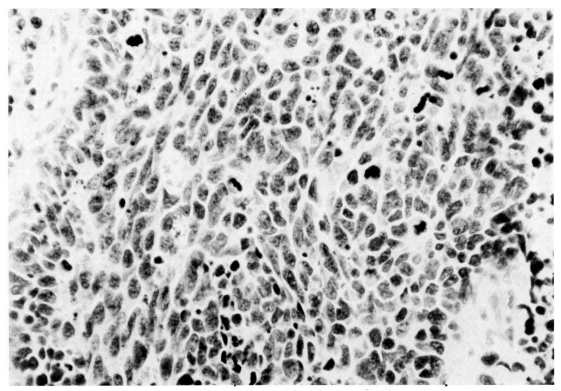

Fig. 686. Poorly differentiated, bronchogenic squamous cell carcinoma, nonkeratinized (60-year-old male, × 310).

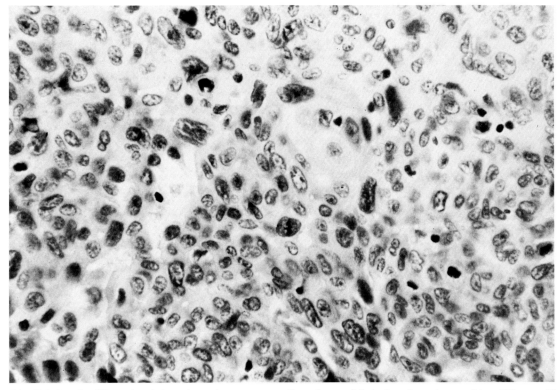

Fig. 687. Poorly differentiated, bronchogenic squamous cell carcinoma: Marked nuclear pleomorphism (49-year-old male, × 310).

691

Squamous cell carcinoma

Treatment

Radiation therapy:
– It is debatable whether radiation therapy should be applied following radical surgery. Radiation therapy is often used to remove bronchial obstruction and superior vena caval obstruction and for the treatment of pain and bleeding [120].
– Dosage according to the applied technique: 40 to 70 Gy in 4 to 6 weeks.

Chemotherapy:
– Squamous cell carcinomas show practically no response to chemotherapy [33, 34].
– Chemotherapy is used for palliation. There are reports of the use of high dose methotrexate with citrovorum factor rescue [40] or adriamycin [21, 44, 84, 110].
– Combined chemotherapy and radiation therapy has been recommended in cases of advanced tumor disease [109, 111].
– The combination of **immunization and chemotherapy** is under investigation following encouraging results due to immunization of the patients [119].

Pancoast tumor:
It may be attempted to resect the tumor or to use radiation therapy for palliation.
There are reports in which a 4-drug chemotherapy (COPP) has been used.

Prognosis

1. Squamous cell carcinoma has the best prognosis of all bronchogenic carcinomas.
   This is due to early symptoms and a relatively slow dissemination.
2. The 5-year survival rate for operated patients is 25%.
   The overall 5-year survival is minimal.
3. The prognosis for inoperable lung cancer is determined by weight loss, supraclavicular metastases, and age, but not by the histological type of the tumor.
4. Survival time of inoperable tumors from the time of first treatment: 5 to 14 months [80].
   About 75% of the patients are inoperable at the time of diagnosis.
5. It seems that marked elevation of the CEA level is linked with a very poor prognosis in bronchogenic carcinoma [38].
   This might be due to a correlation between the CEA blood level and the extension of the tumor [52, 75, 131].

Further Information

1. The mean doubling time for squamous cell carcinoma is about 103 days.
2. The duration of the in situ stage of an infiltrating carcinoma is not known.
   The preclinical stage of squamous cell carcinoma in the lung, including carcinoma in situ, could be of a long duration, perhaps years [27] (Fig. 690).
3. Carcinoma in situ may possibly be observed in about 20% of squamous cell carcinomas.
   The in situ carcinoma may involve the submucosal glands [12].
4. Screening of the sputum of 4000 cigarette-smoking men with normal chest X-rays detected lung cancer in 9 men [11, 86, 91].

[11] Auerbach et al. 1979.
[12] Baker et al. 1979.
[21] Bitran et al. 1978.
[27] Carter et al. 1976.
[33] Cohen 1978.
[34] Cohen and Selawry 1975.
[38] Dent et al. 1978.
[40] Djerassi et al. 1977.
[44] Fetzer et al. 1977.
[52] Gropp et al. 1978.
[75] Krebs et al. 1977.

[80] Lanzotti et al. 1977.
[84] Livingston et al. 1977.
[86] Lukeman et al. 1979.
[91] Melamed et al. 1977.
[109] Sealy 1979.
[110] Seeber and Schmidt 1979.
[111] Seeber et al. 1977.
[119] Stewart et al. 1978.
[120] Sugaar and LeVeen 1979.
[131] Vincent et al. 1979.

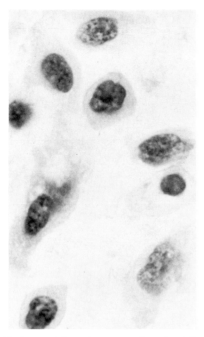

Fig. 688. Sputum cytology in a case of moderately differentiated squamous cell carcinoma: Large nucleus with clumped, coarse chromatin. Well-defined cytoplasm (HE, × 1200).

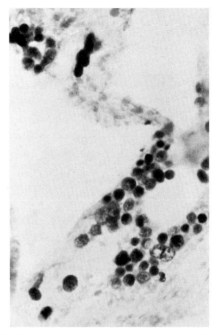

Fig. 689. Cytology sputum: Bronchogenic small cell carcinoma: Group of lymphocyte-like cells with discrete pleomorphism (HE, × 400).

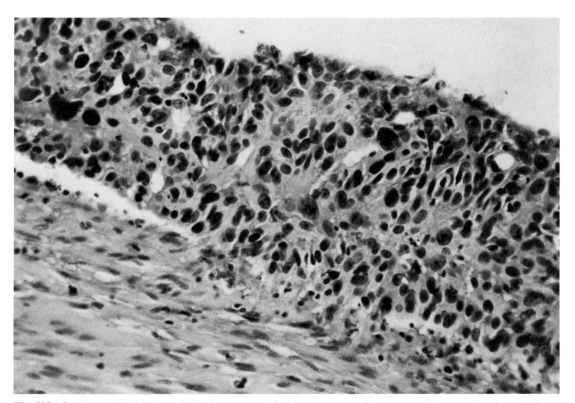

Fig. 690. Carcinoma in situ in the neighborhood of an infiltrating squamous cell carcinoma (56-year-old male, × 200).

M-8140/3
T 162.9

2. Bronchogenic adenocarcinoma (WHO)

**General
Remarks**

Incidence: About 15% of bronchogenic carcinomas are adenocarcinomas.

Age: A large number of patients are in the 5th to 7th decades; however, younger age groups can be affected.

The peak age is the 6th decade; in women this tumor occurs earlier.

Sex: Adenocarcinomas are observed more frequently in men than in women.

About 50% of all bronchogenic carcinomas in females are of the adenocarcinoma type.

About 10% of all bronchogenic carcinomas in males are of the adenocarcinoma type.

Site: About 70% of adenocarcinomas grow in peripheral locations, involving the pleura.

About 30%, however, can arise in the mucus glands of large bronchi.

Further notes:

– There are indications that the incidence of adenocarcinomas is increasing in both sexes [132].

– Smokers are more frequently affected by this tumor than nonsmokers.

– Adenocarcinomas in a peripheral position are rather often related to interstitial fibrosis or scars [9] (Fig. 691).

Macroscopy

Adenocarcinomas are poorly delineated tumors with a yellowish cut surface.

According to the amount of produced mucin, they have a more or less mucoid appearance.

At the time of tumor detection, a large number of peripheral adenocarcinomas have infiltrated the visceral pleura.

Histology

Bronchogenic adenocarcinomas are composed of cells that show different degrees of differentiation and produce different amounts of mucin.

According to the grade of differentiation, the amount of mucin production, and the growth pattern, a subclassification has been recommended [76]:

M-8550/3

a) Acinar type of adenocarcinoma with mucin (WHO):

This adenocarcinoma is characterized by cell growth with a glandular-acinar pattern (Fig. 692).

There are different degrees of mucin production. Occasionally, there is no mucin detectable:

b) Acinar type of adenocarcinoma without mucin (WHO).

[9] Auerbach et al. 1979.
[76] Kreyberg et al. 1967.
[132] Vincent et al. 1977.

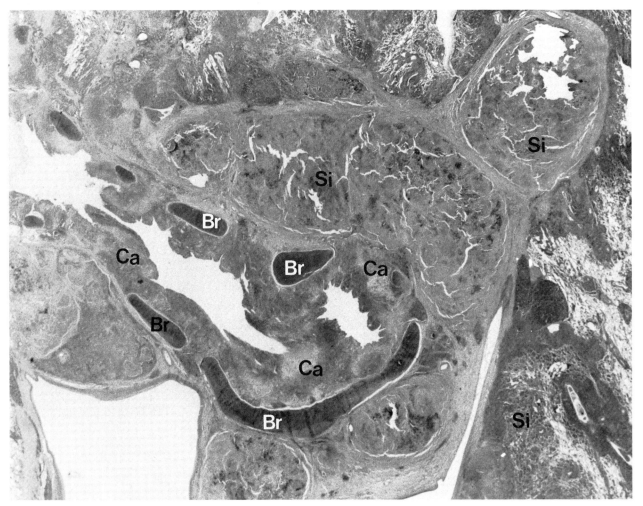

Fig. 691. Scar-induced carcinoma in silicosis (62-year-old male) (Ca = carcinoma, Br = bronchus, Si = silicotic lung tissue).

M-8260/3

c) Papillary type of adenocarcinoma with or without mucin (WHO):

In these cases the tumor cells form papillary structures that grow into the lumen of the tumor glands.

M-8012/3

d) Large cell carcinoma (WHO):

This type of adenocarcinoma is dominated by large cells.
In some of these tumors the large cells produce mucin; in others there is no evidence of mucin production.
These large cells form large complexes without glandular formations:

e) Large cell carcinoma, solid type, with or without mucin-like content (WHO) (Figs. 693 and 694).

f) Large cell carcinoma, giant cell type (WHO) [135]:

A variety of this tumor shows large cells that occasionally form multinucleated giant cells.
Mucin production can be found (Figs. 695 and 696).
Occasionally these tumors show areas with a glandular growth pattern.
Giant cell carcinomas almost always grow in the **periphery** of the lung and are very malignant.

g) Large cell carcinoma, clear cell type (WHO):

This adenocarcinoma is characterized by solid cell complexes. The cells have a large clear cytoplasm and distinct cell borders.
Mucin production can be observed occasionally.
These tumors also grow in the **periphery** of the lung and are very malignant.

Differential Diagnosis

1. Bronchogenic adenocarcinoma **with metastatic adenocarcinoma.**
2. Bronchogenic adenocarcinoma **with poorly differentiated squamous cell carcinoma, nonkeratinized** (see Further information, page 700).

Spread

1. Local extension into the visceral pleura in tumors with peripheral localization.
2. Early lymph node metastases.
3. Early hematogenous metastases into adrenal, brain, bone, liver, and other organs.

---

[135] Wang et al. 1976.

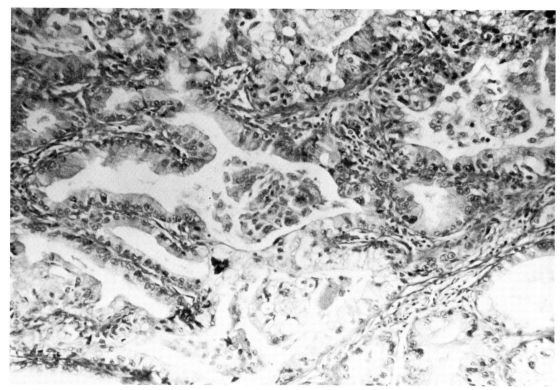

Fig. 692. Bronchogenic adenocarcinoma, mucin-producing (acinar type) (53-year-old male, × 200).

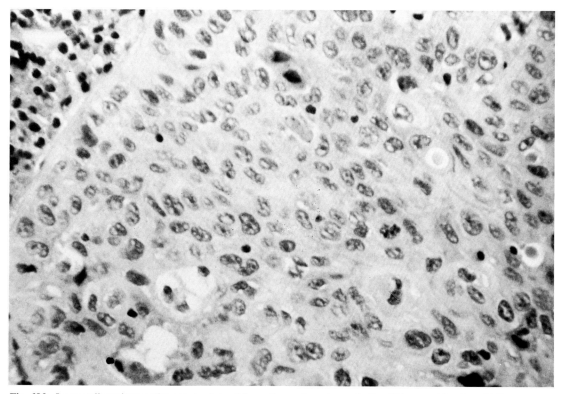

Fig. 693. Large cell carcinoma: Remnants of gland formation and mucin production (72-year-old male, × 310).

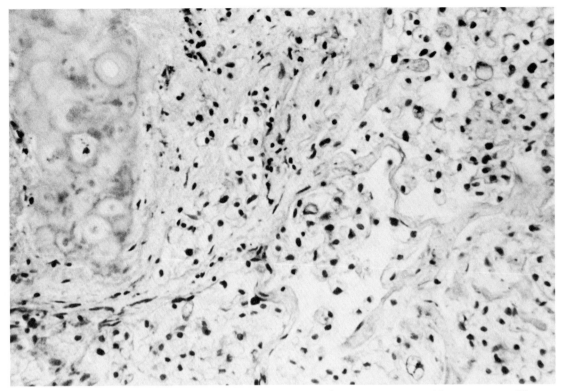

Fig. 694. Large cell (bronchogenic) adenocarcinoma, signet cell type (autopsy case, tumor without metastases, 71-year-old male, × 200).

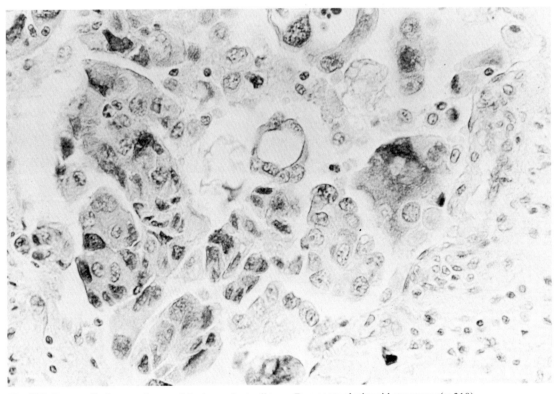

Fig. 695. Large cell adenocarcinoma of the lung, giant cell type: Remnants of adenoid structures (× 310).

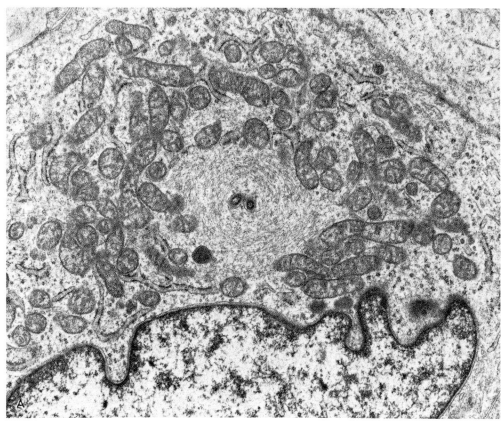

Fig. 696. Large cell carcinoma of the lung, giant cell type: Concentric whorl of filaments, surrounded by mitochondria (× 15,500) (Wang et al. Hum. Pathol. *7* (1976) 3-16).

Adenocarcinoma

**Clinical
Findings**

Most of the adenocarcinomas grow in peripheral locations.

Therefore, clinical symptoms occur late in the course of the disease and are often due to hematogenous metastases.

Treatment

Surgery:

In resectable cases, lobectomy or pneumectomy with removal of lymph node metastases should be tried.

Radiation therapy:

This treatment should be applied for palliation purposes (40 to 50 Gy in 4 to 5 weeks) [59].

Chemotherapy:

Polychemotherapy has been considerd rather effective [4].

Postoperative adjuvant chemotherapy does not seem to be of any benefit [112].

It is debatable whether in cases of unresectable tumors any treatment might increase the survival time [108].

Prognosis

The overall 5-year survival rate for adenocarcinoma is about 10%.

**Further
Information**

In some instances the histological subtyping cannot be determined because there is lack of squamous cell differentiation, glandular growth pattern, or mucin production.

Occasionally some of these tumors contain giant cells:

M-8031/3

h) Undifferentiated giant cell tumor (WHO) (Figs. 697 to 700).

In large cell, undifferentiated carcinoma of the lung, the tumor cells contain desmosomes with tonofilaments and intercellular bridges [29] and glycogen.

It might be possible that some of these undifferentiated tumors were originally adenocarcinomas [24] (Figs. 701 and 702).

[4] Alberto et al. 1976.
[24] Byrd et al. 1968.
[29] Churg 1978.
[59] Heilmann et al. 1976.
[108] Scheer and Wilson 1975.
[112] Shields et al. 1977.

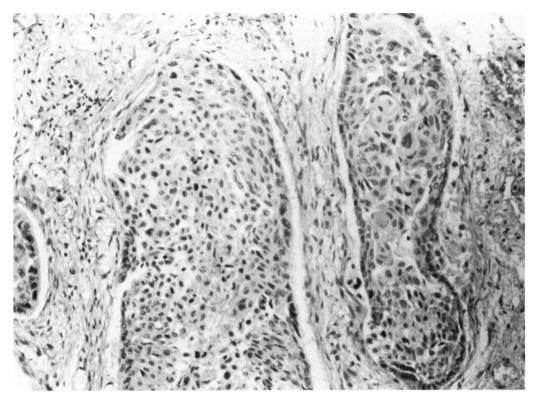

Fig. 697. Keratinizing squamous cell carcinoma of the bronchus (88-year-old male, × 125).

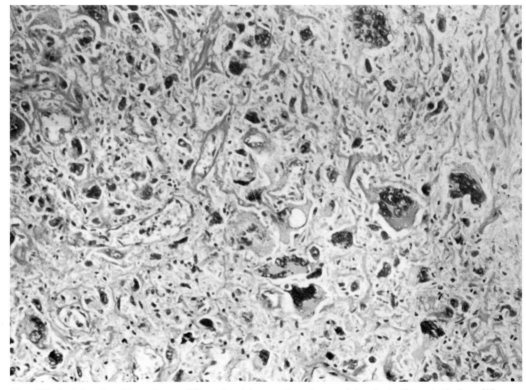

Fig. 698. Peripheral position of an undifferentiated, large cell carcinoma of the giant cell type in the lung (88-year-old male, × 125); same case as Fig. 697).

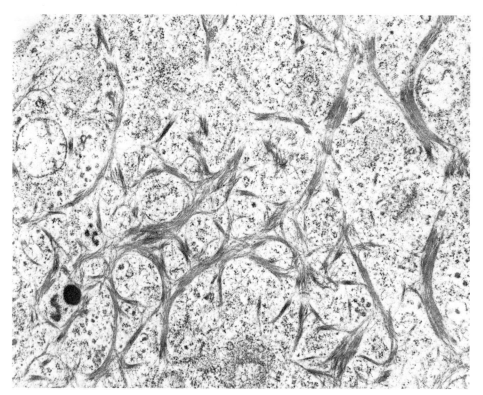

Fig. 699. Undifferentiated carcinoma of the lung: Tumor cell with network of intracytoplasmic microfilaments (× 23,700).

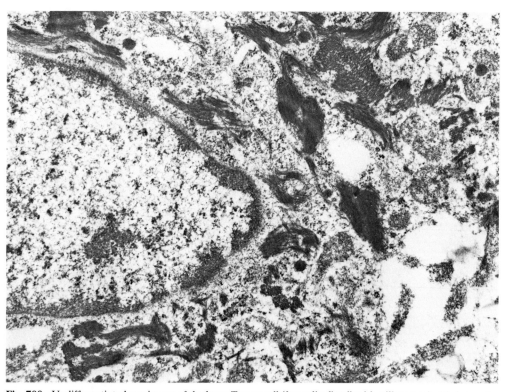

Fig. 700. Undifferentiated carcinoma of the lung: Tumor cell (formalin-fixed) with still recognizable intracytoplasmic microfilaments (× 10,000).

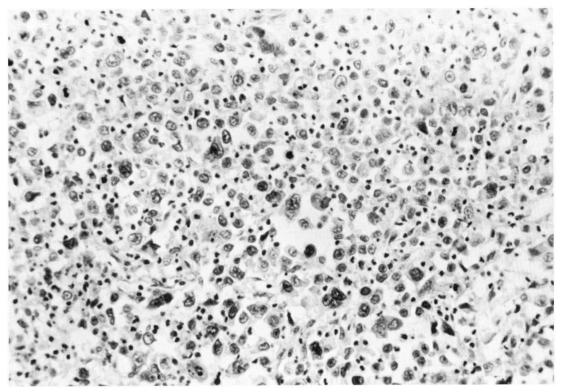

Fig. 701. Undifferentiated giant cell tumor of the bronchus (55-year-old male, × 200).

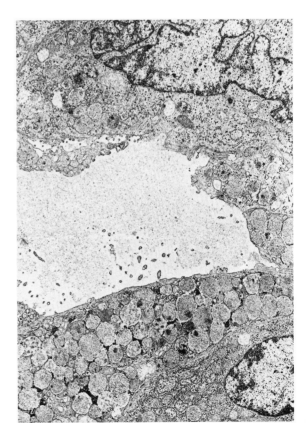

Fig. 702. Poorly differentiated adenocarcinoma of the lung, large cells: Cells with mucin granules around a lumen (× 8000) (Churg, Hum. Pathol. *9* (1978) 143-156).

M-8250/3
T 162.9

3. Bronchioloalveolar carcinoma (WHO)
(bronchiolar cell carcinoma; adenocarcinoma, bronchioloalveolar)

**General
Remarks**

Incidence: About 3% of lung cancers are bronchioloalveolar carcinomas.
Age: This tumor can arise in younger age groups; the peak age is the 6th decade.
Sex: Men and women are equally affected.
Site: The tumor usually grows at multiple sites in peripheral locations.
Further notes: Most probably this tumor originates from the bronchiolar epithelial cells [79].
In many cases bronchioloalveolar carcinomas are assumed to have a multicentric origin.

Macroscopy

Bronchioloalveolar carcinomas are soft tumors with a whitish-yellowish or pinkish cut surface.
According to the amount of mucin produced, the cut surface can be more or less gelatinous.
This tumor can grow diffusely into the lobe of a lung and give the impression of a lobar pneumonia.
In other instances the tumor is rather localized, and these variations of this carcinoma might be rather firm.
Often this bronchioloalveolar carcinoma presents as multiple nodules, which grow in 80% of the cases in both lungs.

Histology

The columnar tumor cells line spaces that often correspond to recognizable alveoli (Fig. 703). These spaces are lined by monolayers of tumor cells; however, the cells can also grow in multilayers.
Often the tumor cells are arranged in a papillary growth pattern (Figs. 704 and 705).
Mucin production can occasionally be detected by special stains. Often this tumor produces large amounts of mucin, which can even dominate the histological picture (Figs. 706 and 707).
The nuclei of the tumor cells are rather small and the nucleoli are large.
The regular lining cells of the bronchioli and alveolar cells can abruptly change into atypical tumor cells [121] (Fig. 708).

**Electron
Microscopy**

Bronchioloalveolar carcinoma contains tumor cells with no mucin-secreting granules, lamellated inclusion bodies, and junctional complexes joining the cells with each other.
The surface has numerous microvilli.
Occasionally the nucleus contains tubular structures [124].

[79] Kuhn 1972.
[121] Tao et al. 1978.
[124] Torikata and Ishiwata 1977.

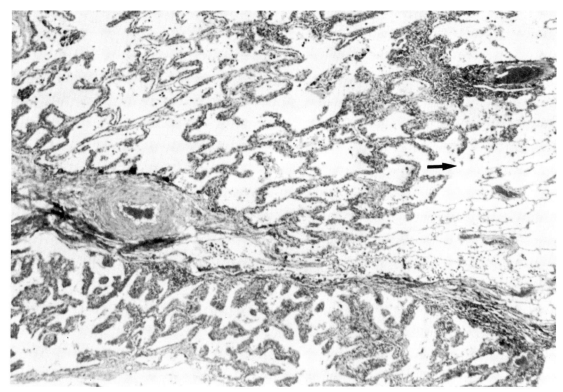

Fig. 703. Bronchioloalveolar carcinoma: Remnants of normal alveoli (53-year-old male, × 40).

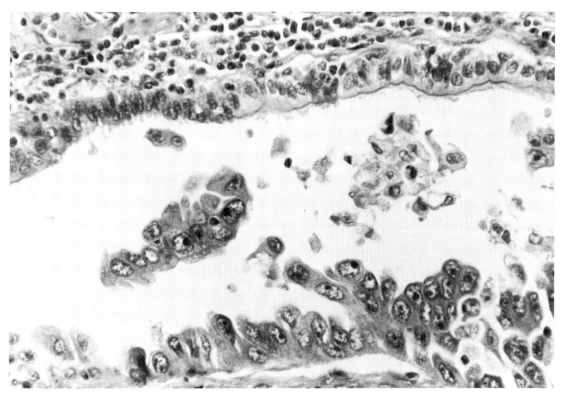

Fig. 704. Bronchioloalveolar carcinoma: Transition of respiratory epithelium (bronchiolus) into malignant cells (× 310).

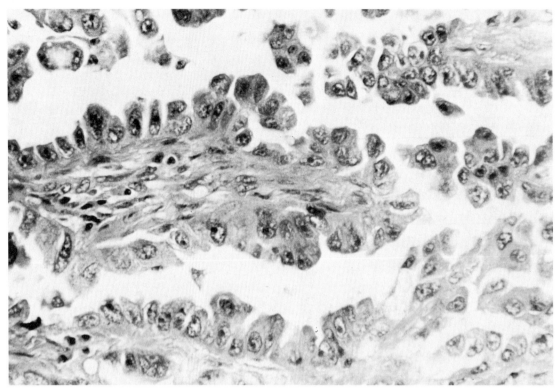

Fig. 705. Bronchioloalveolar carcinoma: Papillary tumor cell growth (×310).

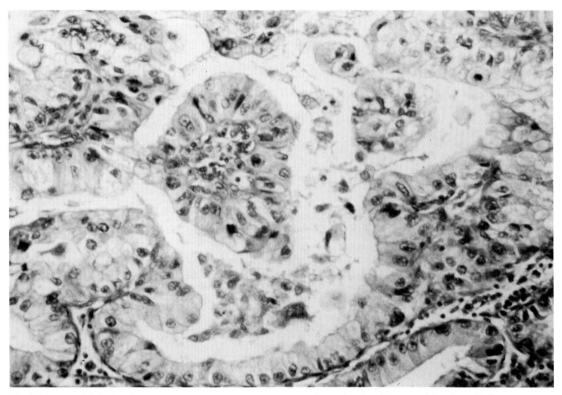

Fig. 706. Bronchioloalveolar carcinoma: Columnar tumor cells, mucin production (53-year-old male, ×200).

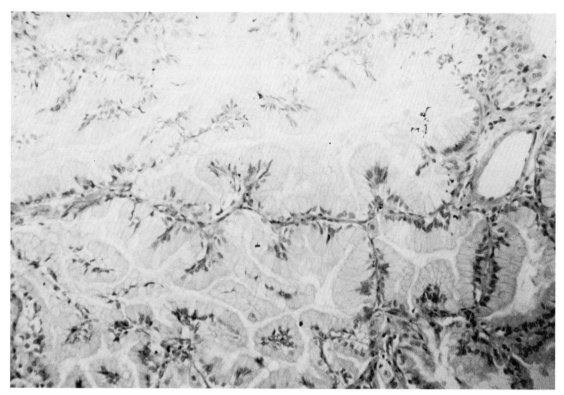

Fig. 707. Bronchioloalveolar carcinoma: Columnar tumor cell lining of the alveoli (53-year-old male, × 125).

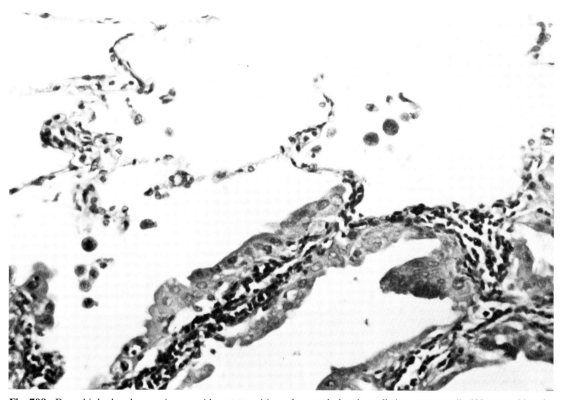

Fig. 708. Bronchioloalveolar carcinoma: Abrupt transition of normal alveolar cells into tumor cells (53-year-old male, × 125).

Bronchioloalveolar carcinoma

Differential Diagnosis

1. Bronchioloalveolar carcinoma **with bronchogenic adenocarcinoma** (Fig. 692):
Proof of a multicentric origin and the abrupt transition of regular bronchiolar cells into tumor cells indicates bronchioloalveolar carcinoma.
In bronchioloalveolar carcinoma, there are never foci of squamous cell differentiation.

M-8250/1
T 162.9

2. Bronchioloalveolar carcinoma **with adenomatosis of the lung:**
It has not been determined whether this entity, adenomatosis of the lung, exists because often an insidious transition into bronchioloalveolar carcinoma is observed.

3. Bronchioloalveolar carcinoma **with metastasizing adenocarcinoma:**
Due to the papillary growth of the tumor, the differential diagnosis with metastases from tumors of the ovary, but also from the gastrointestinal tract, might be difficult.
Again helpful is the detection of abrupt transition of normal cells into tumor cells.

4. Bronchioloalveolar carcinoma **with metastasizing malignant mesothelioma of the pleura:**
If histological differentiation is difficult, the gross appearance might be helpful because the pleural tumor thickens the pleura.
However, the pleura covering bronchioloalveolar carcinoma can be considerably thickened [90].
The differential diagnosis can occasionally be solved by scanning electron microscopy: The surface of bronchioloalveolar cells has stubby microvilli, while the mesothelial tumor cells show shaggy microvilli [39, 128] (Figs. 709 and 710).

Spread

1. About 50% of the cases show lymph node metastases at the time of diagnosis.
2. Hematogenous spread into brain, liver, adrenal, bone, kidney, and other organs.
3. In about 50% of the cases the tumor does not disseminate outside the thorax, although in the lung large tumor masses might have developed.

Clinical Findings

The leading symptoms are dyspnea and cyanosis, while cough and hoarseness are less common.
The sputum is abundant and watery.
Due to the multilocular origin of small tumors, the beginning of the tumor disease might be insidious.
The roentgenogram shows solitary or multiple foci and occasionally can give the impression of pneumonia.

Treatment

Surgery:
In cases of localized tumor, pneumectomy or lobectomy might be tried.
Treatment is very difficult in cases of wide tumor infiltration or dissemination into both lungs.
Radiation therapy:
Radiation therapy should be applied only for palliation purposes.
Chemotherapy:
Chemotherapy does not seem to influence the tumor.

[39] Dionne and Wang 1977.
[90] McCaughey 1965.
[128] Uys 1979.

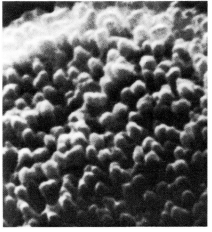

Fig. 709. Bronchioloalveolar carcinoma with stubby microvilli on the surface of the tumor cells (×28,000) (Dionne and Wang, Cancer *40* (1977) 707-715).

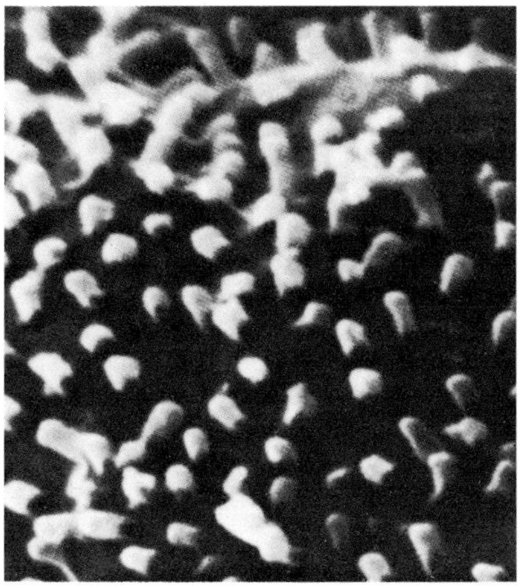

Fig. 710. Pleura mesothelioma: Large microvilli on the surface of the cells (×28,000) (Dionne and Wang, Cancer *40* (1977) 707-715).

Prognosis

The 5-year survival rate is about 5%.

Eighty to 90% of the patients die during the 1st year after diagnosis.

The median survival time is about 3 to 4 years.

Further Information

Rarely a **Clara cell adenocarcinoma** has been observed in the lung. Probably this tumor originates from the terminal bronchiolus [32, 92].

[32] Clara 1937.
[92] Montes et al. 1977.

M-8560/3
T 162.9

4. Combined squamous cell carcinoma and adenocarcinoma
(adenosquamous carcinoma) (WHO)

This tumor is relatively rare (about 10% of all malignant tumors of the lung).

The tumor is composed of foci of adenocarcinoma, in which foci of squamous cell carcinomas grow (Figs. 711 to 713).

The tumor resembles adenocarcinoma: Often it is related to scar tissue and the main location is the periphery of the lung.

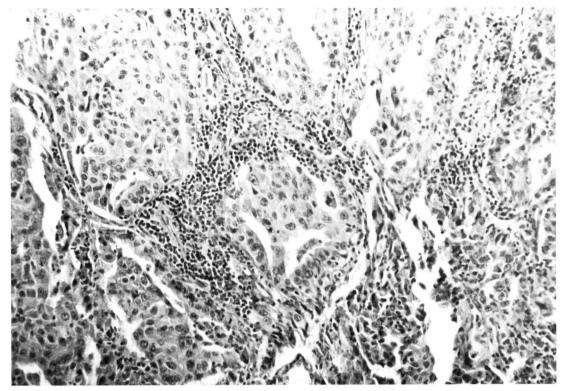

Fig. 711. Combined adeno- and squamous cell carcinoma (71-year-old male, × 125).

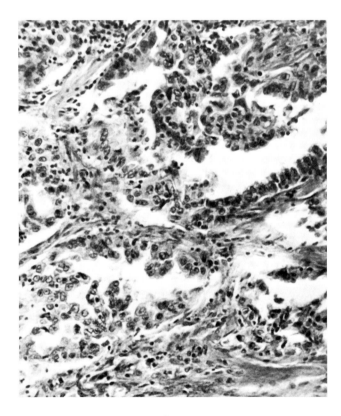

Fig. 712. Combined bronchogenic carcinoma: Area of adenocarcinoma (71-year-old male, × 125).

5. Tumors of the bronchial glands

M-8200/3 **a) Adenoid cystic carcinoma** (WHO)

T 162.2 Almost always this tumor develops in the major bronchi; occasionally it develops in the
T 162.0 trachea.

Histology This tumor is composed of atypical cells that form glandular structures and cysts.
The histological picture is identical to the corresponding tumor of the salivary glands
(Figs. 588 to 592).

Spread The tumor disseminates into the regional lymph nodes, occasionally also causing distant
metastases.

Treatment The tumor is treated by radical pneumectomy.
Radiation therapy can be attempted.

Prognosis The prognosis is poor [88] although the course of the disease is rather slow.

M-8430/3 **b) Mucoepidermoid carcinoma** (WHO) [125]
T 162.9

This tumor shows solid cell complexes with different degrees of glandular-like structures.
Mucin production can be observed (Fig. 714).
This mucoepidermoid carcinoma histologically is identical with the corresponding tumor
in salivary glands (see page 581).

The tumor behaves according to the degree of differentiation with metastases into
regional lymph nodes.

In cases of poor differentiation, the tumor has a very poor prognosis.

---

[88] Markel et al. 1964.
[125] Turnbull et al. 1971.

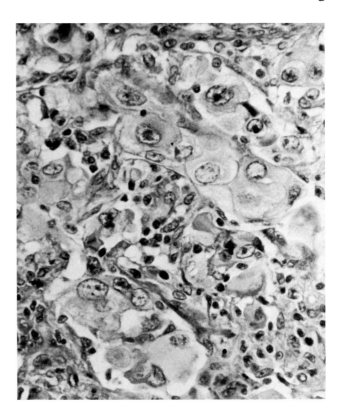

Fig. 713. Combined bronchogenic carcinoma: Area of squamous cell carcinoma (71-year-old male, ×310).

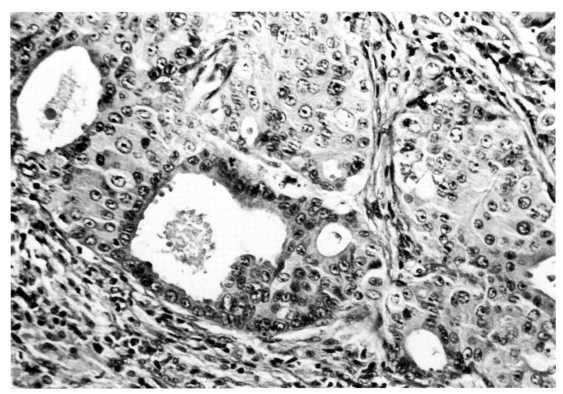

Fig. 714. Mucoepidermoid carcinoma of bronchial glands (×200).

713

M-8240/3
T 162.9

6. Carcinoid tumor (WHO)
(bronchial carcinoid; bronchial adenoma)

**General
Remarks**

Incidence: About 5% of lung tumors are carcinoid tumors.
Age: The peak age is around 40 years.
Sex: Men and women are equally affected.

T 162.0
T 162.2

Site: The main localization is in the trachea, the main stem bronchus, or the lobar bronchus.
Carcinoids in the periphery of the lung are rare [23]. The right lung is more frequently affected than the left lung.

Macroscopy

Carcinoid tumors grow into the lumen of the bronchus, causing obstruction.
There is also infiltration of the wall.
In most instances the epithelial layer covering the carcinoid tumor is not ulcerated.
The cut surface is grayish, and yellowish areas with hemorrhages are often observed.

Histology

This very vascular tumor is composed of cells that have a rather regular, round, and small nucleus, which is centrally located. Mitotic figures are rare (Figs. 715 to 717).
In most instances the small tumor cells are argyrophilic (argentaffin), as observed in the stomach and duodenum.

M-8290/0

Occasionally the tumor cells can be rich in acidophilic granules **(oncocytoma).**
The growth pattern of the tumor cells is quite variable and differs in one tumor from area to area:
– The tumor cells are arranged in solid nests, ribbons, or a trabecular pattern (Figs. 718 and 719).
– Occasionally the carcinoid cells are spindle-shaped and form whorls.
The tumor cells occasionally infiltrate the surrounding tissue and can be found in the lymphatics.

**Electron
Microscopy**

The tumor cells of carcinoid of the lung contain secretory granules [23, 26].

**Tissue
Culture**

Carcinoid cells can be kept for several months in tissue culture without losing the ability to produce large numbers of neurosecretory type granules [17].

**Differential
Diagnosis**

1. Carcinoid tumor **with adenoid cystic carcinoma** (Fig. 589):
   The adenoid growth pattern is rare in carcinoid tumors.
   Adenoid cystic carcinoma shows massive lymphatic infiltration, which is rare in carcinoid tumors.
2. Carcinoid tumor **with mucoepidermoid carcinoma** (Fig. 586):
   The growth pattern in both instances is different. In doubtful cases, a positive reaction for mucin indicates mucoepidermoid carcinoma.

[17] Bensch et al. 1976.
[23] Bonikos et al. 1976.
[26] Capella et al. 1979.

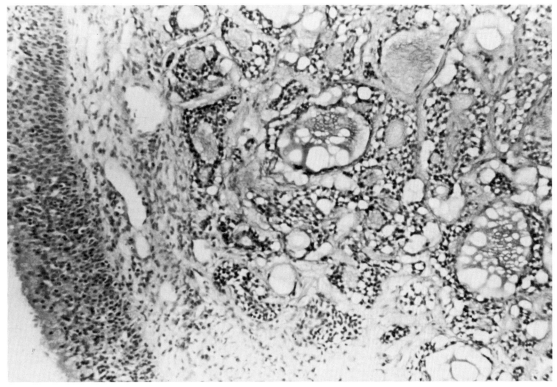

Fig. 715. Bronchial carcinoid: Note cysts (similar to adenoid cystic carcinoma) and solid nests (72-year-old male, left main bronchus, × 125).

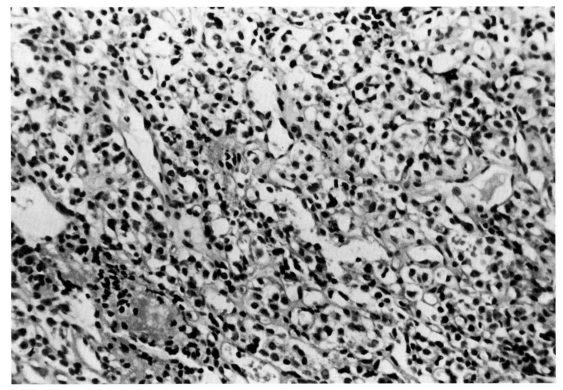

Fig. 716. Bronchial carcinoid: Nests of regular cells, occasionally clear cytoplasm, numerous blood vessels (40-year-old female, × 200).

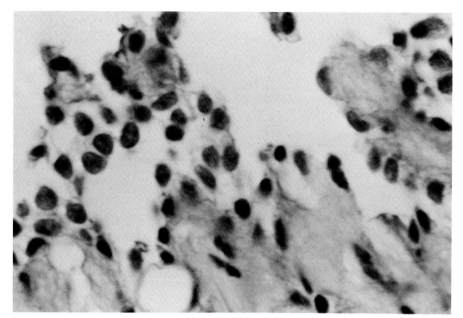

Fig. 717. Bronchial carcinoid (74-year-old male, × 600).

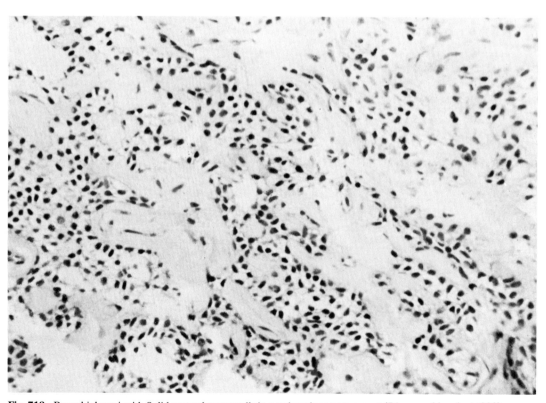

Fig. 718. Bronchial carcinoid: Solid nests of tumor cells in a trabecular arrangement (74-year-old male, × 200).

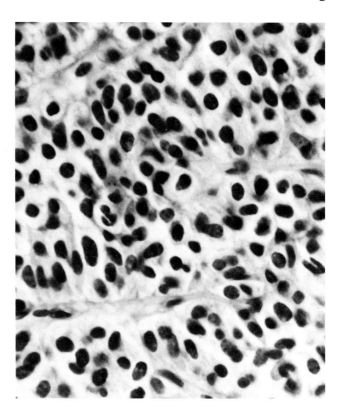

Fig. 719. Bronchial carcinoid (× 400).

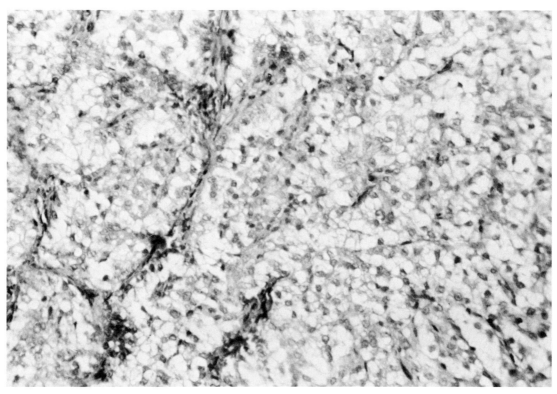

Fig. 720. Clear cell adenoma ("sugar tumor") of the bronchus (71-year-old male, × 310).

Bronchial carcinoid

Differential Diagnosis

3. Carcinoid tumor **with oat cell carcinoma** (Figs. 721 to 724):

Occasionally it might be necessary to differentiate between these two tumors, since transitions have been observed [7].

In case of doubt, the evidence of argentaffin cells solves the problem in favor of carcinoid tumor.

Spread

1. Direct spread into the surrounding tissue can occur.
2. Invasion of the lymphatics with lymph node metastases is possible; occasionally even distant metastases develop [51].

Clinical Findings

Signs of bronchial obstruction with cough, hemoptysis, pneumonia, and tumor atelectasis.

Endocrinology:

Most of the bronchial carcinoids are silent; however, some of them cause a carcinoid syndrome.

Occasionally the carcinoid can produce ACTH, with the subsequent development of Cushing's syndrome [35].

Treatment

The bronchial carcinoid should be treated by **surgery.**

According to the site and the extent of the disease, lobectomy or pneumectomy should be done.

The regional lymph nodes should be removed.

Prognosis

Bronchial carcinoids are slow-growing tumors.

In most instances the tumor can be resected.

The 10-year survival rate for resected tumors: about 80%.

Untreated bronchial carcinoids: 10-year survival, about 10% [137].

Further Information

1. The cell of origin for bronchial carcinoids is the Kulschitzky type cell (Feyrter) [45].
2. In a number of cases the tumor cells contain neurosecretory granules [19].
3. Adenomas of the bronchus **(noncarcinoid tumors)** are relatively rare:

M-8310/0 T 162.9

a) **"Sugar tumor"** (clear cell adenoma) [83]:

This is a small benign tumor that histologically is composed of glycogen-rich cells. This glycogen gives a clear appearance to the tumor cells (Fig. 720).

The glycogen is membrane-bound [16, 103].

M-8290/0 T 162.9

b) **Oncocytoma:**

This adenoma is composed of cells with a large amount of acidophilic cytoplasm [42, 105].

[7] Arrigoni et al. 1972.
[16] Becker and Soifer 1971.
[19] Bensch et al. 1965.
[35] Cohen et al. 1960.
[42] Fechner and Bentinck 1973.
[45] Feyrter 1959.
[51] Graham and Womack 1945.
[83] Liebow and Castleman 1971.
[103] Sale and Kulander 1976.
[105] Santos-Briz et al. 1977.
[137] Wilkins Jr. et al. 1963.

M-8480/0
T 162.9

c) Mucus gland adenoma:
This tumor grows in the bronchial wall and is composed of mucin-producing glandular structures [77].

4. There are other benign tumors that can grow into the lumen of the bronchus and cause bronchial obstruction:

M-9580/0

– **granular cell tumor** [46] (Fig. 123),

M-8050/0
T 162.2
T 162.0

– **benign papilloma.**
The latter tumor can also develop in the trachea (Figs. 537 and 538) [93].

---

[46] Gallivan et al. 1966.
[77] Kroe and Pitcock 1967.
[93] Moore and Lattes 1959.

M-8042/3
T 162.2

7. Small cell carcinoma
(oat cell carcinoma) (WHO) [81]

**General
Remarks**

Incidence: About 10% of all malignant lung tumors are small cell carcinomas.
Age: The peak age is the 5th and 6th decades.
Sex: The great majority of patients are males.
Site: The majority of the tumors grow in the main bronchi.
Further notes: The overwhelming majority of the patients are smokers [69].

Macroscopy

The tumor diffusely thickens the wall of the bronchus, in most instances with only discrete narrowing of the lumen. The whitish, soft tumor mass extends into the surrounding pulmonary parenchyma and is disseminated along the lymphatics underneath the bronchial mucosa.
Often this covering mucosa is nonulcerated.

**Histology
M-8042/3**

a) The majority of small cell carcinoma are of the
"oat cell type" (lymphocyte-like type) (WHO):
These tumor cells are characterized by very hyperchromatic nuclei surrounded by a very sparse, barely visible cytoplasm (Figs. 721 to 724).
Although necroses are relatively rare, these tumor cells are easily deformed by the preparative technical histological procedure (Figs. 725 and 726).

The tumor cells, however, can take different shapes:

b) In some instances the tumor is composed of spindle-shaped cells

M-8043/3
Small cell carcinoma, fusiform cell type (WHO) (Figs. 727 to 729).

c) In other instances the tumor cells are polygonal, with marked nuclear atypias. The nuclei have a nucleolus and are less hyperchromatic than in the lymphocyte-like type.
This variety of small cell carcinoma is called
Small cell carcinoma, polygonal cell type (WHO) [62, 141] (Fig. 730).

d) Occasionally, the tumor cells of a small cell carcinoma are oat cell-like, with zones of marked anaplasia and less hyperchromatic nuclei. These tumor cells cannot be classified in one of the above groups and are called

M-8041/3
Small cell anaplastic carcinoma (WHO) (Figs. 731 and 732).

[62] Hinson et al. 1975.
[69] Kato et al. 1969.
[81] Larsson and Zettergren 1976.
[141] Yesner et al. 1965.

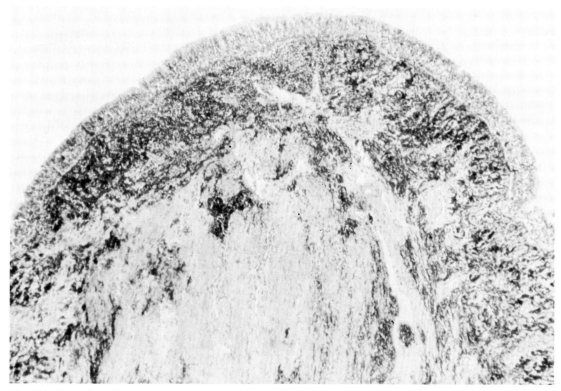

Fig. 721. Oat cell carcinoma of the bronchus growing underneath the epithelial cells by lymphatic spread (66-year-old male, ×40).

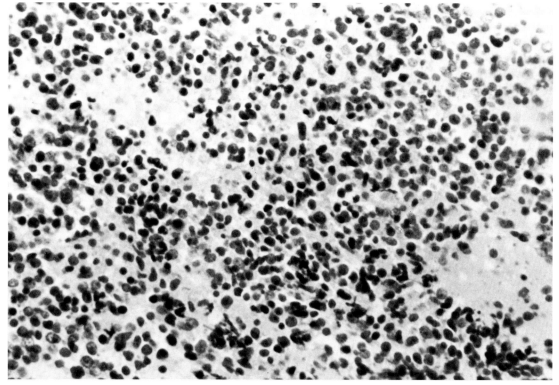

Fig. 722. Small cell carcinoma ("oat cell type") of the bronchus (67-year-old male, ×200).

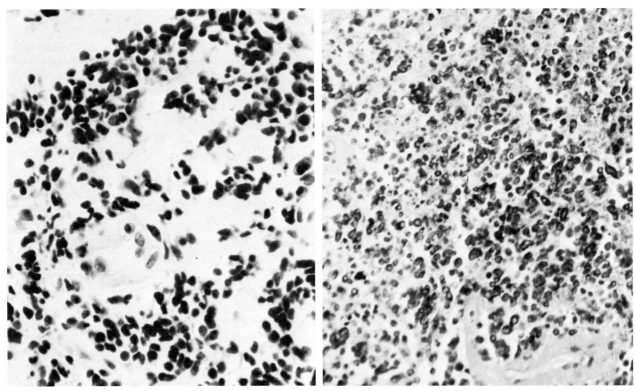

Fig. 723. Small cell carcinoma ("oat cell type") of the bronchus (66-year-old male, ×310).

Fig. 724. Small cell carcinoma ("oat cell type") of the bronchus (43-year-old male, ×200).

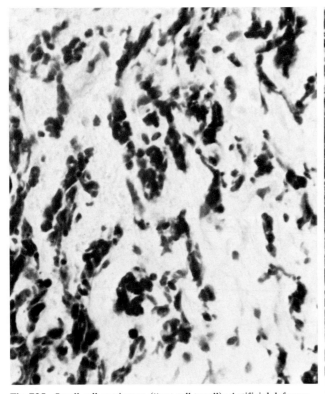

Fig. 725. Small cell carcinoma ("oat cell type"): Artificial deformation of tumor cells (66-year-old male, ×310).

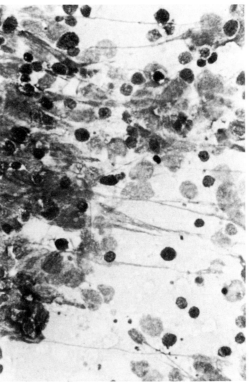

Fig. 726. Small cell anaplastic carcinoma: Destruction of the cells and nuclei by the smear procedure (lymph node biopsy, ×400).

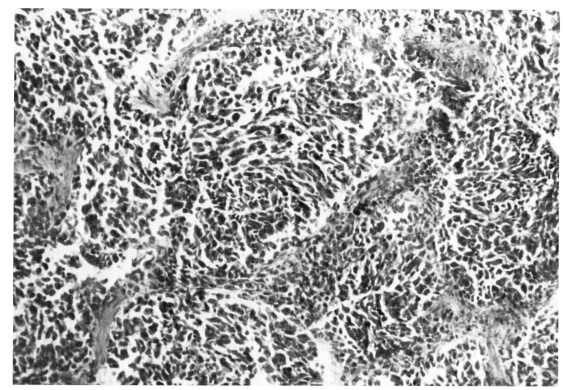

Fig. 727. Small cell carcinoma, fusiform cell type (× 125).

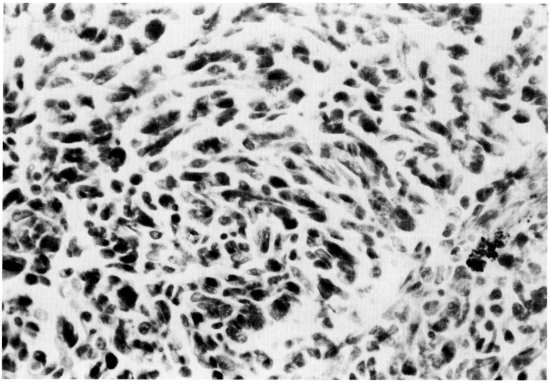

Fig. 728. Small cell carcinoma, fusiform cell type (× 310).

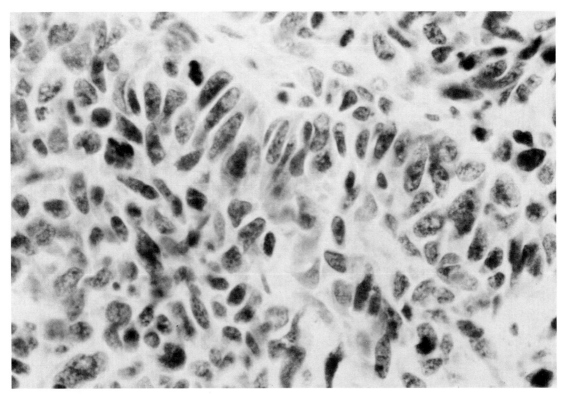

Fig. 729. Small cell carcinoma, fusiform cell type (× 600).

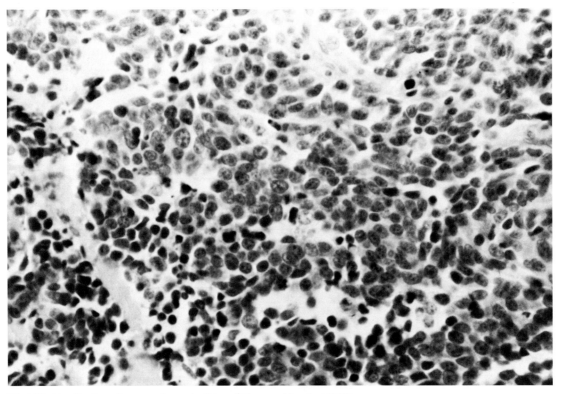

Fig. 730. Small cell carcinoma, polygonal cell type (60-year-old male, × 310).

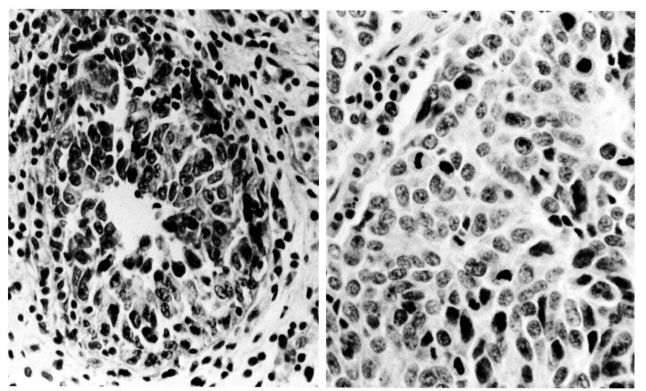

Fig. 731. Small cell anaplastic carcinoma (60-year-old male, ×310).

Fig. 732. Small cell anaplastic carcinoma (60-year-old male, ×310).

Small cell carcinoma

**Differential
Diagnosis**

1. Small cell carcinoma **with poorly differentiated squamous cell carcinoma** (Figs. 686 and 687):

   The separation of these two tumors might be very difficult, especially in cases of fusiform or polygonal cell types of small cell carcinoma [141].

   Occasionally, it might be helpful to use the ultrastructural particularities of squamous cell carcinoma with evidence of tonofibrils.

2. Small cell carcinoma **with bronchial carcinoid** (Figs. 715 to 717):

   Occasionally transitions between both tumors have been observed, which can cause a problem when differentiating these two types.

3. Small cell carcinoma, lymphocyte-like type, **with malignant lymphoma:**

   This distinction can be very difficult, especially in metastatic lesions of the "oat cell" carcinoma.

Spread

1. Early spread into the surrounding tissue with invasion of the lymphatics.
2. Early lymph node metastases.
3. Early hematogenous metastases into adrenal, bone, brain, kidney, liver, bone marrow, and other organs [64].
4. Rarely, the tumor can disseminate by transbronchial spread.

**Clinical
Findings**

1. The symptoms are determined by the extension of the disease.

   Symptoms due to local tumor growth and symptoms due to systemic tumor disease: Hemoptysis, signs of pulmonary inflammation, loss of weight, anorexia, weakness.

2. Oat cell carcinomas occasionally can develop **paraneoplastic syndromes:**
   - Cushing's syndrome,
   - hypernatremia,
   - carcinoid syndrome,
   - gynecomastia,
   - neuropathic and myopathic syndromes,
   - hyperpigmentation (MSH production),
   - hypocalcemia (calcitonin production).

   Occasionally these tumors produce multiple hormones:

   For instance, ADH, ACTH, and beta-MSH [63] (see also Introduction to lung tumors, page 684, and Islet cell tumors, page 424).

Treatment

Surgery:
Due to early lymphatic spread and metastases, the majority of the tumors are unresectable at the time of diagnosis [101].

Radiation therapy:
The cells of small cell carcinomas are radiosensitive:
Radiation therapy reduces the tumor size considerably if applied first.
It seems that the lymphocyte-like cell type of small cell carcinoma is particularly sensitive to radiation therapy.

---

[63] Hirata et al. 1976.
[64] Hirsch et al. 1977.
[101] Rilke et al. 1979.
[141] Yesner et al. 1965.

Treatment

The irradiation of inoperable tumors can be given in split courses [6]: About 50 Gy has been recommended [102].

Because of frequent brain metastases, a prophylactic brain irradiation is hoped to be of benefit [94].

Chemotherapy:

a) It is doubtful if postoperative adjuvant chemotherapy is of benefit for the patient [112].

b) Polychemotherapy has been recommended, for instance, a 4-drug treatment combining cell cycle-nonspecific with cell cycle-specific agents (combination of alkylating agents and antimetabolites).

It has been reported that the combination of cyclophosphamide, methotrexate, vincristine, and bleomycin is not superior to the combination of vincristine and bleomycin; cyclophosphamide and methotrexate; or cyclophosphamide and methotrexate as single agents [106].

c) It has been recommended to start treatment with chemotherapy before initiating radiation therapy so as to observe the responsiveness of the individual tumor [48].

Combination of radiation therapy and chemotherapy:

This combination of treatment procedures has been used [1, 66].

However, it seems that the survival prolongation is minimal [138].

Adjuvant chemotherapy [82] seems to be ineffective.

Nonspecific immunotherapy:

Nonspecific immunotherapy seems to be of no benefit [61, 65].

Generally, small cell carcinoma responds rapidly (within 6 to 12 weeks) to treatment [33].

Prognosis

Very poor, due to extensive metastases.

The overall 5-year survival rate is 1% [69].

Further Information

1. Several observations support the suggestion that the Kulchitzky neuroendocrine cell is the origin of the small cell carcinoma [18, 56], a hypothesis that is not shared by other specialists [49].

2. In a few cases it was possible to extract from undifferentiated carcinomas (some of the small cell variety) catecholamine, vanilylmandelic acid, and 5-hydroxy-3-indole acetic acid [50].

[1] Abeloff et al. 1976.
[6] Aristizabal and Caldwell 1976.
[18] Bensch et al. 1968.
[33] Cohen 1978.
[48] Gilby et al. 1977.
[49] Godwin and Brown 1977.
[50] Gould and Chejfec 1978.
[56] Hattori et al. 1972.
[61] Herberman et al. 1979.

[65] Holoye et al. 1978.
[66] Hornback et al. 1976.
[69] Kato et al. 1969.
[82] Legha and Muggia 1979.
[94] Moore et al. 1978.
[102] Salazar et al. 1976.
[106] Schaerer et al. 1977.
[112] Shields et al. 1977.
[138] Wittes et al. 1977.

M-8980/3
T 162.9

8. Carcinosarcoma (WHO)

Carcinosarcomas are rare.

The tumor is composed of malignant mesenchymal and epithelial cells.

The epithelial cells can grow as small cell carcinoma; more often they are squamous carcinomas.

The sarcomatous component can be a fibrosarcoma, poorly differentiated, or osteosarcoma [85] (see also Figs. 1361 to 1364).

Most of the carcinosarcomas grow in the central bronchi and occlude the lumen by polypoid masses.

Distant metastases occur; however, it might be that in some cases the prognosis is better than in bronchogenic carcinomas [20, 85]

M-8981/3
T 162.9

9. Carcinosarcoma of embryonal type (WHO)
(pulmonary blastoma; malignant mixed tumor in adults) [89]

This tumor usually grows in the periphery of the bronchus.

The tumor is composed of malignant epithelial cells growing in a glandular pattern (Fig. 733).

The tumor seems to have a better prognosis than the carcinosarcoma [118]. Some pulmonary blastomas behaved as a benign tumor after removal.

The mesenchymal part, in which the epithelial cells are embedded, consists of embryonal-looking loose mesenchyma.

The mesenchyma might contain areas with smooth muscle fibers or well-differentiated fibrous tissue.

[20] Bergmann et al. 1951.
[85] Ludwigsen 1977.
[89] Marsden and Scholtz 1976.
[118] Stackhouse et al. 1969.

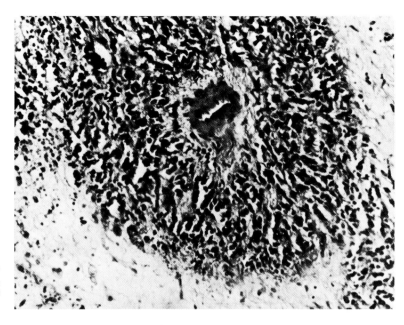

Fig. 733. Pulmonary blastoma with epithelial clefts in tumor aggregates (× 200) (Marsden and Scholz, Virchows Arch. A Path. Anat. and Histol. *372* (1976) 161-165)

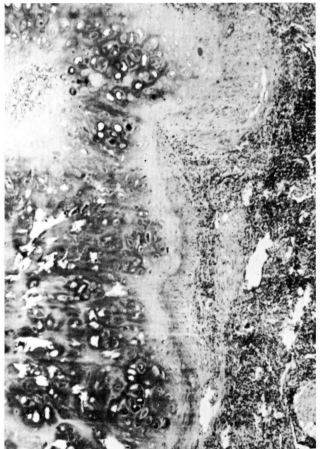

Fig. 734. Pulmonary hamartoma: Cartilage, adjacent pulmonary tissue (68-year-old male, × 50).

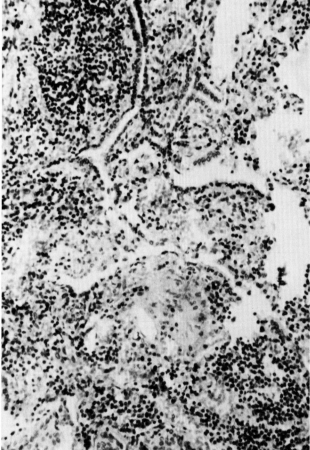

Fig. 735. Pulmonary hamartoma: Lining of spaces by respiratory epithelium (68-year-old male, × 125).

M-9351/0
T 162.9

10. Hamartoma (WHO)

**General
Remarks**

Incidence: This is a rare lesion.
Age: The lesion is mostly found in adult patients.
Site: The site is often subpleural.

Macroscopy

This is usually a small, lobulated, firm, sharply demarcated tumor. The cut surface is cartilagenous.
The tumor can grow into the lumen of a bronchus.

Histology

The tumor is composed of cartilage that can be calcified.
Other areas contain fat cells, spaces lined by epithelial cells (respiratory cells), or smooth muscle fibers (Figs. 734 and 735).

**Differential
Diagnosis**

Rarely, **highly differentiated metastases of a testicular tumor** can mimic hamartomas.

Treatment

The lesion can be resected, which means cure.

**Further
Information**

1. Very rarely hamartomas can consist of **multiple pulmonary leiomyomas** [114].
   There is a report of a hamartoma with rhabdomyomatous dysplasia in a 4-month-old child [100].

M-8832/0
T 162.9

2. **Sclerosing hemangioma of the lung**
   This lesion consists of numerous blood vessels that grow in connective tissue. This connective tissue is arranged in papillary formations, which are covered by atypical epithelial cells.
   In the tumor histiocytes with hemosiderin and a xanthomatous appearance may be observed.
   This is a benign lesion, which clinically can present with hemoptysis [71].

---

[71] Kennedy 1973.
[100] Remberger and Hübner 1974.
[114] Silverman and Kay 1976.

11. Lymphocytoma of the lung (WHO)

This lesion consists of numerous lymphocytes, which can form follicles.
The lesion is considered to be hyperplasia of the lymphatic tissue.
Occasionally giant cells are observed.
The tumor forms large foci that seem to extend into the pulmonary parenchyma, occasionally giving the impression of infiltration (Figs. 736 and 737).
This lymphatic hyperplasia most probably originates in the wall of the bronchi [3, 25, 60, 104].

12. Malignant lymphoma

Malignant non-Hodgkin's lymphomas and Hodgkin's disease can be observed as primary lesions of the lung.
More often, however, the lung is involved while the disease disseminates.
Occasionally, the differential diagnosis between malignant lymphoma and lymphocytoma of the lung is required.
The appearance of follicles indicates the benign lesion [104]; furthermore, the regional lymph nodes are not involved in cases of lymphocytoma.

Rarely **pulmonary plasmacytomas** have been found; occasionally they produce paraproteins [14, 136].

[3] Albertini 1955.
[14] Baroni et al. 1977.
[25] Cain and Kraus 1975.
[60] Heine 1957.
[104] Saltzstein 1963.
[136] Wile et al. 1976.

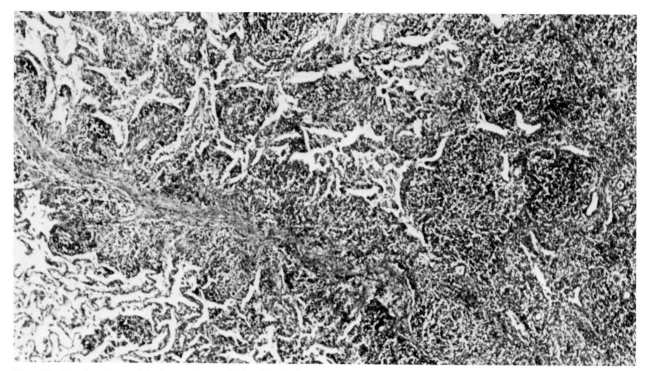

Fig. 736. Lymphocytoma of the lung (65-year-old female, × 50).

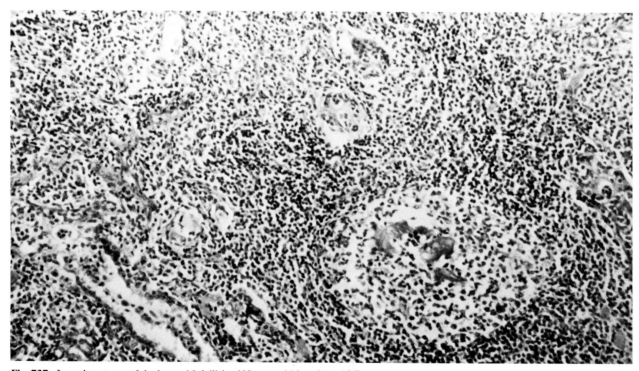

Fig. 737. Lymphocytoma of the lung with follicles (65-year-old female, × 125).

M-8000/6
T 162.9

13. Pulmonary metastases

1. Numerous malignant tumors disseminate into the lung and grow as solitary or multiple metastatic nodules (Fig. 738).
2. The disseminating tumor cells can involve the bronchus by lymphatic spread and occasionally mimic a primary bronchogenic carcinoma.
3. Resection of solitary pulmonary metastases has been recommended [54].

   This **surgical removal** of tumors should be attempted only if the metastasis develops 5 years after the resection of the primary tumor.

   Furthermore, the metastatic lesion should reveal a well-differentiated malignant tumor, originating (for instance) from
   - a malignant teratoma of the testes,
   - carcinoma of the colon (Fig. 739),
   - sarcomas [43],
   - osteosarcoma [41],
   - renal cell carcinoma [70].

   It seems that this procedure might prolong life. The 5-year survival rate has been indicated as 25.8% [87].

   Even cures have been reportet [129]. Other reports indicate that recurrent metastasizing gastric leiomyoblastomas [123] and metastases from an acinic cell carcinoma of the parotid gland have been successfully resected [113].
4. **Resection of metastatic lesions in other organs** has also been attempted: Liver, bone, brain, skin, lymph nodes. About 20% of these patients survived 5 years after resection of the metastases [58, 67].

[41] Dunn and Dehner 1977.
[43] Feldman and Kyriakos 1972.
[54] Habein Jr. et al. 1959.
[58] Hegemann and Mühe 1974.
[67] Huang et al. 1978.
[70] Katzenstein et al. 1978.
[87] Mack et al. 1976.
[113] Sidhu and Forrester 1977.
[123] Tisell et al. 1978.
[129] Vidne et al. 1976.

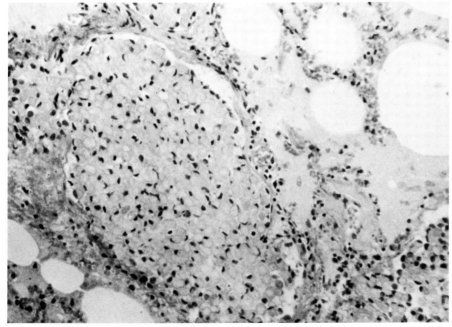

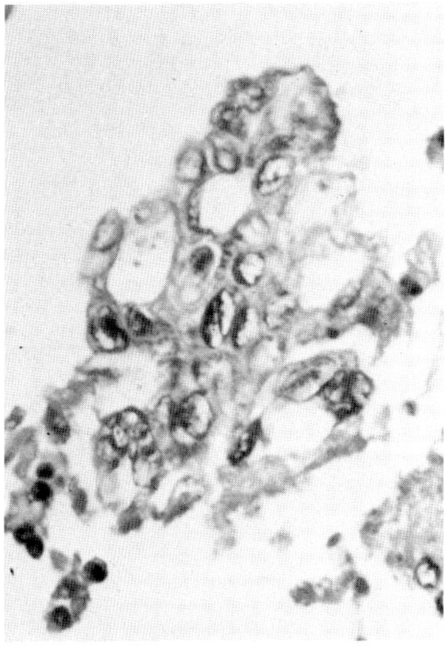

Fig. 739. Bronchial washing: Cells of a metastatic adenocarcinoma of the colon in the lung (× 200).

Fig. 738. Metastasis of signet ring cell carcinoma of the stomach in the lung (× 125).

T 162.9

14. Benign soft tissue tumors of the lung

Infrequently, soft tissue tumors can arise in the lung (page 7).
These diseases can affect younger patients much more than cancer of the lung.

M-8810/0

a) Fibroma
About 10% of the benign pulmonary tumors are fibromas (Figs. 740 and 741).
If the tumor is resected, the patient is cured [68].

M-9120/0
M-9150/0

b) Hemangioma and hemangiopericytoma
These tumors have been reported. They can cause hemoptysis (Fig. 742).

Other soft tissue tumors found in the lung are

M-8840/0

c) myxomas [8],

M-8850/0

d) lipomas [37],

M-9560/0

e) neurofibromas,

M-8890/0

f) leiomyomas [122].

M-9174/1

g) Lymphangiomyomatosis
This lesion affects only women of reproductive age.
The lesion consists of multiple nodules that are composed of smooth muscle fibers (leiomyomas). They are disseminated through the parenchyma of the lung [15, 36].
Due to obstruction of bronchioles, emphysematous lesions develop.
A corresponding lymphangiomyomatosis develops also in abdominal and thoracic lymph nodes.
It is debated whether this lymphangiomyomatosis represents a form fruste of tuberous sclerosis [36].

[8] Ashley 1978.
[15] Basset et al. 1976.
[36] Corrin et al. 1975.
[37] Crutcher et al. 1968.
[68] Justich et al. 1976.
[122] Taylor and Miller 1969.

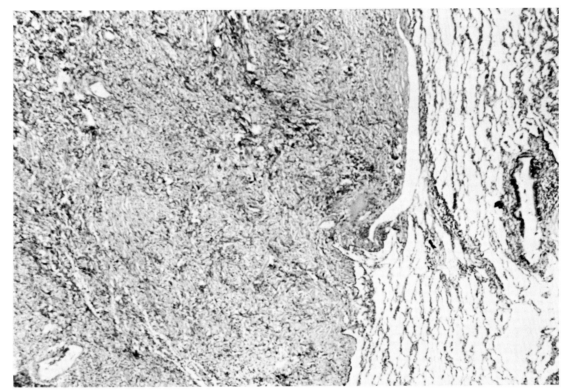

Fig. 740. Pulmonary fibroma (×40).

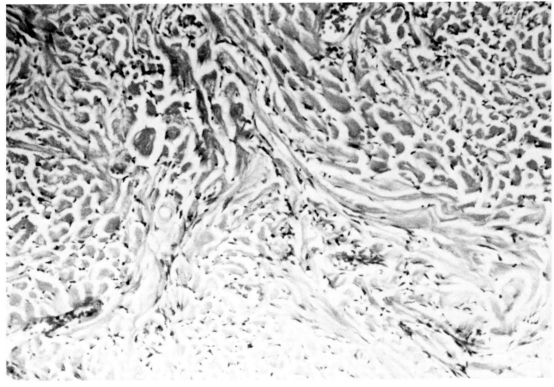

Fig. 741. Pulmonary fibroma (×125).

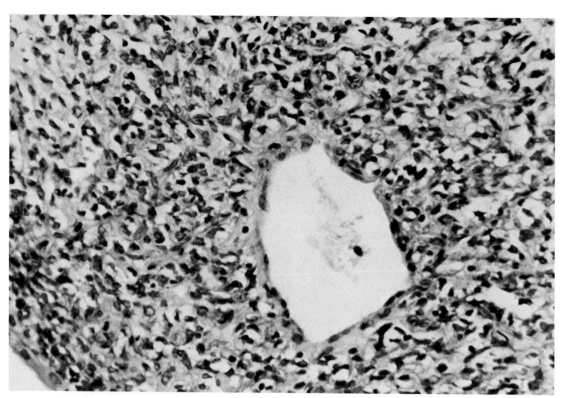

Fig. 742. Hemangiopericytoma of the lung (62-year-old female, death by hemoptysis, × 250).

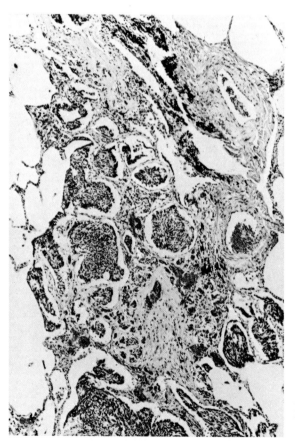

Fig. 743. Chemodectoma: Tumorlet nest near an arterial branch (× 60) (Churg and Warnock, Cancer *37* (1976) 1469-1477).

T 162.9

15. Malignant soft tissue tumors of the lung

These tumors have rarely been reported [2]:

M-8890/3

a) **Leiomyosarcoma** was observed in one case in a 14-month-old boy [98];

M-8810/3

b) **Fibrosarcoma;**

M-8900/3

c) **Rhabdomyosarcoma** including sarcoma botryoides [53, 126];

M-9220/3

d) **Chondrosarcoma;**

e) **Primary sarcoma of the vascular intima** has been observed in one case [5].

M-8693/1
T 162.9

16. Chemodectoma (WHO) [22]

This lesion is composed of chemoreceptor cells.
This lesion (tumorlets) is without clinical significance [74].
The ultrastructure of the cells, however, resembles meningioma cells, not paraganglioma cells [30] (Fig. 743).

M-8040/0
T 162.9

Other authors claim that these cells correspond to carcinoid tumors:
Bronchial carcinoidtumorlet type [31, 99].

[2] Ackerman and Rosai 1974.
[5] Altman and Shelley 1973.
[22] Blessing et al. 1973.
[30] Churg and Warnock 1976.
[31] Churg and Warnock 1976.
[53] Grouls and Helpap 1976.
[74] Korn et al. 1960.
[98] Ownly et al. 1976.
[99] Ranchod 1977.
[126] Ueda et al. 1977.

M-8693/1
T 162.9

17. Tumors resembling nonchromaffin paraganglioma

These tumors are very rare [115].
Clinically they do not show any symptoms.
On electron microscopy, the tumor cells contain neurosecretory granules [115].

M-8720/3
T 162.9

18. Malignant melanoma (see page 1222)

M-9100/3
T 162.9

19. Choriocarcinoma

Exceptionally, primary choriocarcinoma can develop in the pulmonary parenchyma [57].

M-8000/3
T 162.9

20. Unclassified tumors (WHO)

Occasionally tumors grow in such a way that the histological picture does not permit any classification.

---

[57] Hayakawa et al. 1977.
[115] Singh et al. 1977.

M-9050/1
T 163.9

21. Pleural mesothelioma (WHO)

General
Remarks

Incidence: The incidence of pleural mesotheliomas is low.
Further notes: This tumor is usually associated with asbestosis [13, 47, 55, 133].

Macroscopy

Mesotheliomas grow as localized or diffuse tumors.

M-9051/0

a) Benign fibrous mesothelioma:
Circumscribed, encapsulated mesothelioma on the surface of the lung.
The cut surface of these benign fibrous mesotheliomas shows whorls with mostly small cysts.
The cut surface is yellowish.

M-9051/3

b) Malignant fibrous mesothelioma:
This tumor grows diffusely and covers the surface of the lung. The tumor is nonencapsulated.

M-9052/1, 3

c) Malignant epithelioid mesothelioma:
This tumor grows diffusely, covering the surface of the lung. The thickened pleura contains nodules that are whitish on the cut surface (Fig. 744).

Histology

a) Benign fibrous mesothelioma (WHO) [96, 107]:
The tumor is dominated by collagen fibers that form interlacing bundles. Occasionally the tumor contains very few cells; occasionally it contains numerous cells.
Foci of epithelial cells are disseminated among the collagen fibers. These cells grow in a tubular pattern or form small nests.
This benign mesothelioma develops from mesothelial cells [97] (Figs. 745 to 749).

b) Malignant fibrous mesothelioma (WHO):
The tumor is dominated by collagen fibers. However, numerous cells are present. The high cellularity already indicates the malignant potential of this tumor.
One can detect in these cells multiple mitotic figures and signs of malignant nuclei (Figs. 750 to 754).

c) Malignant epithelioid mesothelioma (WHO):
This tumor contains numerous epithelial cells that grow in different patterns: They form nests, papillary structures, tubuli, and glandular formations.
Mitotic figures are observed, and signs of nuclear malignancy are present.
The cytoplasm of the cells is acidophilic.
The cells are embedded in connective tissue; however, it is less well developed than in the previously mentioned forms of mesothelioma (Figs. 755 to 759).
Occasionally the tumor cells contain mucinous substances (positive stain with PAS and mucicarmine) [128].

[13] Baris 1975.
[47] Giese 1960.
[55] Hain et al. 1974.
[96] Okike et al. 1978.
[97] Osamura 1977.
[107] Scharifker and Kaneko 1979.
[133] Wagner et al. 1960.

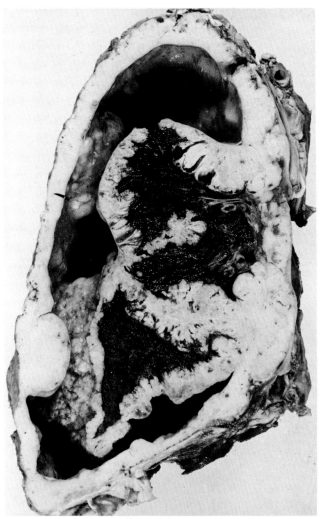

Fig. 744. Malignant epithelioid mesothelioma of the pleura: White tumor tissue compressing the lung parenchyma (56-year-old male).

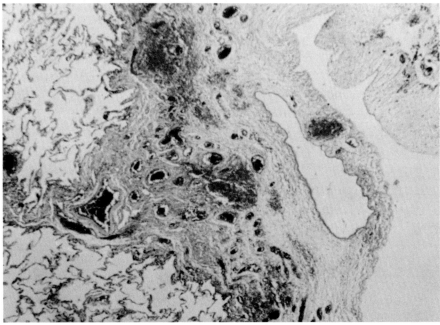

Fig. 745. Benign fibrous mesothelioma of the pleura: Angiomatous areas (×40).

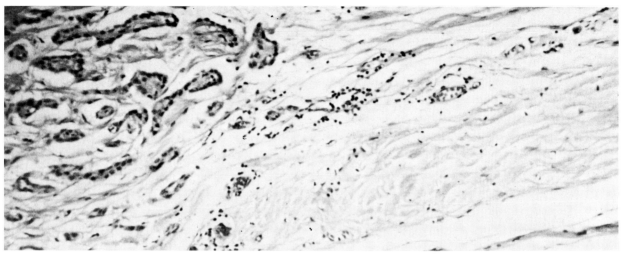

Fig. 746. Benign fibrous mesothelioma of the pleura: Nests of proliferating mesothelial cells (× 125).

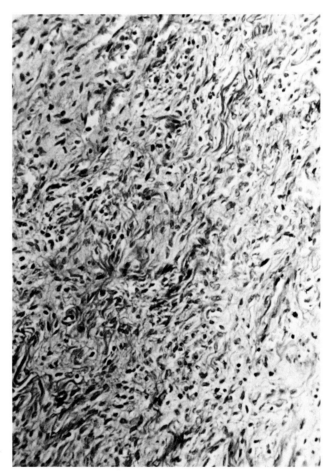

Fig. 747. Benign fibrous mesothelioma of the pleura: Area of interlacing collagen bundles, regular nuclei (× 200).

741

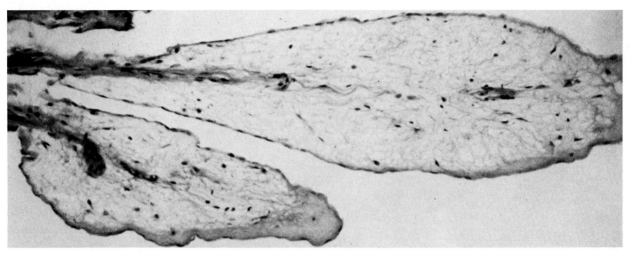

Fig. 748. Benign fibrous mesothelioma of the pleura, papillary form (× 50).

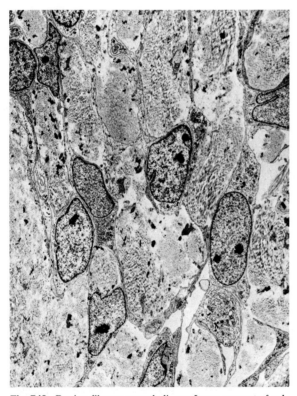

Fig. 749. Benign fibrous mesothelioma: Large amount of collagen fibers in the cytoplasm of tumor cells (× 4000) (Osamura, Cancer *39* (1977) 139-142).

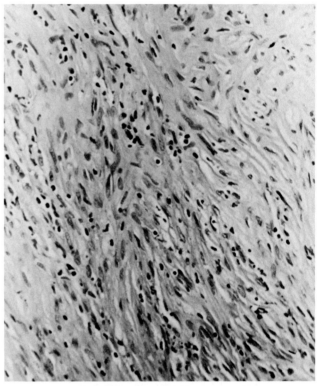

Fig. 750. Malignant fibrous mesothelioma of the pleura: High cellularity, atypical nuclei (58-year-old male, previous exposure to asbestos, × 125).

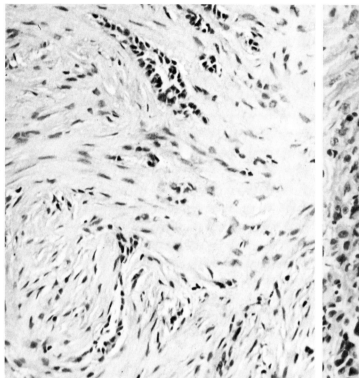

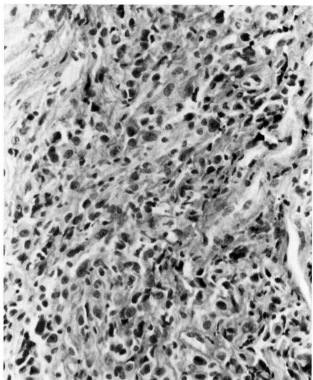

Fig. 751. Malignant fibrous mesothelioma of the pleura: Nests of epithelial cells (67-year-old male, previous exposure to asbestos, ×125).

Fig. 752. Malignant fibrous mesothelioma of the pleura: High cellularity and nuclear atypias (58-year-old male, ×200).

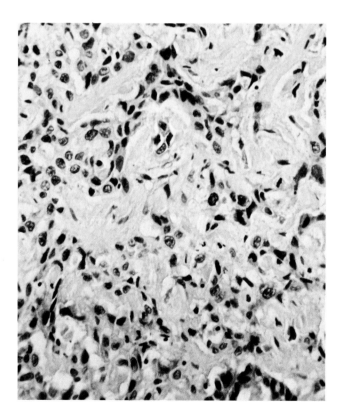

Fig. 753. Malignant fibrous mesothelioma of the pleura: Collagen bundles and small nests of very atypical (epithelial) cells (81-year-old male, ×200).

743

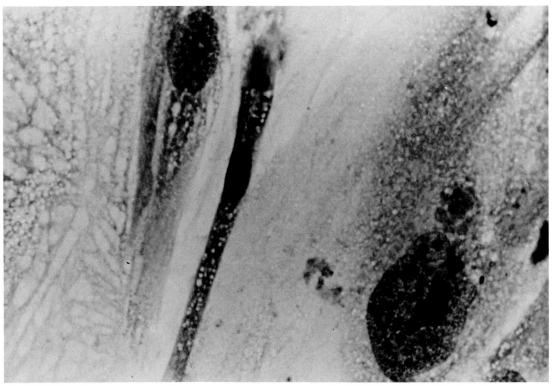

Fig. 754. Large nuclei in mesothelial cells after 15 days of tissue culture, mimicking malignant growth (× 600).

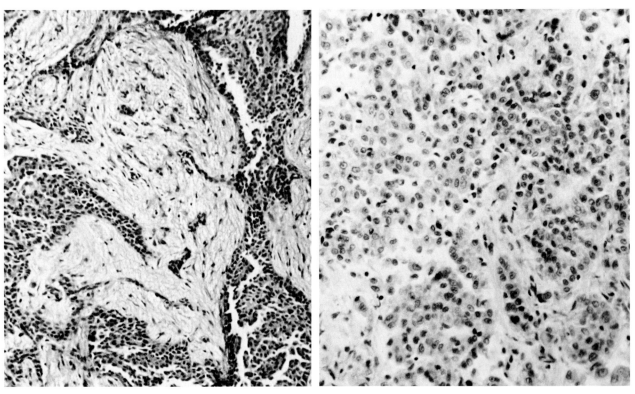

Fig. 755.

Fig. 756.

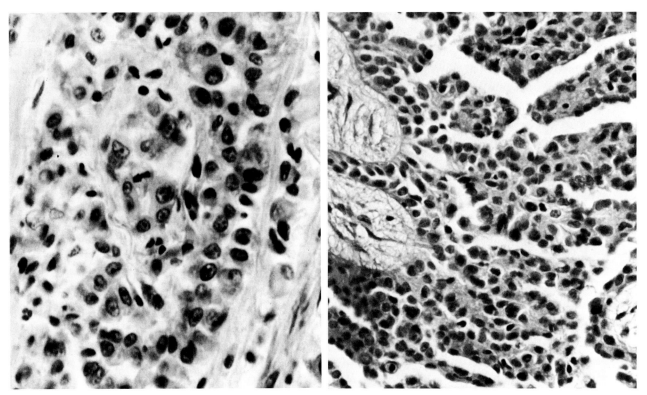

Fig. 757. Malignant epithelioid mesothelioma of the pleura (55-year-old male, × 400).

Fig. 758. Malignant epithelioid mesothelioma of the pleura (67-year-old male, previous exposure to asbestos, × 300).

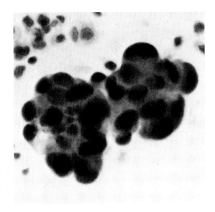

Fig. 759. Pleural mesothelioma: Tumor cells with hyperchromatic nuclei of a rather uniform shape, mulberry-shaped cluster formation by the tumor cells (Papanicolaou's stain, × 400).

◁
Fig. 755. Malignant epithelioid mesothelioma of the pleura: Large nests of epithelial cells separated by loose connective tissue (67-year-old male, × 125).

Fig. 756. Malignant epithelioid mesothelioma of the pleura (55-year-old male, previous exposure to asbestos, × 200).

745

Differential Diagnosis

1. **Malignant mesothelioma with benign mesothelioma:**
   Benign mesotheliomas in most instances are localized.
   - Benign epithelial mesotheliomas are extremely rare.
   - Cellularity and signs of cellular atypias indicate the presence of a malignant mesothelioma.
2. Malignant mesothelioma **with bronchioloalveolar carcinoma** (Figs. 705 to 708).
3. Malignant mesothelioma **with metastatic tumor.**

Spread

1. The tumor extends into the surface of the lung, involving visceral and parietal pleura. Growth can reach the peritoneum and involve the superficial part of the lung.
2. Metastases are relatively rare and might involve lymph nodes.
3. Distant metastases can occur; again, they are rare.
   In cases of distant metastases the growth pattern of mesothelioma becomes less clear, and the recognition of a metastasizing pleural mesothelioma might become difficult.

Clinical Findings

Dyspnea, cough, chest pain.

Treatment

Surgery:
Circumscribed tumors are resectable [73, 134].
In cases of resectable tumors: The resection should include parts of the thoracic wall.
Radiation therapy:
Recommended is the megavoltage therapy for palliation.
Chemotherapy:
Chemotherapy alone or in combination with radiation therapy can be attempted, occasionally combined with pleurectomy.
Treatment with cyclophosphamide, vincristine, methotrexate, and 5-fluorouracil or adriamycin alone has been tried [28, 78, 117, 140].

Prognosis

The prognosis is poor, especially for the epithelial malignant mesothelioma, while the fibrosarcomatous type (malignant fibrous mesothelioma) seems to allow longer survival after resection of the tumor [134].

[28] Chahinian and Holland 1978.
[73] Klima and Gyorkey 1977.
[78] Kuguksu et al. 1976.
[117] Spremulli et al. 1977.
[128] Uys 1979.
[134] Wanebo et al. 1976.
[140] Yap et al. 1978.

Recommendations for differential diagnosis in tumors of the lung and pleura

squamous cell carcinoma	with	– different subtypes (WHO)
poorly differentiated carcinoma	with	– squamous cell carcinoma – adenocarcinoma – small cell carcinoma
bronchioloalveolar carcinoma	with	– bronchogenic adenocarcinoma – carcinoid tumor – adenoid cystic carcinoma – metastatic tumor – metastatic pleura mesothelioma
primary bronchogenic adenocarcinoma	with	– metastatic adenocarcinoma
carcinoid tumor	with	– adenoid cystic carcinoma – small cell carcinoma – mucoepidermoid carcinoma
small cell carcinoma	with	– undifferentiated squamous cell carcinoma – undifferentiated adenocarcinoma – carcinoid tumor – metastatic tumor (neuroblastoma) – malignant lymphoma
hamartoma	with	– metastatic lesions from sarcoma – metastatic lesion from testicular teratoma
pleura mesothelioma, benign	with	– malignant pleura mesothelioma – metastatic adenocarcinoma – chronic inflammation – metastatic synovial sarcoma
malignant mesothelioma	with	– benign mesothelioma – chronic inflammation – bronchioloalveolar carcinoma – metastatic tumor

References

[1] Abeloff, M.D., D.S. Ettinger, S.B. Baylin, and T. Hazra: Management of small cell carcinoma of the lung. Therapy, staging, and biochemical markers. Cancer *38* (1976) 1394-1401.

[2] Ackerman, L.V., and J. Rosai: Surgical pathology. Fifth edition, C.V. Mosby Company 1974.

[3] Albertini, A.V.: Histologische Geschwulstdiagnostik. Thieme, Stuttgart 1955.

[4] Alberto, P., K.W. Brunner, G. Martz, J.-P. Obrecht, and R.W. Sonntag: Treatment of bronchogenic carcinoma with simultaneous or sequential combination chemotherapy, including methotrexate, cyclophosphamide, procarbazine, and vincristine. Cancer *38* (1976) 2208-2216.

[5] Altman, N.H., and W.M. Shelley: Primary intimal sarcoma of the pulmonary artery. Johns Hopkins Med. J. *133* (1973) 214-222.

[6] Aristizabal, S.A., and W.L. Caldwell: Radical irradiation with the split-course technique in carcinoma of the lung. Cancer *37* (1976) 2630-2635.

[7] Arrigoni, M.G., L.B. Woolner, and P.E. Bernatz: Atypical carcinoid tumors of the lung. J. Thoracic Surg *64* (1972) 413-421.

[8] Ashley, D.J.B.: In: Evan's Histological appearances of tumours. Churchill Livingstone, Edinburgh–London–New York 1978.

[9] Auerbach, O., L. Garfinkel, and V.R. Parks: Scar cancer of the lung. Increase over a 21 year period. Cancer *43* (1979) 636-642.

[10] Auerbach, O., J.B. Gere, J.B. Forman, T.G. Petrick, H.J. Smolin, G.E. Muehsam, D.Y. Kassouny, and A.P. Stout: Changes in the bronchial epithelium in relation to smoking and cancer of the lung. N. Engl. J. Med. *256* (1957) 97-104.

[11] Auerbach, O., E.C. Hammond, and L. Garfinkel: Changes in bronchial epithelium in relation to cigarette smoking, 1955-1960, VS. 1970-1977. N. Engl. J. Med. *300* (1979) 381-386.

[12] Baker, R.R., W.C. Ball, D. Carter, J.K. Frost, B.R. Marsh, F.P. Stitik, and M.S. Tockman: Identification and treatment of clinically occult cancer of the lung. In: Lung cancer: Progress in therapeutic research. Raven Press, New York 1979.

[13] Baris, Y.I.: Pleural mesotheliomas and asbestos pleurisies due to environmental exposure in Turkey: An analysis of 120 cases. Hacettepe Bull. Med. Surg. *8* (1975) 165-185.

[14] Baroni, C.D., T.C. Mineo, C. Ricci, S. Guarino, and F. Mandelli: Solitary secretory plasmocytoma of the lung in a 14-year-old boy. Cancer *40* (1977) 2329-2332.

[15] Basset, F., P. Soler, J. Marsac, and B. Corrin: Pulmonary lymphangiomyomatosis: Three new cases studied with electron microscopy. Cancer *38* (1976) 2357-2366.

[16] Becker, N.H., and J. Soifer: Benign clear cell tumor („sugar tumor"). of the lung. Cancer *27* (1971) 712-719.

[17] Bensch, K.G., D.S. Bonikos, and P.E. Hockberger: Pulmonary carcinoid tumors in tissue and organ culture. Cancer *38* (1976) 2006-2016.

[18] Bensch K.G., B. Corrin, R. Pariente, and H. Spencer: Oat-cell carcinoma of the lung; its origin and relationship to bronchial carcinoid. Cancer *22* (1968) 1163-1172.

[19] Bensch, K.G., G.B. Gordon, and L.R. Miller: Electron microscopic and biochemical studies of the bronchial carcinoid tumor. Cancer *18* (1965) 592-602.

[20] Bergmann, M., L.V. Ackerman, and R.L. Kemler: Carcinosarcoma of the lung; review of the literature and report of two cases treated by pneumonectomy. Cancer *4* (1951) 919-929.

[21] Bitran, J.C., R.K. Desser, T. DeMeester, and H.M. Golomb: Metastatic non-oat-cell. bronchogenic carcinoma. Therapy with cyclophosphamide, doxorubicin, methotrexate, and procarbazine (CAMP). JAMA *240* (1978) 2743-2746.

[22] Blessing, M.H., F. Borchard und W. Lenz: Glomustumor (sog. Chemodektom) der Lunge. Pathologisch-anatomische und biochemische Befunde. Virchows Arch. A. Path. Anat. and Histol. *359* (1973) 315-329.

[23] Bonikos, D.S., K.G. Bensch, and R.W. Jamplis: Peripheral pulmonary carcinoid tumors. Cancer *37* (1976) 1977-1998.

[24] Byrd, R.B., W.E. Miller, D.T. Carr, W.S. Payne, and L.B. Woolner: The roentgenographic appearance of large cell carcinoma of the bronchus. Mayo Clin. Proc. *43* (1968) 333-336.

[25] Cain, H., und B. Kraus: Das Lymphocytom der Lunge. Fragen zu Ätiologie, Pathogenese, Differentialdiagnose und Dignität. Virchows Arch. A Path. Anat. and Histol. *365* (1975) 41-62.

[26] Capella, C., M. Gabrielli, J.M. Polak, R. Buffa, E. Solcia, and C. Bordi: Ultrastructural and histological study of 11 bronchial carcinoids. Evidence for different types. Virchows. Arch. A Path. Anat. and Histol. *381* (1979) 313-329.

[27] Carter, D., B.R. Marsh, R.R. Baker, Y.S. Erozan, and J.K. Frost: Relationships of morphology to clinical presentation in ten cases of early squamous cell carcinoma of the lung. Cancer *37* (1976) 1389-1396.

[28] Chahinian, A.P., and J.F. Holland: Treatment of diffuse malignant mesothelioma: A review. Mt. Sinai J. Med. NY *45* (1978) 54-67.

[29] Churg, A.: The fine structure of large cell undifferentiated carcinoma of the lung. Evidence for its relation to squamous cell carcinomas

and adenocarcinomas. Hum. Pathol. *9* (1978) 143-156.

[30] Churg, A., and M.L. Warnock: Pulmonary tumorlet. A form of peripheral carcinoid. Cancer *37* (1976) 1469-1477.

[31] Churg, A.M., and M.L. Warnock: So-called "minute pulmonary chemodectoma". A tumor not related to paragangliomas. Cancer *37* (1976) 1759-1769.

[32] Clara, M.: Zur Histobiologie des Bronchialepithels. Z. Mikrosk. Anat. Fschg. *41* (1937) 321-347.

[33] Cohen, M.H.: Lung cancer: Prognostic factors and adjuvant therapy results. In: Immunotherapy of cancer: Present status of trials in man. Edited by W.D. Terry and D. Windhorst. Raven Press, New York 1978.

[34] Cohen, M.H., and O.S. Selawry: Bronchogenic carcinoma: Prognostic factors and criteria of response. In: Cancer therapy: Prognostic factors and criteria of response. Edited by M.J. Staquet, Raven Press, New York 1975.

[35] Cohen, R.B., G.D. Toll, and B. Castleman: Bronchial adenomas and Cushing's syndrome; their relation to thymomas and oat cell carcinomas associated with hyperadrenocorticism. Cancer *13* (1960) 812-817.

[36] Corrin, B., A.A. Liebow, and P.J. Friedman: Pulmonale lymphangiomyomatose. Am. J. Path. *79* (1975) 348-382.

[37] Crutcher, R.R., T.L. Waltuch, and A.K. Ghosh: Bronchial lipoma. J. Thoracic Surg. *55* (1968) 422-425.

[38] Dent, P.B., P.B. McCulloch, O. Wesley-James, R. Mac Laren, W. Muirhead, and C.W. Dunnett: Measurement of carcinoembryonic antigen in patients with bronchogenic carcinoma. Cancer *42* (1978) 1484-1491.

[39] Dionne, G.P., and N.-S. Wang: A scanning electron microscopic study of diffuse mesothelioma and some lung carcinomas. Cancer *40* (1977) 707-715.

[40] Djerassi, I., J.S. Kim, N.P. Nayak, H. Ohanissian, and S. Adler: High-dose methotrexate with citrovorum factor rescue: A new approach to cancer chemotherapy. In: Recent advances in cancer treatment. Ed. by H.J. Tagnon and M.J. Staquet. Raven Press, New York 1977.

[41] Dunn, D., and L.P. Dehner: Metastatic osteosarcoma to lung. A clinicopathologic study of surgical biopsies and resections. Cancer *40* (1977) 3054-3064.

[42] Fechner, R.E., and B.R. Bentinck: Ultrastructure of bronchial oncocytoma. Cancer *31* (1973) 1451-1457.

[43] Feldman, P.S., and M. Kyriakos: Pulmonary resection for metastatic sarcoma. J. Thoracic Surg. *64* (1972) 784-799.

[44] Fetzer, J., D. Fullenbach und H. Gabel (Hrsg.): Solide Tumoren, Hämoblastosen. In: Adriamycin. Kehrer Offset Kg, 1977.

[45] Feyrter, F.: Über das Bronchuscarcinoid. Virchows Arch. Pathol. Anat. *332* (1959) 25-43.

[46] Gallivan, G.J., C.T. Dolan, R.E. Stam, B.S. Eggertsen Jr., and J.D. Tovey: Granular-cell myoblastoma of the bronchus. Report of a case. J. Thoracic Surg. *52* (1966) 875-881.

[47] Giese, W.: Die Atemorgane. In: Lehrbuch der speziellen pathologischen Anatomie. E. Kaufmann und M. Staemmler, II. Band, 3. Teil. Walter de Gruyter, Berlin 1960.

[48] Gilby, E.D., P.K. Bondy, R.L. Morgan, and T.J. McElwain: Combination chemotherapy for small cell carcinoma of the lung. Cancer *39* (1977) 1959-1966.

[49] Godwin, J.D., and C.C. Brown: Comparative epidemiology of carcinoid and oat-cell tumors of the lung. Cancer *40* (1977) 1671-1673.

[50] Gould, V.e., and G. Chejfec: Ultrastructural and biochemical analysis of "undifferentiated" pulmonary carcinomas. Hum. Pathol. *9* (1978) 377-384.

[51] Graham, E.A., and N.A. Womack: Problem of so-called bronchial adenoma. J. Thoracic Surg. *14* (1945) 106-119.

[52] Gropp, C., K. Haveman, and F.-G. Lehman: Carcinoembryonic antigen and ferritin in patients with lung cancer before and during therapy. Cancer *42* (1978) 2802-2808.

[53] Grouls, V., und B. Helpap: Das Rhabdomyosarkom der Lungen. Thoraxchirurgie *24* (1976) 94-97.

[54] Habein, H.C.Jr., O.T. Clagett, and J.R. McDonald: Pulmonary resection for metastatic tumors. Arch. Surg. *78* (1959) 716-723.

[55] Hain, E., P. Dalquen, H. Bohlig, A. Dabbert und I. Hinz: Katamnestische Untersuchungen zur Genese des Mesothelioms. Int. Arch. Arbeitsmed. *33* (1974) 15-37.

[56] Hattori, S., M. Matsuda, R. Tateishi, H. Nishihara, and T. Horai: Oat-cell carcinoma of the lung; clinical and morphological studies in relation to its histogenesis. Cancer *30* (1972) 1014-1024.

[57] Hayakawa, K., M. Takahashi, K. Sasaki, A. Kawaoi, T. Otsuka, and Y. Murota: Primary choriocarcinoma of the lung. Case report of two male subjekts. Acta. Path. Jap. *27* (1977) 123-135.

[58] Hegemann, G., und E. Mühe: Die Resektion von Metastasen und Rezidiven. Indikation und Ergebnisse. Dtsch. Med. Wschr. *99* (1974) 989-993.

[59] Heilmann, H.-P., E. Doppelfeld, H.-J. Fernholz, R. Birkner, H. Schlicker, G. Becker, L. Gordon-Harris, A. Hackl, W.D. Sager, F. Jentsch, W. Kraft, H. Bünemann, W. Horstmann, E. Hassenstein, H. Kuttig, C. Wieland, N. Schmidt, A. Müller, J. Quäck, L. Buchelt, F. Heß, E.A. Koop, H. von Lieven, H.G. Heinze, W. Castrup, M. Wannenmacher, G. Rey, A.-C. Voss, A. Nüse, E. Eibach, W. Grund, W. Bohndorf und G. Schindler: Ergebnisse der Strahlenbehandlung des Bronchialkarzinoms. Dtsch. Med. Wschr. *101* (1976) 1557-1562.

[60] Heine, J.: Lymphozytom der Lunge und generalisierte Plasmozytose. Zbl. Allg. Path. Anat. *96* (1957) 16-20.

[61] Herberman, R.B., J.L. Weese, R.K. Oldham, G.D. Bonnard, E. Perlin, W. Heim, C. Miller, J.

Reid, and R.J. Connor: Prospects for immunotherapy of lung cancer with specific immunoadjuvants. In: Lung cancer: Progress in therapeutic research, Raven Press, New York 1979.

[62] Hinson, K.F.W., A.B. Miller, and R. Tall: An assessment of the World Health Organization classification of the histologic typing of lung tumors applied to biopsy and resected material. Cancer *35* (1975) 399-405.

[63] Hirata, Y., S. Matsukura, H. Imura, T. Yakura, S. Ihjima, C. Nagase, and M. Itoh: Two cases of multiple hormon -producing small cell carcinoma of the lung. Coexistence of tumor ADH, ACTH and beta-MSH. Cancer *38* (1976) 2575-2582.

[64] Hirsch, F., H.H. Hansen, P. Dombernowsky, and B. Hainau: Bone-marrow examination in the staging of small-cell anaplastic carcinoma of the lung with special reference to subtyping. An evaluation of 203 consecutive patients. Cancer *39* (1977) 2563-2567.

[65] Holoye, P.Y., M.L. Samuels, T. Smith, and J.G. Sinkovics: Chemoimmunotherapy of small cell bronchogenic carcinoma. Cancer *42* (1978) 34-40.

[66] Hornback, N.B., L. Einhorn, H. Shidnia, B.T. Joe, M. Krause, and B. Furnas: Oat cell carcinoma of the lung. Early treatment results of combination radiation therapy and chemotherapy. Cancer *37* (1976) 2658-2664.

[67] Huang, M.N., F. Edgerton, H. Takita, H.O. Douglas, and C. Karahousis: Lung resection for metastatic sarcoma. Ann. J. Surg. *135* (1978) 804-806.

[68] Justich, E., G. Suppan, K.O. Schmid und G. Klepp: Intrapulmonale Fibrome. Thoraxchirurgie *24* (1976) 87-94.

[69] Kato, Y., T.B. Ferguson, D.E. Bennett, and T.H. Burford: Oat cell carcinoma of the lung. A review of 138 cases. Cancer *23* (1969) 517-524.

[70] Katzenstein, A.-L., R. Purvis Jr., J. Gmelich, and F. Askin: Pulmonary resection for metastatic renal adenocarcinoma. Pathologic findings and therapeutic value. Cancer *41* (1978) 712-723.

[71] Kennedy, A.: Sclerosing hemangioma of the lung: An alternative view of its development. J. Clin. Pathol. *26* (1973) 792-801.

[72] Kent, C.H., and J.G. Schwade: Preoperative radiation therapy in carcinoma of the lung. In: Lung cancer: Progress in therapeutic research, Raven Press, New York 1979.

[73] Klima, M., and F. Gyorkey: Benign pleural lesions and malignant mesothelioma. Virchows Arch. A. Path. Anat. and Histol. *376* (1977) 181-193.

[74] Korn, D., K. Bensch, A.A. Liebow, and B. Castleman: Multiple minute pulmonary tumors resembling chemodectomas. Am. J. Path. *37* (1960) 641-672.

[75] Krebs, B., P. Turchi, C. Bonet, M. Schneider, C.M. Lalanne, and N. Namer: Carcino-embryonic antigen assay in breast and bronchus cancers. Eur. J. Cancer *13* (1977) 375-376.

[76] Kreyberg, L., A.A. Liebow, and E.A. Uehlinger: Histological typing of lung tumours. WHO, Geneva 1967.

[77] Kroe, D.J., and J.A. Pitcock: Benign mucous gland adenoma of the bronchus. Arch. Pathol. *84* (1967) 539-542.

[78] Kuguksu, N., W. Thomas, and E.Z. Ezdinli: Chemotherapy of malignant diffuse mesothelioma. Cancer *37* (1976) 1265-1274.

[79] Kuhn, C.: Fine structure of bronchiolo-alveolar cell carcinoma. Cancer *30* (1972) 1107-1118.

[80] Lanzotti, V.J., D.R. Thomas, L.E. Boyle, T.L. Smith, E.A. Gehan, and M.L. Samuels: Survival with inoperable lung cancer. An integration of prognostic variables based in simple clinical criteria. Cancer *39* (1977) 303-313.

[81] Larsson, S., and L. Zettergren: Histological typing of lung cancer. Application of the World Health Organization classification to 479 cases. Acta. Pathol. Microbiol. Scand. Sect. A. *84* (1976) 529-537.

[82] Legha, S.S., and F.M. Muggia: Adjuvant chemotherapy in lung cancer: An appraisal of past studies. In: Lung cancer: Progress in therapeutic research. Raven Press, New York 1979.

[83] Liebow, A.A., and B. Castleman: Bening clear cell ("sugar") tumor of the lung. Yale J. Biol. Med. *43* (1971) 213-222.

[84] Livingston, R.B., L. Heilbrun, D. Lehane, J.J. Costanzi, R. Bottomley, R.L. Palmer, W.J. Stuckey, and B. Hoogstraten: Comparative trial of combination chemotherapy in extensive squamous carcinoma of the lung: A southwest oncology group study. Cancer Treat. Rep. *61* (1977) 1623-1629.

[85] Ludwigsen, E.: Endobronchial carcinosarcoma. A case with osteosarcoma of pulmonary invasive part, and a review with respect to prognosis. Virchows Arch. A. Path. Anat. and Histol *373* (1977) 293-302.

[86] Lukeman, J.M, R.A. Wilson, and R.F. Samuel: Cytologic and histologic correlation of lung tumors. In: Lung cancer: Progress in therapeutic research. Raven Press, New York 1979.

[87] Mack, D., E. Knetsch und A. Harlacher: Das Schicksal der Patienten mit operativ entfernten Lungen- oder Pleurametastasen. Thoraxchirurgie *24* (1976) 353-356.

[88] Markel, S.F., M.R. Abell, C. Haight, and A.J. French: Neoplasms of bronchus commonly designated as adenomas. Cancer *17* (1964) 590-608.

[89] Marsden, H.B., and C.L. Scholtz: Pulmonary blastoma. Virchows Arch. A. Path. Anat. and Histol. *372* (1976) 161-165.

[90] McCaughey, W.T.E.: Asbestos and neoplasia: Diffuse mesothelial tumors. Criteria for diagnosis of diffuse mesothelial tumors. Ann. N.Y. Acad. Sci. *132* (1965) 603-613.

[91] Melamed, M.R., M.B. Zaman, B.J. Flehinger, and N. Martini: Radiologically occult in situ and incipient invasive epidermoid lung cancer. Detection by sputum cytology in a survey of asymptomatic cigarette smokers. Am. J. Surg. Path. *1* (1977) 5-16.

[92] Montes, M., J.P. Binette, A.P. Chaudhry, R.H. Adler, and R. Guarino: Clara cell adenocarcinoma. Light and electron microscope studies. Am. J. Surg. Path. *1* (1977) 245-253.

[93] Moore, R.L., and R. Lattes: Papillomatosis of larynx and bronchi. Case report with 34-year follow-up. Cancer *12* (1959) 117-126.

[94] Moore, T.N., R. Livingston, L. Heilbrun, J. Eltringham, O. Skinner, J. White, and D. Tesh: The effectiveness of prophylactic brain irradiation in small cell carcinoma of the lung. A southwest oncology group study. Cancer *41* (1978) 2149-2153.

[95] Mountain, C.F., and K.E. Hermes: Management implications of surgical staging studies. In: Lung cancer: Progress in therapeutic research. Raven Press, New York 1979.

[96] Okike, N., P.E. Bernatz, and L.B. Woolner: Localized mesothelioma of the pleura. Benign and malignant variants. J. Thoracic Surg. *75* (1978) 363-372.

[97] Osamura, R.Y.: Ultrastructure of localized fibrous mesothelioma of the pleura. Report of a case with histogenetic considerations. Cancer *39* (1977) 139-142.

[98] Ownly, D., G. Lyon, and A. Spock: Primary leiomyosarcoma of the lung in childhood. Am. J. Dis. Child. *130* (1976) 1132-1133.

[99] Ranchod, M.: The histogenesis and development of pulmonary tumorlets. Cancer *39* (1977) 1135-1145.

[100] Remberger, K., and G. Hübner: Rhabdomyomatous dysplasia of the lung. Virchows Arch. A. Path. Anat. and Histol. *363* (1974) 363-369.

[101] Rilke, F., A. Carbone, C. Clemente, and S. Pilotti: Surgical pathology of resectable lung cancer. In: Lung cancer: Progress in therapeutic research. Raven Press, New York 1979.

[102] Salazar, O.M., P. Rubin, J.C. Brown, M.L. Feldstein, and B.E. Keller: Predictors of radiation response in lung cancer. A clinicopathobiological analysis. Cancer *37* (1976) 2636-2650.

[103] Sale, G.F., and B.G. Kulander: Benign clear cell tumor of lung with necrosis. Cancer *37* (1976) 2355-2358.

[104] Saltzstein, S.L.: Pulmonary malignant lymphomas and pseudolymphomas; classification, therapy and prognosis. Cancer *16* (1963) 928-955.

[105] Santos-Briz, A., J. Terrón, R. Sastre, L. Romero, and A. Valle: Oncocytoma of the lung. Cancer *40* (1977) 1330-1336.

[106] Schaerer, R., J.J. Sotto, U. Wiget, A. Perdrix, J.-C. Bensa, and P. Ribaud: Chemotherapy of bronchogenic carcinomas by a combination of cyclophosphamide, methotrexate, vincristine, and bleomycin. Eur. J. Cancer *13* (1977) 425-428.

[107] Scharifker, D., and M. Kaneko: Localized fibrous "mesothelioma" of pleura (submesothelial fibroma). A clinicopathologic study of 18 cases. Cancer *43* (1979) 627-635.

[108] Scheer, A.C., and R.F. Wilson: Cancer of the lung and its response to non-surgical treatment. Z. Krebsforsch. *83* (1975) 1-6.

[109] Sealy, R.: Combined radiotherapy and chemotherapy in non-small cell carcinoma of the lung. In: Lung cancer: Progress in therapeutic research. Raven Press, New York 1979.

[110] Seeber, S., und C.G. Schmidt: Chemotherapie des Bronchialkarzinoms. Dtsch. Med. Wschr. *104* (1979) 76-78.

[111] Seeber, S., C.G. Schmidt, H. Holfeld und E. Scherer: Integrale Behandlung (Chemo- und Radiotherapie) des inoperablen Bronchialkarzinoms. Vorläufige Ergebnisse bei 50 Patienten. Dtsch. Med. Wschr. *102* (1977) 147-152.

[112] Shields, T.W., E.W. Humphrey, C.E. Eastridge, and R.J. Keehn: Adjuvant cancer chemotherapy after resection of carcinoma of the lung. Cancer *40* (1977) 2057-2062.

[113] Sidhu, G.S., and E.M. Forrester: Acinic cell carcinoma: Long-term survival after pulmonary metastases. Light and electron microscopic study. Cancer *40* (1977) 756-765.

[114] Silverman, J.F., and S. Kay: Multiple pulmonary leiomyomatous hamartomas. Report of a case with ultrastructure examination. Cancer *38* (1976) 1199-1204.

[115] Singh, G., R.E. Lee, and D.H. Brooks: Primary pulmonary paraganglioma. Report of a case and review of the literature. Cancer *40* (1977) 2286-2289.

[116] Sobin, L.H.: The WHO histological classification of lung tumors. In: Lung cancer: Progress in therapeutic research. Raven Press, New York 1979.

[117] Spremulli, E., G. Wampler, W. Regelson, D. Borochovitz, and T. Hardy: Chemotherapy of malignant mesothelioma. Cancer *40* (1977) 2038-2045.

[118] Stackhouse, E.M., E.G. Harrison Jr., and F.H. Ellis: Primary mixed malignancies of lung; carcinosarcoma and blastoma. J. Thoracic Surg. *57* (1969) 385-399.

[119] Stewart, T.H.M., A.C. Hollinshead, J.E. Harris, S. Raman, R. Belanger, A. Crepeau, A.F. Crook, W.E. Hirte, D. Hooper, D.J. Klaassen, E.F. Rapp, and H.J. Sachs: Survival Study of immunochemotherapy in lung cancer. In: Immunotherapy of cancer: Present status of trials in man; edited by W.D. Terry and D. Windhorst. Raven Press, New York 1978.

[120] Sugaar, S., and H.H. LeVeen: A histopathologic study on the effects of radiofrequency thermotherapy on malignant tumors of the lung. Cancer *43* (1979) 767-783.

[121] Tao, L.C., N.C. Delarue, D. Sanders, and G. Weisbrod: Bronchiolo-alveolar carcinoma. A correlative clinical and cytologic study. Cancer *42* (1978) 2759-2767.

[122] Taylor, T.L., and D.R. Miller: Leiomyoma of the bronchus. J. Thoracic Surg. *57* (1969) 284-288.

[123] Tisell, L.E., L. Angervall, J. Dahl, C. Merck, and B.F. Zachrisson: Recurrent and metastasizing gastric leiomyoblastoma (epithelioid leiomyosarcoma) associated with multiple pulmonary chondrohamartomas. Long survival of

a patient treated with repeated operations. Cancer *41* (1978) 259-265.

[124] Torikata, C., and K. Ishiwata: Intranuclear tubular structures observed in the cells of an alveolar cell carcinoma of the lung. Cancer *40* (1977) 1194-1201.

[125] Turnbull, A. D., A. G. Huvos, J. T. Goodner, and F. W. Foote Jr.: Mucoepidermoid tumors of bronchial glands. Cancer *28* (1971) 539-544.

[126] Ueda, K., R. Gruppo, F. Unger, L. Martin, and K. Bove: Rhabdomyosarcoma of lung arising in congenital cystic adenomatoid malformation. Cancer *40* (1977) 383-388.

[127] Underwood, G. H. Jr., R. G. Hooper, S. P. Axelbaum, and D. W. Goodwin: Computed tomographic scanning of the thorax in the staging of bronchogenic carcinoma. N. Engl. J. Med. *300* (1979) 777-778.

[128] Uys, C. J.: Observations on the pathology and ultrastructure of mesothelioma. In: Lung cancer: Progress in therapeutic research. Raven Press, New York 1979.

[129] Vidne, B. A., S. Richter, and M. J. Levy: Surgical treatment of solitary pulmonary metastasis. Cancer *38* (1976) 2561-2563.

[130] Viereck, H.-J., G. Viehweger und E. Eckert: Kombination von Bestrahlung und Operation zur Behandlung des Bronchialkarzinoms. Med. Klin. *69* (1974) 1391-1397.

[131] Vincent, R. G., T. M. Chu, W. W. Lane, A. C. Gutierrez, P. J. Stegeman, and S. Madajewicz: Carcinoembryonic antigen as a monitor of successful surgical resection in 130 patients with carcinoma of the lung. In: Lung cancer: Progress in therapeutic research. Raven Press, New York 1979.

[132] Vincent, R. G., J. W. Pickren, W. W. Lane, I. Bross, H. Takita, L. Houten, A. C. Gutierrez, and T. Rzepka: The changing histophathology

of lung cancer. A review of 1682 cases. Cancer *39* (1977) 1647-1655.

[133] Wagner, J. C., C. A. Sleggs, and P. Marchand: Diffuse pleura mesothelioma and asbestos exposure in the North Western Cape Province. Br. J. Int. Med. *17* (1960) 260-271.

[134] Wanebo, H. J., N. Martini, M. R. Melamed, B. Hilaris, and E. J. Beattie Jr.: Pleural mesothelioma. Cancer *38* (1976) 2481-2488.

[135] Wang, N. S., T. A. Seemayer, M. N. Ahmed, and J. Knaack: Giant cell carcinoma of the lung. Hum. Pathol. *7* (1976) 3-16.

[136] Wile, A., G. Olinger, J. B. Peter, and L. Dornfeld: Solitary intraparenchymal pulmonary plasmacytoma associated with production of an M-protein. Report of a case. Cancer *37* (1976) 2338-2342.

[137] Wilkins, E. W. Jr., R. C. Darling, L. Soutter, and R. C. Sniffin: A continuing clinical survey of adenomas of the trachea and bronchus in a general hospital. J. Thoracic Surg. *46* (1963) 279-291.

[138] Wittes, R. E., S. Hopfan, B. Hilaris, R. B. Golbey, M. Melamed, and N. Martini: Oat cell carcinoma of the lung. Combination treatment with radiotherapy and cyclophosphamide, adriamycin, vincristine, and methotrexate. Cancer *40* (1977) 653-659.

[139] Yalow, R. S.: Ectopic ACTH in carcinoma of the lung. In: Lung cancer: Progress in therapeutic research. Raven Press, New York 1979.

[140] Yap, B.-S., R. S. Benjamin, A. Burgess, and G. P. Bodney: The value of adriamycin in the treatment of diffuse malignant pleural mesothelioma. Cancer *42* (1978) 1692-1696.

[141] Yesner, R., B. Gerstl, and O. Auerbach: Application of the World Health Organization classification of lung carcinoma to biopsy material. Ann. Thorac. Surg. *1* (1965) 33-49.

18 Tumors of the brain

1. One to 2% of all malignant tumors grow in the central nervous system [101]. In childhood these neoplasms are the second most frequent malignant tumor.

   About 1% of all deaths are due to primary brain tumors (that is, without metastatic lesions or tumors of the pituitary gland) [73, 102].

2. The cells of tumors of the central nervous system and their growth pattern are unique for this organ system and are not found in other tumors.

3. There are different **classifications** of brain tumors [39, 73, 100-102].

   On the following pages we have tried to follow the proposed classification of the WHO, which can be reproduced in almost all instances by routine staining techniques.

4. Metastases into the brain originating from primary tumors outside the central nervous system are relatively frequent.

   In some instances these metastatic lesions can be treated surgically (see page 733).

   Primary brain tumors rarely disseminate outside the central nervous system.

5. The therapeutic approach to brain tumors is in most instances surgery. The success of treatment depends on tumor type, location, and size.

   Well-differentiated benign tumors like meningiomas, neurilemomas, and astrocytomas can be operated upon with the possibility of cure.

   With other tumors, like glioblastomas, surgery must be complemented by radiation therapy (up to 60 Gy for the brain and 30 to 40 Gy for the medulla, and spinal cord).

   Chemotherapy has little or no benefit. Occasionally, regressions of very malignant tumors have been observed with the use of BCNU and CCNU.

   The overall 5-year survival rate for brain tumors for all histological types is about 25%.

[39] Kernohan and Sayre 1952.
[73] Russell and Rubinstein 1977.
[100] Zülch 1956.
[101] Zülch 1958.
[102] Zülch and Mennel 1974.

Tumors of neuroepithelial tissue (WHO)

Astrocytic tumors (WHO)

M-9400/3

1. Astrocytoma

General Remarks

Incidence: About 1 to 2% of all malignant tumors are brain tumors.
Astrocytoma is the most common tumor of the central nervous system (about 7%) [101].
Age: All ages can be affected; the peak age is the 4th decade.
In **children** 30% of the brain tumors are astrocytomas.
Site: The main locations are the cerebrum, cerebellum, thalamus, optic chiasm, pons, and spinal cord.

Macroscopy

Astrocytomas might have different macroscopic appearances according to the age of the patient and the location.
a) Astrocytomas in **adults** in the **cerebrum** are often ill-defined tumors. The astrocytoma enlarges one or both hemispheres, but does not reveal a clear demarcation from the surrounding tissue. Occasionally this indistinct enlargement is the only sign of the tumor. In other cases, the cut surface of the tumor is spongy.
b) **Cerebellar** astrocytomas in **children** can be well delineated from the surrounding tissue and have a grayish-whitish cut surface. They have a solid consistency, but no cysts.

Clinical Findings

The clinical findings are determined by the tumor site.
The tumor causes general cerebral symptoms, which develop slowly or rapidly, according to the size and the degree of tumor differentiation.

Histology

The histological aspect of astrocytomas varies. This variation includes the number of glial fibrils, the aspect of the tumor cells, and the arrangement of the tumor cells and fibrils.
According to these variations, subtypes have been established.
It is debatable whether this subclassification has clinical and prognostic significance, with the exception of the gemistocytic astrocytoma, which has a poorer prognosis than the other types [44].
More important than the subclassification of the tumor is the degree of malignancy: Nuclear atypias, zones of necroses, and number of mitoses.
In biopsies "benign"-looking astrocytomas can contain in other areas atypical tumor cells.
A biopsy with mature-looking astrocytomas does not rule out a possible malignant behavior of the entire tumor.
However, if in biopsy a poorly differentiated tumor is detected, the prognosis is poor, even if the remaining tumor is well differentiated.

[44] Leibel et al. 1975.
[101] Zülch 1958.

Astrocytoma

M-9400/3   **a) Well-differentiated astrocytoma** (WHO Grade I-II)

This tumor is composed of astrocytes that often look normal. The cells are normal-sized, and the nucleus is oval and occasionally larger than normal, containing a nucleolus.
The tumor is characterized by an increased cellularity of normal-looking astrocytes, which gradually disappear in the adjacent normal brain tissue, the tumor therefore being ill-defined. Other parts, however, might contain (besides normal-looking cells) tumor cells with hyperchromasia and cellular pleomorphism (Figs. 760 to 762).

M-9401/3   **b) Anaplastic (malignant) astrocytoma** (WHO Grade III)

This astrocytoma is characterized by high cellularity and is dominated by atypical cells that reveal severe pleomorphism. The blood vessels react early with proliferation.
Only in zones of better-differentiated tumor cells can the true nature of an astrocytoma be detected (Figs. 763 to 765).
This friable, smooth tumor contains areas of necrosis and bleeding and is found in the **cerebrum.**

M-9420/3   **c) Fibrillary astrocytoma** (WHO Grade II)

This subtype of astrocytoma is dominated by numerous, long neuroglial fibrils (Fig. 766).
This firm tumor does not reveal on histological analysis a proliferation of blood vessels.

M-9410/3   **d) Protoplasmic astrocytoma** (WHO Grade II)

The tumor cells in this subtype of astrocytoma have an abundant cytoplasm with eosinophilic staining (Fig. 767).
Occasionally the tumor cells can form microcysts.
The tumor has few fibrils and is highly cellular.
The **cerebrum** is the main site for this astrocytoma.

M-9411/3   **e) Gemistocytic astrocytoma** (WHO Grade II)

This astrocytoma grows in the **cerebrum** and is soft.
It is composed of closely packed tumor cells, which leave only a discrete amount of intercellular matrix (Fig. 768).
The tumor cells have a nucleus in an eccentric position. The nucleus occasionally contains nucleoli.

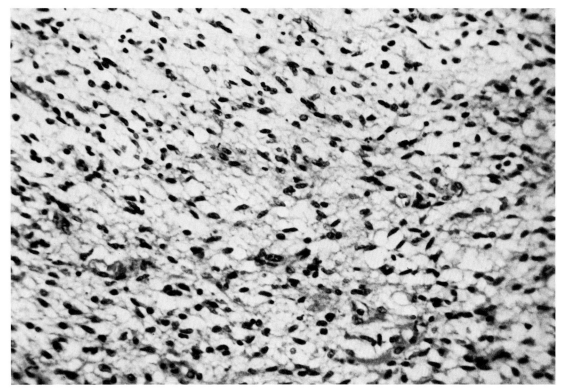

Fig. 760. Astrocytoma, Grade I (× 200).

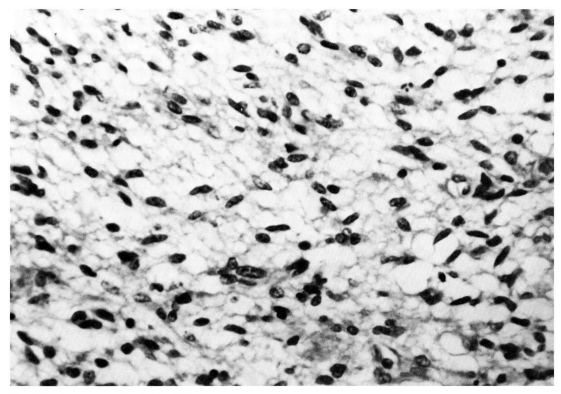

Fig. 761. Astrocytoma, Grade I (× 310).

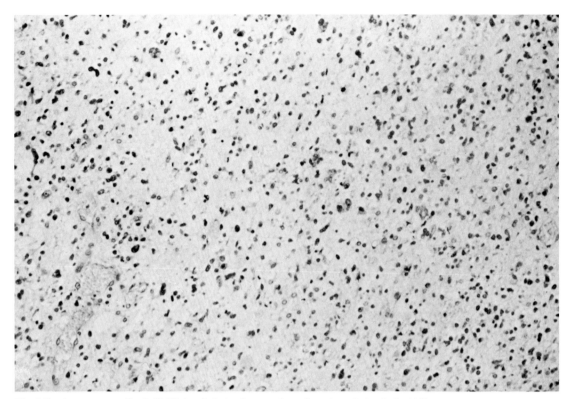

Fig. 762. Astrocytoma, Grade II: High cellularity, increased number of atypical cells (× 125).

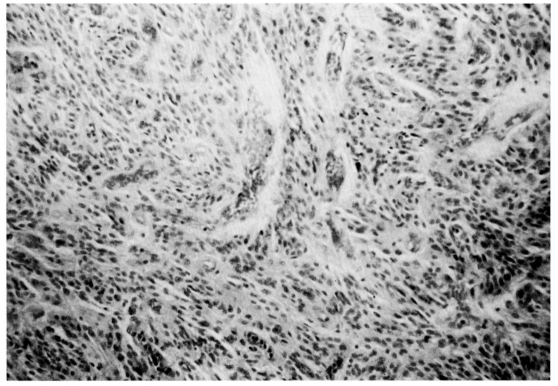

Fig. 763. Astrocytoma, Grade III: Vascular proliferation, atypical cells (× 125).

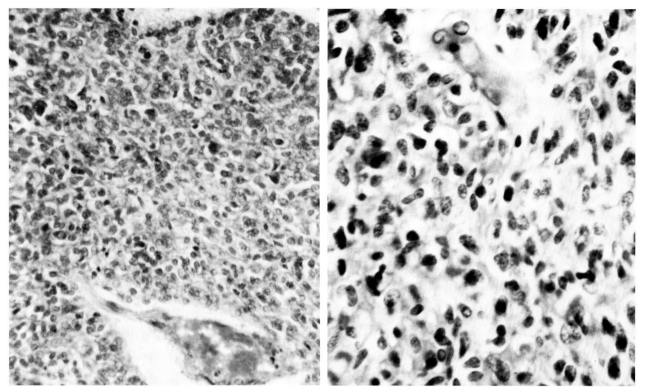

Fig. 764. Astrocytoma, Grade III: Vascular proliferation, numerous atypical cells (15-year-old male, × 200).

Fig. 765. Astrocytoma, Grade III (15-year-old male, × 400).

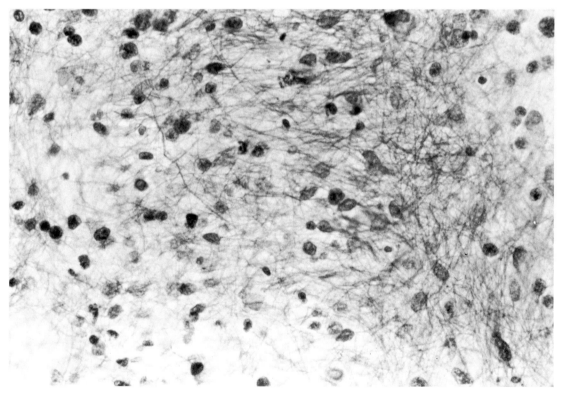

Fig. 766. Fibrillary astrocytoma with numerous neuroglial fibrils (× 310).

761

The most characteristic feature is the abundant hyalin-looking eosinophilic cytoplasm, giving to these tumor cells a resemblance to gangliocytes (Figs. 769 and 770).
There is only a very discrete fibril formation.

M-9421/3   **f) Pilocytic astrocytoma** (WHO Grade I)

The tumor cells are bipolar and spindle-shaped with an elongated cytoplasm. Occasionally "Rosenthal" fibers can be observed as homogeneous, strongly eosinophilic masses (Figs. 771 to 773).
The tumor cells grow in rows with a parallel arrangement. The cells are surrounded by fibrils, which form interlacing structures. This variety of astrocytoma is mainly observed in the **third ventricle.**
This tumor is observed particularly during adolescence and childhood.

M-9381/3   **g) Diffuse astrocytoma**
(gliomatosis cerebri, glioblastosis – WHO)

This tumor does not grow in a circumscribed fashion, but enlarges the cerebral hemisphere.
Only on histological analysis can the tumor cells be detected: They are in most instances well differentiated; the tumor, however, might contain small foci of undifferentiated cells (Figs. 774 to 777).
Gliomatosis cerebri is rare.

M-9430/3   **h) Astroblastoma** (WHO Grade II)

This variety of astrocytoma occurs usually in early adult life and is found in the **cerebrum.**
This well-defined tumor is composed of astrocytes with signs of atypias. The tumor contains necroses and hemorrhages; occasionally cysts are observed. The blood vessels do not proliferate.
The tumor cells are occasionally arranged in a pseudorosette-like fashion in a perivascular position (Figs. 778 and 779).
Astroblastoma can occasionally be observed in an otherwise well-differentiated astrocytoma, which probably reflects the stage of anaplasia in astrocytomas [73].

[73] Russell and Rubinstein 1977.

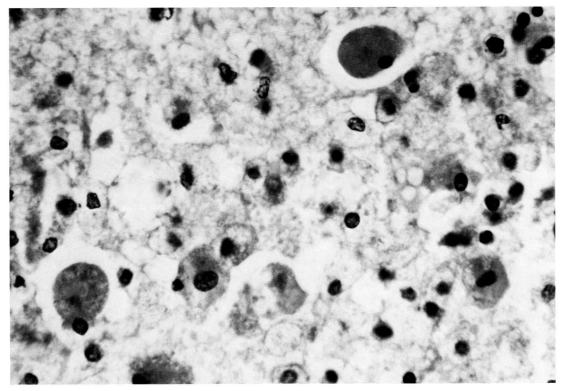

Fig. 767. Protoplasmic astrocytoma: Small microcysts (×400).

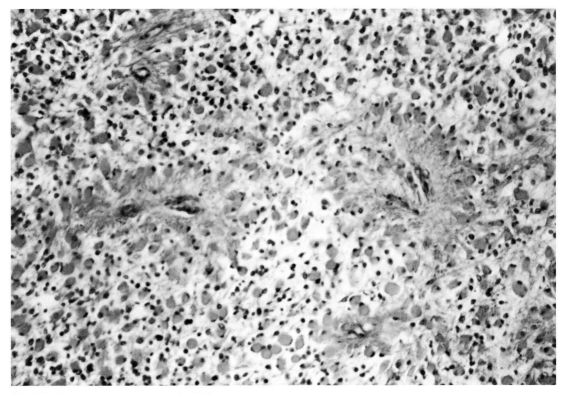

Fig. 768. Gemistocytic astrocytoma (×200).

763

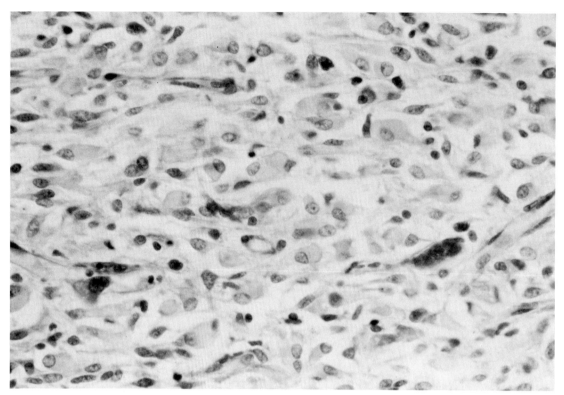

Fig. 769. Gemistocytic astrocytoma (× 310).

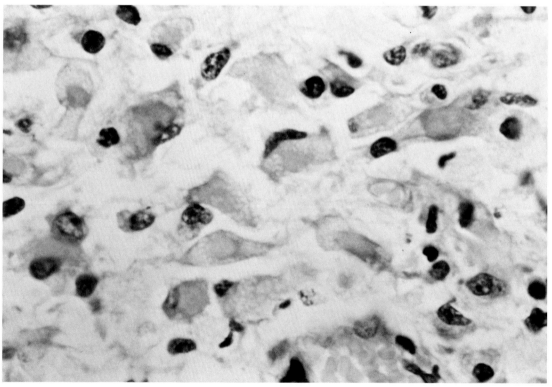

Fig. 770. Gemistocytic astrocytoma (54-year-old male, × 600).

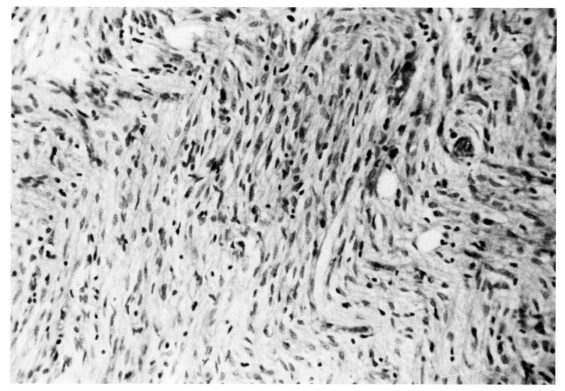

Fig. 771. Pilocytic astrocytoma (× 200).

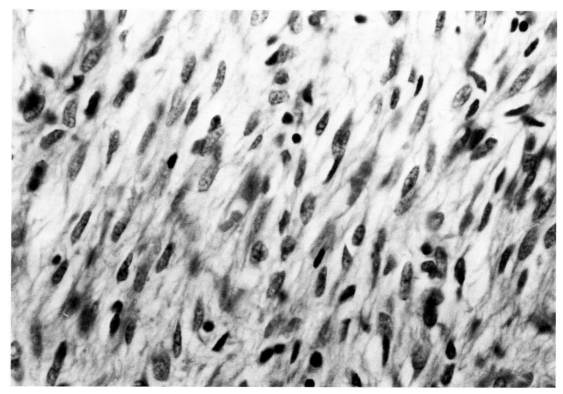

Fig. 772. Pilocytic astrocytoma (× 400).

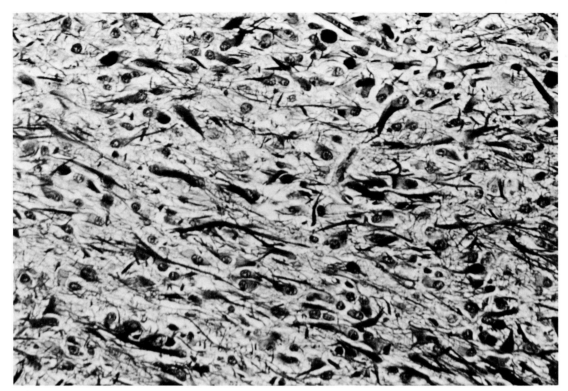

Fig. 773. Pilocytic astrocytoma: Rosenthal fibers (Holzer's stain, × 310).

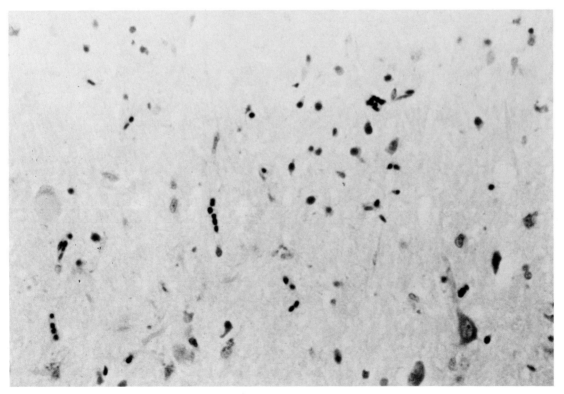

Fig. 774. Diffuse gliomatosis (61-year-old male, × 200).

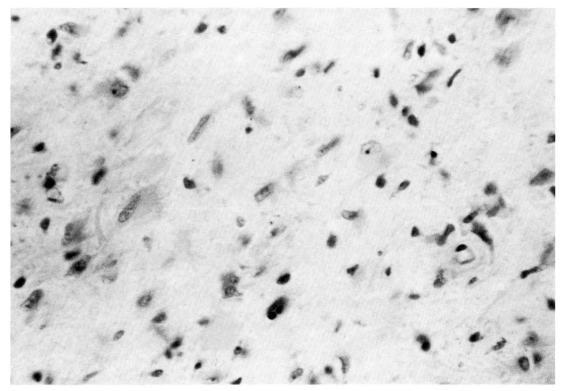

Fig. 775. Diffuse gliomatosis (× 310).

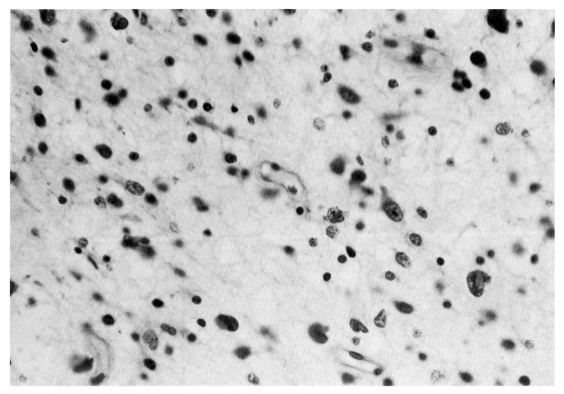

Fig. 776. Diffuse gliomatosis. Some undifferentiated cells (× 200).

Astrocytoma

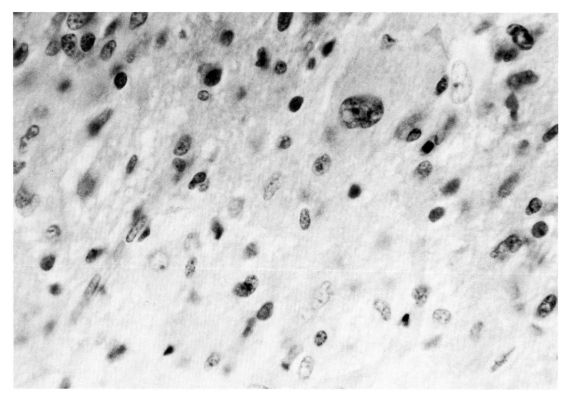

Fig. 777. Diffuse gliomatosis: Atypical cells (65-year-old male, × 400).

768

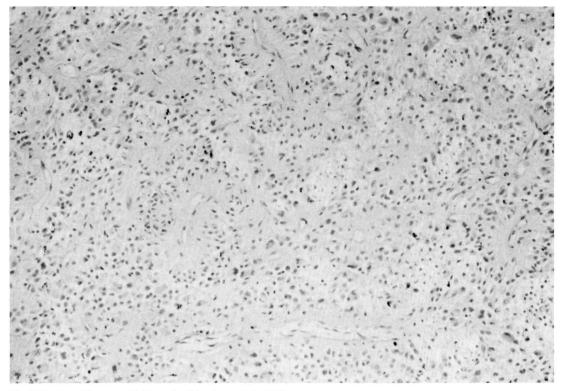

Fig. 778. Astroblastoma: Thick-walled blood vessels (× 125).

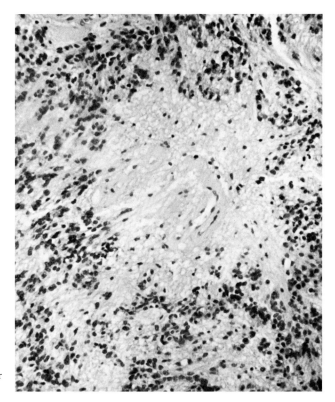

Fig. 779. Astroblastoma: Closely packed tumor cells around blood vessels (× 125).

As mentioned above the different types of astrocytomas are often linked with a particular **age** and **location:**

M-9400/3
T 191.6

Astrocytoma of the cerebellum

Age: This tumor is usually observed in children.
Site: The tumor grows symmetrically in the vermis in the midline, extending into the fourth ventricle.

Macroscopy

The tumor is distinct (and can occasionally be removed surgically).
The tumor can contain cysts on the cut surface.

Histology

The tumor is well differentiated and only rarely shows foci of anaplastic tumor cells. Astrocytomas in this location can occasionally be entirely composed of gemistocytic astrocytoma cells.

Treatment

Surgical removal of the tumor.

Prognosis

This is the most benign variety of astrocytoma, which might be cured by surgery: the 5-year survival rate is 85%.
Megavoltage radiation therapy has been recommended [51].

Further Information

With electron microscopy the cerebellar astrocytomas are identical to optic gliomas [92].

M-9400/3
T 191.7

Astrocytoma of the brain stem, medulla, and pons

Age: This tumor usually occurs in children.

Macroscopy

The involved areas are enlarged by a diffuse tumor infiltration (Fig. 780).

Histology

The tumor shows signs of atypias.
This astrocytoma often grows in the pilocytic variety.

Treatment

Radiation therapy can be attempted: 50 to 60 Gy in 6 to 7 weeks according to the size of the irradiation field.

[51] Marsa et al. 1975.
[92] Walter 1978.

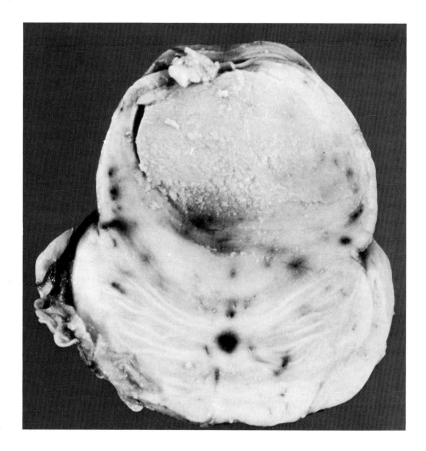

Fig. 780. Pilocytic astrocytoma of the brain stem.

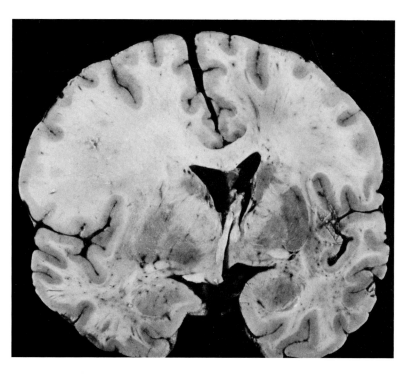

Fig. 781. Large astrocytoma in the left hemisphere (Grade I).

Astrocytoma

M-9400/3
T 191.0

Astrocytoma of the cerebrum

Age: This astrocytoma usually occurs in adults.

Macroscopy

This astrocytoma is in most instances a very large tumor, which is ill-defined (Fig. 781). The tumor might extend into the leptomeninges.

Histology

This cerebral astrocytoma usually grows in the fibrillary and pilocytic variety.
In most instances the tumor is well differentiated; however, considerable variation in the degree of differentiation in different regions of the tumor should be anticipated.
Some areas of the tumor might also be composed of gemistocytic astrocytoma.

Treatment

Surgery.
Megavoltage radiation therapy [35].
Chemotherapy:
BCNU has been reported to be the most active agent [35].

Prognosis

The 5-year survival rate after megavoltage radiation therapy has been reported to be about 40% [35].
Postoperative 5-year survival, 35 to 60%.

M-9400/3
T 192.2

Astrocytoma of the spinal cord

This rare tumor grows mainly in the upper segments: The thoracic and cervical part of the spinal cord.

Macroscopy

In most instances this is a solitary lesion that might be combined with von Recklinghausen's disease.
The tumor is firm and in most instances well circumscribed.

Histology

This spinal astrocytoma in most instances is of the pilocytic or fibrillary type.

Treatment

In cases of nonoperable tumor, radiation therapy can be attempted, as in other astrocytomas of Grade I-II [48].

[35] Jones 1978.
[48] Lütolf et al. 1978.

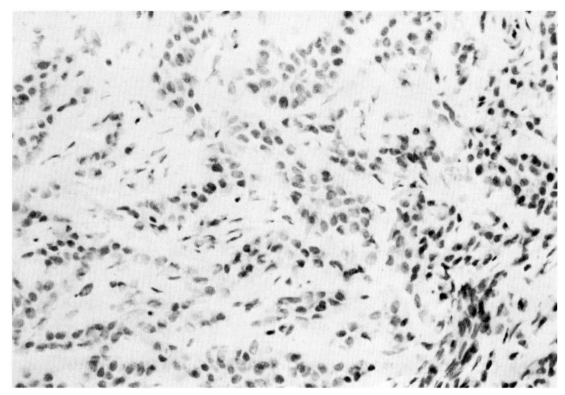

Fig. 782. Spongioblastoma in tuberous sclerosis (13-year-old male, × 125).

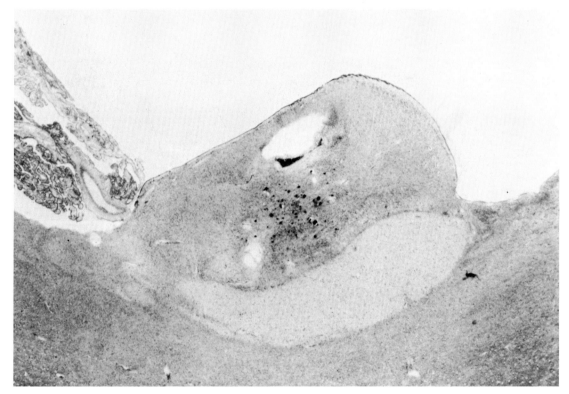

Fig. 783. Ventricular tumor in tuberous sclerosis, calcifications (× 30).

Brain tumors in tuberous sclerosis

In tuberous sclerosis, brain tumors can be observed. They are **giant cell astrocytomas of the protoplasmic type,** or **spongioblastomas,** or both (Fig. 782).

These tumors show calcifications (Figs. 783 and 784) that can be detected on X-rays.

Very rarely, malignant tumors of the glioblastoma type have been reported.

These giant cell astrocytomas in tuberous sclerosis grow in the wall of the **lateral ventricle.** They are sharply defined.

If the tumors are large they can cause obstruction.

The tumor contains areas of angioma.

The tumor cells are very large, having an eosinophilic, glassy cytoplasm. The cytoplasm is sometimes fibrillated or coarse.

It extends into processes. The shape of the tumor cells is fusiform. Giant cells with numerous nuclei are observed.

The nucleoli are in a peripheral or central position. The size of the cells is rather uniform (Fig. 785).

Occasionally the cells are centered around blood vessels.

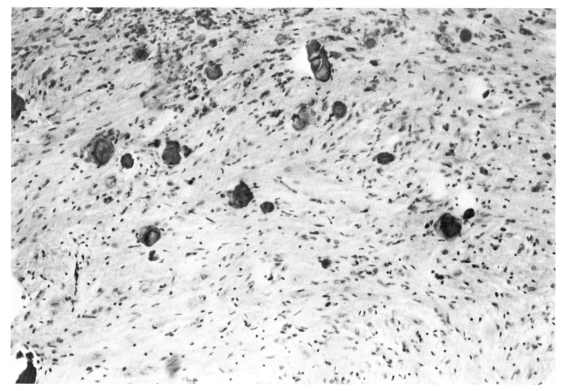

Fig. 784. Calcifications in a tumor in a case of tuberous sclerosis (× 200).

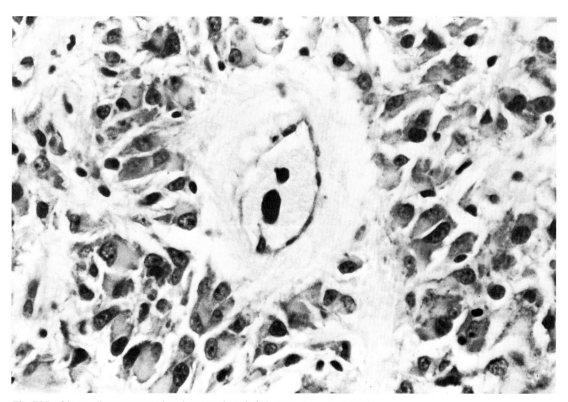

Fig. 785. Giant cell astrocytoma in tuberous sclerosis (13-year-old male, × 310).

Poorly differentiated and embryonal tumors

M-9440/3
T 191.0

2. Glioblastoma (multiforme) (WHO)
(astrocytoma, WHO Grade III-IV; undifferentiated glioma)

General Remarks

Incidence: This is the most frequent tumor of the neuroepithelial tissue (glioma). More than 90% of all gliomas in adults located in the cerebrum are glioblastomas. More than 25% of all intracranial gliomas are glioblastomas.

Age: The main age is about the 5th decade; however, all ages can be affected. Glioblastomas are rare in children: About 10% of brain tumors in children are glioblastomas [21].

Site: About 30% of glioblastomas are bilateral, extending into both hemispheres or having a multicentric origin.

The main sites are cerebrum, cerebral hemisphere, and frontal lobes.

T 191.6   The tumor is rare in the cerebellum.

Further notes: Most of the glioblastomas derive from anaplastic astrocytomas [73].

Macroscopy

The tumor can be small, only a few centimeters in diameter, or extremely large, occupying (for instance) an entire lobe with deformation of the hemisphere (Fig. 786 and 787). On the cut surface the tumor shows a reddish color, dark red zones, cysts, and areas of yellowish necrosis (Fig. 788).

On multiple sections multiple foci of this tumor can be discovered (about 6% of the cases).

The tumor can arise in the corpus callosum and extend into both hemispheres.

Histology

The tumor cells are highly undifferentiated. They show an unusual pleomorphism and unusual multinucleated giant cells.

The cytoplasm of the tumor cells is in most instances well developed and eosinophilic. Occasionally astroblastic foci are encountered in a glioblastoma.

Areas with numerous tumor cells can alternate with necrotic zones (Fig. 789). The tumor cells surrounding these necrotic zones are arranged in a palisading pattern (Figs. 790 and 791), giving the impression of wreath rosettes.

The blood vessels show an unusual proliferation of adventitia cells and endothelial cells. The proliferating blood vessels occasionally resemble renal glomerula (Fig. 792). Occasionally the blood vessels contain thrombi with surrounding ischemic necroses. In other sites the thrombi are recanalized.

---

[21] Farwell et al. 1977.
[73] Russell and Rubinstein 1977.

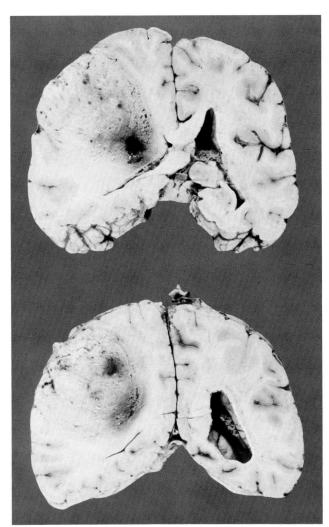

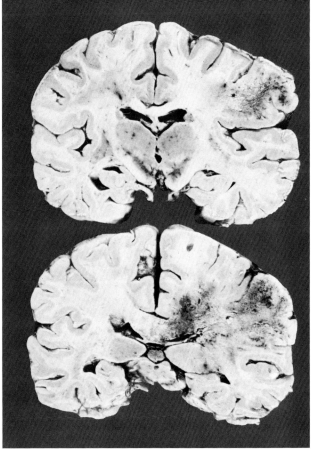

Fig. 786. Glioblastoma multiforme with necroses and hemorrhages of the left hemisphere.

Fig. 787. Large glioblastoma multiforme involving parts of the hemisphere and the corpus callosum.

Glioblastoma multiforme

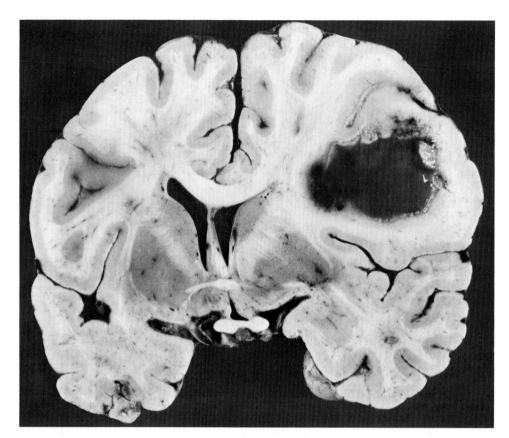

Fig. 788. Glioblastoma multiforme: Necroses and bleeding.

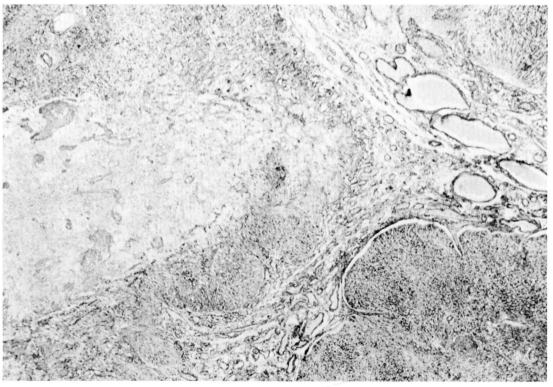

Fig. 789. Glioblastoma multiforme: Necrotic tumor tissue beside intact tumor tissue, numerous blood vessels (× 40).

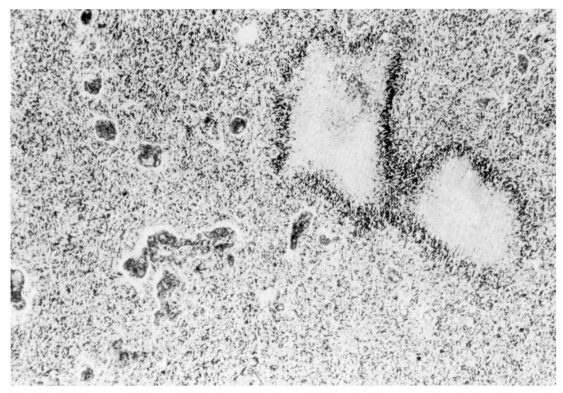

Fig. 790. Glioblastoma multiforme: Proliferation of blood vessels (glomerulus-like structures), palisading of tumor cells around necrotic areas (× 40).

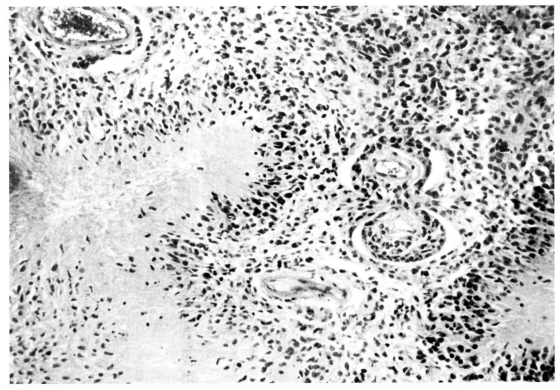

Fig. 791. Glioblastoma multiforme: Proliferation of adventitial and endothelial cells, palisading of tumor cells around necrotic zones (× 125).

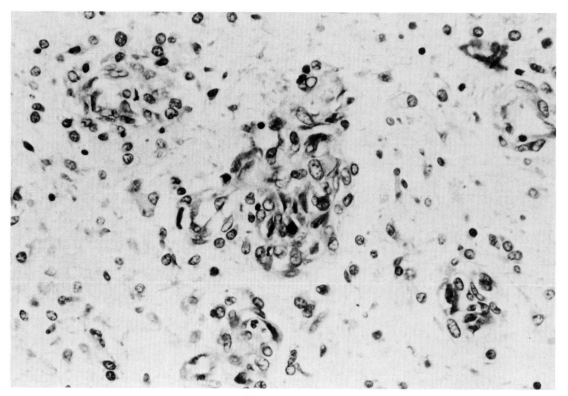

Fig. 792. Glioblastoma multiforme: Glomerulus-like structures due to blood vessel proliferation (× 200).

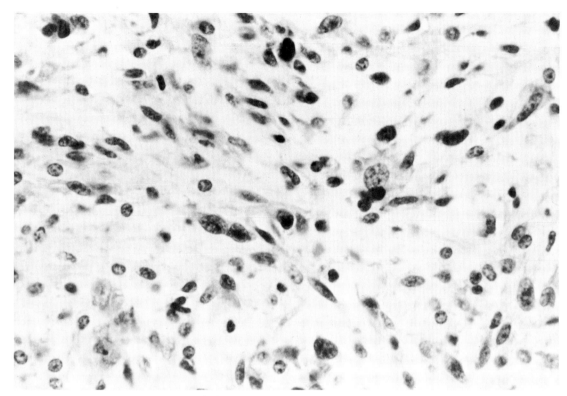

Fig. 793. Moderate anaplasia in an area of glioblastoma multiforme (× 310).

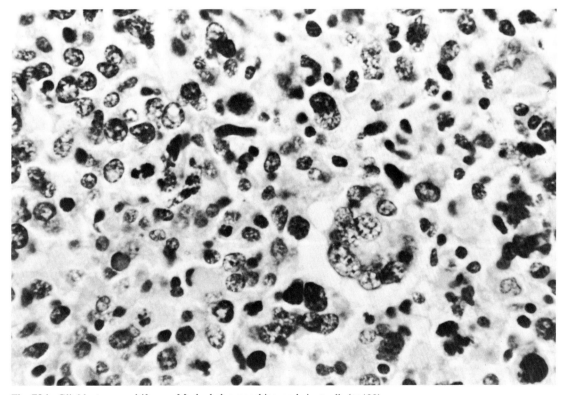

Fig. 794. Glioblastoma multiforme: Marked pleomorphism and giant cells (× 400).

Glioblastoma multiforme

Histology

It is remarkable how extremely pathological the mitoses in this tumor can be.
In pilocytic areas of glioblastoma "Rosenthal" fibers can be found.
The variability of the histological picture is rather important (Figs. 793 and 794).
Occasionally areas with sarcoma-like cells can be observed, even with the production of reticulin fibers.

This tumor is called

M-9442/3

– **Glioblastoma with sarcomatous component** (WHO) [42]
(mixed glioblastoma and sarcoma) (Figs. 795 and 796).

Occasionally the tumor is dominated by giant cells:

M-9441/3

– **Giant cell glioblastoma** (WHO) (Figs. 797 and 798).

Differential Diagnosis

Glioblastoma **with metastatic tumors into the brain:**
The histological diagnosis of glioblastoma is supported by
– palisading of tumor cells around tumor necroses (tumor cells of metastases grow around blood vessels).
– The adventitial and endothelial cell proliferations in the tumor blood vessels are very indicative of glioblastoma.

Spread

1. The tumor grows into the surrounding brain tissue and extends into the meninges [20].
2. Very rarely extraneural metastases can appear before the surgical intervention for the brain tumor [32].
3. Lymph node metastases and metastases into the viscera are extremely unusual.

Clinical Findings

General cerebral symptoms:
– Headache, vomiting, psychic changes, convulsion.
Rarely symptoms can be attributed to a lesion in a lobe.
Symptoms progress rapidly within weeks, and health deteriorates rapidly.

Treatment

Surgery:
Surgery to remove the tumor in most instances is for palliation.
Surgery can be combined with **radiation therapy** of up to 60 Gy.
Chemotherapy:
Chemotherapy is often without effect. However, the benefit of an increased survival time has been reported [96].
Combination chemotherapy with BCNU and CCNU sometimes combined with prednisone has been attempted [68].

[20] Erlich and Davis 1978.
[32] Hulbanni and Goodman 1976.
[42] Lalitha and Rubinstein 1979.
[68] Pouillart et al. 1977.
[96] Wilson 1976.

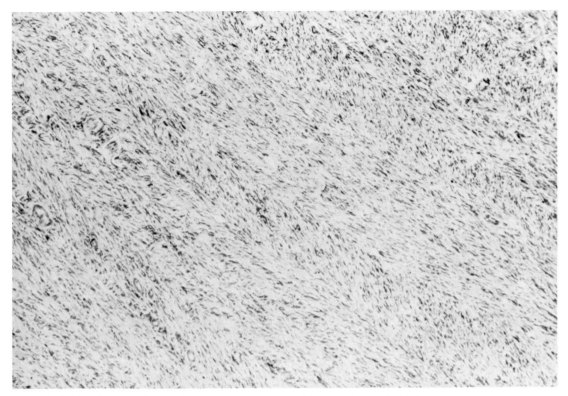

Fig. 795. Glioblastoma multiforme with sarcomatous component: Sarcomatous part (× 40).

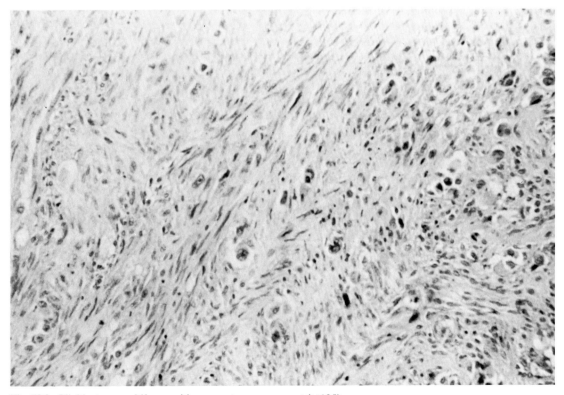

Fig. 796. Glioblastoma multiforme with sarcomatous component (× 125).

Glioblastoma multiforme

Treatment
Surgery or radiation therapy alone do not have curative possibilities [9].
The combination of surgery, irradiation, and chemotherapy occasionally prolongs the life span [89].

Prognosis
Average survival time after surgery: about 6 months.
2-year mortality rate after surgery: about 90%.
The 5-year survival rate after megavoltage radiation therapy: 0% [51].

[9] Bouchard 1973.
[51] Marsa et al. 1975.
[89] Taylor et al. 1975.

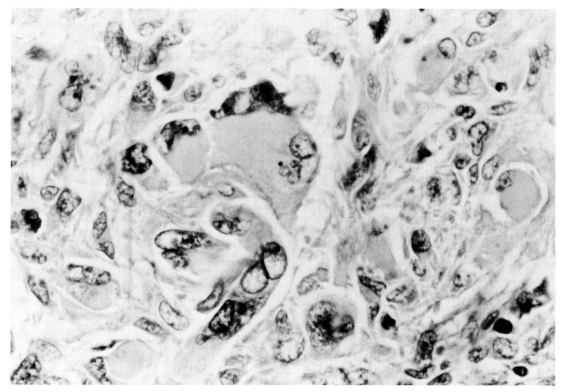

Fig. 797. Giant cell glioblastoma (× 400).

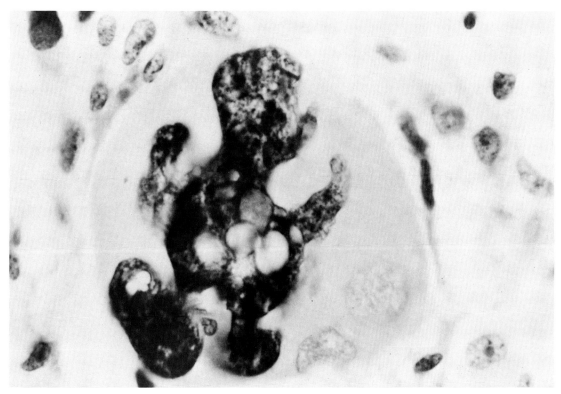

Fig. 798. Giant cell glioblastoma: Bizarre nucleus (× 800).

M-9470/3
T 191.6

3. Medulloblastoma (WHO Grade IV)

**General
Remarks**

Incidence: 25 to 30% of intracranial tumors in children are medulloblastomas.
Age: This is a malignant tumor of childhood. The peak median age is 5 to 9 years; 50% occur in the 1st decade.
Older age groups are very rarely affected, with the peak age in the first half of the 3rd decade.
Site: The main location is the cerebellum, the midline within the vermis.

Macroscopy

Medulloblastomas are grayish-white, soft, friable, and occasionally pinkish.
The tumor is well circumscribed.
The tumor extends from the midline of the vermis into the fourth ventricle, causing an internal hydrocephalus of the third and lateral ventricles.
Occasionally the tumor can reach the surface of the cerebellar hemispheres (Fig. 799).

Histology

This tumor is extremely cellular (Fig. 800).
The tumor cells are small. The nuclei are hyperchromatic, the chromatin is coarse, and the cytoplasm is scanty (Fig. 801).
The growth pattern of the tumor cells is variable:
There are zones with rosette formation, and the center of the rosettes contains neurofibrils, similar to the observations in neuroblastoma (Fig. 802).
In other cases the tumor cells can form solid nests or show a palisade structure in the periphery of the nests.
In other tumors foci of oligodendroglioma are observed (Fig. 803). There are no necroses.

Occasionally the medulloblastoma contains striated myoblasts: This tumor is called

M-9472/3

Medullomyoblastoma (WHO) [57].

A variety of medulloblastoma is characterized by the appearance of collagen fibers that are arranged in whorls:

M-9471/3

Desmoplastic medulloblastoma (WHO) [72].
This variety is a tumor of adults occurring in the cerebellar hemispheres.
This tumor has a better prognosis than medulloblastomas in childhood, since there is a tendency toward neuroblastoma differentiation [67].

[57] Misugi and Liss 1970.
[67] Polak 1967.
[72] Rubinstein and Northfield 1964.

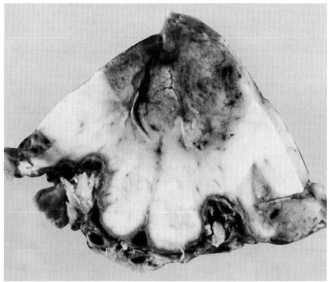
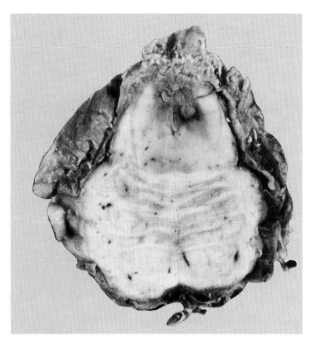

Fig. 799. Medulloblastoma in the medulla oblongata and pons.

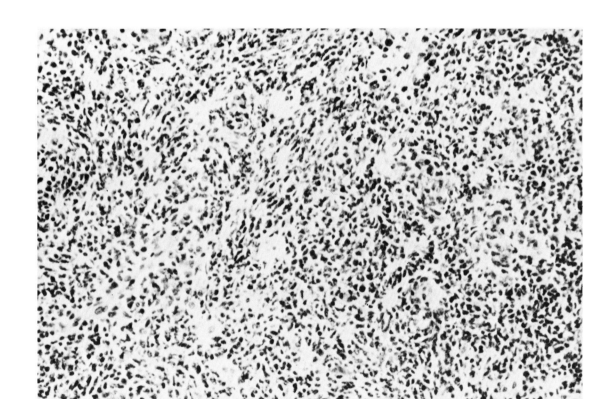

Fig. 800. Medulloblastoma: Closely packed tumor cells (× 125).

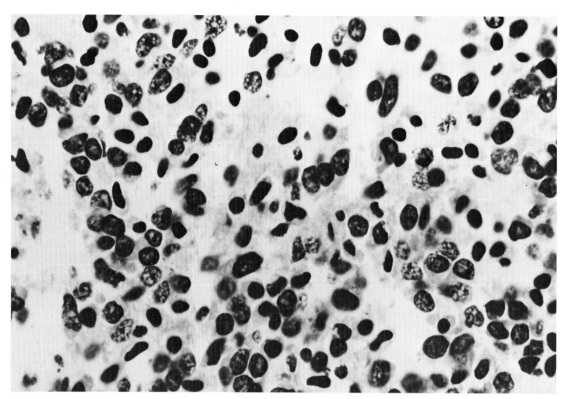

Fig. 801. Medulloblastoma: Hyperchromatic atypical nuclei and sparse cytoplasm (×400).

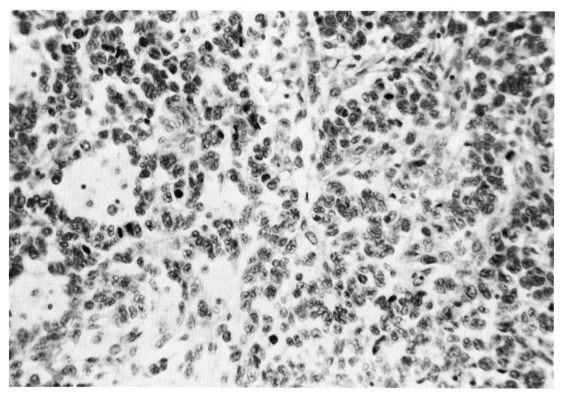

Fig. 802. Medulloblastoma: Bands or rosette-like tumor cell arrangement (15-year-old male, ×200).

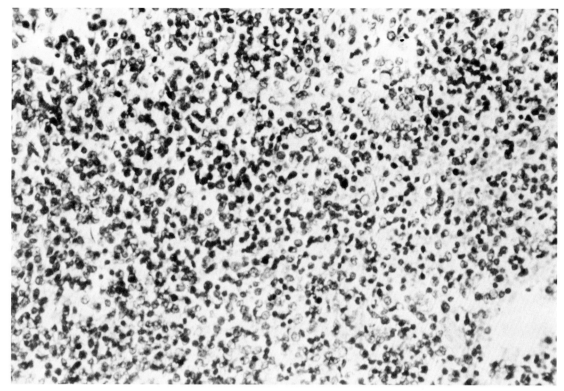

Fig. 803. Medulloblastoma: Hyperchromatic or vesicular nuclei (×200).

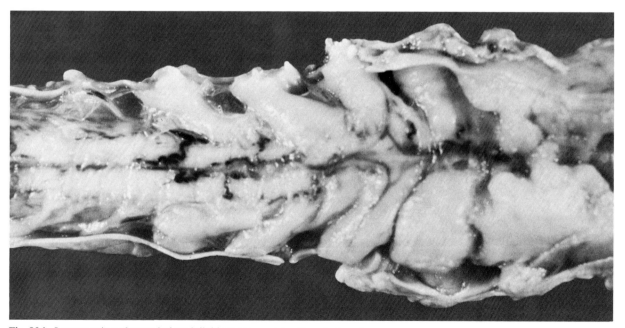

Fig. 804. Leptomeningeal spread of medulloblastoma, covering the spinal cord.

Medulloblastoma

Differential Diagnosis

Medulloblastoma **with cerebellar sarcoma:**
The medulloblastoma reveals reticulin fibers around the blood vessels in increased number, while often the sarcoma cells are individually surrounded by reticulin fibers.

Spread

1. The tumor extends into the subarachnoid space with subpial infiltration and spreads by way of the cerebrospinal path (Fig. 804).
2. Distant metastases can occur in lymph nodes and bone [6, 61].

Clinical Findings

Morning headache, repeated vomiting, nausea, papilledema.

Treatment

Radiation therapy:
Medulloblastoma tumor cells are highly radiosensitive (about 50 Gy in 5 weeks) [25, 90].
The **combination of radiation therapy with surgery** should be attempted [28].
Chemotherapy:
Intrathecal application of vincristine and methotrexate should be tried [19].

Prognosis

This is a very malignant tumor, which can, however, allow a prolonged life for several years after treatment.
The 5-year survival rate after radiation therapy (megavoltage radiation), 32 to 47% [51, 77].
There are even reports of a 5-year survival rate reaching 70% after irradiation therapy [10].
Following therapy the majority of children have mental and physical handicaps [5].
The main reason for failures in treatment are recurrences [12, 28].

Further Information

There is a report of multiple primary tumors of the brain associated with medulloblastoma in the cerebellum [8].

[5] Bamford et al. 1976.
[6] Banna et al. 1970.
[8] Bhangui et al. 1977.
[10] Brown et al. 1977.
[12] Cumberlin et al. 1979.
[19] Duffner et al. 1979.
[25] Glanzmann and Horst 1979.
[28] Harisiadis and Chang 1977.
[51] Marsa et al. 1975.
[61] Oberman et al. 1963.
[77] Sheline 1975.
[90] Tokars et al. 1979.

M-9501/3
T 191.0
T 191.7

4. Medulloepithelioma (WHO Grade IV)

General Remarks

Incidence: This is a very rare tumor.
Age: The tumor occurs in infants and children.
Site: The tumor grows near the ventricle in the cerebral hemispheres, in the midbrain-third ventricle, and the retina (see page 907).

Histology

This exceptional lesion has to be considered an embryonal tumor: The striking histological feature is the palisading and tubular architecture, by which the very primitive-looking cells mimic the medullary canal in its embryonic stage.

M-9502/3

According to these primitive-looking cells, medulloepithelioma can be a component in **malignant teratomas of the brain** (teratoid medulloepithelioma) (see Germ cell tumors, page 842).

Differential Diagnosis

Medulloepithelioma **with malignant ependymoma:**
Both tumors are rather primitive and undifferentiated. Malignant ependymoma is determined by the appearance of blepharoplasts and rosettes (Figs. 814 to 818).

Spread

This is a very malignant tumor with lymph node metastases, extension into the cerebrospinal space, and rapid recurrence.

Prognosis

Extremely poor.

Further Information

Other brain tumors that are considered to originate from embryonal tissue are the neuroblastoma, the polar spongioblastoma, and the ependymoblastoma [71].

---

[71] Rubinstein 1972.

M-9422/3
M-9423/3
T 191.6

5. Polar spongioblastoma
(primitive polar spongioblastoma–WHO Grade IV)

General
Remarks
T 192.0

Incidence: This is a rare tumor.

Age: The main age is childhood.

Site: The main site is the cerebellum, the optic chiasm, or the pons; occasionally the tumor can involve the third and fourth ventricle.

Further notes: Optic chiasm spongioblastomas are associated with von Recklinghausen's disease.

Macroscopy

The tumor is grayish to white, mostly well demarcated, and rather firm (Figs. 805 and 806).

Histology

The tumor cells are arranged in parallel bundles. Between these tumor cells there are neurofibrils and connective tissue with blood vessels.

The tumor cells are spindle-shaped, with a developing uni- or bipolar configuration.

The tumor cells tend to palisade around blood vessels and areas of necroses. Occasionally structures similar to Verocay bodies in neurilemomas are observed (Fig. 807).

The nuclei are small, hyperchromatic, and mostly oval. Rosenthal fibers are frequently found (Fig. 808).

Spread

The tumor infiltrates the meninges, extending into the base of the brain and the spinal cord.

Clinical
Findings

Unspecific symptoms, caused by a slow-growing tumor.

Treatment

Surgery:
Surgery with the intention to remove the entire tumor.

Radiation therapy:
The tumor is not very sensitive to radiation therapy.
Postoperative irradiation has been recommended [41].

Prognosis

The prognosis is doubtful since recurrences often appear many years after the operation. In most instances the complete removal of the tumor is not feasible.

Further
Information

It is still debated whether polar spongioblastoma is an entity or a variety of pilocytic astrocytoma [73, 101].

[41] Koos and Pendl 1975.
[73] Russell and Rubinstein 1977.
[101] Zülch 1958.

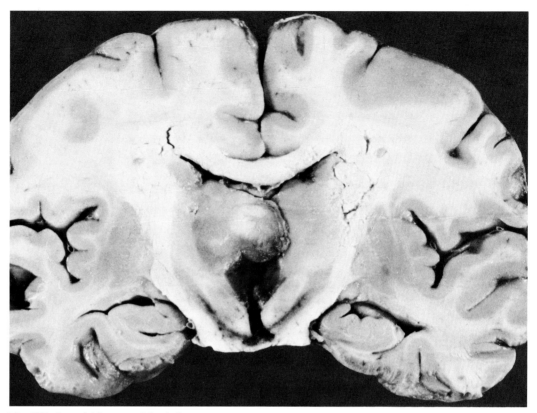

Fig. 805. Spongioblastoma of the thalamus.

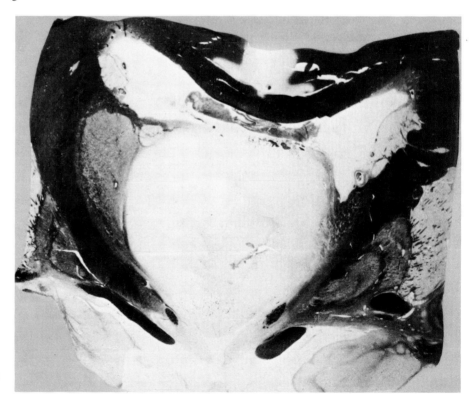

Fig. 806. Bilateral spongioblastoma of the thalamus (Woelke's stain).

Spongioblastoma

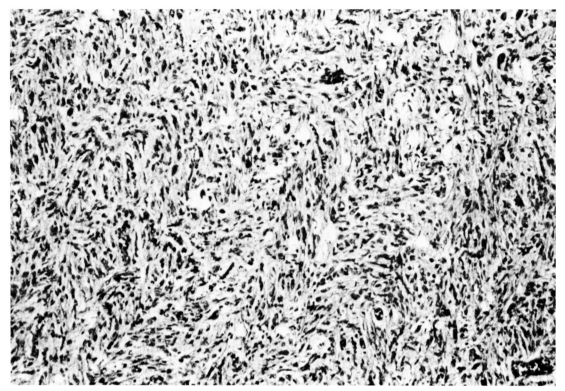

Fig. 807. Spongioblastoma (×125).

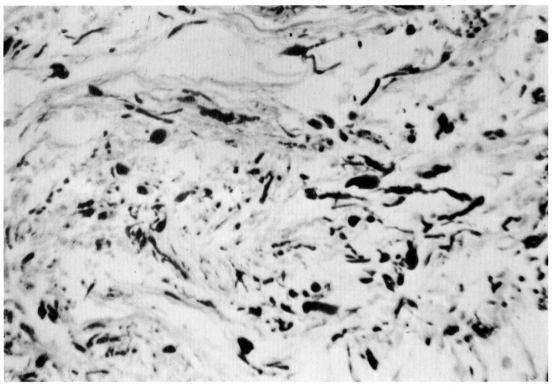

Fig. 808. Spongioblastoma: Rosenthal fibers (×200).

794

Oligodendroglial tumors

M-9450/3

6. Oligodendroglioma (WHO Grade II)

General Remarks

Incidence: About 2 to 6% of all tumors of the neuroepithelial tissue are oligodendrogliomas.

Age: The 3rd to 6th decades can be affected; the main incidence is in the 5th decade.

Sex: Both sexes are equally affected.

T 191.0
T 191.6
T 192.2

Site: The main sites are the cerebrum (frontal region) and cerebellum; the spinal cord can also be involved.

Macroscopy

Often the tumor develops in the central cortex and in the subcortical white matter. The tumor is rather well demarcated and has a grayish color. The tumor is solid and only occasionally reveals cysts on the cut surface.

The extending tumor compresses the brain tissue.

The tumor can contain foci of calcification.

Oligodendrogliomas can be very large and infiltrate the leptomeninges locally.

Histology

The first characteristic impression of this tumor is given by very clear tumor cells. This is due to a pale cytoplasm, which is surrounded by distinct cell borders (Figs. 809 and 810). The tumor cells are rather uniform, having a dark nucleus that contrasts with the clear cytoplasm.

The tumor looks rather uniform due to closely packed cells; between them there is a discrete connective tissue with a few blood vessels.

More than 30% of the tumors show foci of calcification (Fig. 811), which can be detected on X-rays. The tumor contains areas of microcystic degeneration.

Besides solid tumor nests the cells are arranged in sheets.

In oligodendrogliomas, areas can appear containing astrocytomas. These areas sometimes can be recognized by an increased cellularity.

These areas of increased cellularity can, furthermore, show pleomorphism of the cells, malignant nuclei, and numerous mitotic figures. This tumor has been called

M-9460/3

Anaplastic (malignant) oligodendroglioma (WHO Grade III) (oligodendroblastoma) [39, 65].

This tumor might contain foci of mucin, which is laid down extracellulary (Fig. 812).

Electron Microscopy

In oligodendroglioma the cytoplasm of the tumor cells contains bodies with internal structures (autophagic vacuoles), myelin-like figures, and Golgi-like vesicles [87].

Spread

Oligodendrogliomas might extend into the cerebrospinal canal and into the subarachnoidal space.

Distant metastases are extremely rare [84].

---

[39] Kernohan and Sayre 1952.
[65] Pasquier et al. 1978.
[84] Spataro and Sacks 1968.
[87] Takei et al. 1976.

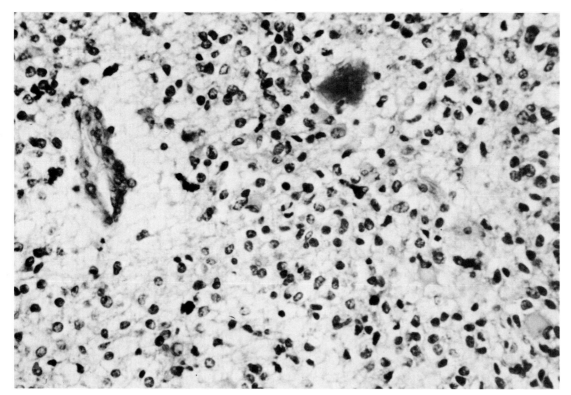

Fig. 809. Oligodendroglioma: Rather regular, pale tumor cells (× 200).

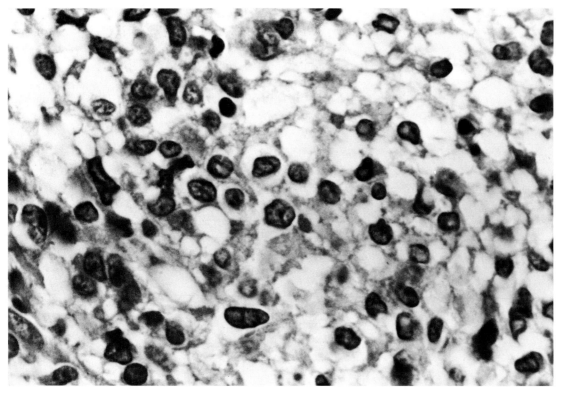

Fig. 810. Oligodendroglioma: Discrete pleomorphism of the nuclei (× 800).

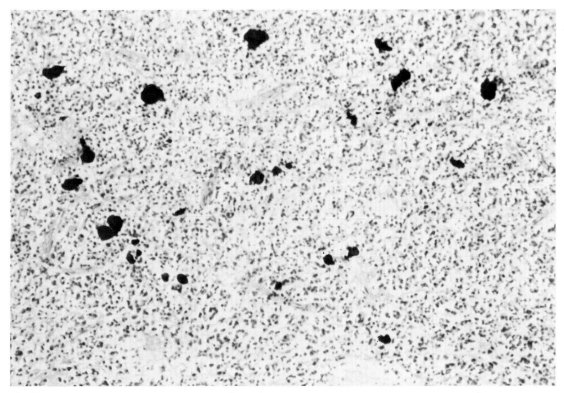

Fig. 811. Oligodendroglioma with calcifications (× 125).

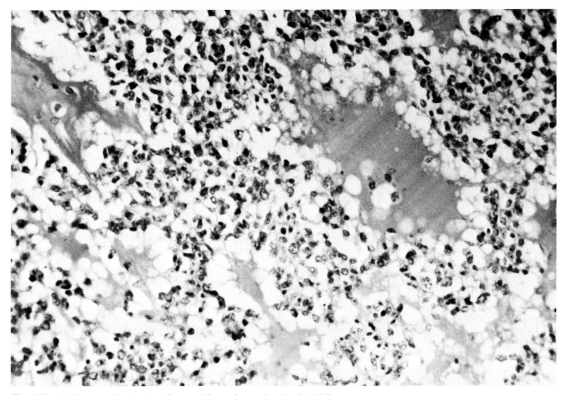

Fig. 812. Malignant oligodendroglioma with mucin production (× 125).

Oligodendroglioma

Clinical Findings

This tumor grows slowly. Often the detection of the tumor is preceded many years by general neurological symptoms.

The calcifications of the tumor can be seen on X-rays.

Treatment

Surgery
Radiation therapy:
60 Gy in about 7 weeks.

Prognosis

This is an unpredictable tumor that can behave for many years as a benign growth. The tumor grows very slowly.

About 50% of the cases, however, show recurrences after surgical treatment [69].

The postoperative 5-year survival rate is 35 to 60%.

Further Information
M-9380/1
T 192.0

Optic nerve glioma:
Incidence: This is a rare tumor.
Age: Optic nerve glioma usually occurs in children but can also be observed in adults.

The tumor is composed of astrocytes (astrocytoma); however, it may be present as an oligodendroglioma or show the combination of both:

M-9382/3

Mixed oligoastrocytoma (WHO Grade II).

The tumor can infiltrate the surrounding tissue; there is no dissemination into the dura.

The tumor can be cured by surgery and radiation therapy (up to 50 Gy) [59], especially in children.

---

[59] Montgomery et al. 1977.
[69] Roberts and German 1966

Ependymal and choroid plexus tumors

M-9391/3

7. Ependymoma (WHO Grade I)

General Remarks

Incidence: 5% of tumors of the neuroepithelial tissue are ependymomas.

Age: All ages can be affected; however, the tumor usually occurs in childhood and adolescence.

In children about 9% of brain tumors are ependymomas.

Site:

T 191.5

a) **Intracranial ependymomas** (ventricles, especially the 4th ventricle) develop most frequently in **children.**

T 192.2

b) In **adults** ependymomas develop in an **intraspinal position,** particularly in the lumbosacral area, arising from the central canal.

Macroscopy

Ependymomas of the cerebrum are large neoplasms well delineated from the brain tissue.

The cut surface is grayish; cysts can appear (Fig. 813).

Ependymomas of the spinal cord are also well demarcated, giving the impression of a capsule. Due to the form of the spinal cord, the tumor is elongated.

Histology

Ependymal tumors are characterized by a great variability of the histological picture. This variability is not only apparent from tumor to tumor, but also is seen in different regions of the same tumor.

The tumor cells are elongated, the cytoplasm may be abundant, and the cell borders are well defined. Occasionally polygonal cells are observed. There is little development of the connective tissue.

Occasionally the nuclei can show pleomorphism and signs of malignancy:

M-9392/3

a) Anaplastic (malignant) ependymoma (WHO Grade III-IV) [70].

Occasionally one can find in the cytoplasm of tumor cells small round or spindle-shaped dense bodies, which represent the basal end of the ciliary shafts: **Blepharoplasts.**

In doubtful cases the evidence of blepharoplasts is important for the diagnosis of ependymoma.

The tumor cells can imitate a glandular formation. These structures are surrounded by **rosettes,** which are similar to rosettes found in medulloblastomas and neuroblastomas (Figs. 814 and 815).

The tumor cells of ependymomas can also form perivascular rosettes (Figs. 816 to 818).

According to the growth pattern and site of the ependymoma, subtypes of this tumor have been defined (see page 804):

---

[70] Rubinstein 1970.

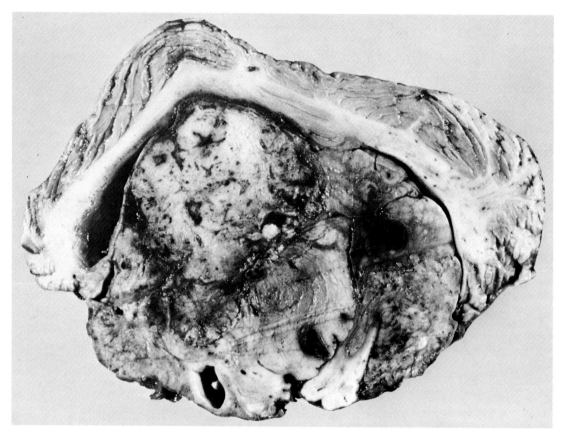

Fig. 813. Ependymoma filling the 4th ventricle.

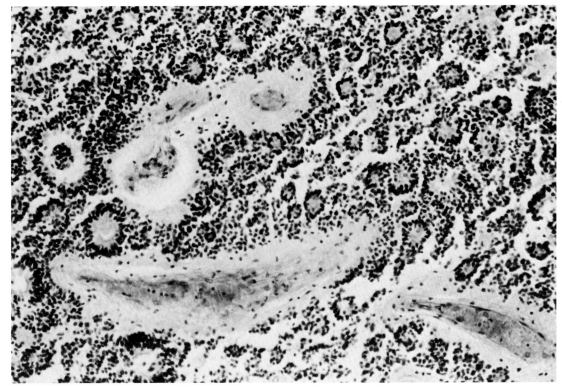

Fig. 814. Microrosette formation in ependymoma (× 125).

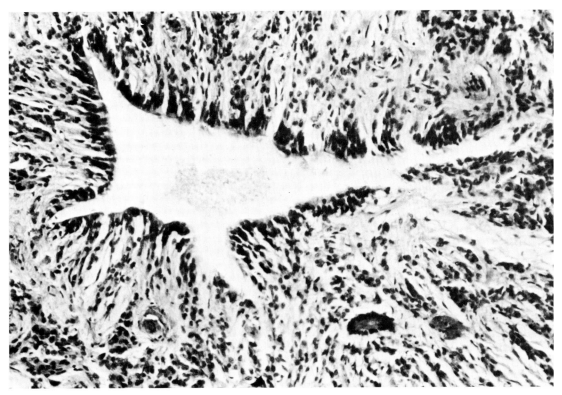

Fig. 815. Duct-like structure with rosette formation in ependymoma (× 200).

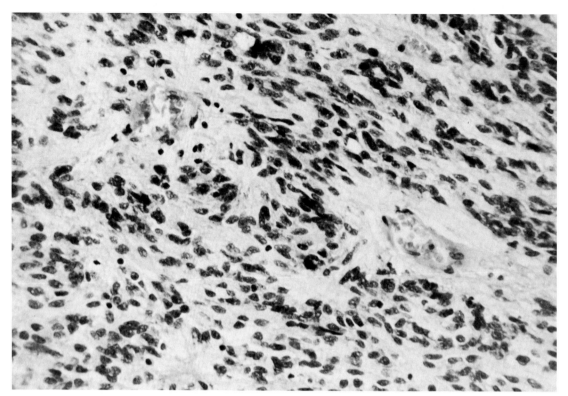

Fig. 816. Ependymoma: Perivascular rosette formation (× 200).

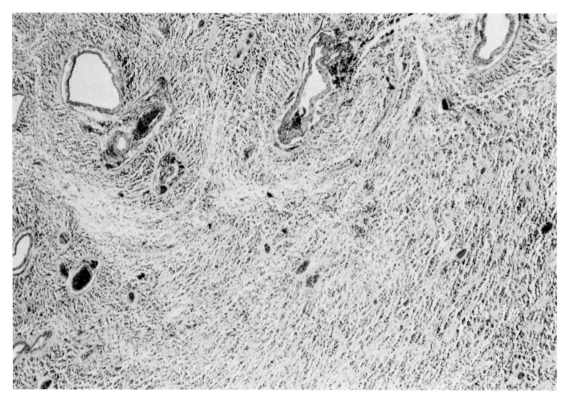

Fig. 817. Cellular ependymoma: Perivascular rosettes (× 40).

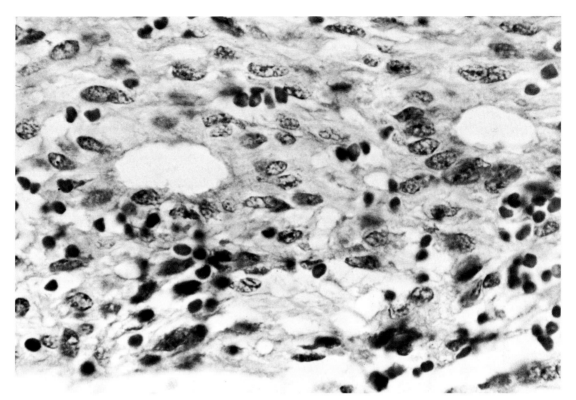

Fig. 818. Ependymoma: Perivascular rosettes and marked pleomorphism of the tumor cells (× 400).

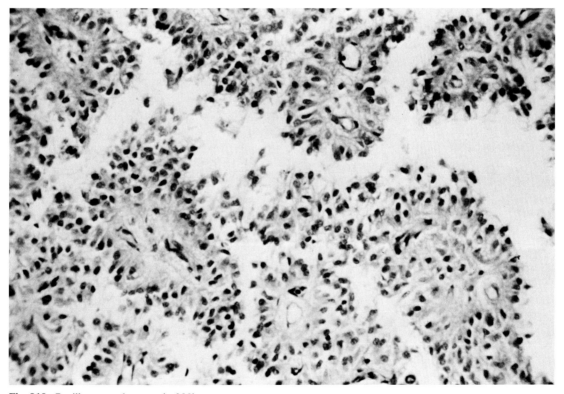

Fig. 819. Papillary ependymoma (× 200).

Ependymoma

M-9393/1

b) Papillary ependymoma (WHO Grade I)

The arrangement of the tumor cells shows distinct papillary structures (Fig. 819).

M-9394/1

c) Myxopapillary ependymoma (WHO Grade I-II)

This variety is found especially in the spinal cord (conus medullaris and filum terminale). Besides papillary formations the stroma is myxomatous. It contains mucoproteins (PAS-positive staining).

M-9383/1

d) Subependymoma (WHO Grade I)
(subependymal gliomas)

This ependymoma grows beneath the ependymal cells.
It arises in adults and grows mostly in the 4th ventricle. On histological analysis this lesion is a mixed tumor composed of ependymal cells and astrocytes, sometimes with numerous fibrils (fibrillary astrocytoma).
This tumor is not always in connection with the ependyma.
The tumor is small and slow-growing and does not obstruct the lumen of the 4th ventricle entirely.

Differential Diagnosis

1. Ependymoma **with astrocytoma** (Figs. 763 and 764).
2. Ependymoma **with medulloblastoma** (Fig. 802).
3. Ependymoma **with astroblastoma** (Fig. 778):
   Especially important for the histological diagnosis of ependymoma are
   – evidence of blepharoplasts
   – rosette formation similar to neuroblastoma and medulloblastoma: In ependymomas the rosette cells have their nucleus in the basal part of the cell;
   – perivascular rosettes.
     These rosettes can also appear in astroblastomas.
     In ependymomas one might find blepharoplasts in these perivascular cells.
     The cytoplasm of the rosette-forming cells in astroblastomas reaches the wall of the blood vessels in foot-plates (which is not the case in ependymoma) (silver impregnation stain might be helpful to differentiate both).

Spread

The malignant anaplastic ependymoma spreads into the subarachnoidal space.
Spread into the extravertebral tissue has also been observed.

Clinical Findings

The symptoms depend on the site of growth:
Ependymoma of the 4th ventricle induces secondary hydrocephalus and increased intracranial pressure. There are general symptoms of cerebral disease.

Treatment

Surgery:
It should be attempted to remove the tumor or to perform a ventriculoatrial shunting for palliation purposes.

Radiation therapy:
The ependymoma of the 4th ventricle is not very sensitive to radiation therapy. However, an extension of life for several months has been observed: Up to 50 Gy in about 5 weeks [41].

Chemotherapy:
Chemotherapy (BCNU, CCNU, for instance) has been applied together with surgery and radiation therapy [1].

Prognosis

Mean survival time: 3 years.
Combined surgery, radiation therapy, and chemotherapy increases the mean survival time by about 18 months [1, 75].
Intraspinal ependymoma: 10-year survival, 75% [58].

[1] Adams and Webster 1977.
[41] Koos and Pendl 1975.
[58] Mørk and Løken 1977.
[75] Salazar et al. 1975.

805

M-9390/0
T 191.5

8. Choroid plexus papilloma (WHO Grade I)

**General
Remarks**

Incidence: 0.5 to 0.6% of intracranial tumors are choroid plexus papillomas [100].
Age: People in the 1st and 2nd decades are mainly affected by papillomas of the lateral ventricle.
Papillomas in the 4th ventricle occur mainly in adults.
Sex: There is no sex preference.
Site: The main site is the 4th ventricle (50%), followed by the lateral ventricles and the 3rd ventricle (less than 10%).
The left ventricle is involved twice as often as the right ventricle.

Macroscopy

The tumor presents as a pink mass, which has a "papillary" surface (cauliflower-like).
The tumor is firm; calcifications can be found.
The size of the tumor varies considerably; it can be very large in the lateral ventricle. The tumor is attached to the plexus.

Histology

The tumor is composed of cuboidal or columnar cells that are arranged in a papillary fashion. The papillary structures are supported by a vascularized stroma, which is covered by the epithelial cells, mostly in monolayers.
The papillomatous structures imitate the normal pattern of the plexus (Figs. 820 and 821).
Very rarely the plexus papillomas show cellular signs of malignancy with hyperchromasia and numerous mitotic figures:

M-9390/3

Anaplastic (malignant) choroid plexus papilloma (WHO Grade III-IV)
This malignant tumor is very rare also in children [73, 79]. In most instances the "choroid carcinoma" is in reality a metastatic lesion; this is especially true for adults.

Spread

Benign papilloma:
Papillomatous cell implantations occur in the subarachnoid space of the spinal cord and the leptomeninges.
Malignant papilloma:
a) Implantation in the wall of the ventricular system.
b) Dissemination into the cerebrospinal leptomeninges.
c) Distant metastases probably do not occur.

**Clinical
Findings**

The symptoms are related to the site and the size of the tumor:
Internal hydrocephalus might occur.
Due to bleeding of the tumor the cerebrospinal fluid can be xanthochromic or blood-stained.

---

[73] Russell and Rubinstein 1977.
[79] Shuangshoti et al. 1971.
[100] Zülch 1956.

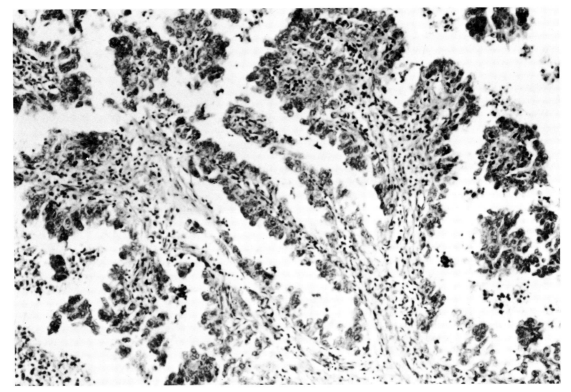

Fig. 820. Papilloma of the choroid plexus (× 125).

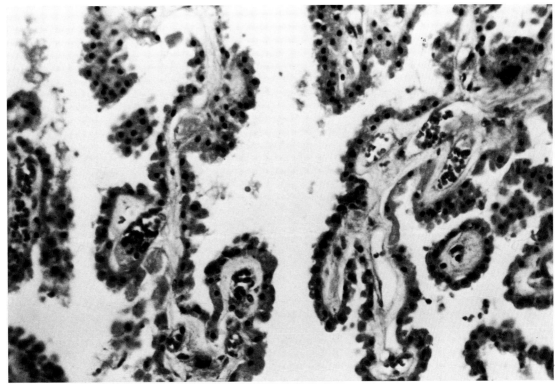

Fig. 821. Plexus papilloma (× 200).

Treatment

Surgery:
Removal of the tumor.
Radiation therapy:
Postoperative radiation therapy should be applied if the tumor cannot be entirely removed.

Prognosis

In cases of complete removal, cure.
Doubtful prognosis in cases of incomplete removal.
The prognosis is also determined by the degree of internal hydrocephalus at the time of surgical intervention.

9. Tumor-like lesions of the choroid plexus

M-4404/0
T 191.5

a) Xanthogranuloma of the choroid plexus

This lesion is characterized by histiocytes with a foamy cytoplasm. These cells grow in the connective tissue of the plexus, forming small granulomas.
In the stroma, cholesterol crystals are deposited between the histiocytes.

M-9395/0
T 191.5

b) Colloid cyst of the third ventricle (WHO)

This cyst growing in the 3rd ventricle is of different sizes; the maximal diameter is 4 cm.
The cyst contains clear fluid.
This cyst is observed mainly in the 3rd and 4th decades.
The unilocular cyst is lined by cuboidal epithelium.
Clinical findings: Acute hydrocephalus.
Treatment: Surgical removal.
Extremely seldom, squamous cell carcinoma develops from such a cyst [97].

---

[97] Wong et al. 1976.

Tumors of meningeal and related tissue

M-9530/0
T 192.1

10. Meningioma (WHO Grade I)

**General
Remarks**

Incidence: 13 to 18% of all primary intracranial tumors are meningiomas [100].
Age: The peak age is the 5th decade.
Meningiomas during adolescence are rare.
Sex: Females are more frequently affected than males.
Site: Main locations are
– parasagittal, associated with the falx,
– at the base of the sphenoid ridge,
– around the sella turcica,
– in the cerebellopontine angle.
Less frequently observed locations are petrous ridge of the temporal lobe, olfactory grooves, intraventricular position.
About 25% of the meningiomas grow in the spinal meninges [39].
The main site in this location is the thoracic region; rarely meningiomas are observed below the level of the conus medullaris.
Further notes: 1 to 2% of the brain tumors in childhood and adolescence are meningiomas [13, 62].

Macroscopy

Meningiomas are firm, round to ovoid tumors with a gray cut surface. The cut surface has a whorl-like structure with calcifications.
The well-circumscribed tumor does not invade the brain, but pushes it aside.
The bone at contact with the meningioma can be thickened (hyperosteosis).

Histology

The meningiothelial tumor cells are spindle-shaped or round.
The cytoplasm is well developed and pale.
The round nuclei are uniform, often vesicular. Mitotic divisions are rarely observed.
The tumor cells can have a foamy cytoplasm (xanthomatous area) or form giant cells.
Occasionally melanin pigment is observed in the tumor cells.
The tumor cells occasionally resemble fibroblasts. They can be surrounded by different amounts of collagen fibers. Tumor cells and fibers grow in a whorled pattern. In the center of these whorls psammoma bodies can be found [30].
A subclassification of meningiomas has been established according to the prevalent histological structures [33, 71]:

[13] Cuneo and Rand 1952.
[30] Horten et al. 1979.
[33] Humeau et al. 1979.
[39] Kernohan and Sayre 1952.
[62] Odom et al. 1956.
[71] Rubinstein 1972.
[100] Zülch 1956.

M-9531/0   **a) Meningiotheliomatous type**
(endotheliomatous; syncytial; arachnotheliomatous) (WHO Grade I)

This form is dominated by cells that rarely form a whorl-like pattern. The cells grow in sheets; the cytoplasm is well developed, finely granular, and pale (Figs. 822 and 823).

M-9532/0   **b) Fibrous (fibroblastic) meningioma** (WHO)

This tumor contains numerous collagen fibers. The tumor cells are spindle-shaped and relatively small.
Whorl formation can be observed, occasionally psammoma bodies are found (Fig. 824).
Due to the high amount of collagen fibers (and reticulin fibers) the tumor is very firm.

M-9533/0   **c) Transitional (mixed; psammomatous) meningioma** (WHO Grade I)

This meningioma is dominated by whorl formation and numerous psammoma bodies (Figs. 825 and 826).

M-9534/0   **d) Angiomatous meningioma** (WHO) [4]

This tumor contains numerous blood vessels separated by the tumor cells.
Occasionally structures similar to von Hippel-Lindau disease can be observed:
M-9535/0   **Hemangioblastic meningioma** (WHO Grade II) (Fig. 827).
In other areas the adventitial cells of the numerous blood vessels are increased, giving a picture similar to hemangiopericytoma:
M-9536/0   **Hemangiopericytic meningioma** (WHO Grade II) (Fig. 828).

M-9538/1   **e) Papillary meningioma** (WHO Grade II-III)
(see Malignant meningioma, page 815)

f) Meningioma en plaque

Grossly, these multiple small tumors cover the convexity of the brain.

M-9530/1   **g) Meningeal meningiomatosis**
T 192.1

This is a rare disease in which numerous soft, fleshy tumors originate at multiple sites.
The tumor develops mostly in adolescents and children.
This tumor tends to infiltrate the brain (Fig. 829).
These tumors can resemble on histological analysis fibrosarcomas:

M-9539/3   **h) Primary meningeal sarcomatosis** (WHO Grade IV)
T 192.1   (diffuse meningeal sarcoma, primary leptomeningeal sarcomatosis)

---

[4] Bailey et al. 1928.

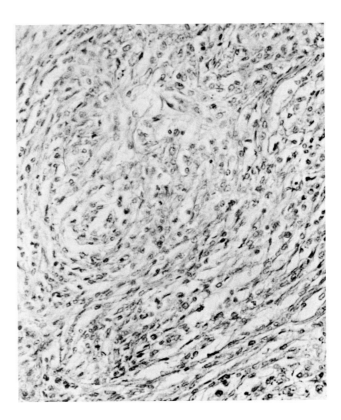

Fig. 822. Meningioma, meningotheliomatous type (× 200).

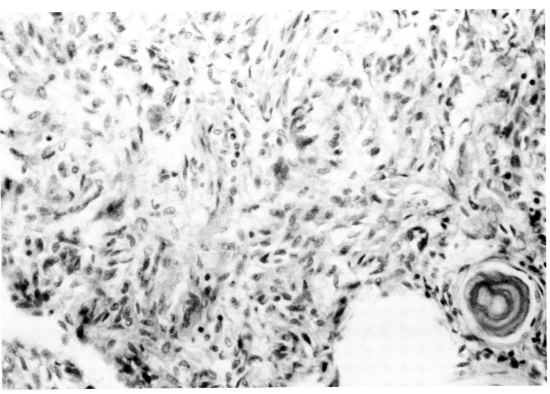

Fig. 823. Meningioma, meningotheliomatous type. Psammoma body formation (× 250).

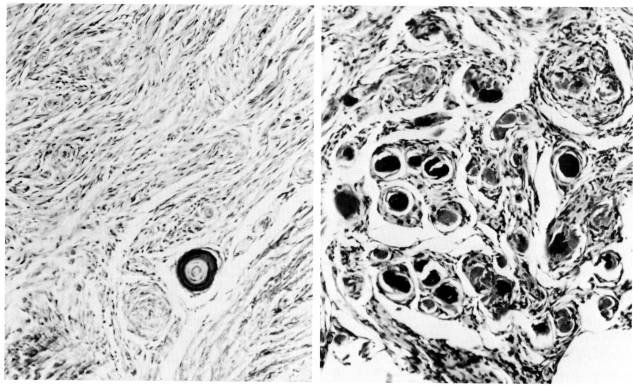

Fig. 824. Fibrous meningioma with psammoma body (× 125).

Fig. 825. Transitional (mixed) meningioma (× 200).

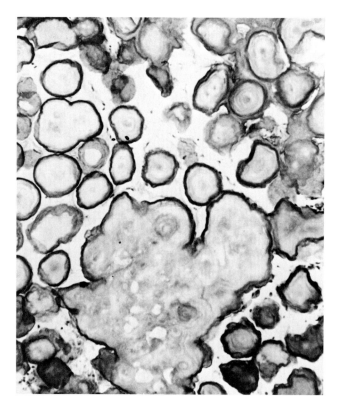

Fig. 826. Psammomatous (transitional) meningioma (× 125).

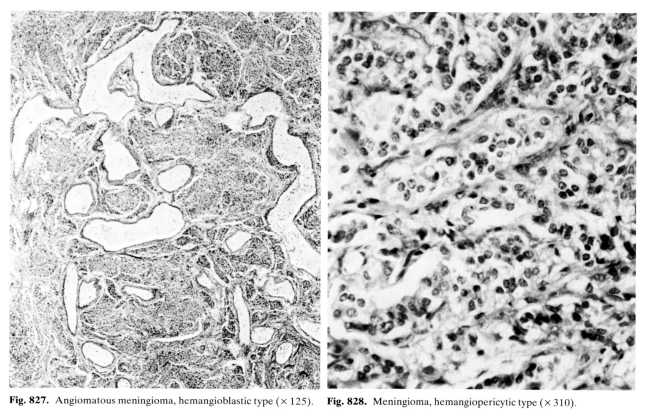

Fig. 827. Angiomatous meningioma, hemangioblastic type (× 125).

Fig. 828. Meningioma, hemangiopericytic type (× 310).

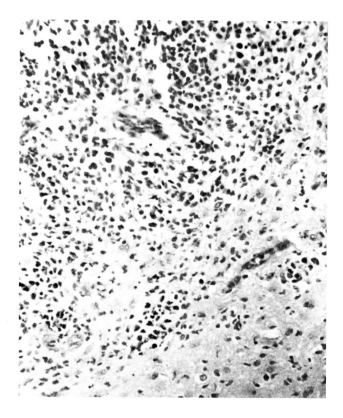

Fig. 829. Meningeal meningiomatosis: Infiltration of tumor cells into the brain tissue (× 200).

Meningioma

Differential Diagnosis

The meningioma grows with different histological appearances.

Most characteristic is the whorled architecture of this tumor.

Differential diagnosis for whorled tumor structure may be necessary between meningioma and **medulloblastoma, gliobastoma multiforme, melanomas,** or eventually **carcinomas** [37].

Spread

1. Direct spread:

   4 to 10% of meningiomas extend into the skull, the dura mater, and the major sinuses (exceptionally into the brain).

   These infiltrations of tumor cells probably explain the recurrences, in about 10% after surgical removal [81].

2. Direct spread of the tumor over the inner dural surface with invasion of the cranium is observed in

Clinical Findings

The symptoms are determined by the site and the size of the tumor as well as by the histological structure (for instance, numerous psammoma bodies or an angioblastic variety shown on arteriogram or CT scan).

Treatment

Surgery:

The tumor should be removed.

About 10% of the operated cases show recurrences.

The rate of recurrence is higher for angioblastic meningiomas and very high for meningeal meningiomatosis.

Radiation therapy:

In cases of incomplete removal or for meningiomas in children, radiation therapy should be applied [24, 45].

Prognosis

Complete removal of the meningioma means cure.

Further Information

1. The psammoma bodies are most probably due to calcifications of extracellular material [91].
2. Extracranial meningiomas are rare: They occur in the paranasal sinuses, the bone of the skull, the nasal cavity, the orbit, the ear, and on the surface of the temporal bone [3].
3. Occasionally meningioma can occupy the cerebellopontine angle. This tumor can be mistaken by gross inspection for a neurilemoma.

[3] Ashley 1978.
[24] Friedman 1977.
[37] Kepes 1976.
[45] Leibel et al. 1976.
[81] Simpson 1957.
[91] Virtanen et al. 1976.

M-9530/3
T 192.1

11. Anaplastic (malignant) meningioma (WHO Grade II-III)
(malignant meningioma; sarcomatous meningioma)

**General
Remarks**

Incidence: Malignant meningiomas are rare.

Histology

On histological analysis the malignant variety of meningioma is of high cellularity with tumor cells showing signs of malignancy (Figs. 830 to 832).
Mitotic figures are numerous.
The malignant tumor shows a papillary arrangement of the cells; this is why papillary meningiomas indicate malignancy [47].

Spread

The tumor invades the adjacent brain.
Cerebrospinal metastases and extracranial metastases are very rare [73, 78, 103].

---

[47] Ludwin et al. 1975.
[73] Russell and Rubinstein 1977.
[78] Shuangshoti et al. 1970.
[103] Zülch et al. 1954.

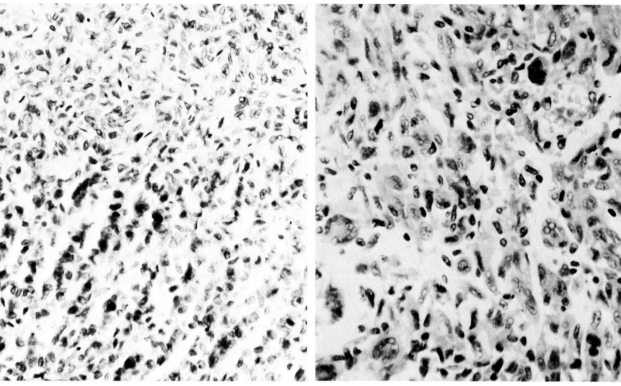

Fig. 830. Sarcomatous meningioma (×200).

Fig. 831. Sarcomatous meningioma: Numerous atypical cells and giant cells (×310).

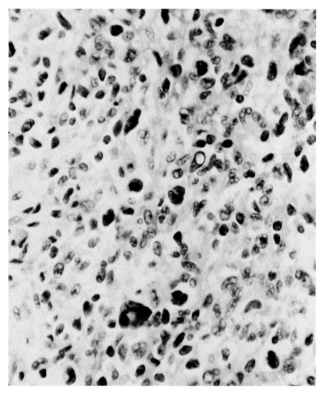

Fig. 832. Sarcomatous meningioma. Numerous malignant cells (×310).

M-8800/3
T 192.1

12. Meningeal sarcomas (WHO)
("primary sarcomas", intracranial sarcomas)

**General
Remarks**

Incidence: Meningeal sarcomas are rare.
Age: They are usually observed in children and infants [40].
Site: In most cases the meningeal sarcoma arises from the dura. However, it can also develop from the leptomeninges.

Macroscopy

These are soft tumors that infiltrate the brain. In the brain they are ill-defined.
The cut surface shows cysts, areas of hemorrhage, and necroses.

Histology

The histological picture varies according to the differentiation of the malignant mesenchymal cells:

M-8810/3

a) Fibrosarcoma (WHO Grade III-IV)

In these instances the tumor is composed of cells that are surrounded by reticulin fibers; numerous collagen fibers are present.

M-8802/3

b) Polymorphic cell sarcoma (WHO Grade III-IV)

This tumor consists of tumor cells that are composed in nests and sheets and infiltrate the surrounding tissue.
Reticulin fibers can be found but they are considerably less well developed than in fibrosarcoma varieties.

M-9539/3

c) Primary meningeal sarcomatosis (WHO) (see page 810).

d) Occasionally meningeal sarcomas have been observed with **chondrosarcomatous** [76] **and myxosarcomatous** [27] **components,** as well as parts of **rhabdomyosarcoma** [43, 55]

**Differential
Diagnosis
M-9640/3**

Meningeal sarcoma **with malignant lymphoma** (reticulosarcoma) [46] (Figs. 833 to 835):
Cells of malignant lymphomas have the cytological features of this malignant tumor.
Malignant lymphomas of the central nervous system are mostly of a multifocal origin [31].

---

[27] Guccion et al. 1973.
[31] Horvat et al. 1969.
[40] Kernohan and Uhlheim 1962.
[43] Lam and Colah 1979.
[46] Littman and Wang 1975.
[55] Min et al. 1975.
[76] Scheithauer and Rubinstein 1978.

Treatment

Surgery:
According to the extent of the disease, surgery has been recommended [46].
Radiation therapy:
This treatment is applied after surgical removal of the tumor.
It is not yet known how sensitive these sarcomatous tumors are [41].

Further Information M-9140/3

1. Meningeal sarcomas can be induced by therapeutic irradiation [26, 73, 93].
2. There is a report of **Kaposi's sarcoma** of the brain [74].
3. Exceedingly rare are reports of primary **intraparenchymal brain sarcomas,** which are occasionally called fibrosarcomas [54].

[26] Gonzales-Vitale et al. 1976.
[41] Koos and Pendl 1975.
[46] Littman and Wang 1975.
[54] Mena and Garcia 1978.
[73] Russell and Rubinstein 1977.
[74] Rwomushana et al. 1975.
[93] Waltz and Brownell 1966.

M-9590/3
T 192.1

13. Primary malignant lymphoma of the brain

General Remarks

Incidence: About 0.2 to 2% of non-Hodgkin's lymphomas have their primary site in the central nervous system [23, 29].

Site: Malignant lymphomas are of a multifocal origin (Fig. 833).

They can involve the leptomeninges and the skull.

M-9650/3 Very rare are **Hodgkin's lymphomas** in the brain.

M-9730/3 Exceedingly rare are primary solitary **plasmacytomas** of the brain substance [36, 95] and of the meninges [49].

Histology

The histological appearance of malignant lymphomas corresponds to those observed outside the central nervous system (Figs. 834 and 835) [88].

M-8831/1, 3

Fibroxanthoma and malignant fibroxanthoma (xanthosarcoma) (WHO):

These tumors are considered varieties of malignant lymphomas, histiocytic type.

The tumor cells have a foamy cytoplasm and giant cells of a Touton type have been observed [38].

Treatment

Surgery:

In cases of circumscribed unilocular malignant lymphoma (reticulosarcoma), surgery combined with postoperative irradiation of at least 45 Gy has been recommended [46].

Radiation therapy:

In cases of multilocular tumors radiation therapy can be tried: The reticulosarcoma is highly radiosensitive (up to 40 Gy in 5 weeks).

---

[23] Freeman et al. 1972.
[29] Herman et al. 1979.
[36] Kamin and Hepler 1972.
[38] Kepes et al. 1973.
[46] Littman and Wang 1975.
[49] Mancilla-Jimenez and Tavassoli 1976.
[88] Taylor et al. 1978.
[95] Weiner et al. 1966.

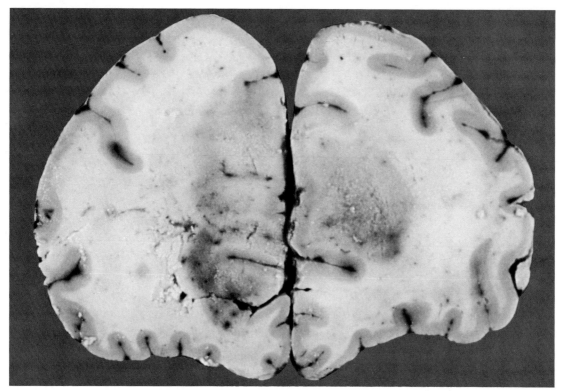

Fig. 833. Primary malignant lymphoma of the brain.

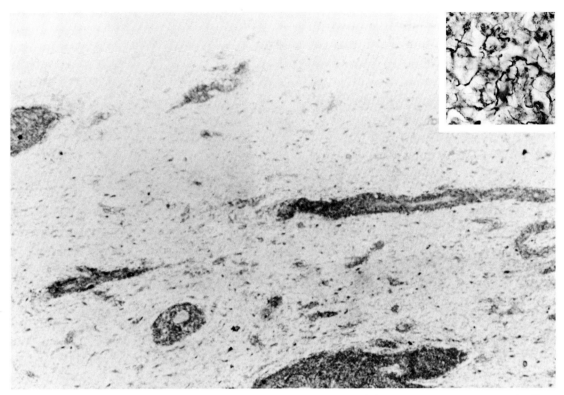

Fig. 834. Primary malignant lymphoma of the brain (reticulum cell sarcoma) (× 40; inset: Reticulin fiber stain, fibers surround the individual tumor cells, × 800).

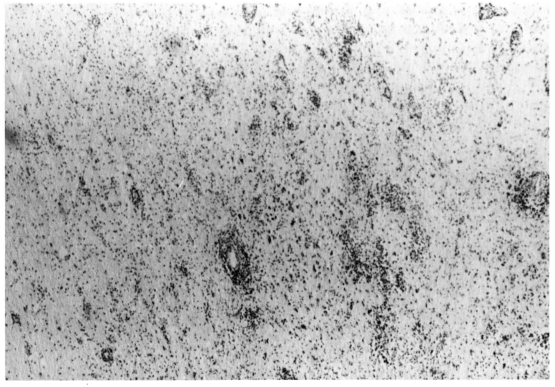

Fig. 835. Primary (lymphocytic) malignant lymphoma of the brain: Perivascular and diffuse infiltration (× 50).

821

Primary melanotic tumors (WHO) (see page 1222)

M-8720/3
T 192.1

14. Melanoma (WHO Grade IV)

Primary melanoma is rare in the brain.
The tumor diffusely infiltrates the meninges.
The prognosis is poor.

15. Meningeal melanomatosis (WHO Grade IV)

The meninges, which cover the brain substance and the spinal cord, are involved by meningeal melanomatosis.
This lesion is usually observed in infants and children.
Very rarely, primary intracranial melanomas can disseminate outside the central nervous system [64].
The origin of these melanotic tumors seems to be the melanocytes of the leptomeninges, shown by ultrastructural observations [80].
Rarely melanin has been observed as a component of cerebral gliomas [52].

M-9363/0
T 192.1

16. Neurocutaneous melanosis (WHO) [15]

This is a benign familial condition, in which melanotic pigmentation of the leptomeninges is combined with large cutaneous nevi.
Occasionally it has been reported that this lesion is combined with peripheral neurofibromas [82].

[15] Dehner et al. 1979.
[52] McCloskey et al. 1976.
[64] Pasquier et al. 1978.
[80] Silbert et al. 1978.
[82] Slaughter et al. 1969.

Neuronal tumors

M-9490/0

17. Gangliocytoma (WHO Grade I)

M-9505/1

18. Ganglioglioma (WHO Grade I-II)

**General
Remarks**

Incidence: These tumors are rare in the central nervous system.
Age: Usually children and people under 30 years old are affected.
Site: The main sites are the third ventricle, temporal lobe, and hypothalamus [86].

Macroscopy

The tumors grow as single lesions or are multiple.
They are well circumscribed and firm and have a granular cut surface. The tumors are small.
The tumors contain areas of calcification.

Histology

Gangliocytoma (ganglioneuroma) [2]:
This tumor is composed of cells of a neuronal origin. It can show abnormalities such as binucleation, multinucleation, and a bizarre shape (Figs. 836 and 837). There are no mitotic figures.
There is no astrocytic proliferation.
Occasionally this tumor can contain lymphocyte-like infiltration, which has a predominance in the perivascular regions.
Calcospherites can be found.

Ganglioglioma:
This tumor is composed of bizarre ganglion cells combined with a proliferation of glioma cells (astrocytoma).
This astrocytic component can be fibrillary or protoplasmic.
Occasionally foci of the gemistocytic or oligodendroglial type are encountered.
Also in this variety foci of lymphocytic infiltration can be observed.
Again foci of calcification might exist.

---

[2] Ahdevaara et al. 1977.
[86] Steegmann and Winer 1961.

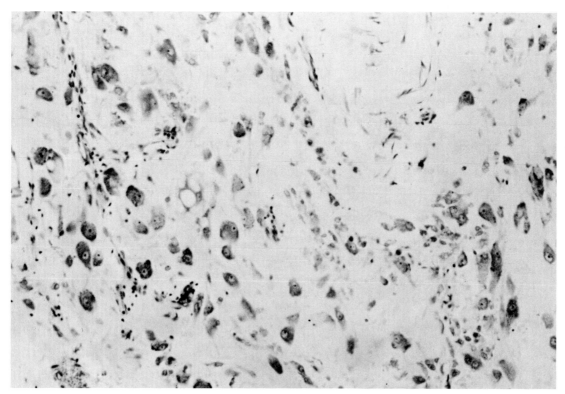

Fig. 836. Gangliocytoma: Bizare-shaped tumor cells (× 125).

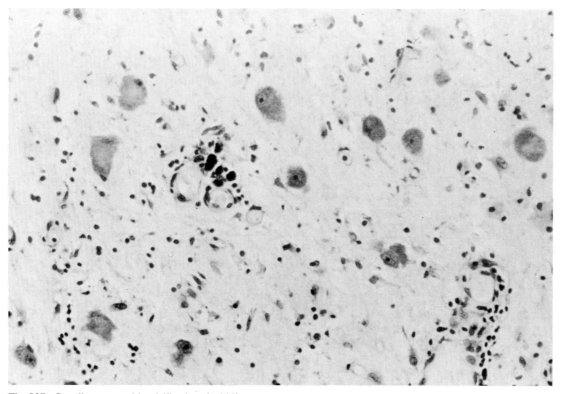

Fig. 837. Gangliocytoma with calcifications (× 200).

M-9490/1

19. Ganglioneuroblastoma (WHO Grade III)

M-9490/3

20. Anaplastic (malignant) gangliocytoma and ganglioglioma (WHO Grade III-IV)

These tumors contain neuronal cells that lack maturation and areas of malignant cells, which can be anaplastic neuronal cells with axons, atypical astrocytes, or cells of a neuroblastoma [22, 66, 73].

Further Information

Hypothalamic neuronal hamartoma (WHO):
This lesion shows gray matter at the site of the corpora mamillaria and the tuber cinerium.
The lesion is very rare.
Almost always males are affected.
Clinically this lesion frequently induces pubertas precox.
On histological examination the lesion is composed of cerebral gray matter [73].
Occasionally, similar hamartomas can be observed in other sites of the brain. Usually they are not clinically important and are accidental findings on autopsy.
Occasionally, they might cause epilepsy.

---

[22] Feigin and Budzilovich 1974.
[66] Pearson et al. 1976.
[73] Russell and Rubinstein 1977.

21. Neuroblastoma (WHO Grade IV)

**General
Remarks**

T 191.0

Incidence: This tumor is very rare in the central nervous system.
Age: This is a tumor of childhood, with a peak incidence in the first decade.
Site: Most of the tumors develop in the cerebral hemispheres, usually in the frontal and frontoparietal areas.

Macroscopy

These are usually large tumors, well differentiated from the surrounding tissue, with a granular cut surface.
Regressive changes with hemorrhage or cysts can be observed.
Usually the tumor is rather firm.

Histology

The tumor is composed of small cells that are closely packed.
The cells are round or oval, and mitoses are frequently encountered.
The tumor cells have hyperchromatic nuclei.
The tumor cells form rosettes with neurofibrils in the center (Homer-Wright rosettes). These rosettes correspond to those found in peripheral neuroblastomas (Figs. 1730 to 1732).
The degree of connective tissue reaction in these tumors varies and determines the firmness of the tumor.
This connective tissue reaction distinguishes the central neuroblastoma from the peripheral tumor [73].

**Differential
Diagnosis**

Neuroblastoma **with malignant lymphoma:**
The appearance of rosettes and the degree of connective tissue reaction indicates neuroblastoma.

Spread

1. Occasionally extraneural metastases can occur.
2. Tumor dissemination can develop in the cerebrospinal path.

Treatment

Surgery.
Radiation therapy:
Neuroblastomas are radiosensitive [16, 17].
Chemotherapy:
Effective drugs are: Adriamycin, dactinomycin, vincristine, and cyclophosphamide.
The response rate is about 40 to 65%; the remission rate is about 20% [16, 17].

Prognosis

The prognosis is determined by the great rate of recurrences, which can appear several years following operation.

[16] DeVita, Jr. 1977.
[17] Dold and Sack 1976.
[73] Russell and Rubinstein 1977.

M-9510/3
T 190.5

22. Retinoblastoma

(see page 906)

M-9522/3
T 160.0

23. Olfactory neuroblastoma

(esthesioneuroepithelioma) (WHO) (Figs. 503 to 505)
(see page 500)

Tumors of blood vessel origin and vascular malformations

M-9161/1
T 191.6

24. Hemangioblastoma (WHO Grade I)
(papillary hemangioblastoma)

**General
Remarks**

Incidence: About 2% of intracranial tumors are hemangioblastomas.
Age: All ages can be affected.
Sex: The tumors occur more often in males than in females.
Site: The tumor in most instances is localized in the cerebellum, especially in a paramedian position.
The tumor might also occur in the vermis, the medulla oblongata, and the spinal cord.
Hemangioblastoma is exceedingly rare in a supratentorial location.

Macroscopy

Hemangioblastomas can occur as solitary tumors; however, occasionally they are multiple.
The tumor is well delineated from the surrounding tissue.
The cut surface is yellowish-brownish.
The tumor induces cyst formation. The cysts can be so large that it might be difficult to find the hemangioblastoma initiating the cyst (Fig. 838).

Histology

The tumor is composed of small capillary blood vessels, which are lined by regular endothelial cells. Between the capillary spaces pericytes are found which occasionally can have hyperchromatic nuclei (Figs. 839 to 842).
These cells, furthermore, can have a xanthomatous cytoplasm.
Occasionally these stroma cells are multinucleated.
The tumor can contain foci of calcification, which become visible on X-rays.

**Electron
Microscopy**

Hemangioblastoma of the cerebellum is composed of stroma cells containing numerous, membrane-bound lipid inclusions and nuclear bodies. The tumor is, furthermore, composed of endothelial cells and pericytes [11].

**Differential
Diagnosis**

Hemangioblastoma **with angioblastic meningioma** (Fig. 827):
Especially with supratentorial tumors it might be difficult to decide whether the tumor is meningioma or hemangioblastoma.
This diagnostic matter is still a topic of controversial discussion.

**Clinical
Findings**

The clinical signs depend on the size and site of the hemangioblastoma.
X-rays might show calcifications in the tumor.

Treatment

Surgery:
Surgical removal of the tumor.

---

[11] Chaudhry et al. 1978.

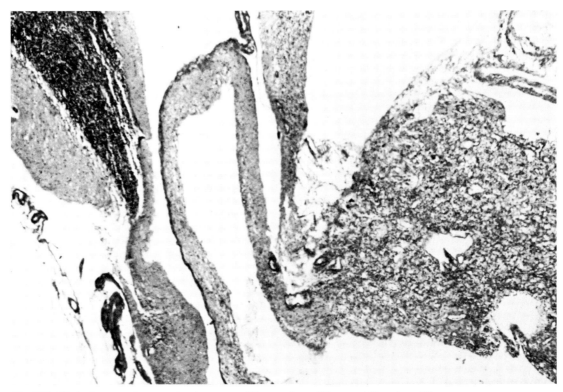

Fig. 838. Lindau's tumor: Large cyst and a very small hemangioma (39-year-old female, × 50).

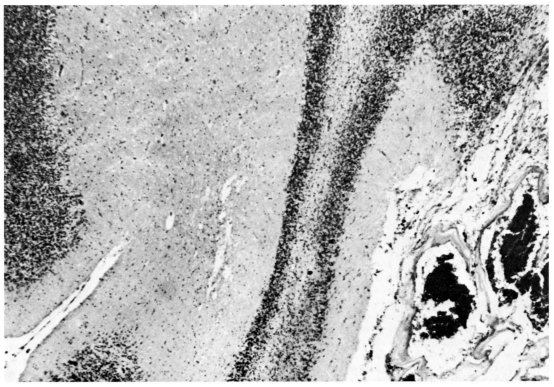

Fig. 839. Angiomatosis in the cerebellum (× 40).

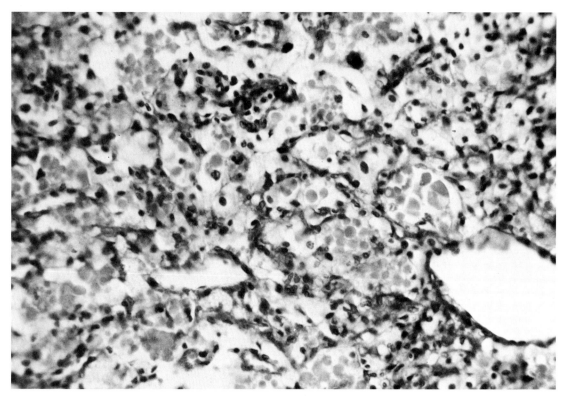

Fig. 840. Capillary hemangioma in Lindau's tumor (39-year-old female, × 200).

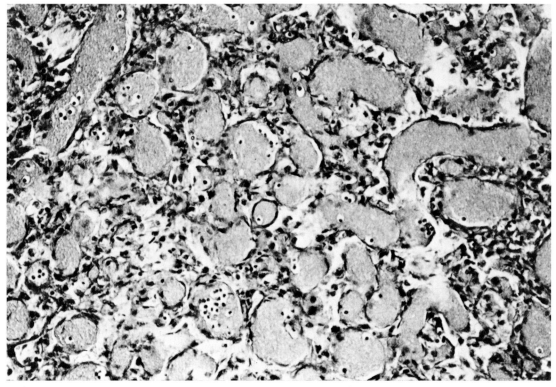

Fig. 841. Dilated numerous blood vessels in Lindau's tumor (× 125).

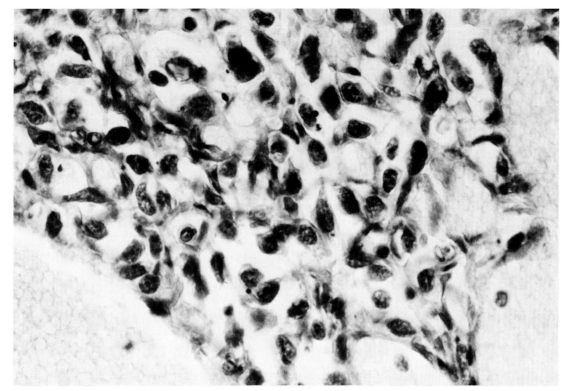

Fig. 842. Hyperchromatic endothelial cells in Lindau's tumor (× 400).

Hemangioblastoma

Prognosis

In cases of solitary hemangioblastoma, resection means cure.

Recurrences might appear. However, they are most probably a sign of the multifocal origin of hemangioblastomas.

Further Information
M-9161/1
T 191.6

1. The hemangioblastoma with cyst formation in the cerebellum **(Lindau's tumor)** may be associated with other lesions:
   - Angiomas in the retina **(von Hippel's disease);** syringomyelia, hydromyelia,
   - cysts of the liver, lung, pancreas, and kidney,
   - renal adenoma and renal cell carcinoma,
   - pheochromocytoma [53].

   Clinical findings in Lindau's tumor:

   Appearance for the first time in the 3rd decade: Headache, cerebellar ataxia, papilledema.

   Often polycythemia is observed (probably due erythropoietin production in the tumor).

   Lindau's disease is hereditary (autosomal-dominant).

   The origin of this tumor might be within the pia [73].

   It seems that endothelial cells and pericytes, stroma sells, and occasionally hematopoietic cells contribute to the formation of this tumor, based on evidence by electron microscopy and organ culture studies [85].

2. Occasionally hemangioblastomas can grow as malignant tumors with giant cells, which might occasionally be difficult to distinguish from a glioblastoma:

M-9481/3
T 191.6

Monstrocellular sarcoma (WHO Grade IV).

---

[53] Melmon and Rosen 1964.
[73] Russell and Rubinstein 1977.
[85] Spence and Rubinstein 1975.

M-9131/0
T 191.7

25. Capillary teleangiectasia
(WHO – vascular malformation)

General Remarks

Incidence: The tumor is seldom of functional importance and is usually detected at autopsy. The true incidence is difficult to determine.
Age: When the tumor is found, the patients are in the 5th to 8th decades.
Sex: Both sexes are equally affected.
Site: The main location is the pons.
The hamartoma is rarely found in the spinal cord.

Macroscopy

This is a discrete lesion, which is in most instances solitary. The lesion is not well delineated from the surrounding brain tissue.
The cut surface is reddish.

Histology

The tumor contains capillaries that are very dilated. However, the lumen of these blood vessels is not uniform: Small and large vessels are observed (Fig. 843).
The blood vessels do not contain muscle fibers or elastic fibers.
The capillaries are surrounded by neural tissue.

Clinical Findings

Occasionally these hamartomas can cause cerebral bleeding.

Further Information

This capillary teleangiectasia may rarely be associated with Osler's disease.

M-9121/0
T 191.0

26. Cavernous hemangioma
(WHO – vascular malformation)

General Remarks

Incidence: This is a rare lesion.
Age: The tumor is detected in the 3rd to 6th decades.
Sex: Males are affected more often than females.
Site: The main site is in the cerebrum (subcortical position), followed by the pons and the spinal cord.

Macroscopy

In most instances this is a solitary tumor, which might be rather large.
The tumor is well delineated from the surrounding tissue and shows a reddish cut surface.
Areas of calcification can be detected on gross inspection.

Histology

The tumor is composed of cavernous blood vessels (cavernoma) that are closely packed together (Fig. 844).
On histological analysis the foci of calcification can be detected; occasionally regression with hyalinization and ossification is seen.

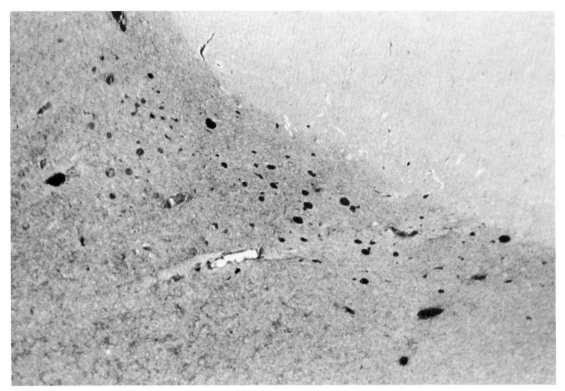

Fig. 843. Capillary teleangiectasia with calcifications (× 40).

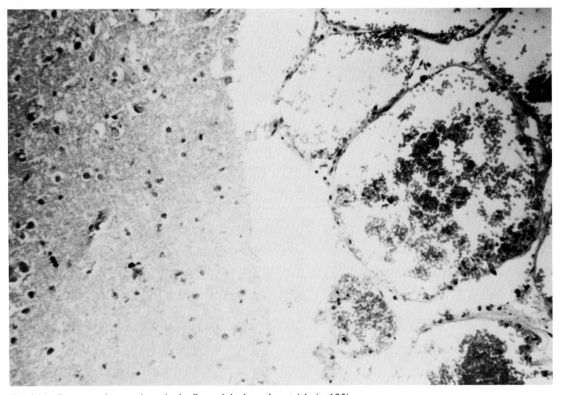

Fig. 844. Cavernous hemangioma in the floor of the lateral ventricle (× 125).

M-9123/0
T 191.0

27. Arteriovenous malformation (WHO)
(cirsoid angioma)

**General
Remarks**

Incidence: About 0.5% of intracranial tumors are arteriovenous hamartomas [73].
Age: The tumor appears with clinical symptoms usually during the 2nd decade.
Sex: Males are more often affected than females.
Site: The majority of these tumors are supplied by the middle cerebral artery (Fig. 845).
This tumor is rarely observed in the spinal cord and the cerebellum.

Macroscopy

The tumor is grossly composed of convoluted, large blood vessels in the meninges and occasionally in the center of the brain.
The lesion extends between the cortical convolutions and might penetrate into the substance of the brain.
Foci of hyalinization and calcification can be detected.

Histology

The tumor is composed of large blood vessels. The walls of the blood vessels show signs of arterial origin (muscle fibers and elastic fibers) or the wall of a vein.
Areas of collagen fibers with calcifications and hyalinizations are found (Fig. 846).
The blood vessels can be occluded by thrombi (Fig. 847).
Formations of aneurysmatic changes in the wall may occur.

**Clinical
Findings**

These hamartomas can cause focal seizures.
Arteriovenous angiomas can be the cause of cerebral or subarachnoid bleeding.

---

[73] Russell and Rubinstein 1977.

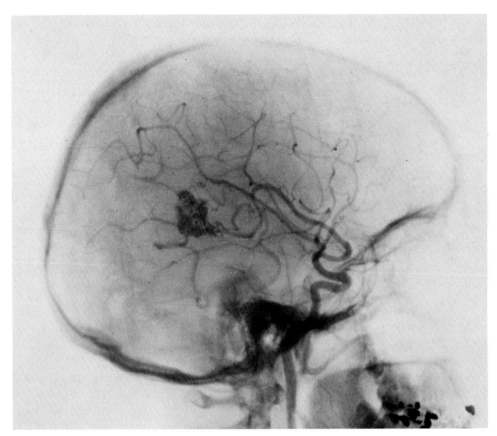

Fig. 845. Angioma racemosum (a. cerebri media).

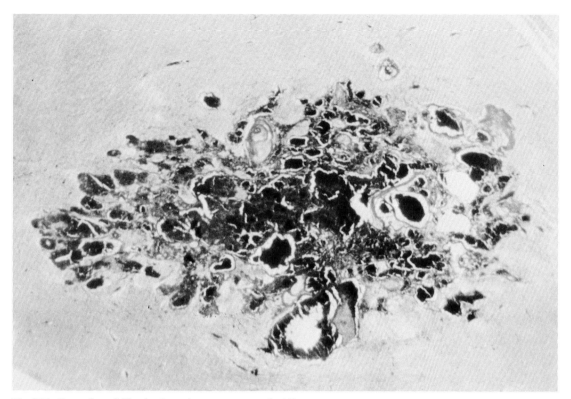

Fig. 846. Extensive calcification in angioma racemosum (× 40).

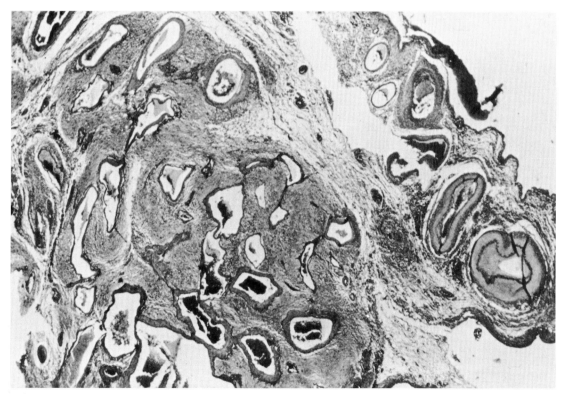

Fig. 847. Angioma racemosum with organized thrombi (× 40).

M-9122/0
T 192.2

28. Venous malformations (WHO)

General
Remarks

Incidence: The tumor is very rare in the brain and more often is observed in the spinal cord, including its meninges.

This hamartoma can also be observed in the choroid plexus.

Macroscopy

This hamartoma is composed of large veins, which might be on the surface of the spinal cord.

Histology

The tumor is composed of large veins.

The wall of the blood vessels can show hyalinizations of the connective tissue.

The blood vessels can be occluded by thrombi.

M-7631/0
T 191.0

29. Sturge-Weber disease (WHO)
(cerebrofacial or cerebrotrigeminal angiomatosis)

General Remarks

Incidence: This is a rare hamartomatous lesion, most probably a subgroup of arteriovenous hamartomas.

Site:

a) The hamartoma affects one cerebral hemisphere.

b) Superficial cavernous angioma of a port wine color (nevus flammeus, localized in the trigeminal nerve region).

c) Choroidal hemangioma with glaucoma and retina degeneration.

Macroscopy

The hamartoma is situated in the leptomeninges, which are thickened.

The brain underneath the leptomeninges is atrophied and contains numerous blood vessels.

Calcifications can be seen.

Histology

This hamartoma is composed of small blood vessels: Small veins and capillaries.

These blood vessels are found in the pia mater and in the underlying cortex.

Calcifications develop in the blood vessel wall, which is thickened due to regressive changes in the connective tissue of the wall.

Clinical Findings

Nevus flammeus combined with focal seizures (on the side opposite the skin hamartoma).

Visual field defects due to choroid hemangioma.

The calcifications can be seen on X-rays in a double contour.

Treatment

In most instances surgical intervention is technically difficult due to the extension of the hamartoma.

In cases of intractable epilepsy, hemispherectomy has been advised.

Anticonvulsant drugs are indicated.

Further Information

1. Occasionally arteriovenous angiomas can develop in the spinal cord in association with cutaneous hemangiomas [18].

2. There are form fruste of Sturge-Weber disease, in which the calcifications may be lacking.

---

[18] Doppman et al. 1969.

Tumors of nerve sheath cells (see page 163)

M-9560/0
T 192.0

30. Neurilemoma (WHO Grade I)
(schwannoma, neurinoma)

Intracranial neurilemomas have their most important site at the acoustic nerve in the cerebellopontine angle.
This tumor is observed in adults as a solitary lesion.

M-9550/0, 1

31. Nerve sheath tumors associated with von Recklinghausen's disease

Neurilemomas and neurofibromas can develop in an intracranial or spinal position in von Recklinghausen's disease (Figs. 848 to 850).
Multiple neurofibromas or bilateral neurilemomas (neurofibromas) in the cerebellopontine angles are observed.
Occasionally these nerve sheath tumors are associated with meningiomas, astrocytomas, ependymomas, and optic nerve gliomas in von Recklinghausen's disease [71].
The treatment of neurilemoma in the cerebellopontine angle is surgical removal.

M-9540/3

32. Anaplastic (malignant) neurilemoma (WHO Grade II)
(Figs. 169 to 172).

M-9540/3

33. Anaplastic (malignant) neurofibroma (WHO Grade III-IV)
(neurofibrosarcoma, neurogenic sarcoma)
(see page 168).

---

[71] Rubinstein 1972.

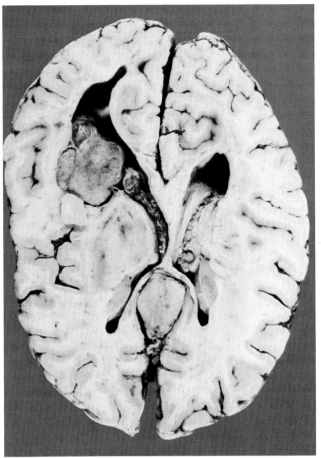

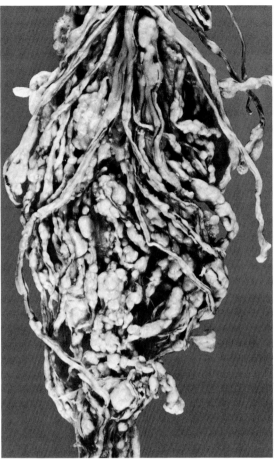

Fig. 848. Intracerebral tumors in von Recklinghausen's disease (29-year-old male) (intraventricular tumor = neurinoma; anterior tumor = meningioma).

Fig. 849. Cerebellopontine angle tumor in von Recklinghausen's disease (29-year-old male).

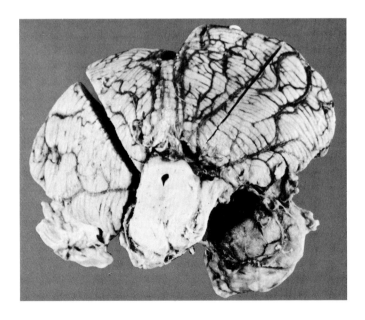

Fig. 850. Numerous tumors in the cauda equina (von Recklinghausen's disease) (29-year-old male).

M-8850/0   # 34. Lipoma

Lipomas in the central nervous system are very rare.
They are mainly observed in the spinal cord and over the corpus callosum.

M-9360/1
T 194.4

35. Tumors of the pineal gland (WHO)
(pinealoma)

Tumors of the pineal gland occur in about 0.4 to 1% of intracranial tumors [100].
The following tumors can develop in the pineal gland:

I. Cysts
Epidermoid cysts and dermoid cysts; non-neoplastic cysts [73].

II. Tumors of the neuroepithelial tissue
For instance, astrocytic tumors, chemodectoma [83], meningioma, ependymoma
[50, 63], malignant melanoma [73] (see corresponding pages) (Fig. 856 a-d).

III. Metastatic tumors

M-9080/1, 3
T 194.4

IV. Germ cell tumors (WHO)
(see also page 1474).

General
Remarks

Incidence: Germ cell tumors in the central nervous system are rare.
Age: The tumors develop in young adults [14].
Sex: Males are more affected than females.
Site: The majority of germ cell tumors develop in the pineal gland or in a suprasellar or
intrasellar position.
The growth of the germ cell tumor can extend into the 3rd ventricle.

---

[14] Dayan et al. 1966.
[50] Markesbery et al. 1976.
[63] Oswald and Hedinger 1972.
[73] Russell and Rubinstein 1977.
[83] Smith et al. 1966.
[100] Zülch 1956.

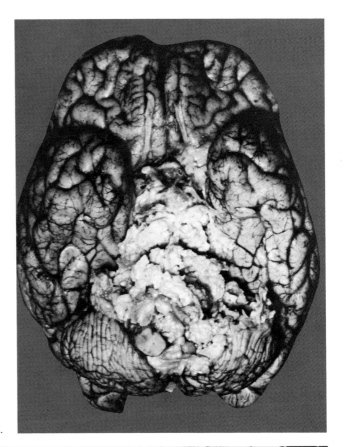

Fig. 851. Cholesteatoma at the base of the brain.

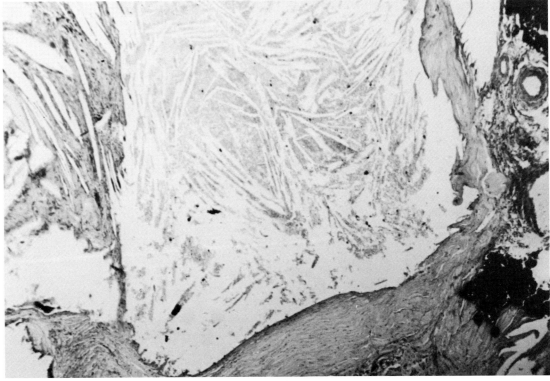

Fig. 852. Cholesteatoma: Scar tissue and calcifications (76-year-old male, × 40).

843

Pineal gland

Macroscopy

Germ cell tumors are well-defined, often lobulated tumors, which are friable and soft. According to the degree of differentiation, they might contain hair, bone, or cartilage.

Histology

Germ cell tumors show different degrees of differentiation.

M-9084/0
T 194.4

a) Dermoid cyst (WHO):

This germ cell tumor contains the three germ cell layers [39] with squamous cell epithelium, hair follicles, sweat glands, and sebaceous glands.
The dermoid cysts are rarely observed in the pineal gland, but more often are in midline position in the vermis or in the 4th ventricle.
Occasionally spinal cord cyst can be lined by intestinal epithelium:
Enterogenous cyst (WHO).

M-7290/0
T 192.9

b) Epidermoid cyst (WHO)
(cholesteatoma):

These cysts can occur in any age group. The first clinical symptoms appear between the 3rd and 6th decades.
Site: Cholesteatomas are found in the cerebellopontine angle (Figs. 851 and 852), in parapituitary position, and in the spinal cord, whereas they are rarely observed in the cerebral hemispheres.

c) Malignant germ cell tumors occur in the pineal gland and in suprasellar or intrasellar position:

- **choriocarcinoma,**
- **embryonal carcinoma,**
- **yolk sac tumor** [98],
- **seminoma** (dysgerminoma) [7, 60].
(For details on germ cell tumors, see Tumors of the testes, page 1469).

Therapy

Surgery, radiation therapy [34, 94].

[7]   Bestle 1968.
[34] Jenkin et al. 1978.
[39] Kernohan and Sayre 1952.
[60] Nishiyama et al. 1966.
[94] Wara et al. 1979.
[98] Yoshiki et al. 1976.

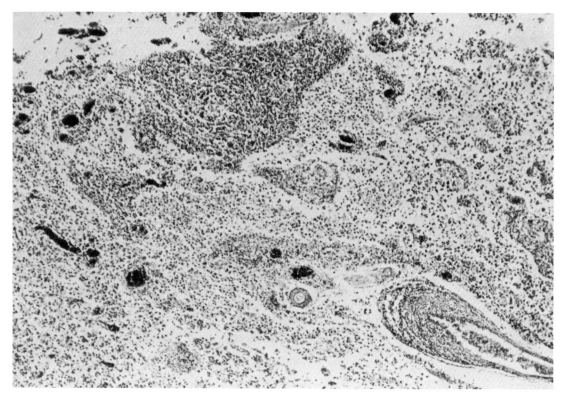

Fig. 853. Pinealoma: Nests of small tumor cells, rosette formation, and perivascular arrangement (× 40).

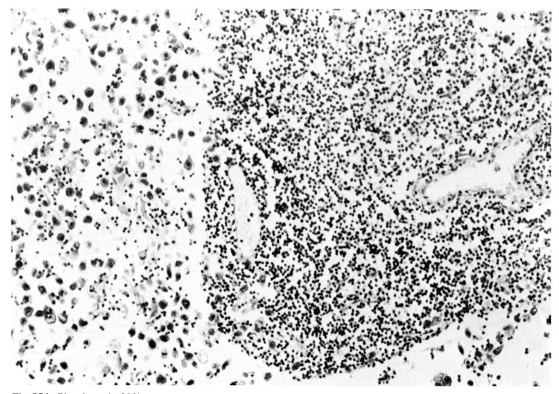

Fig. 854. Pinealoma (× 200).

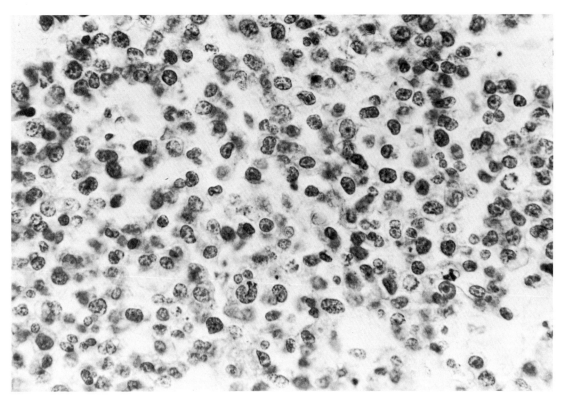

Fig. 855. Pinealoma composed of two different cells (anisomorphous pinealoma) (×400).

V. Pineal cell tumors

M-9361/1
T 194.4

a) Pineocytoma (WHO)
(pinealocytoma)

Incidence: Pineocytomas are exceedingly rare tumors.

They are composed of cells with a dark nucleus, which grow in small nests. These nests are surrounded by connective tissue.
Occasionally the tumor cells are arranged in rosettes.
Pineocytomas can be composed of one cell type with dense nuclei:
Isomorphous pineocytoma (WHO Grade I-III) (Figs. 853 and 854)
or of two different cell types, one with loose clear nuclei:
Anisomorphous pineocytoma (WHO Grade III-IV) (Figs. 855 and 856 a-d).

M-9362/3
T 194.4

b) Pinealoblastoma (WHO Grade IV)

This tumor is extremely cellular and consists of densely packed cells with a hyperchromatic nucleus.
The histological picture resembles neuroblastomas or medulloblastomas.
Radiotherapy of up to 60 Gy seems to be the treatment of choice [56].

---

[56] Mincer et al. 1976.

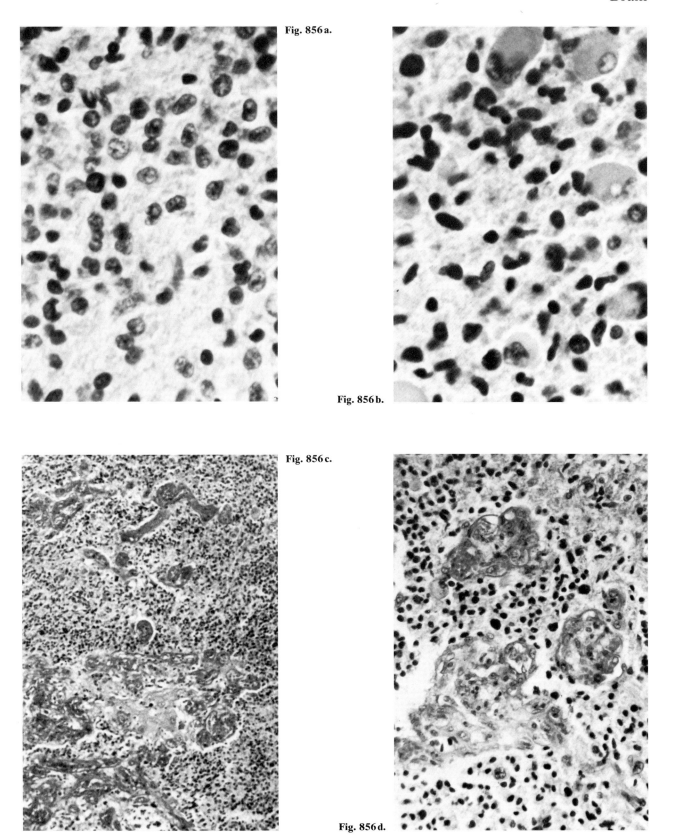

Fig. 856 a.

Fig. 856 b.

Fig. 856 c.

Fig. 856 d.

Fig. 856 a-d. Anisomorphous pineocytoma (a) combined with gemistocytic astrocytoma (b) and glioblastoma multiforme (c, d) (50-year-old male; a, b, × 310; c, × 50; d, × 200).

36. Metastases into the brain

a) Hematogenous metastases:

Metastatic growth in the brain can be solitary or multiple.
Any site of the brain can be affected; only exceptionally is the spinal cord involved.
The metastatic growth is usually well circumscribed.
Metastases are often surrounded by extensive edema (Fig. 857).
Besides the involvement of the brain, the metastatic growth can also develop in the leptomeninges (Figs. 858 to 861).

b) Tumor extension into the brain from surrounding structures:

– Tumors from the skull can involve the brain: for instance, sarcomas, carcinomas of the ear and the mastoid, chordoma (in the majority of cases developing in the vertebral column),
– Chondroma,
– Osteoma,
– Orbital tumors,
– Olfactory neuroblastoma.

c) Occasionally **adenomas of the pituitary gland** can involve the third ventricle.

d) Extension of **glomus jugulare tumors** reaching the cerebellopontine angle.

e) Neurological and psychiatric symptoms as paraneoplastic syndromes [99]
   (see page 424).

---

[99] Zangemeister et al. 1978.

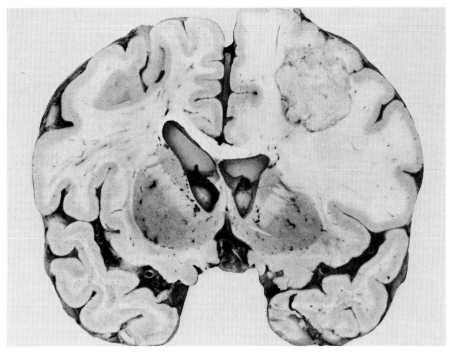

Fig. 857. Major edema around a metastatic lesion in the right hemisphere.

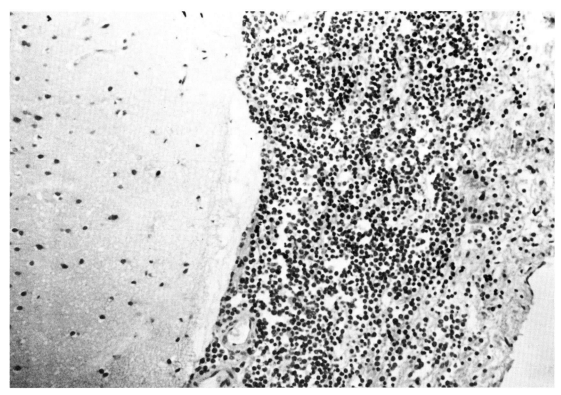

Fig. 858. Meningeosis leukemia (× 200).

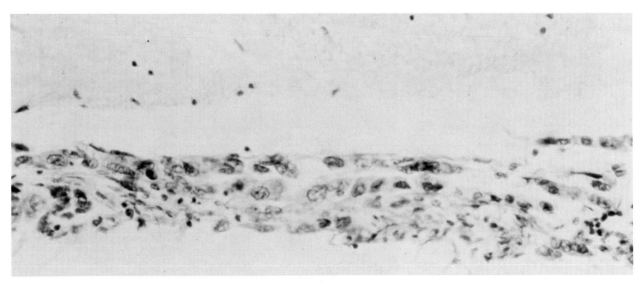

Fig. 859. Carcinomatous spread into the spinal leptomeninges (× 200).

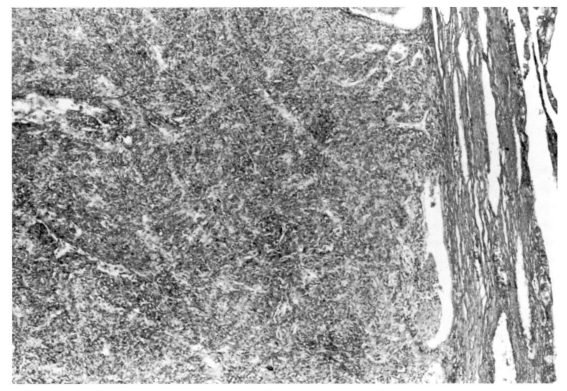

Fig. 860. Metastasis of hemangiopericytoma in the dura (51-year-old female, × 50).

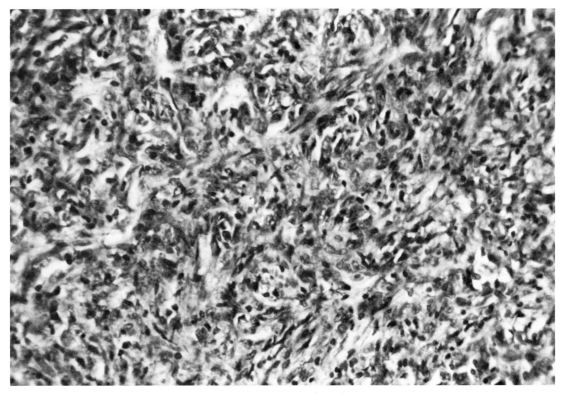

Fig. 861. Metastasis of malignant hemangiopericytoma in the dura (× 200).

References

[1] Adams, R.D., and H. de F. Webster: Neoplastic diseases of the brain. In: Harrison's Principles of internal medicine. Eighth edition. McGraw-Hill Book Company. New York–Düsseldorf etc. 1977.

[2] Ahdevaara, P., H. Kalimo, T. Törmä, and M. Haltia: Differentiating intracerebral neuroblastoma. Report of a case and review of the literature. Cancer *40* (1977) 784-788.

[3] Ashley, D.J.B.: In: Evan's histological appearance of tumours. 3rd. Ed. Churchill Livingstone, Edinburgh–London–New York 1978.

[4] Bailey, P., H. Cushing, and L. Eisenhardt: Angioblastic meningiomas. Arch. Pathol. *6* (1928) 953-990.

[5] Bamford, F.N., P.M. Jones, D. Pearson, G.G. Ribeiro, S.M. Shalet, and C.G. Beardwell: Residual disabilities in children treated for intracranial space-occupying lesions. Cancer *37* (1976) 1149-1151.

[6] Banna, M., L.P. Lassman, and G.W. Pearce: Radiological study of skeletal metastases from cerebellar medulloblastoma. Br. J. Radiol. *43* (1970) 173-179.

[7] Bestle, J.: Extragonadal endodermal sinus tumours originating in the region of the pineal gland. Acta Pathol. Microbiol. Scand. *74* (1968) 214-222.

[8] Bhangui, G.R., G. Roy, and P.N. Tandon: Multiple primary tumors of the brain including a medulloblastoma in the cerebellum. Cancer *39* (1977) 293-297.

[9] Bouchard, J.: Radiation therapy of tumours and diseases of the nervous system. In: G.H. Fletcher (Editor): Textbook of radiotherapy. Lea & Febiger, Philadelphia 1973.

[10] Brown, R.C., L. Gunderson, and H.P. Plenk: Medulloblastoma. A review of the LDS-Hospital experience. Cancer *40* (1977) 56-60.

[11] Chaudhry, A.P., M. Montes, and G.A. Cohn: Ultrastructure of cerebellar hemangioblastoma. Cancer *42* (1978) 1834-1850.

[12] Cumberlin, R.L., K.H. Luk, W.M. Wara, G.E. Sheline, and C.B. Wilson: Medulloblastoma. Treatment results and effect on normal tissues. Cancer *43* (1979) 1014-1020.

[13] Cuneo, H.M., and C.W. Rand: Brain tumours of childhood. C.C. Thomas, Springfield/Ill. 1952.

[14] Dayan, A.D., A.H.E. Marshall, A.A. Miller, F.J. Pick, and N.E. Rankin: Atypical teratomas of the pineal and hypothalamus. J. Path. Bact. *92* (1966) 1-28.

[15] Dehner, L.P., R.K. Sibley, J.J. Sauk, R.A. Vickers, M.E. Nesbit, A.S. Leonard, D.E. Waite, J.E. Neeley, and J. Ophoven: Malignant melanotic neuroectodermal tumor of infancy. A clinical, pathologic, ultrastructural and tissue culture study. Cancer *43* (1979) 1389-1410.

[16] DeVita, V.T. Jr.: In Harrison's "Principles of internal medicine". Eighth edition. McGraw-Hill Book Company. New York–Düsseldorf etc. 1977.

[17] Dold, U.W., und H. Sack: Praktische Tumortherapie. Die Behandlung maligner Organtumoren und Systemerkrankungen. Thieme, Stuttgart 1976.

[18] Doppman, J.L., F.P. Wirth Jr., G. Di Chiro, and A.K. Ommaya: Value of cutaneous angiomas in the arteriographic localization of spinalcord arteriovenous malformations. N. Engl. J. Med. *281* (1969) 1440-1444.

[19] Duffner, P.K., M.E. Cohen, P.R.M. Thomas, L.F. Sinks, and A.I. Freeman: Combination chemotherapy in recurrent medulloblastoma. Cancer *43* (1979) 41-45.

[20] Erlich, S.S., and R.L. Davis: Spinal subarachnoid metastasis from primary intracranial glioblastoma multiforme. Cancer *42* (1978) 2854-2864.

[21] Farwell, J.R., G.J. Dohrmann, and J.T. Flannery: Central nervous system tumors in children. Cancer *40* (1977) 3123-3132.

[22] Feigin, I., and G.N. Budzilovich: Tumors of neurons and their precursors. J. Neuropathol. Exp. Neurol. *33* (1974) 483-506.

[23] Freeman, C., J.W. Berg, and S.J. Cutler: Occurrence and prognosis of extranodal lymphomas. Cancer *29* (1972) 252-260.

[24] Friedman, M.: Irradiation of meningioma: A prototype circumscribed tumor for planning high-dose irradiation of the brain. Int. J. Radiat. Oncol. Biol. Phys. *2* (1977) 949-958.

[25] Glanzmann, C., und W. Horst: Strahlentherapie des Medulloblastoms: Entwicklung der Methodik und Ergebnisse bei 30 Patienten aus dem Zeitraum 1963 bis 1976. Strahlentherapie *155* (1979) 307-310.

[26] Gonzales-Vitale, J.C., R.E. Slavin, and J.D. McQueen: Radiation-induced intracranial malignant fibrous histiocytoma. Cancer *37* (1976) 2960-2963.

[27] Guccion, J.C., R.L. Front, F.M. Enzinger, and L.E. Zimmermann: Extraskeletal mesenchymal chondrosarcoma. Arch. Pathol. *95* (1973) 336.

[28] Harisiadis, L., and C.H. Chang: Medulloblastoma in children: A correlation between staging and results of treatment. Int. J. Radiat. Oncol. Biol. Phys. *2* (1977) 833-841.

[29] Herman, T.S., N. Hammond, S.E. Jones, J.J. Butler, G.E. Byrne Jr., and E.M. McKelvey: Involvement of the central nervous system by non-Hodgkin's lymphoma. The southwest oncology group experience. Cancer *43* (1979) 390-397.

[30] Horten, B.C., H. Urich, and D. Stefoski: Meningiomas with conspicuous plasma cell-lymphocytic components. A report of five cases. Cancer *43* (1979) 258-264.

[31] Horvat, B., C. Pena, and E.R. Fisher: Primary reticulum cell sarcoma (microglioma) of brain. Arch. Pathol. *87* (1969) 609-616.

[32] Hulbanni, S., and P.A. Goodman: Glioblastoma multiforme with extraneural metastases in the absence of previous surgery. Cancer *37* (1976) 1577-1583.

[33] Humeau, C., P. Vic, P. Sentein, and B. Vlahovitch: The fine structure of meningiomas: An attempted classification. Virchows Arch. A Path. Anat. and Histol. *382* (1979) 201-216.

[34] Jenkin, R.D., W.J. Simpson, and C.W. Keen: Pineal and suprasellar germinomas. Results of radiation treatment. J. Neurosurg. *48* (1978) 99-107.

[35] Jones, A.: Cerebral astrocytomata – trends in radiotherapy and chemotherapy: A review. Proc. R. Soc. Med. *71* (1978) 669-674.

[36] Kamin, D.F., and R.S. Hepler: Solitary intracranial plasmocytoma mistaken for retrobulbar neuritis. Am. J. Ophthalmol. *73* (1972) 584-586.

[37] Kepes, J.J.: Cellular whorls in brain tumors other than meningiomas. Cancer *37* (1976) 2232-2237.

[38] Kepes, J.J., M. Kepes, and F. Slowik: Fibrous xanthomas and xanthosarcomas of the meninges and the brain. Acta Neuropath. (Berl.) *23* (1973) 187-199.

[39] Kernohan, J.W., and G.P. Sayre: Tumors of the central nervous system. Atlas of tumor pathology, A.F.I.P. Washington, D.C. 1952.

[40] Kernohan, J.W., and A. Uhlheim: Sarcomas of the brain. C.C. Thomas, Springfield Illinois 1962.

[41] Koos, W.T., und G. Pendl: Zentrales und peripheres Nervensystem. In: Krebsbehandlung als interdisziplinäre Aufgabe. Herausgegeben von K.H. Kärcher. Springer, Berlin–Heidelberg–New York 1975.

[42] Lalitha, V.S., and L.J. Rubinstein: Reactive glioma in intracranial sarcoma: A form of mixed sarcoma and glioma ("sarcoglioma"). Report of eight cases. Cancer *43* (1979) 246-257.

[43] Lam, R.M.-Y., and S.A. Colah: Atypical fibrous histiocytoma with myxoid stroma. A rare lesion arising from dura mater of the brain. Cancer *43* (1979) 237-245.

[44] Leibel, S.A., G.E. Sheline, W.M. Wara, E.B. Boldrey, and S.L. Nielsen: The role of radiation therapy in the treatment of astrocytomas. Cancer *35* (1975) 1551-1557.

[45] Leibel, S.A., W.M. Wara, G.E. Sheline, J.J. Townsend, and E.B. Boldrey: The treatment of meningiomas in childhood. Cancer *37* (1976) 2709-2712.

[46] Littman, P., and C.C. Wang: Reticulum cell sarcoma of the brain. A review of the literature and a study of 19 cases. Cancer *35* (1975) 1412-1420.

[47] Ludwin, S.K., L.J. Rubinstein, and D.S. Russell: Papillary meningioma: A malignant variant of meningioma. Cancer *36* (1975) 1363-1373.

[48] Lütolf, U.M., C. Glanzmann, H.G. Aberle und W. Horst: Ergebnisse der Radiotherapie bei 68 inoperablen Hirntumoren (1950 bis 1975). Strahlentherapie *154* (1978) 8-10.

[49] Mancilla-Jimenez, R., and F.A. Tavassoli: Solitary meningeal plasmocytoma. Report of a case with electron microscopic and immunohistologic observations. Cancer *38* (1976) 798-806.

[50] Markesbery, W.R., W.H. Brooks, L. Milsow, and R.H. Mortara: Ultrastructural study of the pineal germinoma in vivo and in vitro. Cancer *37* (1976) 327-337.

[51] Marsa, G.W., D.R. Goffinet, L.J. Rubinstein, and M.A. Bagshaw: Megavoltage irradiation in the treatment of gliomas of the brain and spinal cord. Cancer *36* (1975) 1681-1689.

[52] McCloskey, J.J., J.C. Parker Jr., W.H. Brooks, and H.M. Blacker: Melanin as a component of cerebral gliomas. The melanotic cerebral ependymoma. Cancer *37* (1976) 2373-2379.

[53] Melmon, K.L., and S.W. Rosen: Lindau's disease; review of the literature and study of a large kindred. Am. J. Med. *36* (1964) 595-617.

[54] Mena, H., and J.H. Garcia: Primary brain sarcomas. Light and electron microscopic features. Cancer *42* (1978) 1298-1307.

[55] Min, K.-W., F. Gyorkey, and B. Halpert: Primary rhabdomyosarcoma of the cerebrum. Cancer *35* (1975) 1405-1411.

[56] Mincer, F., J. Meltzer, and C. Botstein: Pinealoma. A report of twelve irradiated cases. Cancer *37* (1976) 2713-2718.

[57] Misugi, K., and L. Liss: Medulloblastoma with cross-striated muscle: A fine structural study. Cancer *25* (1970) 1279-1285.

[58] Mørk, S.J., and A.C. Løken: Ependymoma. A follow-up study of 101 cases. Cancer *40* (1977) 907-915.

[59] Montgomery, A.B., T. Griffin, R.G. Parker, and A.J. Gerdes: Optic nerve glioma: The role of radiation therapy. Cancer *40* (1977) 2079-2080.

[60] Nishiyama, R.H., J.G. Batsakis, D.K. Weaver, and J.H. Simrall: Germinal neoplasms of the central nervous system. Arch. Surg. *93* (1966) 342-347.

[61] Oberman, H.A., W.C. Hewitt Jr., and A.J. Kalivoda: Medulloblastomas with distant metastases. Am. J. Clin. Pathol. *39* (1963) 148-160.

[62] Odom, G.L., C.H. Davis, and B. Woodhall: Brain tumors in children – clinical analysis of 164 cases. Pediatrics *18* (1956) 856-869.

[63] Oswald, U., und C. Hedinger: Intrakranielle Keimzelltumoren (Teratome und Seminome). Virchows Arch. A Path. Anat. and Histol. *357* (1972) 281-298.

[64] Pasquier, B., P. Couderc, D. Pasquier, M.H. Panh, and J.P. Arnould: Primary malignant melanoma of the cerebellum. A case with metastases outside the nervous system. Cancer *41* (1978) 344-351.

[65] Pasquier, B., P. Couderc, D. Pasquier, M.H. Panh, and A. N'Golet: Sarcoma arising in oligodendroglioma of the brain. A case with intramedullary and subarachnoid spinal metastases. Cancer *42* (1978) 2753-2758.

[66] Pearson, J., M. Milstoc, J. Harris, G. Budzilo-

853

vich, and I. Feigin: Anaplastic neuronal tumours of brain. Cancer *38* (1976) 1424-1437.

[67] Polak, M.: On the true nature of the so-called medulloblastoma. Acta Neuropath. (Berl.) *8* (1967) 84-95.

[68] Pouillart, P., G. Mathe, T. Palangie, J. Lheritier, M. Poisson, P. Huguenin, H. Gautier, P. Morin, and R. Parrot: Treatment of malignant gliomas and brain metastases in adults using a combination of adriamycin, VM 26, and CCNU. Results of a type II trial. Recent Results Cancer Res. *62* (1977) 17-28.

[69] Roberts, M., and W.J. German: A long-term study of patients with oligodendrogliomas; follow-up of 50 cases, including Doctor Harvey Cushing's series. J. Neurosurg. *24* (1966) 697-700.

[70] Rubinstein, L.J.: The definition of ependymoblastoma. Arch. Pathol. *90* (1970) 35-45.

[71] Rubinstein, L.J.: Tumors of the central nervous system. Atlas of tumor pathology. A.F.I.P., Washington, D.C. 1972.

[72] Rubinstein, L.J., and D.W.C. Northfield: The medulloblastoma and the so-called "arachnoidal cerebellar sarcoma": A critical re-examination of a neurologic problem. Brain *87* (1964) 379-412.

[73] Russell, D.S., and L.J. Rubinstein: Pathology of tumours of the nervous system. Fourth edition. Edward Arnold (1977).

[74] Rwomushana, R.J.W., I.C. Bailey, and S.K. Kyalwazi: Kaposi's sarcoma of the brain. A case report with necropsy findings. Cancer *36* (1975) 1127-1131.

[75] Salazar, O.M., P. Rubin, D. Bassano, and V.A. Marcial: Improved survival of patients with intracranial ependymomas by irradiation: Dose selection and field extension. Cancer *35* (1975) 1563-1573.

[76] Scheithauer, B.W., and L.J. Rubinstein: Meningeal mesenchymal chondrosarcoma. Report of 8 cases with review of the literature. Cancer *42* (1978) 2744-2752.

[77] Sheline, G.E.: Radiation therapy of tumors of the central nervous system in childhood. Cancer *35* (1975) 957-964.

[78] Shuangshoti, S., C. Hongsaprabhas, and M.G. Netsky: Metastasizing meningioma. Cancer *26* (1970) 832-841.

[79] Shuangshoti, S., P. Tangchai, and M.G. Netsky: Primary adenocarcinoma of chorioid plexus. Arch. Pathol. *91* (1971) 101-106.

[80] Silbert, S.W., K.R. Smith Jr., and S. Horenstein: Primary leptomeningeal melanoma. An ultrastructural study. Cancer *41* (1978) 519-527.

[81] Simpson, D.: The recurrence of intracranial meningiomas after surgical treatment. J. Neurol. Neurosurg. Psychiatry *20* (1957) 22-39.

[82] Slaughter, J.C., J.M. Hardman, L.G. Kempe, and K.M. Earle: Neurocutaneous melanosis and leptomeningeal melanomatosis in children. Arch. Pathol. *88* (1969) 298-304.

[83] Smith, W.T., B. Hughes, and R. Ermocilla: Chemodectoma of the pineal region, with observations of the pineal body and chemoreceptor tissue. J. Path. Bact. *92* (1966) 69-76.

[84] Spataro, J., and O. Sacks: Oligodendroglioma with remote metastases; case report. J. Neurosurg. *28* (1968) 373-379.

[85] Spence, A.M., and L.J. Rubinstein: Cerebellar capillary hemangioblastoma: Its histogenesis studied by organ culture and electron microscopy. Cancer *35* (1975) 326-341.

[86] Steegmann, A.T., and B. Winer: Temporal lobe epilepsy resulting from ganglioglioma; report of an unusual case in an adolescent boy. Neurology *11* (1961) 406-412.

[87] Takei, Y., S.S. Mirra, and M.L. Miles: Eosinophilic granular cells in oligodendrogliomas. An ultrastructural study. Cancer *38* (1976) 1968-1976.

[88] Taylor, C.R., R. Russell, R.J. Lukes, and R.L. Daves: An immunohistological study of immunoglobulin content of primary central nervous system lymphomas. Cancer *41* (1978) 2197-2205.

[89] Taylor, IV, S.G., L. Nelson, D. Baxter, C. Rosenbaum, R.W. Sponzo, T.J. Cunningham, K.B. Olson, and J. Horton: Treatment of grade III and IV astrocytoma with dimethyl triazeno imidazole carboxamide (DTIC, NSC-45388) alone and in combination with CCNU (NSC-79037) or methyl CCNU (MeCCNU, NSC-95441). Cancer *36* (1975) 1269-1276.

[90] Tokars, R.P., H.G. Sutton, and M.L. Griem: Cerebellar medulloblastoma. Results of a new method of radiation treatment. Cancer *43* (1979) 129-136.

[91] Virtanen, I., E. Lehtonen, and J. Wartiovaara: Structure of psammoma bodies of a meningioma in scanning electron microscopy. Cancer *38* (1976) 824-829.

[92] Walter, G.F.: Kleinhirnastrocytome und Opticusgliome – eine vergleichende feinstrukturelle Untersuchung. Virchows Arch. A Path. Anat. and Histol. *380* (1978) 59-79.

[93] Waltz, T.A., and B. Brownell: Sarcoma: A possible late result of effective radiation therapy for pituitary adenoma – report of two cases. J. Neurosurg. *24* (1966) 901-907.

[94] Wara, W.M., R.D.T. Jenkin, A. Evans, I. Ertel, R. Hittle, J. Ortega, C.B. Wilson, and D. Hammond: Tumors of the pineal and suprasellar region: Childrens cancer study group treatment results 1960-1975. A report from childrens cancer study group. Cancer *43* (1979) 698-701.

[95] Weiner, L.P., P.N. Anderson, and J.C. Allen: Cerebral plasmocytoma with myeloma protein in the cerebrospinal fluid. Neurology *16* (1966) 615-618.

[96] Wilson, C.B.: Chemotherapy of brain tumors. In: Advances in neurology, Vol. 15, edited by R.A. Thompson and J.R. Green, Raven Press, New York 1976.

[97] Wong, S.W., T.B. Ducker, and J.M. Powers: Fulminating parapontine epidermoid carcinoma in a four-year-old boy. Cancer *37* (1976) 1525-1531.

[98] Yoshiki, T., T. Itoh, T. Shirai, T. Noro, Y. To-

mino, I. Hamajima, and T. Takeda: Primary intracranial yolk sac tumor. Immunofluorescent demonstration of alpha-fetoprotein synthesis. Cancer *37* (1976) 2343-2348.

[99] Zangemeister, W. H., G. Schwendemann, and H. J. Colmant: Carcinomatous encephalomyelopathy in conjunction with encephalomyeloradiculitis. J. Neurol. *218* (1978) 63-71.

[100] Zülch, K. J.: Biologie und Pathologie der Hirngeschwülste. Handbuch der Neurochirugie, edited by H. OLivecrona and W. Tönnis, Springer, Berlin (1956).

[101] Zülch, K. J.: Biologie und Pathologie der Ge-

schwülste des Gehirns, des Rückenmarks, der peripheren Nerven und Sympathikus. In: Lehrbuch der speziellen pathologischen Anatomie Band III, 1. Teil. Kaufmann-Staemmler. Walter de Gruyter, Berlin 1958.

[102] Zülch, K. J., and H. D. Mennel: The biology of brain tumors. Handbook of clinical neurology, edited by P. J. Vinken and G. W. Bruyn. North-Holland Publishing Co., Amsterdam 1974.

[103] Zülch, K. J., F. Pompeu, and F. Pinto: Über die Metastasierung der Meningeome. Zbl. Neurochir. *14* (1954) 253.

19 Tumors of the pituitary gland

1. The morphological classification of pituitary tumors is based on routine stain and light microscopic findings:

   Chromophobe adenoma, acidophilic adenoma, basophilic (mucoid cell adenoma), and mixed acidophilic-basophilic adenoma (WHO).

   In recent years, however, the morphological description of pituitary gland tumors has been expanded by electron microscopic and immunohistochemical findings [18, 32]. It may be possible to correlate these new morphological observations with the functional behavior of the tumors, at least to a certain degree. Therefore, it seems justified to establish a new classification that takes into account the ultrastructural and immunohistochemical evidence:

   Adenoma of ACTH cell type,

   Adenoma of TSH cell type,

   Adenoma of prolactin cell type,

   Adenoma of GH cell type.

   The application of this new classification depends on the application of these new techniques. Therefore, the old classification still prevails (see WHO) [1, 31].

   In the following pages the new classification overlaps the classical typing.

2. The clinical symptoms of pituitary adenomas are provoked by the expansion of the adenoma, which compresses the surrounding tissue, and by the functional activity of the hormone-producing cells of which the tumor is composed:

   a) hypopituitarism,

   b) defects in visual field,

   c) headaches,

   d) hyperendocrine function, in most instances characterized by the production of one single hormone (acromegaly, hyperthyreosis, hyperprolactinemia, Cushing's syndrome).

   Occasionally, however, the symptomatology of a polyhormonal hyperproduction is apparent (polyadenomatous endocrine syndrome) [24, 36].

3. The pituitary gland tumors are treated by surgery or radiation therapy, sometimes with a supervoltage irradiation [21].

   A rare complication of radiation therapy is pituitary apoplexia with massive hemorrhage into the pituitary gland: Fever, headache, and blindness.

[1] Ashley 1978.
[18] Kruseman et al. 1976.
[21] Mayer et al. 1976.
[24] O'Neal et al. 1968.
[31] Russell and Rubinstein 1977.
[32] Saeger 1977.
[36] Wermer 1954.

M-8270/0
T 194.3

1. Chromophobe adenoma (WHO)

General Remarks

Incidence: About 70% of pituitary adenomas are chromophobe adenomas.
About 5% of pituitary tumors are chromophobe adenomas.
Age: This tumor affects adults between the 4th and 7th decades.
Sex: Males are more frequently affected than females.
Further notes: In some instances a chromophobe adenoma corresponds to the TSH cell adenoma [18].

Macroscopy

Chromophobe adenomas are soft and solid with a reddish cut surface.
The greater part of the tumor is in a suprasellar position and grows in front of or behind the optic chiasm.
The tumor can encroach on the brain.

Histology

The tumor cells are spindle-shaped and polygonal or round and appear in most instances "chromophobe."
Only rarely are the tumor cells acidophilic.
The growth pattern of the tumor cells varies:
The tumor can grow in solid nests or form perivascular rosettes.
In other fields or in other tumors the tumor cells are arranged in a papillary fashion or show sinusoidal structures. Occasionally the tumor cells can be large or small and can diffusely infiltrate the pituitary gland (diffuse type of adenoma) [16] (Figs. 862 to 865).

Electron Microscopy

The cytoplasm contains ergastoplasmic reticulum, which is arranged in a concentric pattern.
There are few and small secretory granules (300 to 400 mμ [19]) (Fig. 866).

Clinical Findings

1. The growing tumor compresses the normal pituitary parenchyma: Therefore, the symptoms are dominated by a depression of the pituitary gland function.
2. Rarely, this tumor is composed of endocrine-active cells. In these cases acromegaly or gigantism (see Acidophilic adenoma, page 864), as well as occasionally Cushing's syndrome (ACTH cell adenoma, see page 863) or thyrotoxicosis can develop.

Treatment

Surgery combined with **radiation therapy.**
For small adenomas, megavoltage radiation therapy (proton beam irradiation or gamma irradiation) has been recommended [3, 28] (40 to 50 Gy in 3 to 5 weeks).

Further Information

Occasionally adenomas composed of oncocytes are observed [17, 32].
Very rarely, they can be associated with adrenal hypercorticism [12].

[3] Bloom 1977.
[12] Gjerris et al. 1978.
[16] Kernohan and Sayre 1956.
[17] Kovacs and Horvath 1973.
[18] Kruseman et al. 1976.
[19] Lewis and Van Noorden 1972.
[28] Pistenma et al. 1975.
[32] Saeger 1977.

859

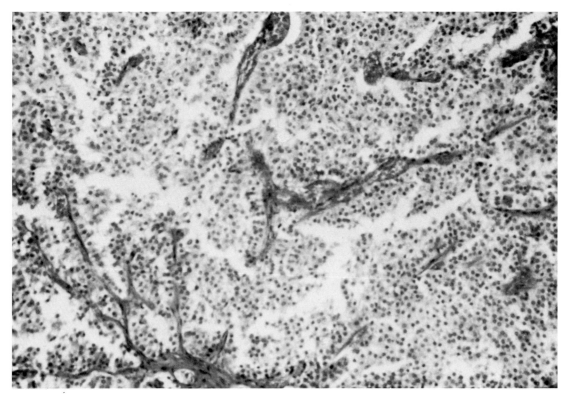

Fig. 862. Chromophobe (papillary) adenoma of the pituitary gland (× 125).

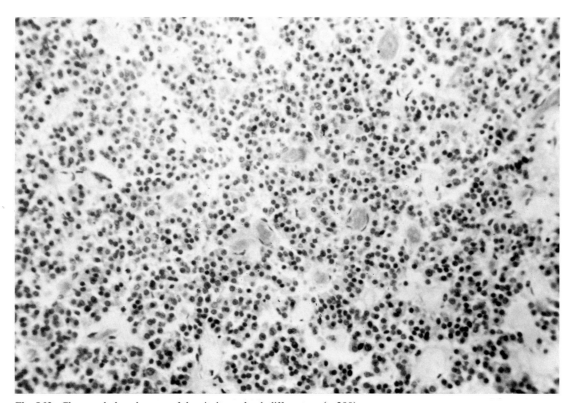

Fig. 863. Chromophobe adenoma of the pituitary gland, diffuse type (× 200).

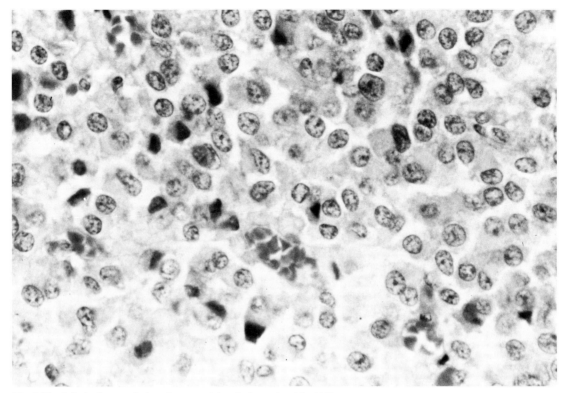

Fig. 864. Cells in chromophobe adenoma of the pituitary gland (× 400).

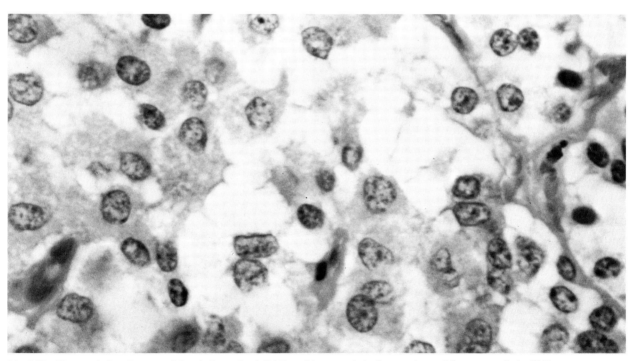

Fig. 865. Chromophobe adenoma of the pituitary gland: PAS-positive granule in the cytoplasm of the tumor cells (× 800).

Chromophobe adenoma

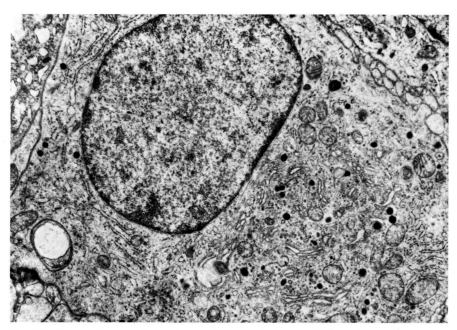

Fig. 866. Large cell chromophobe adenoma: Rough endoplasmic reticulum, pleomorphic secretory granules, mitochondria of different sizes (× 7960).

2. ACTH cell adenoma

General Remarks

Incidence: About 7% of pituitary adenomas are ACTH cell adenomas [22].
Age: This is a tumor of adults in the 4th to 6th decades, but occurs also in childhood.
Sex: Females are more frequently affected than males.
Site: In most instances the tumor grows in the central or posterior region of the pituitary gland.

Histology

Most of these tumors are "chromophobe adenomas":
The tumor cells are uniform, the nuclei are round, and mitotic figures are lacking.
The cytoplasm of the tumor cells contains PAS-positive granules.
The growth pattern of the tumor cells is trabecular or solid.

Electron Microscopy

The tumor cells contain many free ribosomes; the rough endoplasmic reticulum is sparse. Secretory granules are arranged in most instances along the cell membrane. Their size varies from 100 to 600 mµ.

Clinical Findings

Cushing's syndrome.
About 10% of Cushing's syndrome cases are due to ACTH cell adenomas.
The development of ACTH cell adenomas is enhanced by adrenalectomy (Nelson's syndrome; Nelson's tumors) [23, 32].

Treatment

Surgical excision.
The **surgery** can be completed by **radiation therapy** (up to 50 Gy in about 6 weeks) (proton beam irradiation or gamma irradiation).
It has been reported that pituitary irradiation without surgery can be used for tumors during childhood in about 70% of the cases [14].

[14] Jennings et al. 1977.
[22] McCornick and Halmi 1971.
[23] Nelson et al. 1960.
[32] Saeger 1977.

863

M-8280/0
T 194.3

3. Acidophilic (eosinophilic) adenoma (WHO)

**General
Remarks**

Incidence: About 35% of pituitary adenomas are of this type.
Age: This tumor occurs in adult life; however, it can appear also in younger age groups.
Sex: Males are slightly more frequently affected than females.

Macroscopy

In most instances this adenoma is confined to the sella turcica because it is smaller than chromophobe adenoma. If this adenoma reaches diameters of several centimeters, regressive changes and cyst formations can occur.
The tumor is soft and has a reddish color.

Histology

The tumor cells are polygonal with a distinct cell membrane.
They grow in large complexes.
The cytoplasm of these cells contains granules that are coarse and acidophilic. The PAS stain is negative.
Besides these acidophilic cells, areas can be found that contain chromophobe cells.

**Electron
Microscopy**

The tumor cells contain secretory granules that measure 300 to 500 mµ in diameter. However, smaller granules can be observed (Fig. 867).

**Clinical
Findings**

This tumor can induce acromegaly (in about 3% of the cases [22]).
Galactorrhea and amenorrhea can also be induced by this tumor [10].

M-8300/0
T 194.3

4. Basophilic adenoma (WHO)
(mucoid cell adenoma)

**General
Remarks**

Incidence: This tumor is relatively rare. About 7% of pituitary adenomas are of this type.
Age: This tumor is often observed in childhood and adolescence.
Sex: Females are more frequently affected than males.

Macroscopy

This is a small tumor that remains in the sella turcica, which is not enlarged.

Histology

This adenoma is also composed of large cells, which have clear cell borders and are polygonal.
The cytoplasm contains granules that are basophilic. These granules show (contrary to the acidophilic adenoma) a PAS-positive staining reaction [4].
Occasionally an adenoma contains basophilic PAS granules as well as cells that show a PAS-negative reaction of their acidophilic granules:
Mixed acidophilic-basophilic adenoma (WHO).

[4] Capella et al. 1979.
[10] Forbes et al. 1957.
[22] McCornick and Halmi 1971.

Electron Microscopy Immunohisto-chemistry

Both methods reveal that basophilic adenomas can be composed of ACTH cells (Fig. 868) or TSH cells (Fig. 869).

Clinical Findings

This is determined by the endocrine production.

In most instances this tumor induces Cushing's syndrome.

Occasionally it has been reported that massive hemorrhage into the adenomas causing Cushing's syndrome can occur [30].

Treatment

Surgery and/or **radiation therapy.**

Further Information

Electron microscopic findings and immunohistochemical observations reveal that the light microscopic **classification** of the adenomas contains for each of these tumors different endocrine possibilities.

In other words, only the use of these ultrastructural and immunohistochemical techniques can reveal the hormone-producing cells that compose the adenoma:

- **GH cell adenoma:** Gigantism, acromegaly.

- **ACTH cell adenoma:** Cushing's syndrome.

- **Prolactin cell adenoma** (Fig. 870) [26]: Galactorrhea, amenorrhea (Forbes-Albright syndrome) [9].

- **TSH cell adenoma** [4, 27]: Hyperthyroidism.

There is no final evidence for the existence of gonadotropin cell adenomas [32].

Hormone-producing cell adenomas have been described in animals: TSH cells, prolactin cell (LTH), FSH cells, and LH cells [32].

No definite disorders are associated with LH or FSH adenomas. Occasionally sexual precocities are observed. Multiple endocrine neoplasia (MEN) [7].

[4] Capella et al. 1979.
[7] Dralle and Altenähr 1979.
[9] Finn and Mount 1971.
[26] Peake et al. 1969.
[27] Phifer and Spicer 1973.
[30] Rovit and Duane 1969.
[32] Saeger 1977.

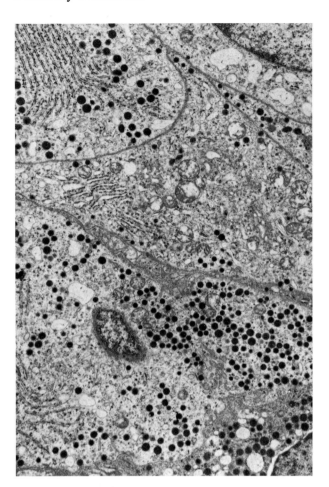

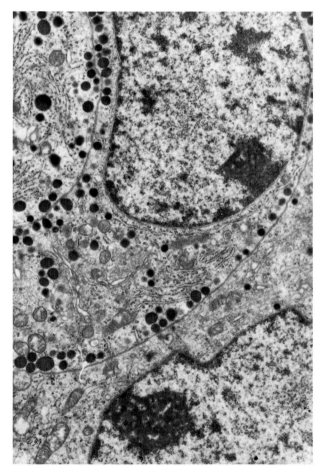

Fig. 867. Undifferentiated acidophil adenoma: Rough endoplasmic reticulum, microtubules, numerous large secretory granules (×6720).

Fig. 868. Highly differentiated ACTH cell adenoma: Peripherally located secretory granules, rough endoplasmic reticulum (×8230).

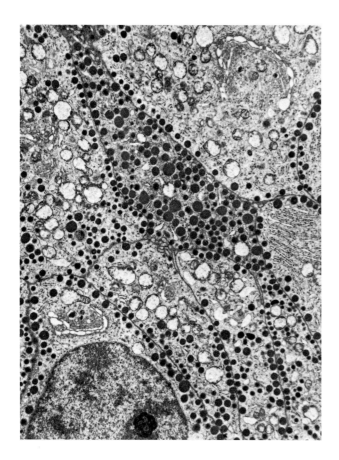

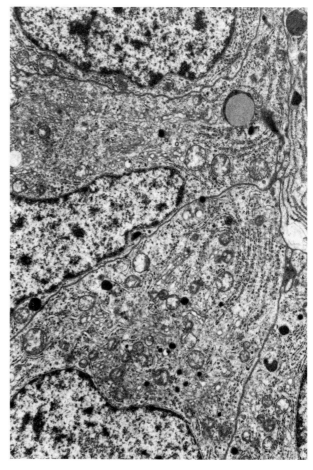

Fig. 869. Highly differentiated GH cell adenoma: Numerous, densely packed secretory granules, vacuolated organelles (× 5680).

Fig. 870. Highly differentiated prolactin cell adenoma: Rough endoplasmic reticulum, medium-sized Golgi apparatus, sparse granulation (× 7760).

867

**M-8270/3
(chromophobe)
M-8280/3
(acidophilic)
M-8300/3
(basophilic)
T 194.3**

5. Pituitary adenocarcinoma (WHO)
(carcinoma [malignant adenoma] of the pituitary gland)

**General
Remarks**

Incidence: It is difficult to assess the incidence of malignant growth in these pituitary tumors.

There are estimates that about 3% of pituitary tumors are aggressive [1].

Macroscopy

Malignant tumors in this region are soft and enlarge the sella turcica. The tumor might extend into the surrounding tissue.

Histology

The tumor cells show a certain degree of pleomorphism. There are some mitotic figures. Besides these discrete indications of possible malignancy, other areas show cells that do not reveal any evidence of the malignant nature of the tumor.

The malignant behavior, however, can be determined if the tumor invades the adjacent structures.

**Differential
Diagnosis**

Pituitary adenocarcinoma **with metastatic tumors into the pituitary gland:**
Metastases into the pituitary gland derive mainly from the lung and breast. In these instances the posterior lobe is more frequently affected than the anterior lobe [34].

Spread

1. The tumor extends into the surrounding tissue: Nasopharynx, cavernous sinus, anterior-middle-posterior fossae, optic nerve, and chiasm.
2. Very rarely, distant metastases occur [8, 20], which are even functionally active [30].
3. Very rarely, extension into the cerebrospinal area can occur.

**Clinical
Findings**

According to the involved structures.

[1] Ashley 1978.
[8] Epstein et al. 1964.
[20] Madonick et al. 1963.
[30] Rovit and Duane 1969.
[34] Teears and Silverman 1975.

6. Tumors of the posterior lobe of the pituitary gland
(neurohypophysis)

The **incidence** of these tumors is very low.

M-9400/3
T 194.3

a) Astrocytoma
The majority of these tumors are of the pilocytic type (Fig. 773).

M-9352/0
T 194.3

b) Choristoma (WHO)
These choristomas contain granulated cells with PAS-positive staining of the granules [1]. They can be considered pituicytes [31] (Fig. 871).

M-9352/0
T 194.3

c) Granular cell tumor (WHO)
This tumor can occur in the stalk or the posterior lobe of the pituitary gland and very rarely causes clinical symptoms by its size.

---

[1] Ashley 1978.
[31] Russell and Rubinstein 1977.

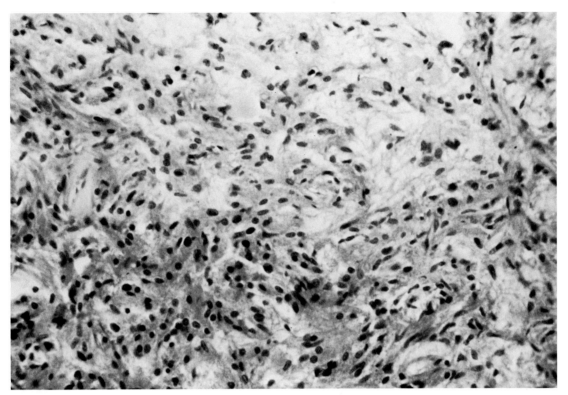

Fig. 871. Choristoma in neurohypophysis: Strands of cells with PAS-positive granules in the cytoplasm (×200).

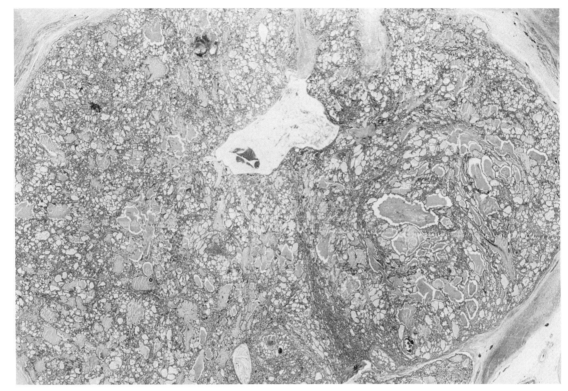

Fig. 872. Craniopharyngioma (× 30).

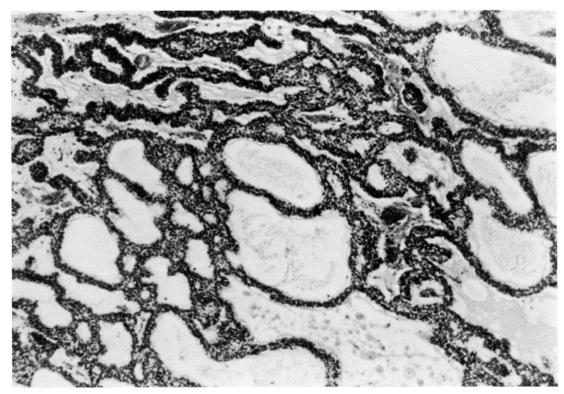

Fig. 873. Craniopharyngioma: Cystic part (× 125).

M-9350/1
T 194.3

7. Craniopharyngioma (WHO)

General Remarks

Incidence: About 3% of all intracranial tumors are craniopharyngiomas [2].
In children, 9% of the intracranial tumors are craniopharyngiomas.
Age: This lesion can affect children and adults as well, with a peak age in the 2nd and 3rd decades.
The incidence increases in the older age groups [37].
Site: The majority of craniopharyngiomas grow in a suprasellar position above the pituitary gland, within the circle of Willis and behind the chiasm.
Craniopharyngiomas in an intrasellar position are rare.

Macroscopy

Craniopharyngiomas are spherical, large tumors. The cut surface is grayish-whitish, reddish, or granular-pale.
Besides calcifications (important for radiography) the tumor contains cysts filled with yellowish fluid and containing cholesterol crystals.

Histology

The tumor is composed of cysts and epithelial cells.
The cystic spaces are lined by squamous epithelium, which grows on a basement membrane (Figs. 872 to 875). These cysts develop in strands of epithelial cells, which are surrounded by cells in a palisade formation, thus giving the tumor a resemblance to adamantinoma [31]. These basal cells can also line the wall of the cysts.
The strands of cells form a network in which occasionally a whorled structure is observed.
Keratinizations are rarely found.
The stroma can show foci of calcification, histiocytes, fibroblasts, and collagen fibers.
This composition of epithelial strands, degeneration of the connective tissue with calcifications, and cyst formations differs from one tumor to another.
The encapsulated craniopharyngioma can induce a gliosis in the surrounding tissue.

Clinical Findings

The symptoms are determined by the size of the tumor and the degree of compression of the pituitary gland:
Diabetes insipidus, visual malfunctions, hydrocephalus, headaches.
On X-rays the calcifications can be found in about 70% of the cases.

Treatment

Surgical excision of the tumor, eventually combined with **radiation therapy** [3, 6, 11, 21, 25] (up to 70 Gy in 8 weeks).

Prognosis

Total removal of the tumor means cure.
Partial removal of the tumor might allow reccurrences due to reformation of the cysts.
Surgical removal of the recurrences is recommended.

[2] Bingas and Wolter 1968.
[3] Bloom 1977.
[6] Claussen et al. 1977.
[11] Garcia-Uria 1978.
[21] Mayer et al. 1976.
[25] Onoyama et al. 1977.
[31] Russell and Rubinstein 1977.
[37] Zülch 1957.

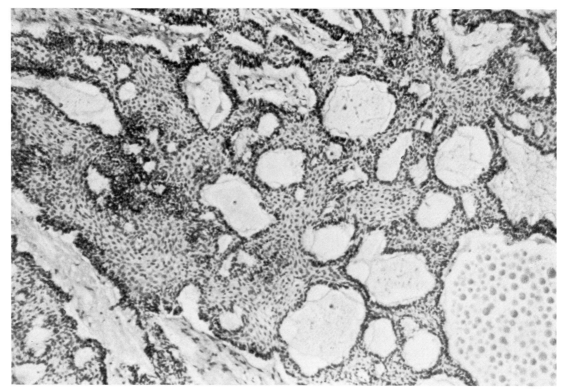

Fig. 874. Craniopharyngioma: Solid nests and cysts (× 125).

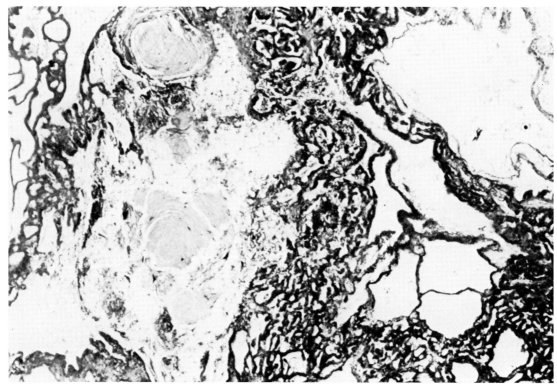

Fig. 875. Craniopharyngioma with keratinization (× 40).

Craniopharyngioma

Further Information

1. The origin of craniopharyngioma is still debated:
   - The tumor could derive from epithelial nests of Rathke's pouch [33, 35].
   - Craniopharyngioma could originate from part of the embryonic enamel organ. Rudimentary tooth structures have been observed in craniopharyngiomas [33].
   - The appearance of a pituitary adenoma associated with craniopharyngioma could also be interpreted as an adenomatous origin (metaplasia) of craniopharyngioma [5, 13].

M-2650/0
T 194.3

2. **Intrasellar cyst**
   (**Rathke's cleft cyst** – WHO)
   These cysts are very rare, originating probably from squamous cell remnants of Rathke's pouch.
   These cysts are small and limited to the sella turcica. The lining epithelium might be cuboidal or can be destroyed.
   The cysts occasionally contain a clear fluid or residues of hemorrhages.
   Other variations of epithelium might line these cysts; one case has been reported with transitional cell layers in Rathke's cleft cyst, causing the picture of a **transitional cell tumor** [15].

M-8120/3
T 194.3

3. Occasionally small **cysts in the suprasellar area** can be found. They are lined by cuboidal epithelium (colloid cysts).

[5] Cheetham 1963.
[13] Hunter 1955.
[15] Kepes 1978.
[33] Seemayer et al. 1972.
[35] Timperley 1968.

8. Tumors at the site of the sella turcica

T 194.3

In the **intrasellar** or **suprasellar** region, other lesions can occur:

M-9080/0

a) Teratomas

M-9084/0

– **Dermoid cysts,** lined by squamous cell layers, containing hair follicles and sweat glands in the wall.
Dermoid cysts are very rare.

M-3341/0

– **Epidermoid cysts**
These cysts are lined by squamous cells or cuboidal cell layers (Figs. 876 and 877).

b) Metastatic carcinoma (Figs. 878 and 879)

M-9370/1, 3

c) Chordoma (see page 1087)
About 30% of these malignant tumors grow at the base of the skull in the spheno-occipital region (Figs. 880 and 881).

M-9530/0

d) Meningioma
(Figs. 822 to 828).

M-7791/0

e) Histiocytosis X as part of the systemic disease (Fig. 1272).

M-9730/3

f) Plasmacytoma [29].

g) Tumor-like lesions
Occasionally granulomatous inflammations can mimic a tumor in that area: Tuberculosis, sarcoidosis.

---

[29] Poon et al. 1979.

Epidermoid cyst

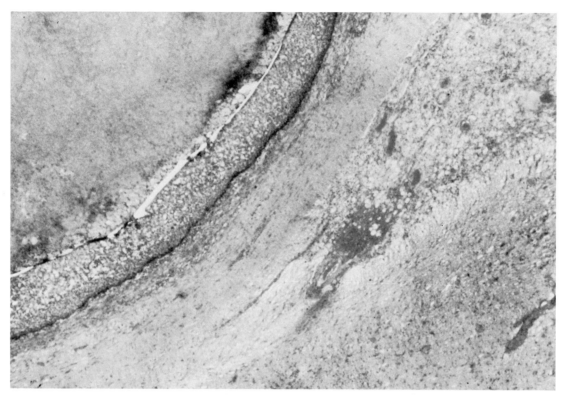

Fig. 876. Epidermoid cyst in the pituitary gland (49-year-old female, × 50).

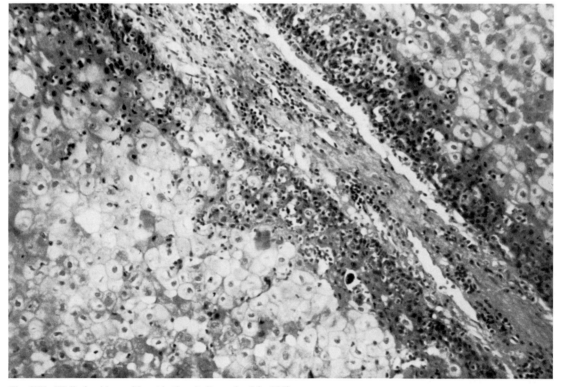

Fig. 877. Wall of epidermoid cyst in the pituitary gland (× 125).

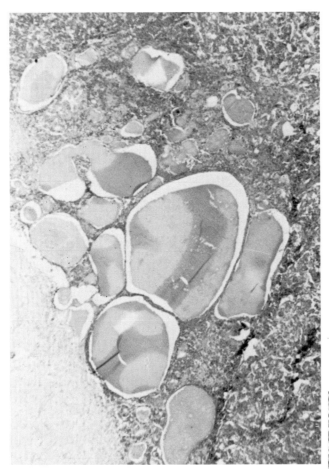

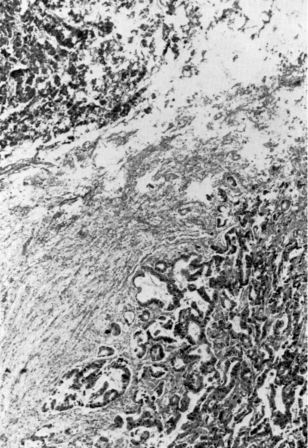

Fig. 878. Metastasis of thyroid carcinoma in the pituitary gland (× 40).

Fig. 879. Metastasis from adenocarcinoma in the pituitary gland (56-years-old male, × 50).

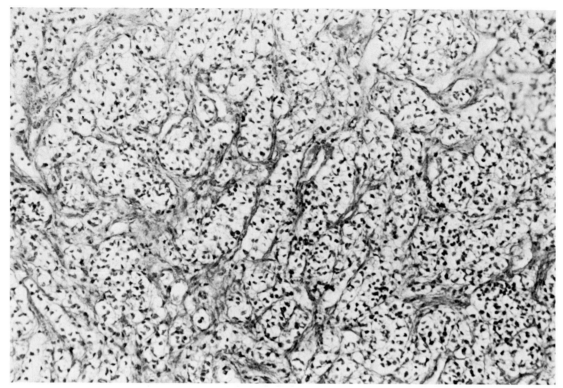

Fig. 880. Chordoma in the pituitary gland (× 125).

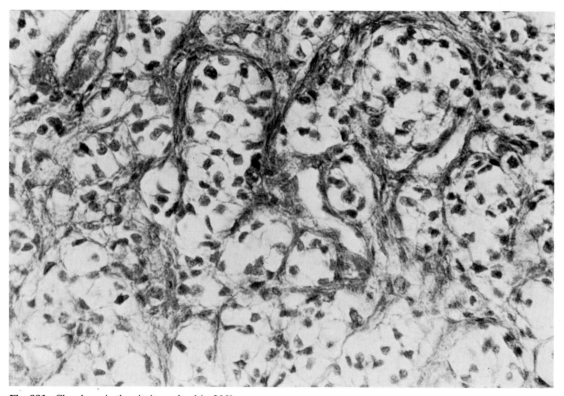

Fig. 881. Chordoma in the pituitary gland (× 200).

References

[1] Ashley, D.J.B.: In: Evans' histological appearances of tumours. 3rd. ed. Churchill Livingstone, Edinburgh–London–New York 1978.

[2] Bingas, B., und M. Wolter: Das Kraniopharyngiom. Fortschr. Neurol. Psychiatr. *36* (1968) 117-195.

[3] Bloom, H.J.: The role of radiotherapy in the management of chiasmal compression. Proc. R. Soc. Med. *70* (1977) 319-326.

[4] Capella, C., L. Usellini, B. Frigerio, R. Buffa, P. Fontana, and E. Solcia: Argyrophil pituitary tumors showing TSH cells or small granule cells. Virchows Arch. A Path. Anat. and Histol. *381* (1979) 295-312.

[5] Cheetham, H.D.: Experimental squamous metaplasia in squamous epithelioma formation in the pituitary of the rat. Br. J. Cancer *17* (1963) 657-662.

[6] Claussen, C., F. Lohkamp, W. Rebien und H. Kuttig: Computertomographische Diagnostik, Therapieplanung und Verlaufskontrolle beim Kraniopharyngeom. Strahlentherapie *153* (1977) 744-753.

[7] Dralle, H., and E. Altenähr: Pituitary adenoma, primary parathyroid hyperplasia and papillary (non-medullary) thyroid carcinoma. A case of multiple endocrine neoplasia (MEN). Virchows Arch. A Path. Anat. and Histol. *381* (1979) 179-187.

[8] Epstein, J.A., B.S. Epstein, L. Molho, and H.M. Zimmerman: Carcinoma of the pituitary gland with metastases to the spinal cord and roots of the cauda equina. J. Neurosurg. *21* (1964) 846-853.

[9] Finn, J.E., and L.A. Mount: Galactorrhea in males with tumors in the region of the pituitary gland. J. Neurosurg. *35* (1971) 723-727.

[10] Forbes, A.P., P.H. Henneman, G.C. Griswold, and F. Albright: Syndrome characterized by galactorrhea, amenorrhea and low urinary FSH: Comparison with acromegaly and normal lactation. J. Clin. Endocr. *14* (1957) 265-271.

[11] Garcia-Uria, J.: Surgical experience with craniopharyngioma in adults. Surg. Neurol. *9* (1978) 11-14.

[12] Gjerris, A., J. Lindholm, and J. Riishede: Pituitary oncocytic tumor with Cushing's disease. Cancer *42* (1978) 1818-1822.

[13] Hunter, I.J.: Squamous metaplasia of cells of the anterior pituitary gland. J. Path. Bact. *69* (1955) 141-145.

[14] Jennings, A.S., G.W. Liddle, and D.N. Orth: Results of treating childhood Cushing's disease with pituitary irradiation. N. Engl. J. Med. *297* (1977) 957-962.

[15] Kepes, J.J.: Transitional cell tumor of the pituitary gland developing from a rathke's cleft cyst. Cancer *41* (1978) 337-343.

[16] Kernohan, J.W., and G.P. Sayre: Tumors of the pituitary gland and infundibulum. Atlas of tumor pathology. A.F.I.P., Washington, D.C. 1956.

[17] Kovacs, K., and E. Horvath: Pituitary "chromophobe" adenoma composed of oncocytes. A light and electron microscopic study. Arch. Pathol. *95* (1973) 235-239.

[18] Kruseman, A.C.N., G.T.A.M. Bots, J. Lindeman, and A. Schaberg: Use of immunohistochemical and morphologic methods for the identification of human growth hormone-producing pituitary adenomas. Cancer *38* (1976) 1163-1170.

[19] Lewis, P.D., and S. Van Noorden: Pituitary abnormalities in acromegaly. Arch. Pathol. *94* (1972) 119-126.

[20] Madonick, M.J., L.J. Rubinstein, M.R. Dacso, and H. Ribner: Chromophobe adenoma of pituitary gland with subarachnoid metastases. Neurology *13* (1963) 836-840.

[21] Mayer, E.G., L.M. Boone, and S.A. Aristizabal: Role of radiation therapy in the management of neoplasms of the central nervous system. In: Advances in neurology, Vol. 15, edited by R.A. Thompson and J.R. Green, Raven Press, New York 1976.

[22] McCornick, W.F., and N.S. Halmi: Absence of chromophobe adenomas from a large series of pituitary tumors. Arch. Pathol. *92* (1971) 231-238.

[23] Nelson, D.H., J.W. Meakin, and G.W. Thorn: ACTH-producing pituitary tumors following adrenalectomy for Cushing's syndrome. Ann. Int. Med. *52* (1960) 560-569.

[24] O'Neal, L.W., D.M. Kipnis, S.A. Luse, P.E. Lacy, and L. Jarett: Secretion of various endocrine substances by ACTH-secreting tumors – gastrin, melanotropin, norepinephrine, serotonin, parathormone, vasopressin, glucagon. Cancer *21* (1968) 1219-1232.

[25] Onoyama, Y., K. Ono, E. Yabumoto, and J. Takeuchi: Radiation therapy of craniopharyngioma. J. Radiology *125* (1977) 799-803.

[26] Peake, G.T., D.W. MacKeel, L. Jarett, and W.H. Daughaday: Ultrastructural, histologic, and hormonal characterization of a prolactin-rich human pituitary tumor. J. Clin. Endocr. *29* (1969) 1383-1393.

[27] Phifer, R.F., and S.S. Spicer: Immunohistochemical and histologic demonstration of thyrotropic cells of the human adenohypophysis. J. Clin. Endocr. *36* (1973) 1210-1221.

[28] Pistenma, D.A., D.R. Goffinet, M.A. Bagshaw, J.W. Hanbery, and J.R. Eltringham: Treatment of chromophobe adenomas with megavoltage irradiation. Cancer *35* (1975) 1574-1582.

[29] Poon, M.-C., J.T. Prchal, T.M. Murad, and J.G. Galbraith: Multiple myeloma masquerading as chromophobe adenoma. Cancer *43* (1979) 1513-1516.

[30] Rovit, R.L., and T.D. Duane: Cushing's syndrome and pituitary tumors; pathophysiology and ocular manifestation of ACTH-secreting pituitary adenomas. Am. J. Med. *46* (1969) 416-427.

[31] Russell, D.S., and L.J. Rubinstein: Pathology of tumors of the nervous system. Fourth edition. Edward Arnold (1977).

[32] Saeger, W.: Pituitary tumours. Fischer, Stuttgart–New York 1977.

[33] Seemayer, T.A., J.S. Blundell, and F.W. Wiglesworth: Pituitary craniopharyngioma with tooth formation. Cancer *29* (1972) 423-430.

[34] Teears, R.J., and E.M. Silverman: Clinicopathologic review of 88 cases of carcinoma metastatic to the pituitary gland. Cancer *36* (1975) 216-220.

[35] Timperley, W.R.: Histochemistry of Rathke pouch tumours. J. Neurol. Neurosurg. Psychiatry *31* (1968) 589-595.

[36] Wermer, P.: Genetic aspects of adenomatosis of endocrine glands. Am. J. Med. *16* (1954) 363-371.

[37] Zülch, K.J.: Brain tumours. Their biology and pathology. Editor Springer, New York 1957.

20 Tumors of the eye and adnexa

T 190.3
T 190.4

Tumors of the conjunctiva and cornea

M-8070/3
T 190.3

1. Squamous cell carcinoma

The majority of these tumors grow at the limbus. Squamous cell carcinoma can also be observed at the bulbar conjunctiva.

This tumor is rare and, due to its site, is detected early. Occasionally, squamous cell carcinomas can contain pigment [16].

M-8081/2

2. Bowen's disease

M-8070/2

3. Carcinoma in situ

T 190.4
T 190.3

Both lesions are very rare.

The preferred site is again the limbus. The tumor can appear at the cornea or conjunctiva.

Histologically, the tumor contains atypical cells that thicken the epithelial layer. There is no infiltration of tumor cells into the underlying tissue (Figs. 1114 to 1117).

M-8050/0
T 190.3
T 190.4

4. Papilloma

This benign lesion can be observed at the conjunctiva and the cornea. This tumor also occurs most often at the limbus.

This papilloma shows histologically thickened epithelial layers; the cells are of regular appearance.

The underlying tissue often contains inflammatory cells. Often the papillary epithelial formations are covered by abundant keratin (Fig. 1111).

---

[16] Jauregui and Klintworth 1976.

883

5. Nevi

The majority of nevi appear at the limbus.

Grossly, the tumor can have a slightly papillary surface.

Occasionally these lesions remain unpigmented for a time, followed by a rather rapid pigmentation. This might lead to the assumption of malignant transformation.

M-8740/0
M-8760/0

Most of the nevi are **junctional or compound nevi** (Figs. 1184 to 1186).

M-8780/0
T 190.3

Occasionally **blue nevus** has been reported to occur in the conjunctiva (Figs. 1195 to 1197).

M-8741/2
T 190.3

6. Precancerous melanosis
(aquired melanosis) (Fig. 1202).

The preferred location for this lesion is again at the limbus or near the limbus.

Grossly, the tumor might be larger than the nevi and occasionally it has a slightly nodular appearance.

Precancerous melanosis has its peak age in the 5th decade.

On histological analysis the nevus cells grow in clusters and infiltrate the epithelial layer. Often these nevus cells can be observed at the basal cell layer.

In small biopsies it is occasionally difficult to differentiate this precancerous melanosis from atypical cells of the compound nevus.

M-8741/3
T 190.3

7. Malignant melanosis (Figs. 1202 to 1220)

Compared with the benign nevi, malignant melanosis is a rare tumor at this location.

This tumor occurs extremely rarely in blacks.

The main site is the bulbar conjunctiva.

The tumor can develop during many years as a benign melanosis. Occasionally, however, malignant melanoma can also appear spontaneously.

Due to the location, this malignant melanoma is detected early and has a better prognosis than, for instance, malignant melanoma of the eyelids.

Treatment: Surgery or beta irradiation of up to 100 to 150 Gy.

M-9590/3
T 190.3

8. Malignant lymphoma

The conjunctiva can be the site of growth for all types of malignant lymphomas, including Hodgkin's disease, and also for infiltrates of leukemia and plasmacytoma (Figs. 882 and 883).

M-7229/0
T 190.3

9. Pseudolymphoma

This lesion is usually small, measuring about 0.5 to 1 cm in diameter.
On histological analysis the combination of lymphoid cells with other inflammatory cells like granulocytes and plasma cells and the observation of lymphoid follicles prove the benign nature of this lymphoid hyperplasia (pseudolymphoma) (Fig. 892).

M-9140/3
T 190.3

10. Kaposi's sarcoma (Figs. 84 to 88)

Occasionally, this tumor can be observed in the conjunctiva when the disease has disseminated.

M-8090/3
T 190.3
T 190.4

11. Basal cell carcinoma (Figs. 1118 to 1125)

This tumor can develop in the conjunctiva and the cornea. Since occasionally these tumors can contain pigment, sometimes the differential diagnosis with melanoma becomes necessary.
About 3.5% of the affected patients die from this tumor [7].

---

[7] Collin 1976.

M-9352/0
T 190.4
T 190.3

12. Choristoma

This is a tumor-like lesion, in which ectopic tissue has been deposited into the cornea and conjunctiva.

These choristomas contain fat and connective tissue. This lesion is covered by intact surface epithelium.

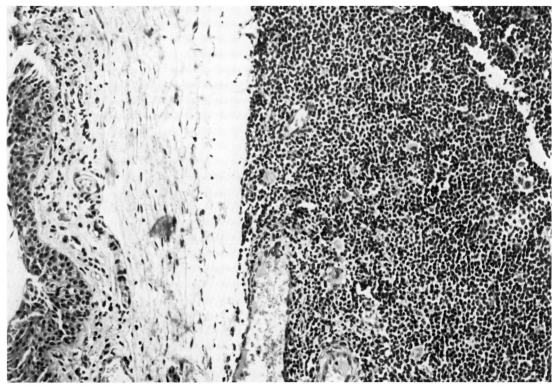

Fig. 882. Malignant lymphoma of the conjunctiva (75-year-old female, × 125).

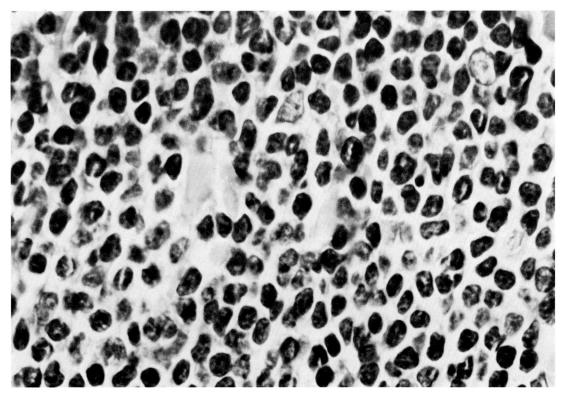

Fig. 883. Malignant lymphoma of the conjunctiva (× 600).

T 190.2

Tumor of the lacrimal glands
(see also Tumors of the salivary glands, page 561)

M-8940/0
T 190.2

13. Pleomorphic adenoma

Pleomorphic adenomas (mixed tumors) are in most instances benign.
The tumor seems to have a capsule.
The tumor is composed of epithelial proliferations interlacing with a matrix of connective tissue.
The tumor corresponds to those observed in the salivary glands (Figs. 572 to 576).

M-8200/3
T 190.2

14. Adenoid cystic carcinoma
(cylindroma)

The tumor corresponds to carcinoma of the salivary glands (Fig. 884).
In the lacrimal gland this is the most frequently observed malignant tumor [26].
This tumor is not encapsulated and shows a very strong tendency for invasion into the lymphatics.
In this way the tumor can invade the bone of the orbit and extend intracranially.
Besides infiltration into the lymphatics, the blood vessels are also affected.

---

[26] Reese 1956.

M-8940/3
T 190.2

15. Carcinoma in pleomorphic adenoma

Rarely, a malignant tumor can develop in a pleomorphic adenoma.
The variety of this carcinoma corresponds to those observed in the salivary glands (Fig. 581).
Carcinomas in pleomorphic adenomas comprise about 5% of lacrimal gland tumors.

M-8430/3
M-8020/3
T 190.2

16. Mucoepidermoid carcinoma

This tumor is exceedingly rare in the lacrimal gland.
It is a malignant tumor that can show different degrees of differentiation, reaching the picture of a poorly differentiated carcinoma in which the remnants of mucoepidermoid carcinoma can be detected with difficulty.
This tumor corresponds to those of the salivary glands (Figs. 582 to 587).

M-9590/3
T 190.2

17. Malignant lymphoma

Lacrimal glands can also be involved by the different types of malignant lymphomas, including Hodgkin's disease.
As in tumor of the conjunctiva and cornea, the differential diagnosis with

M-7229/0

pseudolymphoma
might be occasionally necessary.
The appearance of other inflammatory cells and the evidence of follicles indicate the benign lesion (Figs. 885 and 886).

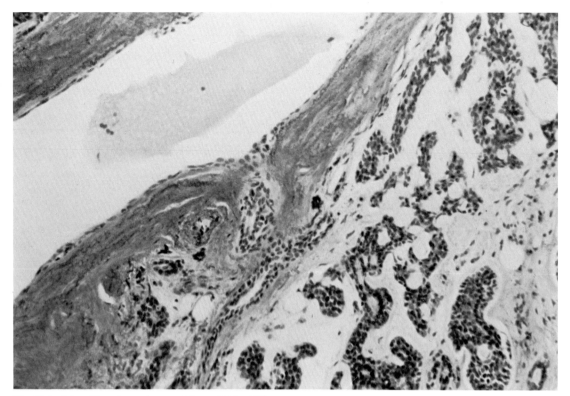

Fig. 884. Adenoid cystic carcinoma of the eyelid (×125).

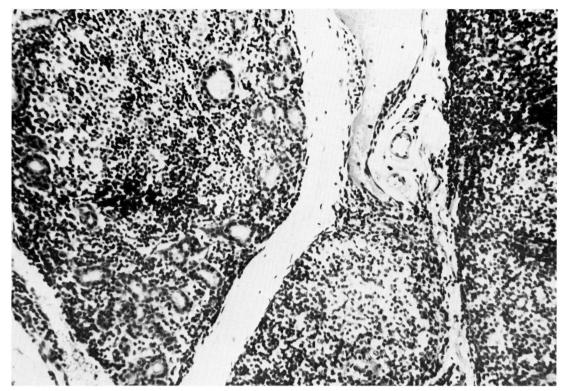

Fig. 885. Pseudolymphoma of the lacrimal gland (Sjögren's syndrome) (× 125).

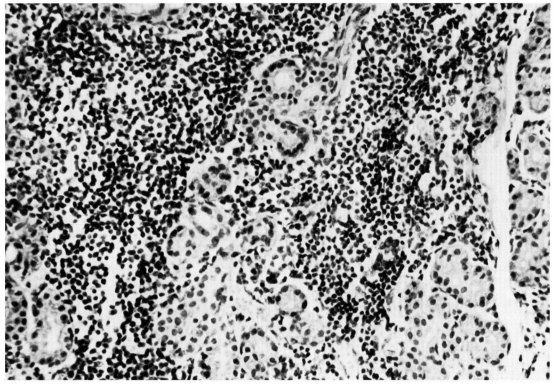

Fig. 886. Pseudolymphoma of the lacrimal gland (Sjögren's syndrome) (× 200).

T 190.7

Tumors of the lacrimal passages

Benign and malignant tumors in this location are very rare.

M-8050/0
T 190.7

18. Papilloma

This epithelial tumor may occur within the lacrimal duct.
It grows into the lumen and causes obstruction.
In other instances the tumor grows toward the underlying tissue, however, without destroying the basement membrane and infiltrating the connective tissue:

M-8053/0

Inverted papilloma [9].

M-3320/0
T 190.7

19. Mucocele

This lesion is due to a chronic inflammation that extends into the lacrimal sac.

20. Malignant tumors of the lacrimal passages

The occurrence of malignant tumors at this site is exceedingly rare.

M-8070/3
T 190.7

The tumor can be a **squamous cell carcinoma,** which in most instances grows into the lumen of the ducts.

M-8430/3
T 190.7

Very rarely **mucoepidermoid carcinoma** has been observed [25].

---

[9] Fechner and Sessions 1977.
[25] Rao and Font 1976.

Tumors of the eyelids

M-8140/0
M-8140/3
T 173.1

21. Adenoma and adenocarcinoma of the meibomian glands [37]

General Remarks

Incidence: These tumors are rare.

Histology

The meibomian glands are variations of sebaceous glands. Tumors originating in these glands can grow as adenocarcinomas that are highly differentiated and still contain signs of sebaceous cells.

However, in other instances this tumor loses the original sebaceous gland structure and is poorly differentiated. The tumor cells then are arranged in a tubular pattern or more often in adenoid-cystic spaces that are disseminated by necrotic areas, causing a cribriform aspect.

M-8542/3

The cells of this adenocarcinoma can grow in the epithelial layer: **Extramammary Paget's disease** (Figs. 1642 and 1643).

Differential Diagnosis

Adenoma and adenocarcinoma **with chalazion** (Figs. 890 and 891):
This inflammatory lesion of the meibomian glands is characterized by the appearance of epithelioid granulomas with giant cells. These granulomas can be surrounded and infiltrated by numerous lymphocytes.

Since this inflammation is probably due to retention of the secretion of the meibomian glands, the glandular structures might be destroyed and disseminated into the inflammatory tissue.

A poorly differentiated carcinoma of the meibomian glands on the other side can induce a similar inflammatory reaction due to the destruction of the glands and liberation of the secretion.

Therefore, one should look carefully for carcinoma of the meibomian glands in cases of recurrent chalazion with necroses.

Spread

Adenocarcinoma of the meibomian glands invades the orbit in about 17% of the cases and causes lymph node metastases in about 28% of the cases.

Treatment

Surgical removal of the tumor.
Radiation therapy has been recommended (up to 60 Gy) [30].

Prognosis

About 14% of the patients die of this disease [5].

Further Information

A very unusual case has been reported in which a sebaceous carcinoma developed in the eyelid 11 years after curative radiation therapy for bilateral retinoblastoma [19].

---

[5] Boniuk and Zimmerman 1968.
[19] Lemos et al. 1978.
[30] Scherer and Schietzel 1976.
[37] Zimmerman 1962.

M-8140/3
T 173.1

22. Adenocarcinoma of Moll's glands

Moll's glands are the sweat glands of the eyelid.
The appearance of an adenocarcinoma in this location is exceedingly rare.
This tumor can appear as Paget's disease in the epidermis of the eyelid.

M-8400/1, 3
T 173.1

Exceedingly rare are **tumors of the eccrine sweat glands.**
These tumors are composed of clear cells and might involve the eyelid [28].

M-8090/3
T 173.1

23. Basal cell carcinoma

Most of the tumors of the eyelid are basal cell carcinomas.
The histology corresponds to the basal cell carcinoma of the skin at any other site (Figs. 1118 to 1125).
Due to the pigmentation of basal cell carcinoma, occasionally the differential diagnosis with malignant melanoma becomes necessary.
In other instances the basal cell carcinoma can grow in such a way that it mimics pilomatrixoma.
On gross inspection a basal cell carcinoma can be taken for a papilloma or a seborrheic acanthosis.
The treatment of basal cell carcinoma is complete surgical removal and/or radiation therapy.

---

[28] Rosen et al. 1975.

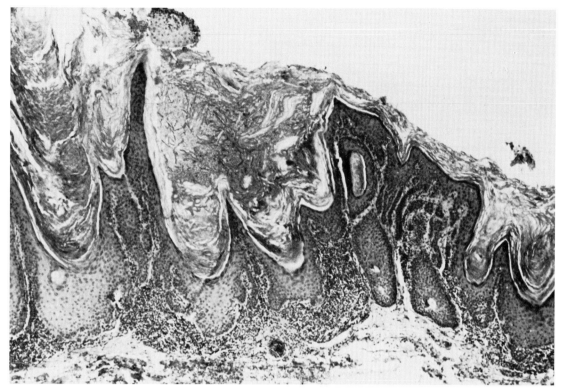

Fig. 887. Benign squamous keratosis of the eyelid (67-year-old male, × 50).

M-8052/0
T 173.1

24. Squamous cell papilloma with keratosis

This tumor in the eyelid is characterized by epithelial cells that do not show signs of atypia. The papillary epithelial formations are covered by abundant keratin.
The underlying tissue often contains an inflammatory cell population (Fig. 887).

M-8070/3
T 173.1

25. Squamous cell carcinoma

This tumor is rare in the eyelid [4].

[4] Bertelsen and Gadeberg 1978.

M-9120/0
T 173.1

26. Hemangioma

Hemangiomas in the eyelid can be capillary. In most instances they are, however, cavernous hemangiomas (Fig. 71).
They can have a pseudocapsule.
Hemangioma in association with other vascular malformations in Sturge-Weber disease is characterized by a very closely packed arrangement of multiple blood vessels, which have different sizes.
Hemangiomas can be treated by irradiation very well (recommended dosis of up to 10 to 15 Gy) [3].

M-7275/0
T 173.1

27. Seborrheic keratosis

This lesion corresponds to the disease observed in other parts of the skin (Figs. 1094 to 1097).
On gross inspection the differential diagnosis with melanoma occasionally cannot be solved and requires histological examination.

M-7660/0
T 173.1

28. Warts

This skin lesion consists of epithelial cells with basophilic inclusion bodies in their cytoplasm and occasionally in the nuclei (Fig. 1098).

M-9540/0
T 171.1

29. Neurofibroma

Neurofibromas can be observed in the eyelids and, in this location, are occasionally associated with von Recklinghausen's disease (Fig. 178).

---

[3] Bamberg and Scherer 1978.

M-8720/0
M-8720/3
T 171.1

30. Nevi and malignant melanoma

The histological appearance of this tumor corresponds to those observed at other sites (Figs. 1202 to 1220).
The prognosis of malignant melanoma in the eyelid is poor, since this tumor disseminates early.

T 171.1

31. Other tumors of the skin and soft tissue

can rarely be observed in the eyelids (Figs. 888 and 889):

M-8850/0   – **lipoma,**

M-8810/0   – **fibroma,**

M-8110/0   – **pilomatrixoma** (Figs. 1137 to 1139),

M-7666/0   – **molluscum contagiosum** (Figs. 1100 and 1101),

M-8407/0   – **syringoma** (Figs. 1147 to 1149),

M-8940/0   – **pleomorphic adenoma** [18].

M-8000/6
T 171.1

32. Metastases of malignant tumors into the eyelid

a) Tumors from the surrounding tissue can extend into the eyelids.

b) Eyelids can be involved by **leukemias** and **malignant lymphomas.**

c) Malignant tumors from different organs can disseminate into the eyelids.

[18] Kreibig 1961.

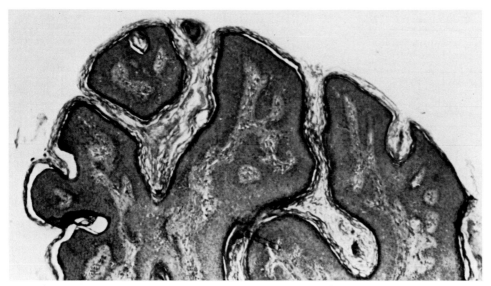

Fig. 888. Fibropapilloma of the eyelid (51-year-old female, × 50).

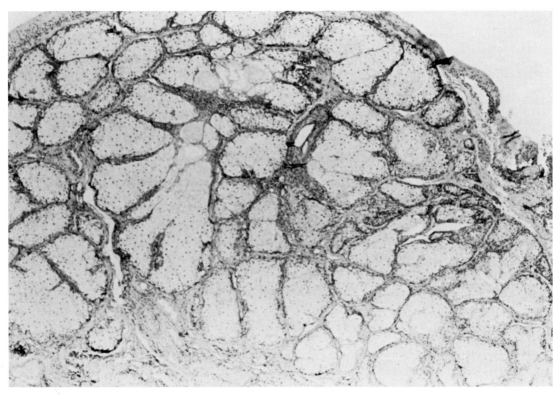

Fig. 889. Sebaceous nevus of the eyelid (47-year-old male, × 50).

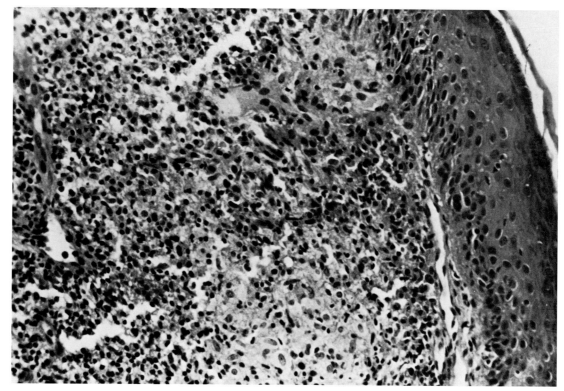

Fig. 890. Chalazion (69-year-old male, × 200).

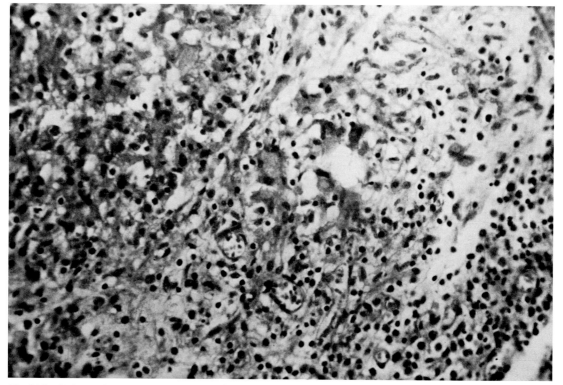

Fig. 891. Chalazion (× 200).

33. Tumor-like lesions of the eyelid

a) Xanthelasma

This yellowish lesion can occur on both eyelids. Xanthelasmas are usually observed in patients in the 5th and 6th decades.
Histologically, the tumor contains foamy histiocytes, which are packed closely together and are sometimes surrounded by a discrete lymphocytic infiltration (Figs. 33 and 34).

M-4300/0
T 173/1

b) Chalazion

This epithelioid granulomatous inflammation is induced by the secretion of the meibomian glands.
Besides the epithelioid cells, histiocytic giant cells are present.
In the granulomas there are no necroses (Figs. 890 and 891) (see Differential diagnosis with adenocarcinoma of the meibomain glands, page 893).

M-9084/0
T 173.1

c) Dermoid cyst

The cysts are histologically lined by squamous cells. The wall contains hairs; the lumen is filled with keratin.
By rupture of the wall, the cysts can induce an inflammation with foreign body reaction in the surrounding tissue.
This dermoid cyst occurs in most instances at the upper eyelid.

d) Cysts of Moll's glands

These cysts occur at the margin of the eyelids.
Histologically the cysts are lined by cuboidal cells. Probably the cysts develop by extension of the ducts of Moll's glands.

T 190.1

Tumors of the orbit

The orbit can be involved by tumors originating in the surrounding areas and extending into the orbit.
Primary tumors in the orbit originate from the optic nerve or the soft tissue.

M-9380/0
T 192.0

34. Glioma of the optic nerve [22]

General Remarks

Incidence: Gliomas of the optic nerve comprise about 1% of all intracranial tumors.
Age: Most of these tumors develop during the 1st decade.
Site: In most instances this is a unilateral tumor arising in the orbital part of the optic nerve.

Macroscopy

The nerve has a fusiform deconfiguration, which might expand within the skull.
On the cut surface one sees that the tumor infiltrates the enveloping sheath.
Occasionally cysts are observed.

Histology

The tumor shows a considerable variability in the histological picture:
The tumor is very cellular. Most of the cells exhibit signs of malignancy. The tumor cells often have a spindle shape.
Mitoses are rare. Reticulin fibers can be deposited. Occasionally the tumor cells form perivascular pseudorosettes.
Cysts can exist, and occasionally they contain mucin.
The tumor cells infiltrate the pial sheath and thicken the arachnoidea.
This tumor can be composed of astrocytes (pilocytic astrocytoma). This tumor can also be combined with an oligodendroglioma.

Clinical Findings

Exophthalmus with or without signs of inflammation in the orbital tissue.
Glioma of the optic nerve can be a component or a solitary manifestation of von Recklinghausen's disease.

Treatment

Surgical excision.
Radiation therapy:
Megavoltage photon irradiation has been recently recommended [21].

[21] Montgomery et al. 1977.
[22] Naumann 1968.

M-9530/0
T 192.1

35. Meningioma (Figs. 822 to 828)

This tumor can originate from the meninges of the optic nerve or extend from a meningioma originating in the sphenoidal ridge.

M-9120/0
T 190.1

36. Angioma (Figs. 70 to 76)

Angiomas are the most common soft tissue tumors in the orbit. They almost always occur in infancy and childhood.

M-8900/3
T 190.1

37. Rhabdomyosarcoma

Rhabdomyosarcomas occur in infancy and childhood and are relatively rare malignant soft tissue tumors (Figs. 111 to 122).
Differential diagnostic problems can be posed with metastatic lesions, especially with neuroblastomas.

T 190.1

38. Other soft tissue tumors of rare occurrence

M-9150/0   – **hemangiopericytoma,**

M-9180/3   – **osteosarcoma,**

M-8832/0   – **histiocytoma,**

M-8850/0   – **lipoma,**

M-8810/0   – **fibroma,**

M-8840/0   – **myxoma,**
(see Soft tissue tumors, page 7).

M-9080/0
T 190.1

39. Cystic teratoma

Very rarely, benign cystic teratomas of the orbit have been observed.

M-8693/1
T 190.1

40. Chemodectoma [27]

M-9560/0
M-9540/0
T 190.1

41. Neurilemoma and neurofibroma (Figs. 165 to 168 and 178)

Both tumors can occur in association with von Recklinghausen's disease.

M-9590/3
M-9650/3
T 190.1

42. Malignant lymphoma, Hodgkin's disease [32]

Malignant lymphoma can involve the orbit as well as other parts of the eye.

M-7229/0

Here again, differential diagnosis with **pseudolymphoma** might be required: Inflammatory cells and lymphoid follicles indicate the benign lesion [32] (Fig. 892).

M-8000/6
T 190.1

43. Metastatic lesions [10]

M-9930/3

Different tumors might disseminate into the orbit, including leukemia, which occasionally grows in the orbit as a **granulocytic sarcoma** (chloroma).

---

[10] Font and Ferry 1976.
[27] Reese 1963.
[32] Schwarze et al. 1976.

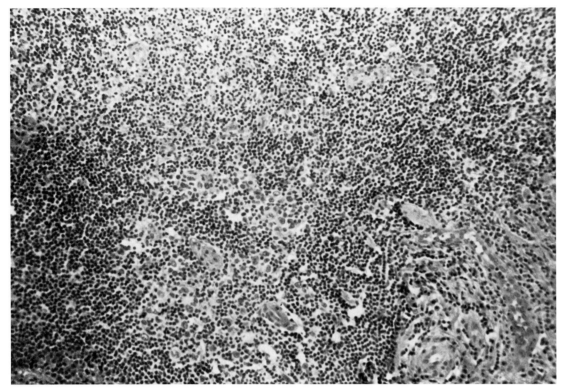

Fig. 892. Lymphocytic inflammation of the orbit (62-year-old male, × 125).

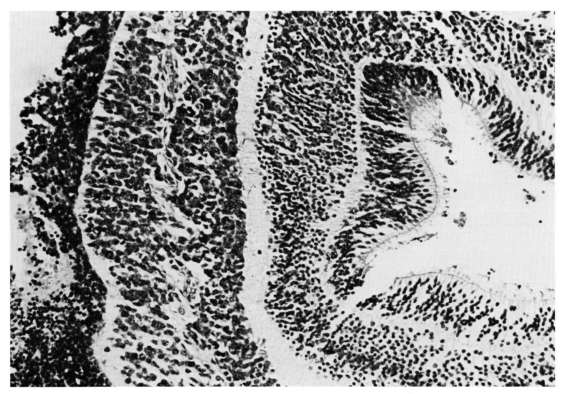

Fig. 893. Retinoblastoma (× 125).

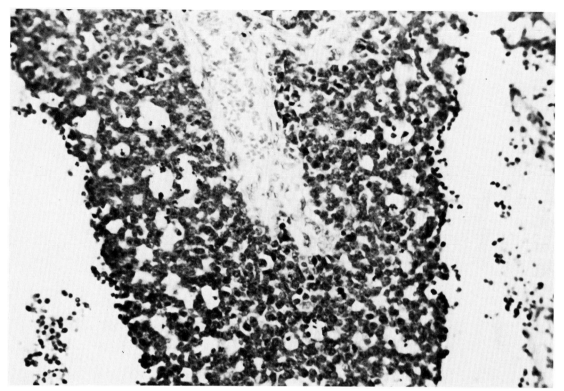

Fig. 894. Retinoblastoma: Rosette formation (× 200).

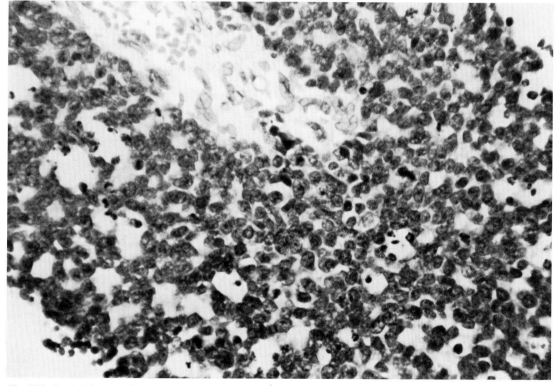

Fig. 895. Retinoblastoma: Large nuclei, sparse cytoplasm (× 310).

Intraocular tumors

M-9510/3
T 190.5

44. Retinoblastoma

General
Remarks

Incidence: Retinoblastoma is a very rare tumor. It is observed in about 1 child in 30,000 births.
Age: Retinoblastoma is the most frequent ocular tumor in children:
The great majority are found in children before the age of 3 years (more than 75%).
Occasionally, the tumor is seen at birth; very rarely by 6 years; exceedingly rarely in adult life.
Sex: Both sexes are equally affected.
Site: 75% of the tumors are unilateral.
Further notes: It seems that some of retinoblastomas are inherited tumors [11, 17].

Macroscopy

Retinoblastoma often grows in a multifocal fashion: Small, barely visible, white nodules are seen, resembling tuberculosis.
The solitary tumor is a whitish nodule, which can finally form a mass in the posterior chamber or extend through the retina.

Histology

The tumor cells have large hyperchromatic nuclei that are surrounded by a scanty cytoplasm. There are numerous mitotic figures.
The tumor growth is interrupted by large areas of necroses.
Tumor cells in such necrotic areas are still visible in a perivascular arrangement.
Occasionally tumor cells form rosettes that are not arranged around blood vessels. The center of the rosettes contains fibrillar structures (Figs. 893 to 895).
It is important to check the surgical margin of the optic nerve since the tumor tends to grow preferentially along that structure.

Spread

1. Local invasion of the tumor:
   The tumor infiltrates the orbital tissue.
   The tumor extends into the anterior extraocular region.
   The tumor infiltrates the skull.
   The tumor grows along the optic nerve and infiltrates the chiasm and the leptomeninges.
2. The tumor infiltrates into the lymphatics and causes distant lymph node metastases.
3. Hematogenous metastases into liver, pancreas, and bone.

Clinical
Findings

Glaucoma, enlargement of the globe.
In cases of bilateral retinoblastoma, the tumors can grow at the same time or with a time lag of weeks or months.

[11] François et al. 1975.
[17] Knudson Jr. 1975.

Treatment

Surgery:
Enucleation of the eye [33].
Radiation therapy:
The cells of retinoblastomas are radiosensitive.
In cases of involvement of the optic nerve, postoperative radiation of up to 50 Gy in about 5 weeks has been recommended.
In case of bilateral retinoblastoma, irradiation of one eye and enucleation of the other could be tried [12].

Prognosis

Overall 5-year survival rate for all stages: 60 to 80% [8].
Rarely spontaneous regressions of retinoblastoma have been reported [29].

Further Information

1. Very exceptionally, retinoblastomas can be associated with secondary intracranial malignancies [14].
2. Two other tumors of the retina should be mentioned, which are exceedingly rare:

**M-9501/3
T 190.5**

a) Medulloepithelioma
(diktyoma) [38]
This exceedingly rare tumor affects young children and is often present at birth.
This is a slow-growing tumor, which grows as a flat white cover, finally filling the eye.
The tumor imitates the structure of the retina: The tumor cells are arranged in rows, which can anastomose with each other. In the rows the spindle-shaped nuclei have a palisading pseudoretina arrangement [2, 39].
The tumor infiltrates the surrounding tissue.
Metastases do not occur.
The tumor is treated by enucleation of the eye.

**M-9400/3
T 190.5**

b) Exceedingly rare are **astrocytomas** of the retina.
The majority are associated with tuberous sclerosis [23].

---

[2] Andersen 1962.
[8] Ellsworth 1968.
[12] Gaitan-Yanguas 1978.
[14] Jakobiec et al. 1977.
[23] Orton and Willis 1944.
[29] Russell and Rubinstein 1977.
[33] Seydel 1976.
[38] Zimmerman 1971.
[39] Zimmerman et al. 1972.

M-8720/3
T 190.0

45. Malignant melanoma of the uveal tract

**General
Remarks**

Incidence: With the exception of retinoblastomas in children, malignant melanoma is the most frequent ocular malignant tumor.
Age: The majority of these malignant melanomas occur during the 5th to 6th decades.
Site: Most of the melanomas originate in the choroid, followed by the ciliary body.
Further notes: Probably malignant melanoma develops from a preexistent nevus [36] (Fig. 896).

Macroscopy

Malignant melanoma of the uveal tract can be very small or large. Therefore, about 10% of these tumors are found only after enucleation of the eye.

Histology

This tumor contains the usual cellular composition, with the great variety of appearances in the tumor cells (Figs. 897 to 901).
However, these malignant melanomas of the uveal tract often contain spindle cells, which can be large or small. Often both types are combined. Occasionally, foci of epithelioid-like cells are observed.

Spread

1. The tumor extends into the surrounding tissue.
2. Hematogenous metastases are early and occur in all distant organs.
3. Relatively rare, however, are lymph node metastases.

Treatment

Surgery:
Enucleation of the eye or iridectomy (small tumors of the iris).
Postoperative **irradiation** or in cases of incomplete removal of the tumor: 60 to 70 Gy in 6 to 7 weeks.

Prognosis

The overall 5-year survival rate is about 50 to 70%.
It has been reported that the prognosis in the individual case is also determined by the type of tumor cells: Callender's classification [6].
Small cells carry a better prognosis than larger cells, mixed cellularity, or epithelioid cells.
The individual prognosis is also determined by the site of the tumor:
Melanomas of the iris are detected early and have an excellent prognosis.
Melanomas of the posterior uvea are clinically silent for a long time and have a bad prognosis [24, 34].

[6] Callender 1931.
[24] Paul et al. 1962.
[34] Smith 1974.
[36] Yanoff and Zimmerman 1967.

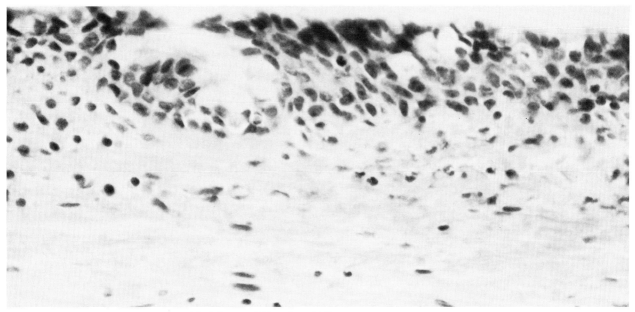

Fig. 896. Precancerous melanosis of the iris (18-year-old female, × 310).

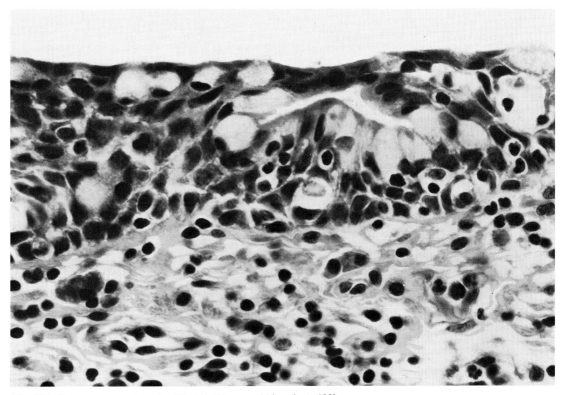

Fig. 897. Precancerous melanosis of the iris (18-year-old female, × 400).

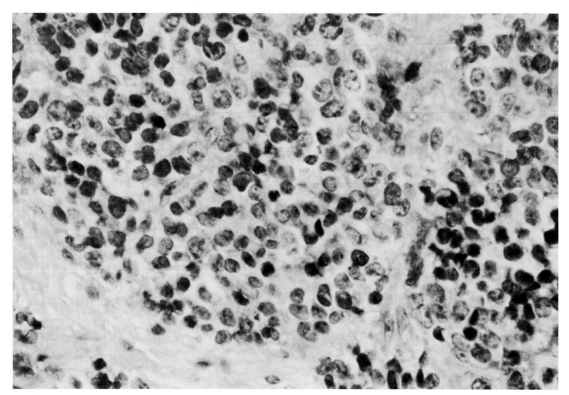

Fig. 898. Malignant melanoma of the uvea: Round cell type (18-year-old female, × 400).

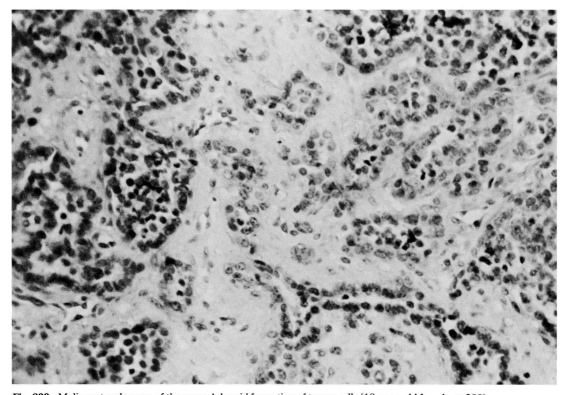

Fig. 899. Malignant melanoma of the uvea: Adenoid formation of tumor cells (18-year-old female, × 200).

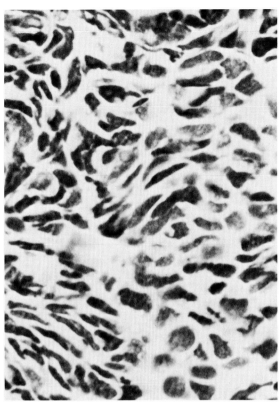

Fig. 900. Malignant melanoma of the uvea: Spindle cell type (18-year-old female, × 600).

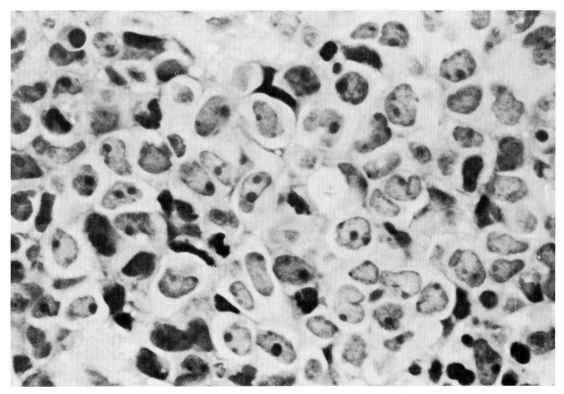

Fig. 901. Malignant melanoma of the uvea: Large cell type (18-year-old female, × 800).

M-7631/0
T 190.5

46. Angiomatosis retinae

Angiomatosis retinae is part of von Hippel's disease and is associated with cerebellar hemangiomatosis in about 25% of the cases [13].

M-9590/3
T 190.5

47. Primary malignant lymphoma of the retina

All types of lymphoma can occur. This is, however, very rare [35] and includes leukemias and Hodgkin's disease.

48. Mesectodermal leiomyoma

A case has been reported in which mesectodermal leiomyoma developed in the ciliary body [15].

M-8010/0, 2, 3
T 190.0

49. Epithelial tumors of the ciliary body [20]

M-8000/6
T 190.0

50. Metastases

Metastases of malignant epithelial or mesenchymal tumors into the intraocular part of the eye are very rare [1].
The most frequently observed epithelial tumors metastasizing into this region originate from the breast or the lung. Occasionally adenocarcinoma of the colon has been reported to disseminate into the eye [31].

[1] Albert et al. 1967.
[13] Jakobiec et al. 1976.
[15] Jakobiec et al. 1977.
[20] Lommatzsch et al. 1979.
[31] Schneider and Bosshard 1978.
[35] Völcker et al. 1977.

Recommendations for differential diagnosis in tumors of the eye

adenocarcinoma of the meibomian glands	with	– chalazion – noninfiltrating adenoma
malignant melanosis	with	– precancerous melanosis
primary tumor	with	– metastatic tumor
malignant lymphoma	with	– chronic inflammation (pseudolymphoma) – Hodgkin's disease
retinoblastoma	with	– poorly differentiated malignant tumor (metastatic) – malignant lymphoma – leukemic infiltration
basal cell carcinoma	with	– pilomatrixoma – papilloma

References

[1] Albert, D.M., R.A. Rubenstein, and H.G. Scheie: Tumor metastasis to the eye. Part I. Incidence in 213 adult patients with generalized malignancy. Am. J. Ophthalmol. *63* (1967) 724-726.

[2] Andersen, S.R.: Medulloepithelioma of the retina. Internat. Ophth. Clin *2* (1962) 1483-1497.

[3] Bamberg, M., und E. Scherer: Zur Strahlentherapie der blastomatösen Hämangiome unter besonderer Berücksichtigung von 44 Lidhämangiomen. Strahlentherapie *154* (1978) 233-239.

[4] Bertelsen, K., and C. Gadeberg: Carcinoma of the eyelid. Acta Radiol. Oncol. *17* (1978) 58-64.

[5] Boniuk, M., and L.E. Zimmerman: Sebaceous carcinoma of the eyelid, eyebrow, caruncle, and orbit. Tr. Am. Acad. Ophthalmol. Otolaryngol. *72* (1968) 619-642.

[6] Callender, G.R.: Malignant melanotic tumors of the eye: A study of histologic types in 111 cases. Tr. Am. Acad. Ophthalmol. Otolaryngol. *36* (1931) 131-142.

[7] Collin, J.R.O.: Basal cell carcinoma in the eyelid region. Brit. J. Ophthal. *60* (1976) 806-809.

[8] Ellsworth, R.M.: Treatment of retinoblastoma. Am. J. Ophthalmol. *66* (1968) 49-51.

[9] Fechner, R.E., and R.B. Sessions: Inverted papilloma of the lacrimal sac, the paranasal sinuses and the cervical region. Cancer *40* (1977) 2303-2308.

[10] Font, R.L., and A.P. Ferry: Carcinoma metastatic to the eye and orbit. III. A clinicopathologic study of 28 cases metastatic to the orbit. Cancer *38* (1976) 1326-1335.

[11] François, J., M.T. Matton, S. DeBie, Y. Tanaka, and D. van den Bulcke: Genesis and genetics of retinoblastoma. Ophthalmologica Basel *170(5)* (1975) 405-425.

[12] Gaitan-Yanguas, M.: Retinoblastoma: Analysis of 235 cases. Int. J. Radiat. Oncol. Biol. Phys. *4* (1978) 359-365.

[13] Jakobiec, F.A., R.L. Font, and F.B. Johnson: Angiomatosis retinae. An ultrastructural study and lipid analysis. Cancer *38* (1976) 2042-2056.

[14] Jakobiec, F.A., M.O.M. Tso, L.E. Zimmerman, and P. Danis: Retinoblastoma and intracranial malignancy. Cancer *39* (1977) 2048-2058.

[15] Jakobiec, F.A., R.L. Font, M.O.M. Tso, and L.E. Zimmerman: Mesectodermal leiomyoma of the ciliary body. A tumor of presumed neural crest origin. Cancer *39* (1977) 2102-2113.

[16] Jauregui, H.O., and G.K. Klintworth: Pigmented squamous cell carcinoma of cornea and conjunctiva. A ligh microscopic, histochemical, and ultrastructural study. Cancer *38* (1976) 778-788.

[17] Knudson, A.G. Jr.: The genetics of childhood cancer. Cancer *35* (1975) 1022-1026.

[18] Kreibig, W.: Das Auge und sein Hilfsapparat. In: Handbuch der speziellen pathologischen Anatomie. Kaufmann-Staemmler. III/2, Walter de Gruyter, Berlin 1961.

[19] Lemos, L.B., D.J. Santa Cruz, and N. Baba: Sebaceous carcinoma of the eyelid following radiation therapy. Am. J. Surg. Path. *2* (1978) 305-311.

[20] Lommatzsch, P., K. Vorpahl, G. Bauke und H. Klug: Über epitheliale Tumoren des Ziliarkörpers – klinische, histologische und elektronenmikroskopische Beobachtungen. Klin. Mbl. Augenheilk. *174* (1979) 34-40.

[21] Montgomery, A.B., T. Griffin, R.G. Parker, and A.J. Gerdes: Optic nerve glioma: The role of radiation therapy. Cancer *40* (1977) 2079-2080.

[22] Naumann, G.: Tumoren der Augen der Augenhöhle. Handbuch der Kinderheilkunde. VIII/2. Springer-Verlag, Berlin–Heidelberg–New York 1968.

[23] Orton, R.H., and R.A. Willis: Rare retinal tumour probably derived from Müller's fibres. J. Path. Bact. *56* (1944) 255-257.

[24] Paul, E.V., B.L. Parnell, and M. Fraker: Prognosis of malignant melanoma of the chorioid and ciliary body. Int. Ophthalmol. Clin. *2* (1962) 387-402.

[25] Rao, N.A., and R.L. Font: Mucoepidermoid carcinoma of the conjunctiva. A clinicopathologic study of five cases. Cancer *38* (1976) 1699-1709.

[26] Reese, A.B.: Tumors of the eye and adnexa. Atlas of tumor pathology, A.F.I.P., Washington, D.C. 1956.

[27] Reese, A.B.: Tumors of the eye. Hoeber Ed., New York 1963.

[28] Rosen, Y., B. Kim, and V.A. Yermakov: Eccrine sweat gland tumor of clear cell origin involving the eyelids. Cancer *36* (1975) 1034-1041.

[29] Russell, D.S., and L.J. Rubinstein: Pathology of tumours of the nervous system. Fourth edition. Edward Arnold (1977).

[30] Scherer, E., und M. Schietzel: Die Strahlentherapie der Augenlidkarzinome. Strahlentherapie *151* (1976) 144-150.

[31] Schneider, P.A., und C. Bosshard: Aderhautmetastasen bei Kolonkarzinom. Klin. Mbl. Augenheilk. *172* (1978) 513-516.

[32] Schwarze, E.-W., T. Radaszkiewicz, G. Pülhorn, M. Goos und K. Lennert: Maligne und benigne Lymphome des Auges, der Lid- und Orbitalregion. Virchows Arch. A Path. Anat. and Histol. *370* (1976) 85-96.

[33] Seydel, H.G.: Retinoblastoma. In: Trends in childhood cancer. Donaldson M.H., H.G. Seydel, eds. New York; John Wiley & Sons. (1976).

[34] Smith, M.E.: Eyes and ocular adnexa. In: Surgical pathology, Ackerman, L.V. and J. Rosai. Fifth edition, Mosby Company, St. Louis, 1974.

[35] Völcker, H.E., G.O.H. Naumann, F. Rentsch und J. Wollensak: "Primäres" Retikulumzellsarkom der Retina. I. Eine klinisch-pathologische Studie und Literaturübersicht. Klin. Mbl. Augenheilk. *171* (1977) 489-499.

[36] Yanoff, M., and L.E. Zimmerman: Histogenesis of malignant melanomas of the uvea. II. The relationship of uveal nevi to malignant melanomas. Cancer *20* (1967) 493-507.

[37] Zimmerman, L.E.: Tumors of the eye and adnexa. Int. Ophthalmol. Clin. *2* (1962) 239-264.

[38] Zimmerman, L.E.: Verhoeff's "terato-neuroma"; a critical reappraisal in light of new observations and current concepts of embryonic tumors. The fourth Frederick H. Verhoeff lecture. Am. J. Ophthalmol. *72* (1971) 1039-1057.

[39] Zimmerman, L.E., R.L. Font, and S.R. Andersen: Rhabdomysarcomatous differentiation in malignant intraocular medulloepitheliomas. Cancer *30* (1972) 817-835.

Topography – numerical list

140 lip
140.0   upper lip, NOS
140.1   lower lip, NOS
140.3   mucosa of upper lip
140.4   mucosa of lower lip
140.5   mucosa of lip, NOS
140.6   commissure of lip
140.9   lip, NOS

141 tongue
141.0   base of tongue, NOS
141.1   dorsal surface of tongue, NOS
141.2   border of tongue
141.3   ventral surface of tongue, NOS
141.4   anterior 2/3 of tongue, NOS
141.5   junctional zone of tongue
141.6   lingual tonsil
141.9   tongue, NOS

142 major salivary glands
142.0   parotid gland
142.1   submandibular gland
142.2   sublingual gland
142.9   major salivary gland, NOS

143 gum
143.0   upper gum
143.1   lower gum
143.8   gum, NOS

144 floor of the mouth
144.0   anterior floor of the mouth
144.1   lateral floor of the mouth
144.9   floor of the mouth, NOS

**145 other and unspecified parts
     of the mouth**
145.0   cheek mucosa
145.1   vestibule of the mouth

145.2   hard palate
145.3   soft palate, NOS
145.4   uvula
145.5   palate, NOS
145.6   retromolar area
145.9   oral cavity

146 oropharynx
146.0   tonsil, NOS
146.1   tonsillar fossa
146.2   tonsillar pillar
146.3   vallecula epiglottica
146.4   anterior surface of epiglottis
146.5   junctional region of oropharynx
146.6   lateral wall of oropharynx
146.7   posterior wall of oropharynx
146.8   other parts of oropharynx
146.9   oropharynx, NOS

147 nasopharynx
147.0   superior wall of nasopharynx
147.1   posterior wall of nasopharynx
147.2   lateral wall of nasopharynx
147.3   anterior wall of nasopharynx
147.9   nasopharynx, NOS

148 hypopharynx
148.0   postcricoid region
148.1   pyriform sinus
148.2   aryepiglottic fold, NOS
148.3   posterior wall of hypopharynx
148.9   hypopharynx, NOS

**149 pharynx and ill-defined sites
     in lip, oral cavity, and pharynx**
149.0   pharynx, NOS
149.1   Waldeyer's ring, NOS
149.9   ill-defined sites in lip, oral cavity,
        and pharynx

150 esophagus

150.0 cervical esophagus
150.1 thoracic esophagus
150.2 abdominal esophagus
150.3 upper third of esophagus
150.4 middle third of esophagus
150.5 lower third of esophagus
150.9 esophagus, NOS

151 stomach

151.0 cardia, NOS
151.1 pylorus
151.2 pyloric antrum
151.3 fundus of stomach
151.4 body of stomach
151.5 lesser curvature of stomach, NOS
151.6 greater curvature of stomach, NOS
151.8 other parts of stomach
151.9 stomach, NOS

152 small intestine

152.0 duodenum
152.1 jejunum
152.2 ileum
152.3 Meckel's diverticulum
152.9 small intestine

153 colon

153.0 hepatic flexure of colon
153.1 transverse colon
153.2 descending colon
153.3 sigmoid colon
153.4 cecum
153.5 appendix
153.6 ascending colon
153.7 splenic flexure of colon
153.9 colon, NOS

**154 rectum, rectosigmoid junction,
     anal canal, and anus, NOS**

154.0 rectosigmoid junction
154.1 rectum, NOS
154.2 anal canal
154.3 anus, NOS
154.8 other parts of rectum

155 liver and intrahepatic bile ducts

155.0 liver
155.1 intrahepatic bile duct

**156 gallbladder and extrahepatic
     bile ducts**

156.0 gallbladder
156.1 extrahepatic bile duct
156.2 ampulla of Vater
156.9 biliary tract, NOS

157 pancreas

157.0 head of pancreas
157.1 body of pancreas
157.2 tail of pancreas
157.3 pancreatic duct
157.4 islets of Langerhans
157.9 pancreas, NOS

158 retroperitoneum and peritoneum

158.0 retroperitoneum
158.8 specified parts of peritoneum
158.9 peritoneum, NOS

**159 other and ill-defined sites within
     digestive organs and peritoneum**

159.0 intestinal tract, NOS
159.9 gastrointestinal tract, NOS

160 nasal cavity, accessory sinuses, middle ear, and inner ear
160.0 nasal cavity
160.1 middle ear
160.2 maxillary sinus
160.3 ethmoid sinus
160.4 frontal sinus
160.5 sphenoid sinus
160.9 accessory sinuses, NOS

161 larynx
161.0 glottis
161.1 supraglottis
161.2 subglottis
161.3 laryngeal cartilage
161.9 larynx, NOS

162 trachea, bronchus, and lung
162.0 trachea
162.2 main bronchus
162.3 upper lobe, lung
162.4 middle lobe, lung
162.5 lower lobe, lung
162.8 other parts of lung or bronchus
162.9 lung, NOS

163 pleura
163.0 parietal pleura
163.1 visceral pleura
163.9 pleura, NOS

164 thymus, heart, and mediastinum
164.0 thymus
164.1 heart
164.2 anterior mediastinum
164.3 posterior mediastinum
164.9 mediastinum, NOS

165 other and ill-defined sites within respiratory system and intrathoracic organs
165.0 upper respiratory tract
165.9 ill-defined sites within respiratory system

169 hematopoietic and reticuloendothelial systems
169.0 blood
169.1 bone marrow
169.2 spleen
169.3 reticuloendothelial system, NOS
169.9 hematopoietic system, NOS

170 bones, joints, and articular cartilage
170.0 bones of skull and face and associated joints (excludes mandible-T 170.1)
170.1 mandible
170.2 vertebral column
170.3 rib, sternum, clavicle, and associated joints
170.4 long bones of upper limb, scapula, and associated joints
170.5 short bones of upper limb and associated joints
170.6 pelvic bones, sacrum, coccyx, and associated joints
170.7 long bones of lower limb and associated joints
170.8 short bones of lower limb and associated joints
170.9 bone, NOS

171 connective, subcutaneous, and other soft tissues
(includes adipose tissue, aponeuroses, artery, autonomic nervous system, blood vessels, bursa, connective tissue, fibrous tissue, fascia, fatty tissue, ganglia, ligament, lymphatics, muscle, nerve parasympathetic nervous system, peripheral nerves, skeletal muscle, spinal nerves, subcutaneous tissue, sympathetic nervous system, tendon sheath, vein, vessel)
171.0 connective, subcutaneous, and other soft tissues of head, face, and neck
171.1 head, face, and neck
171.2 connective, subcutaneous, and other soft tissues of upper limb and shoulder
171.3 connective, subcutaneous, and other soft tissues of lower limb and hip
171.4 connective, subcutaneous, and other soft tissues of thorax
171.5 connective, subcutaneous, and other soft tissues of abdomen

171.6 connective, subcutaneous,
and other soft tissues of pelvis
171.7 connective, subcutaneous,
and other soft tissues of trunk
171.9 connective, subcutaneous,
and other soft tissues, NOS

173 skin
173.0 skin of lip, NOS
173.1 eyelid
173.2 external ear
173.3 skin of other and unspecified parts
of face
173.4 skin of scalp and neck
173.5 skin of trunk
173.6 skin of arm and shoulder
173.7 skin of leg and hip
173.9 skin, NOS

174 female breast
174.0 nipple
174.1 central portion of breast
174.2 upper inner quadrant of breast
174.3 lower inner quadrant of breast
174.4 upper outer quadrant of breast
174.5 lower outer quadrant of breast
174.6 axillary tail of breast
174.8 inner breast
174.9 female breast, NOS

175 male breast
175.9 male breast, NOS

179 uterus, NOS
179.9 uterus, NOS

180 cervix uteri
180.0 endocervix (internal os)
180.1 endocervix (external os)
180.8 other parts of cervix
180.9 cervix uteri, NOS

181 placenta
181.9 placenta, fetal membranes

182 corpus uteri
182.0 corpus uteri
182.1 isthmus uteri

**183 ovary, fallopian tube,
and broad ligament**
183.0 ovary
183.2 fallopian tube
183.3 broad ligament
183.4 parametrium
183.5 round ligament
183.8 other parts of uterine adnexa
183.9 uterine adnexa, NOS

**184 other and unspecified female
genital organs**
184.0 vagina, NOS
184.1 labium majus
184.2 labium minus
184.3 clitoris
184.4 vulva, NOS
184.9 female genital tract, NOS

185 prostate gland
185.9 prostate gland

186 testis
186.0 undescended testis
186.9 testis, NOS

187 penis and other male genital organs
187.1 prepuce
187.2 glans penis
187.3 body of penis
187.4 penis, NOS
187.5 epididymis
187.6 spermatic cord
187.7 scrotum, NOS
187.8 other parts of male genital organs
187.9 male genital organs, NOS

188 urinary bladder
188.0 trigone of urinary bladder
188.1 dome of urinary bladder
188.2 lateral wall of urinary bladder
188.3 anterior wall of urinary bladder
188.4 posterior wall of urinary bladder
188.5 bladder neck
188.6 ureteric orifice
188.7 urachus
188.9 urinary bladder, NOS

189 kidney and other urinary organs

189.0 kidney, NOS
189.1 renal pelvis
189.2 ureter
189.3 urethra
189.4 paraurethral gland
189.9 urinary system, NOS

190 eye and lacrimal gland

190.0 eyeball
190.1 orbit, NOS
190.2 lacrimal gland
190.3 conjunctiva
190.4 cornea, NOS
190.5 retina
190.6 choroid
190.7 lacrimal duct, NOS
190.9 eye, NOS

191 brain

191.0 cerebrum
191.1 frontal lobe
191.2 temporal lobe
191.3 parietal lobe
191.4 occipital lobe
191.5 ventricle, NOS
191.6 cerebellum, NOS
191.7 brain stem
191.8 other parts of brain
191.9 brain, NOS

**192 other and unspecified parts
of nervous system**

192.0 cranial nerve
192.1 cerebral meninges
192.2 spinal cord
192.3 spinal meninges
192.9 nervous system, NOS

193-194 endocrine glands

193 thyroid gland

193.9 thyroid gland

194 other endocrine glands

194.0 suprarenal gland
194.1 parathyroid gland
194.3 pituitary gland
194.4 pineal gland
194.5 carotid body
194.6 aortic body and other paraganglia
194.8 multiple endocrine glands
194.9 endocrine gland, NOS

195 other ill-defined sites

195.0 head, face, or neck, NOS
195.1 thorax, NOS
195.2 abdomen, NOS
195.3 pelvis, NOS
195.4 upper limb, NOS
195.5 lower limb, NOS
195.8 other ill-defined sites

196 lymph nodes

196.0 lymph nodes of head,
        face, and neck
196.1 intrathoracic lymph nodes
196.2 intra-abdominal lymph nodes
196.3 lymph nodes of axilla or arm
196.5 lymph nodes of inguinal region or leg
196.6 pelvic lymph nodes
196.8 lymph nodes of multiple regions
196.9 lymph nodes, NOS

199 unknown primary site

199.9 unknown primary site

Index

Index

2*

Index

Index

Index

Index

Index

Index

Index

Index

Index

Index

Index